PRIMARY AND SECONDARY PREVENTIVE NUTRITION

NUTRITION ◊ AND ◊ HEALTH
Adrianne Bendich, Series Editor

SERIES INTRODUCTION

The *Nutrition and Health* series has been very fortunate to have each of the volumes recognized by rating services, such as Doody's, as valuable contributions for health professionals and individuals interested in the most up-to-date and balanced information from the experts in nutrition. These independent accolades may have occurred because the *Nutrition and Health* series has as its overriding mission to provide health professionals with texts that are considered essential because each book includes: (1) a synthesis of the state of the science, (2) timely, in-depth reviews by the leading researchers in their respective fields, (3) extensive, up-to-date fully annotated reference lists, (4) a detailed index, (5) relevant tables and figures, (6) identification of paradigm shifts and the consequences, (7) virtually no overlap of information between chapters, but targeted, inter-chapter referrals, (8) suggestions of areas for future research, and (9) balanced, data-driven answers to patient questions, which are based upon the totality of evidence rather than the findings of any single study.

The series volumes are not the outcome of a symposium. Rather, each editor has the potential to examine a chosen area with a broad perspective, both in subject matter as well as in the choice of chapter authors. The international perspective, especially with regard to public health initiatives, is emphasized where appropriate. The editors, whose trainings are both research and practice oriented, have the opportunity to develop a primary objective for their book; define the scope and focus, and then invite the leading authorities from around the world to be part of their initiative. The authors are encouraged to provide an overview of the field, discuss their own research, and relate the research findings to potential human health consequences. Because each book is developed de novo, the chapters can be coordinated so that the resulting volume imparts greater knowledge than the sum of the information contained in the individual chapters.

Primary and Secondary Preventive Nutrition, edited by Richard J. Deckelbaum and me, represents the latest series volume and clearly exemplifies the mission of the *Nutrition and Health* series. This book includes 24 new chapters on the role of diet, dietary factors, nutrients, and their components in optimizing health, and reducing the risk of specific disease conditions in healthy individuals (primary prevention) as well as those with a pre-exisiting condition (secondary prevention). The text includes critically important chapters that discuss topics which are particularly relevant to consumers and patients concerned with nutrition issues frequently appearing in the press. By providing in-depth, balanced reviews of the current science behind questions related to topics such as soy, vitamin supplements, fat substitutes, DHA, trans-fatty acids, and numerous other dietary components, this volume provides health care professionals and students with excellent, well-referenced answers. Medically oriented professionals will certainly find the chapters related to obesity across the age span and including the genetic components of related diseases, of particular importance to their practice. Additional chapters provide in-depth reviews of the functions of vitamins and minerals and other dietary factors in the endocrine, cardiovascular, gastrointestinal, immune, skeletal, and ocular systems of the body. The volume is of particular importance because it includes understandable chapters in highly technical areas written by the leading authorities of their fields of research.

Of added value to health care professionals who are interested in public health is the exceptional introductory chapter that places preventive nutrition in its historic perspective and goes on to project the enormous potential for preventive strategies to reduce human suffering. This volume includes unique chapters that examine the nutritional consequences of ethnicity and socioeconomic status in the US, as well as on a global basis. An often-overlooked dietary component, alcohol, is critically examined, since it can well be a double-edged sword. Other chapters examine the national differences in the consumer messages that are permitted for dietary factors, the current status of nutrition education in medical schools, and the health economics of preventive nutrition.

Thus, *Primary and Secondary Preventive Nutrition* represents a comprehensive, up-to-date resource for undergraduate, graduate, and medical students, nutrition and public health educators, practicing physicians, and other health care providers, as well as clinical researchers.

Adrianne Bendich, PhD
SmithKline Beecham
Consumer HealthCare,
Parsippany, NJ

FOREWORD

This new text synthesizes a wealth of information on what is and what is not known about the benefits of nutritional strategies for the primary and secondary prevention of disease and the promotion of health. It could not be more timely. Health professionals regularly interact with patients who are totally ignorant about appropriate nutrition and exhibit the worst dietary behavior. Increasingly, however, they also encounter patients who are ill informed, responding in Pavlovian fashion to the latest tabloid headlines extolling the alleged value of some food or supplement du jour to prevent aging, increase libido, regrow hair, and otherwise dramatically improve their quality of life. These problems will become more pervasive, since the FDA has recently ruled that health claims for foods and supplements addressing natural conditions of life (e.g., memory, menopause, aging, energy, and libido) will no longer undergo scrutiny and review.

It is the health professional's responsibility to educate those who are ignorant and have grossly unhealthy dietary behaviors as much as it is to help the anxious well place every new nutritional panacea in context and recognize the value and certainty of the evidence.

Definitive data on the value of specific diets and supplements are largely confined to classical nutritional deficiencies (e.g., scurvy, rickets, and xerophthalmia) and limited areas of over- or underindulgence. The growing prevalence of obesity reduces life expectancy; reduced consumption of red meat and saturated fats has dramatically curtailed the epidemic of coronary artery disease in the US; limited salt intake helps to control hypertension; increased folate consumption prior to pregnancy reduces the risk of neural tube defects, and is the reason cereal grains are now fortified with folic acid; calcium supplements can mitigate osteoporosis.

On the other hand, though many observational studies have strongly suggested that beta carotene should reduce the risk of lung cancer, and fiber the risk of colon cancer, gold-standard randomized trials proved that these expectations were unfounded. Unfortunately, most of the nutritional breakthroughs breathlessly touted by the popular press represent selected associations culled from large and complex observational studies. The health professional needs to explain that these apparent associations may arise by chance, may be real, but noncausal, and even if causal, may have little relevance past a certain age or chronicity of disease. Though it is difficult to conduct a randomized trial for every possible nutrient and dietary supplement, it is equally difficult to tease out exactly what dietary component, if any, might have been responsible for purported health outcomes observed in large observational studies.

The well-educated health professional will be thoughtful about these matters, will follow the literature for definitive data that provide a firm basis for counseling their patients, and will be prepared to place the patient's and the population's concerns, anxieties, or what they believe to be the latest elixir of health, in proper perspective.

Primary and Secondary Preventive Nutrition, combined with its predecessor (*Preventive Nutrition*), helps establish the present state of knowledge, and thereby advances the art and science of preventive nutrition.

Alfred Sommer, MD
School of Hygiene and Public Health,
Johns Hopkins University,
Baltimore, MD

PREFACE

Our major objective in developing *Primary and Secondary Preventive Nutrition* is to highlight and critically review the key recent research findings that are topical issues for health care professionals and their clients, faculty and students of nutritional sciences, and educated consumers who also seek a reliable source of nutrition information. In order to reach this goal, we have invited the leading expert researchers to share their findings in a historical context to provide readers with clear recommendations that are based upon the totality of evidence rather than the findings of a single study. By doing so, we have included chapters that are balanced, data dense, and, at the same time, easy to understand.

Preventive nutrition incorporates dietary practices and interventions directed towards the reduction in disease risk (primary prevention), improvements in diseases already manifest (secondary prevention), and/or improvement in health outcomes. Preventive nutrition is a critical component not only of preventive medicine, but also of therapeutic medicine and provides approaches to prevent disease and reduce its impact once it occurs. Our first volume, *Preventive Nutrition: The Comprehensive Guide for Health Professionals,* contributed to the concept that nutritional strategies are a very cost effective way of decreasing morbidity and mortality, and improving individual functioning. This new volume, *Primary and Secondary Preventive Nutrition* focuses on more recent information about optimizing human health. Comprehensive, the book provides 24 new, relevant reviews by international medical authorities and research experts on the complex role of nutrition throughout the entire life cycle. This new text includes expanded insights into the role of nutrition in the etiology of the major chronic diseases underpinned by the most significant findings of current nutrition research, including both epidemiological and clinical intervention studies. The public health implications and economic consequences of author-recommended appropriate dietary modifications are clearly spelled out. The emphasis of each chapter is balance: discussions and recommendations are based on the totality of the evidence and authors have included comprehensive tables and figures to clarify the current state of the research in their fields of expertise.

With the recent recognition that obesity and type 2 diabetes are emerging as major public health problems worldwide, these conditions are the primary or a major emphasis of one third of the chapters in this volume. Material is presented relevant to these conditions in both the pediatric and adult age groups. The authors comprehensively review not only prevention, but also potential modes of therapy. These chapters are especially of value as the authors are internationally recognized authorities with hands-on experience in the care of affected patients. The importance of nutritional strategies in the areas of insulin resistance, diabetes, and obesity is thus a major focus of this volume.

Overall, the book contains well-organized and -referenced reviews by respected scientists in areas including the primary prevention of cancer, cardiovascular disease, obesity, osteoporosis, and osteoarthritis. Additionally, of equal importance are the new data on the critical role of specific nutrients in the prevention of further damage and slowing of disease progression in individuals with cancer, cardiovascular disease, renal disease, obesity, diabetes, osteoporosis, and/or autoimmune diseases. Recent reports of great consumer interest on the roles of soy, fiber, and retinoids, as well as the contrasting effects of trans- vs long-chain fatty acids, are also clearly presented. Each of the chapters concludes with the authors' assessment of the current state of the science and includes recommendations for professional health care providers and their patients.

Moreover, the significance of exposure to key nutrients early in life, even before birth, and the influence of environmental factors are examined in depth. New to this volume is the insightful chapter considering lifestyle factors such as alcohol consumption. Emphasis is also given to chapters that explore the nutritional consequences of economic crises in underdeveloped countries, relevant findings from countries in nutritional transition, and the status of preventive nutrition in developed countries, with an emphasis on the role of socioeconomic status on the nutritional status of the population

This volume also contains a key chapter that describes the current status of approaches for incorporating preventive nutrition into the curriculum in medical schools. The education of health care providers is critical to the dissemination of balanced, well-documented information in any health-related field; unfortunately, there exists a major gap in nutrition education in many medical school curricula today. *Primary and Secondary Preventive Nutrition* can serve as an important reference tool for medical and other students interested in the importance of nutrition in advancing human health, but a text cannot take the place of focused emphasis as part of a curriculum.

In emphasizing the major economic benefits to be obtained via nutritional approaches, the first and last chapters of this volume undertake an extensive examination of the cost effectiveness of preventive nutrition and have shown that disease prevention, rather than treatment alone, not only makes sense, but also saves cents… and dollars. Thus, this volume adds to the major contribution of the previous volume, *Preventive Nutrition,* by including a strong body of added evidence of the economic as well as health value of preventive nutrition strategies.

Each chapter is generally organized to provide an overview of the field, the authors' own research, and how these findings fit with the overview. Extensive summary tables and figures illustrate the depth of knowledge in the area and recommendations for various population and patient groups. There is an extensive index. Also included is a list of journals that specialize in publishing clinical studies in preventive nutrition, a bibliography of recent, relevant books, and web sites providing most up-to-date information in a variety of nutrition fields. By addressing the nutrition questions most often raised and by examining the issues based on disease as well as age, it is hoped that this volume will serve as a critical resource for health professionals interested in enhancing their ability to utilize nutrition to improve health outcomes of individuals and to assist in the planning of national disease prevention programs for enhancing the health status of populations.

We hope that this book serves as an added resource for the spectrum of health professionals including physicians, nutritionists, dentists, pharmacists, nurses, dietitians, health educators, policy makers, and research investigators by providing reliable, useful, balanced, and well-documented approaches to frequently asked questions and problems. We anticipate that this volume will enhance discussions on the public health implications of preventive nutrition strategies to improve human health and at the same time reduce health care costs. As editors, we continue to be excited by the evolving field of preventive nutrition that is so clearly represented by the excellent chapters contained within this and our previous volume.

Adrianne Bendich
Richard J. Deckelbaum

CONTENTS

CONTRIBUTORS

DAVID B. ALLISON • *Obesity Research Center, St. Luke's–Roosevelt Hospital, Institute of Human Nutrition, Columbia University College of Physicians and Surgeons, New York, NY*

ANDREA BELLUZZI • *Via Vizzani, Bologna*

ADRIANNE BENDICH, PHD • *SmithKline Beecham Consumer Healthcare, Parsippany, NJ*

ERIK BERGSTRÖM • *Epidemiology, Department of Public Health and Clinical Medicine, Umea University, Umea, Sweden*

MARTIN W. BLOEM • *Helen Keller International, Jakarta, Indonesia*

IAN DARNTON-HILL • *Helen Keller International, New York, NY*

RICHARD J. DECKELBAUM • *Institute of Human Nutrition and Department of Pediatrics, Columbia University, New York, NY*

TAMÁS DECSI • *Department of Paediatrics, University Medical School of Pécs, Pécs, Hungary*

SRIDEVI DEVARAJ • *Division of Clinical Biochemistry and Human Metabolism, University of Texas Southwestern Medical Center, Dallas, TX*

ANNETTE DICKINSON • *Council for Responsible Nutrition, Washington, DC*

RICHARD EASTELL • *Division of Clinical Sciences (NGHT), Section of Medicine, Bone Metabolism Group, Northern General Hospital, The University of Sheffield, Sheffield, UK*

JOHN W. ERDMAN, JR. • *Division of Nutritional Sciences, University of Illinois at Urbana-Champaign, Urbana, IL*

NANCY D. ERNST • *National Heart, Lung, and Blood Institute, National Institutes of Health, Bethesda, MD*

MYLES S. FAITH • *Obesity Research Center, St Luke's–Roosevelt Hospital, Columbia University, College of Physicians and Surgeons, New York, NY*

DAVID B. FOURNIER • *Clinical Oncology and Chemoprevention, G. D. Searle & Co., Skokie, IL*

HENRY I. FRIER • *Slim Fast Foods Company, West Palm Beach, FL*

AMY FUNKHOUSER • *Obesity Research Center, St. Luke's–Roosevelt Hospital, Institute of Human Nutrition, Columbia University, College of Physicians and Surgeons, New York, NY*

ALLAN GELIEBTER • *Obesity Research Center, St. Luke's–Roosevelt Hospital, Columbia University, College of Physicians and Surgeons, New York, NY*

GARY B. GORDON • *Clinical Oncology and Chemoprevention, G. D. Searle & Co., Skokie, IL*

HARRY L. GREENE • *Slim Fast Foods Company, West Palm Beach, FL*

OLLE HERNELL • *Department of Clinical Sciences and Paediatrics, Umea Univeristy, Umea, Sweden*

STEVEN B. HEYMSFIELD • *Obesity Research Center, St. Luke's–Roosevelt Hospital, Institute of Human Nutrition, Columbia University, College of Physicians and Surgeons, New York, NY*

HOWARD N. HODIS • *Division of Cardiology, University of Southern California School of Medicine, Los Angeles, CA*

ELLEN K. HOOGEVEEN • *Department of Internal Medicine, University Medical Centre St. Radboud, Nijmegen, The Netherlands*

WOLFGANG J. ISSING • *Ludwig Maximilians Universität München, München, Germany*

ISHWARLAL JIALAL • *Division of Clinical Biochemistry and Human Metabolism, University of Texas Southwestern Medical Center, Dallas, TX*

BERTHOLD KOLETZKO • *Kinderklinik and Kinderpoliklinik, Dr. Von Haunersches Kinderspital, Ludwig-Maximilians–University of Munich, München, Germany*

SUSAN M. KREBS-SMITH • *Risk Factor Monitoring and Methods Branch, National Cancer Institute, National Institutes of Health, Bethesda, MD*

ALAN R. KRISTAL • *Cancer Prevention Research Program, Fred Hutchinson Cancer Research Center, Seattle, WA*

SHIRIKI K. KUMANYIKA • *Department of Biostatistics and Epidemiology, University of Pennsylvania School of Medicine, Philadelphia, PA*

WILLIAM E. M. LANDS • *National Institute on Alcohol Abuse and Alcoholism, National Institutes of Health, Bethesda, MD*

WENDY J. MACK • *Department of Preventive Medicne, University of Southern California School of Medicine, Los Angeles, CA*

PATTY E. MATZ • *Obesity Research Center, St. Luke's–Roosevelt Hospital, Columbia University, College of Physicians and Surgeons, New York, NY*

TIMOTHY E. McALINDON • *Arthritis Center, Boston University School of Medicine, Boston, MA*

J. MICHAEL McGINNIS • *The Robert Wood Johnson Foundation, Princeton, NJ*

RONALD P. MENSINK • *Department of Human Biology, Maastricht University, Maastricht, The Netherlands*

MARIAN L. NEUHOUSER • *Cancer Prevention Research Program, Fred Hutchinson Cancer Research Center, Seattle, WA*

RUTH E. PATTERSON • *Cancer Prevention Research Program, Fred Hutchinson Cancer Research Center, Seattle, WA*

CLAUDIA A. PEREDA • *Bone Metabolism Group, Division of Clinical Sciences, Section of Medicine, Northern General Hospital, The University of Sheffield, Sheffield, UK*

ANGELO PIETROBELLI • *Obesity Research Center, St. Luke's–Roosevelt Hospital, Columbia University, College of Physicians and Surgeons, New York, NY*

CLAUDIA S. PLAISTED • *School of Public Health and School of Medicine, University of North Carolina at Chapel Hill, Chapel Hill, NC*

KENNETH J. ROTHMAN • *Section of Preventive Medicine, Department of Medicine, Boston University School of Medicine, and Department of Epidemiology and Biostatistics, Boston University School of Public Health, Boston, MA*

ALEX SEVANIAN • *Department of Molecular Pharmacology and Toxicology, University of Southern California School of Pharmacy, Los Angeles, CA*

BARBARA A. UNDERWOOD • *Institute of Medicine, Washington, DC*

SUSANNE H. F. VERMUNT • *Department of Human Biology, Maastricht University, Maastricht, The Netherlands*

CHRISTINE L. WILLIAMS • *Department of Pediatrics and Institute of Human Nutrition, Columbia University, New York, NY*

RAFFAELLA ZANNOLLI • *Department of Pediatrics, University of Siena, Siena, Italy*

STEVEN H. ZEISEL • *Department of Nutrition, University of North Carolina at Chapel Hill, Chapel Hill, NC*

I INTRODUCTION

1
Preventive Nutrition
A Historic Perspective
and Future Economic Outlook

J. Michael McGinnis and Nancy D. Ernst

1. INTRODUCTION

For the two out of three adult Americans who do not smoke and do not drink excessively, one personal choice seems to influence long-term health prospects more than any other; what we eat.

This statement, taken from the 1988 *Surgeon General's Report on Nutrition and Health (1)*, offers an indication of both the challenge and the opportunity facing the nutrition community for the twenty-first century. These are times of unprecedented change. In a historical sense, changes in the nutritional challenges that have occurred in this century have been more dramatic than those that occurred over the entire course of the previous millennium, as the dominant nutritional issues have shifted from those of nutrient deficiency to nutrient excess in the developed world.

Four major points underlie the discussion in this chapter. First, the contribution of the nutrition sciences will assume increasing and compelling importance in the prevention of disease in the twenty-first century. Second, the greatest challenge to constructive engagement of these issues is dealing with the uncertainty attendant to change. Third, in the face of uncertainty, the role of policy is to bring focus to the points of social and scientific convergence. Finally, in the face of change, the role of the clinician is to bring focus to the individual. These are discussed below as underlying factors and policy implications.

2. FACTORS INFLUENCING NUTRITION AND CHRONIC DISEASE PREVENTION

The factors most likely to influence the nutrition policy agenda of the new century include the national disease profile, demographic profiles, economics, changing meal patterns, changing meal sources, public awareness, professional awareness, the development of scientific insights, and the advent of new technologies.

2.1. National Disease Profile

Fundamentally, any public health agenda is driven to a substantial extent by the population's profile of disease and disability, the nature of the problems at hand, and the rates at which they are changing. The most concrete indicator of the disease profile for

From: *Primary and Secondary Preventive Nutrition*
Edited by: A. Bendich and R. J. Deckelbaum © Humana Press Inc., Totowa, NJ

Table 1
Leading Causes of Death, 1996

Heart disease	733,834
Cancer	544,278
Cerebrovascular disease	160,431
Chronic lung disease	106,146
Accidents	93,874
Pneumonia and influenza	82,579
Diabetes	61,559
HIV infection	32,655
Suicide	30,862
Chronic liver disease/cirrhosis	25,135

Adapted from ref. 2.

Table 2
Real Causes of Death, 1990

Tobacco	400,000
Diet/inactivity patterns	300,000
Alcohol	100,000
Certain infections	90,000
Toxic agents	60,000
Firearms	35,000
Sexual behavior	30,000
Motor vehicles	25,000
Drug use	20,000

Adapted from ref. 3.

Americans is found in the mortality tables. In 1996, approx 2.2 million Americans died. Their death certificates state that the top five causes of death were heart disease (HD), cancer, cerebrovascular disease, chronic lung diseases, and accidents (Table 1). The next five conditions, listed in order of magnitude, are pneumonia and influenza, diabetes, HIV infection, suicide, and chronic liver disease/cirrhosis. Since 1990, both chronic lung disease and HIV infection have moved higher on the list (2).

Currently, five of the ten leading causes of death have important dietary links, including three—HD, cancer, and stroke—which account for almost 70% of all deaths in the United States. As a result of a generation of biomedical research, it is known that diet-related factors, including relationships with physical activity and overweight, account for a large proportion of these diseases. Studies have variously associated dietary factors or sedentary lifestyles with between one-fifth and one-third of cardiovascular deaths, 20–60% of fatal cancers, and 50–80% of diabetes mellitus cases, including 30% of diabetes deaths (3). Drawing on available studies to assign responsibility for deaths on the vital statistics ledgers, to what is now known to be their root causes, reveals just how important dietary factors are to the health of Americans (Table 2). Together, diet and the prevailing pattern of inactivity contribute 300,000–500,000 deaths annually, according them the dubious distinction of either the first or second ranking as actual causes of death for Americans, depending on whether one looks to the higher or the lower end of the estimated range, and the only one that is a daily factor for the entire population (3).

Table 3
Annual Burden of Preventable Conditions

Condition	Annual burden
Coronary heart disease	14 million cases
Certain cancers	1.2 million yearly
Stroke	600,000 yearly
Diabetes	16 million cases
Many injuries	2.6 million hospitalized
Chronic lung disease	28 million cases
Alcoholic liver disease	14 million alcoholics
HIV and other STDs	16 million yearly
Low weight babies	285,000 yearly
Many neural tube defects	2500 yearly
Vaccine-preventable diseases	55,000 yearly

Adapted from ref. *4.*

But moving beyond the mortality tables, to the issue of the aggregate burden of preventable conditions (Table 3), is enlightening. Manifest here is the fact that dietary factors predispose, to varying degrees, to many of these conditions. Included are contributions to the 14 million annual cases of coronary heart disease (CHD), 1.2 million cancer cases, 600,000 strokes, 16 million cases of diabetes (almost 80% of which are maturity-onset), some 285,000 low-weight births, and 2500 neural tube defects (NTDs) *(4)*. For some of these, solid nutrition-related risk factors have been identified, and discernible progress is already manifest for application of the information in disease control, albeit far short of what ought to be possible. Certain of the most intractable, like cancers or low birth weight, have nutrition components that are suggestive, but the mechanisms are less clear. A more fulsome rendition of serious health challenges to the American population would also include a number that are growing rapidly, such as AIDS, Alzheimer's, and arthritis, but are without clearly defined nutritional components. As new understanding is gained about the relationship between dietary patterns and disease outcomes, the role of nutrition is likely to grow as a public policy priority.

2.2. Demographic Profiles

Public policy is generally more responsive to groups whose numbers are growing than to those whose numbers are shrinking. Over the course of this century, the median age of the population increased by nearly 16 yr, from 23 to 39 yr, with a 1200% increase in the share over age 85 yr, and a 40% decrease in the share under age 25 yr. If projected to the year 2040, the population over age 85 yr will have nearly doubled again, relative to the year 2010, and will represent 4.2% of the total. The nutrition concerns of older people are going to move quickly up the public health agenda. Clearly contributing to the sense of urgency will be the aging of the population (Table 4).

In the period from 1970 to 2020, the population over age 65 yr will more than double, growing from approx 20 million to approx 53 million people (Table 4). In this period, those over age 65 yr will grow from 10% to nearly 20% of the population. Those over age 85 yr will almost quadruple in that same period, growing from just under 2 million to almost 7 million by 2020. Indeed, if projected to the year 2040, the population over age

Table 4
Aging of the Population

No. people 65 yr + (in millions)						
1900	1920	1940	1960	1980	2000	2020
3.1	4.9	9.0	16.6	25.6	35.3	53.3

Adapted from ref. 5.

85 yr will have nearly doubled again, relative to the year 2010, and will then represent over 4% of the total population (5).

With the cost of treatments that often accompany the aging experience (not only coronary bypass procedures, chemotherapy, stroke rehabilitation, and joint replacements, which can range from $25,000 to $250,000 each, but also the day-to-day management of problems such as congestive heart failure and diabetes) it is apparent that the aggregate cost of potentially preventable conditions has already become an urgent societal concern that is likely to worsen.

Whether from the perspective of individual citizens seeking help or that of policymakers seeking solutions, the demands for sound nutritional interventions, already substantial, can be expected to increase in the years ahead.

2.3. Economics

Economics is an undeniable determinant of public policy. It is in fact not uncommon for advocacy organizations to define policy strictly in budgetary terms. Nutrition and disease prevention are influenced by several forces of economics, including the economics of eating patterns, which influence the development of disease, and the economics of food production and marketing.

Estimates on the potential effects of diet on the development of chronic diseases have been used to estimate the benefit of improved dietary patterns. The economic impact analysis for the Nutrition Labeling and Education Act (NLEA) estimated that the benefits of the amendments to require mandatory food labeling for virtually all foods would result in beneficial changes in food purchases that would be associated with over 39,000 fewer cancer and CHD cases. The economic benefit of the total NLEA proposals (changes in the information panel, including new nutrient and ingredient information, as well as changes such as new definitions for nutrient content claims and health claims) were estimated to be $4.4–$26.5 billion over a 20-yr period (6,7). This analysis was based primarily on an estimated 1% reduction in intake of fat and saturated fatty acids (SFAs) and a 0.1% reduction in consumption of cholesterol (6,7).

A later economic impact analysis, prepared for regulations that require fortification of cereal-grain products with folate at 0.14 mg/100 g, also provided estimates of economic benefit. These analyses, based on the occurrence of 2500 cases of NTDs/yr, of which a proportion are folate-related, estimates 116 NTDs and 25 infant deaths would be prevented per year, and result in economic benefits, calculated to the "willingness to pay" methodology, in the range of an estimated $651–$788 million/yr (8).

A recent analysis provided estimates of the total economic costs associated with U.S. food consumption patterns and the predicted economic benefit from dietary change. This projection estimated that healthier diets could prevent $71 billion/yr in medical costs, lost productivity, and the value of premature deaths associated with four of these conditions: CHD, cancer, stroke, or diabetes. Specifically, medical costs account for 47% of the total, premature deaths for 39%, and lost productivity associated with morbidity accounts for the remaining 13%. These estimates did not include diet related costs associated with osteoporosis, hypertension, overweight, and NTDs *(9)* (*see* Chapter 24).

Federal initiatives, such as the 1969 White House Conference on Nutrition *(10)*, focused national attention on the need for food assistance programs to address poverty-related hunger and nutrition. As a result, federal obligations for food assistance programs increased by over 500% from fiscal 1990 to 1994. These food assistance programs, primarily administered by U.S. Department of Agriculture (USDA), provide different types of food benefits to various target recipients. Three of these programs account for 85% of the total $33.6 billion spent on food assistance in 1998: the Food Stamp Program ($18.8 billion), the National School Lunch Program ($5.8 billion), and the Women, Infants, and Children Program ($3.8 billion) *(11)*. In recent years, expansion of the food assistance programs has slowed, decreasing about 18% from fiscal 1994 to fiscal 1998 *(11)*. The primary intent of the programs is to provide an adequate quantity of food, not to assure that the quality of the food choices is optimal for the prevention of chronic diseases. However, USDA provides reimbursement to states for half of the cost of approved Food Stamp Program education and promotion activities. Thus, there is an opportunity to influence food choices. Currently, 46 states have approved nutrition education plans *(11)*. Also, in 1995, USDA published the final rules on School Meals for Healthy Children, regulations to ensure that school meals comply with the Dietary Guidelines for Americans, making available meals that are reduced in fat, SFAs, cholesterol, and sodium (Na), and that provide nutrient adequacy *(12)*. Do food assistance programs affect the nutrient quality of diets consumed by the program recipients? The clearest evidence is that the programs increase the quantity of food consumed. Otherwise, the cross-sectional data provide no certain conclusion regarding the effect of the programs on the quality of the recipients' diets *(11)*. The above look at examples of federal food-related initiatives demonstrates that economic benefits may be achieved by dietary change.

Food is an $800 billion U.S. industry. The objective of the food industry is to encourage people to eat more food, not less. In contrast, the intent of the dietary guidance for health promotion is to emphasize the selection of certain foods, to advise limits on serving sizes, and, indeed, to encourage people to eat less food and calories, to prevent overweight. The food industry will seek to sell more food, spending $30 billion/yr on food advertising ($10 billion/yr in direct media advertising and $20 billion on point-of-purchase campaigns and development of new food products *(13)*. Despite the different objectives of dietary guidance policy, compared with the food industry, the availability of leaner meats and reduced fat food, and the increased diversity of fruits and vegetables in the marketplace, demonstrate the potential to achieve improved dietary intake when industry responds to government recommendations and consumer demands.

2.4. Changing Meal Patterns

The forces of change are dramatic for food and nutrition today, as is the pace of that change. Certainly, important changes have occurred in the choices people make. The notion that behavior is immutable has long since been put to rest. From food disappearance data (the foods available for consumption) it is evident that the type of food on the American menu is changing (Table 5). Since 1970, the availability of red meat is down about one-sixth, fish is up by about one-third, and poultry has increased almost twofold.

Table 5
Food Consumption (lb per capita)

	1970	1980	1997
Red meat	132	126	111
Fish	12	12	15
Poultry	34	41	65
Eggs (#)	309	271	239
Whole milk	214	142	70
Skim milk	12	12	34
Cheese	11	17	28
Flour/cereal	136	145	200
Fresh fruits	101	105	133
Fresh vegetables	153	149	186

Adapted from ref. *14*.

On the other hand, summing the pounds per capita in these three components of the meat group suggests that the combined total poundage available for consumption is up 7%. The largest increase occurred in the period after 1980. Coincidentally, egg availability (reported as shell eggs) has declined by almost one-quarter. However, use of egg products (liquid or dried) has nearly doubled since 1983, and is expected to increase, as consumers choose to use more prepared foods. Whole milk is down by two-thirds; skim milk (nonfat) has increased by more than 275%. Per capita consumption of cheese is up 2.5× the 1970 level *(14)*. Also, food supply nutrient data show that total fat and SFAs provided by dairy products has remained constant since 1970 *(15)*. The availability of grain and cereal products and fresh fruits and vegetables is also up, in the range of 20–50% *(14)*. These are considerable changes to have occurred in a relatively short period of time, and, in general, in the direction of lower saturated fat/total fat products that health officials have been encouraging.

Also, in response to the nature of dietary guidance recommendations, has been a change in the food products available. Supermarket shelves are simply not the same places that they were two decades, or even one decade, ago (Table 6). They are now jammed with low-fat, reduced-Na, high-fiber, high-calcium, nutrient-fortified, and organic foods, as well as nutritionals and other health-oriented products of every size and shape. In the year 1980, over 9000 new food products were introduced into the marketplace; in 1994, that number was even higher. More recently, some slowing has occurred in the introduction of new products. In 1998, new food product introductions declined approx 12% with 10,932 new foods introduced, compared with 12,147 in 1997. Six of the food categories posted increases in 1998 (dairy, desserts, breakfast cereals, entrees, processed meat, and soup) *(16)*. Few low-fat or fat-free products were introduced, suggesting a slowing of the trend for fat-focused foods.

In 1998, the combined snack bar/snack mix and fruit bar subcategories posted the largest (25%) increase in the food product category over the previous year *(16)*. These products included special features, such as nutritional snacks for the physically active, or dietary supplements in a snack food form. Bar and snack formulations meet the needs of the quick-paced U.S. lifestyle. Quickly prepared foods are going up in popularity; 3/4 households have microwave ovens used to prepare a new generation of prepackaged

Table 6
New Food Product Introductions, 1989–1998

Category	1989	1990	1991	1992	1993	1994	1995	1996	1997	1998
Baby foods	53	31	95	53	7	45	61	25	53	35
Bakery foods	1155	1239	1631	1508	1420	1636	1855	1340	1200	1178
Bakery ingredients	233	307	335	346	383	544	577	419	422	295
Beverages	913	1143	1367	1538	1842	2250	2854	2033	1606	1547
Breakfast cereals	118	123	104	122	99	110	128	121	83	84
Candy/gum/snacks	1355	1486	1885	2068	2043	2450	2462	2310	2505	2065
Condiments	1701	2028	2787	2555	3147	3271	3698	2815	2631	1994
Dairy	1,348	1,327	1,111	1,320	1,099	1,328	1,614	1,345	862	940
Desserts	69	49	124	93	158	215	125	100	109	117
Entrees	694	753	808	698	631	694	748	597	629	678
Fruits and vegetables	214	325	356	276	407	487	545	552	405	375
Processed meat	509	663	798	785	453	565	790	637	672	728
Side dishes	489	538	530	560	680	980	940	611	678	597
Soups	215	159	265	211	248	264	292	270	292	299
Total	9,066	10,171	12,196	12,133	12,617	14,845	16,702	13,245	12,147	10,932

Adapted from ref. 16.

9

Table 7
Expenditures for Food Purchases, 1980–1998

	1980	1997	% Change
Grocery stores	205	403	+ 96
Food service units	80	236	+ 195

Adapted from ref. *17*.

meals. These facts suggest a rapid change in what consumers are demanding and purchasing, and, presumably, what they are eating and metabolizing. It will probably be some time before the full range of nutritional implications of these changes are known.

2.5. Changing Meal Sources

Compounding the analytic challenge is the fact that the supermarket is not the only place in which these changes are occurring (Table 7). Increasingly, people are also eating out or purchasing prepared food or food that requires minimal preparation before consumption. In 1980, food purchases at grocery stores outstripped purchases of prepared foods from food service facilities by 2.5 to 1. But over the succeeding decade and a half, the growth in the proportion of meals taken outside the home was about twice that for grocery store purchases (17). Accordingly, now nearly 40% of the food dollar is spent on food away from home (18).

The nutritional implications of these trends are not fully determinable. However, a recent analysis, based on national food consumption data, calculated that, if food away from home had the same average nutritional densities as food at home in 1995, U.S. consumers would have consumed 197 fewer calories per day, reduced their fat intake to 31.5% of calories (instead of 33.6%), and reduced their SFAs intake to 10.9% of calories (instead of 11.5%). In addition, the consumption of calcium would have increased by 7% and their consumption of fiber and iron by 9% each (19). Na intakes would not have changed significantly, possibly because most Na is added to food prior to its entry into the households. The preceding data raise concerns, especially for those in certain socio-economic categories, about the potential of a lower intake of fresh fruits and vegetables and higher caloric, and probably higher fat, especially saturated fat, patterns of consumption, relative to what would be consumed at home.

Despite consumer interest in purchasing lower-fat, lower-calorie products, their aggregate purchases have continued, and enhanced the twentieth-century pattern of excess. The result has been a 15% increase in average daily calories available in the food supply, from 3300 per capita in 1970 to 3800 in 1994 (20). And, of immediate concern from the perspective of the nation's health profile, an increase in the prevalence of obesity has occurred. The prevalence of overweight among Americans has increased from 24% in 1960 to 33% in 1994 (21).

It is clear that a practical consideration for public health programs in nutrition is the places people eat. Both as a determinant of nutrient intake profiles, and as a possible locus for education and intervention on those profiles, the ways in which meals are taken present special opportunities. Increasingly, patterns are determined according to convenience.

2.6. Public Awareness

There is little question that the public is increasingly interested in nutrition, and aware of the central issues. Over the decade from 1975 to 1985, there was about a threefold increase in awareness of the relation between Na and high blood pressure *(22)*, and almost a doubling in knowledge of the link between fat and HD *(23)*.

In contrast, in this same time period, there was little change in the awareness of SFAs as the major dietary influence on blood cholesterol levels, and thus on the risk of CHD. By 1995, over 60% of consumers identified total fat, but only about 10% identified saturated fat, as a dietary factor related to HD *(23)*. A possible explanation may be that, for consumers, the application of a simple message (total fat) obfuscates important scientific nuances, e.g., SFAs and *trans* FAs—not total fat—raise blood cholesterol level, and thus the risk of CHD, and lower fat is not synonymous with lower calorie intake.

No longer are the major messages those that reflect the carefully distilled products of scientific and public health consensus. Today's messages include the latest findings from the latest study. They arrive piecemeal. There is no question about the value of new data, even if it is at odds with prevailing views: This is, after all, how research proceeds. Nonetheless, public health policymakers and other leading health groups must be vigilant to recognize the potential for confusion of the public with the latest research news.

A major challenge must be faced in helping people sort out the central tendencies of new information released to the public from scientific research, in effect, helping people understand what is important for them, given their particular circumstances.

2.7. Professional Awareness

Throughout the past two decades, physician awareness and interest in nutritional issues has lagged behind that of the public. In 1983, nearly twice as many of those in the general public believed in a salutary effect of reducing high blood cholesterol, compared with physicians. There are indications, however, that the treatment guidelines of the National Cholesterol Education Program (NCEP) have influenced clinical practice. In 1995, more than 90% of physicians surveyed said they were aware of the guidelines, and almost 90% said they used the guidelines in their practice. In 1995, the percentage of physicians who reported that they routinely measured blood cholesterol levels of new patients ranged from about 60–90%, depending on the age and sex of the patient. In 1983, the median range of cholesterol level at which physicians reported initiating dietary therapy for high blood cholesterol was 219–260 mg/dL; in 1995, it had dropped to 200–219 mg/dL *(24)*. The NCEP convened, in late 1999, an expert committee to update the existing guidelines. The expert group will examine several scientific and educational issues, and will disseminate recommendations to physicians and other health professionals. The topics include nontraditional CHD risk factors, antioxidants, and other nutrients *(25)*.

Health care provider attitudes have changed substantially in recent years, but nutrition education in medical schools is still weak: particularly when considered against the translational challenge physicians will have to face in the future.

Public policy can do much to turn these developments into positive influences on the health of the public, but, if the full potential is to be reached, a close partnership will be required with the scientific and medical/health provider communities.

2.8. Development of Scientific Insights Coupled with New Technologies

Clearly, new scientific insights can change the role of nutrition in prevention, especially the public policy aimed at chronic disease prevention. A good example is what has already happened with the NCEP, based on more than a half century of research about the relationship between blood lipids and cardiovascular disease.

The future will undoubtedly hold much more, as the nutritional sciences incorporate the lessons from molecular biology and genetics. The priority categories of the Federal Interagency Committee on Human Nutrition Research indicate areas in which advances may be expected: nutrient requirements throughout the life cycle; nutrient interactions and bioavailability; nutrition and chronic diseases; energy regulation, obesity, and eating disorders; nutrition surveillance and monitoring methodology; and nutrition education techniques.

Impressive change is also occurring in the science and technology base. These advances have contributed to important developments in the epidemiology of nutrition and chronic diseases, in the understanding of nutrient action at the molecular level, and about individual variation in response to nutrient challenges. Perhaps the most dramatic developments, if only in terms of the pace of change, are coming from the increasing understanding of how people vary.

The Human Genome Project is likely to make a large difference in terms of expectations for nutrition and prevention in 10 years' time *(26)*. The project's target of having a genetic linkage map in hand by 1995 was exceeded by a year. The goal for completing a physical map of the genome is now already essentially completed. Sequencing is rapidly progressing, with nine megabases now characterized, and the full genome sequencing anticipated to be completed by 2003, two years ahead of schedule, with myriad implications for understanding individual variation in response to dietary patterns. Recent reports also indicate progress toward a genetic linkage map for human obesity *(27)*.

The notion of using genetic engineering to alter an offending gene may lag, often by decades, but already the techniques of engineering genetic change are being put to work in the development of new types of food products. Plant primary and secondary metabolites are estimated to number over 20,000 unique chemical structures *(28)*. Potentially, these could be cultivated and harvested commercially in species, through the transfer of genes within a metabolic path. The current knowledge of plant FA biosynthesis genes indicates that many of the genes to alter lipid biosynthesis are available. It is now possible to alter lipid metabolism in plants, for example, to reduce high levels of SFAs in vegetable oils *(29)*.

Or, if specific vitamins are shown to affect the development of cancer, the vitamin content could be enhanced in foods through gene manipulation techniques *(30)*. Beyond genetics, food and ingredient synthesis technology will obviously bring other new trends to market, as those mentioned earlier continue to grow.

Advances in the instruments to measure health status, i.e., to assess body composition, to assay serum and tissue levels of micronutrients, and efforts to utilize technology such as double-labeled water as an objective measure of energy intake, and nitrogen balance as an objective measure of protein intake, will all improve and provide new and better information. As a result of these technological developments, those concerned with dietary guidance recommendations are dealing with the complexities of multiple developments, compelling a change of perspectives, if not strategies, on many dimensions.

3. POLICY IMPLICATIONS

In the face of uncertainty, the role of policy is to bring focus to the points of social convergence. Policy is fundamentally targeted to wielding levers that address common denominators. Virchow, in saying in 1509 that "medicine is the purest form of politics" *(31)*, could well have had the challenge of dietary guidance in mind. In this matter of great importance to the health of the American people, the task is reminiscent of the basic challenge of any policy process: the task of finding the right balance in the dialectic of the debate between the dictum "the greatest good for the greatest number" and the Hippocratic admonition "first, do no harm."

A convergence is emerging from the often disparate vantage points of studies of different disease processes in the American population. From studies of CHD etiology comes the lesson that intake levels of FAs and cholesterol are correlated with higher serum cholesterol levels, and therefore higher risk of CHD *(32)*. From studies of cancers of the breast, colon, and prostate, indications are offered of the increased risk attendant to higher consumption patterns of animal fat and total energy *(32)*.

Beyond the question of separating the independence of the effects of dietary fat and total energy consumption, clarity is elusive with respect to the differing roles of different types of fats: How do different SFAs act variably? How do the effects of SFAs in beef differ from those in peanut oil? With emerging concerns about *trans* FAs (about 2–3% of calories) and the known cholesterol-raising effect of SFAs (12% of calories), what role can the federal government play to help achieve economic health benefits? Are monounsaturated FAs protective against elevated levels of cholesterol, triglycerides, and insulin resistance? The list of questions is a long one. But, especially given the fact that fat delivers twice as many calories as carbohydrates or proteins, the general recommendation that emphasizes reduced consumption of the major sources of SFAs, cholesterol and *trans* FAs, and moderation in sources of total fat, and to couple this emphasis with a recommendation for healthier weight, should offer minimal scientific controversy for the U.S. population as a whole.

Offering little opposition for the general population, especially given the current trends in the wrong direction, should be the twin recommendations to reduce energy intake and increase energy expenditure. The relationships between obesity and increased risk for high blood pressure, HD, stroke, diabetes, various cancers, and osteoarthritis, are now well established *(1,32)*. In the face of this information, all indications suggest ever-larger amounts of food consumed by people, ever-more-sedentary lifestyles shaped by emerging patterns of work and leisure activity, and only a slight increase, on a population-wide basis, in the number of people engaging in regular physical activity programs.

Also well established are the merits of diets with ample representation of vegetables, fruits, cereals, and whole grains *(32)*. Whether from the perspective of their ability to deliver vital micronutrients, their fiber content, or their potential to displace high fat/saturated-fat sources from the diet, an expanded role for these staples could contribute to reduced risk for HD, cancers, stroke, and diabetes, yet these foods are substantially underrepresented in the American diet.

Other convergences could be discussed, but these few in themselves can provide sufficient focus for recommendations to the general public. How do they stack up against the USDA/Department of Health and Human Services *Dietary Guidelines for Americans* *(33*; Table 8)? Reasonably well, on the whole. Yet it is not clear that the messages

Table 8
Dietary Guidelines for Americans (33)

Aim for a healthy weight and be physically active each day.
Let the pyramid guide your food choices.
Choose a variety of grains daily, especially whole grain.
Choose a variety of fruits and vegetables daily.
Choose a diet that is low in salt, saturated fat, cholesterol, and moderate in total fat.
Choose beverages and foods to moderate sugar intake.
If you drink alcoholic beverages, do so in moderation.

Adapted from ref. *33*.

Table 9
Public Health Nutrition Interventions

Nutrition goals
Dietary guidelines
Food assistance
Food safety regulation
Food labeling
Tax policies
Linkage to other sectors

formulated have been direct enough. The 1995 fat recommendation offers an example. Rather than indicating in a straightforward manner that most people should reduce their intake of fatty foods, and, in particular, should reduce their consumption of foods from animal sources, the wording left more interpretive license than is perhaps nutritionally desirable. In 2000, the emphasis is a diet that is low in SFAs and cholesterol to reduce the risk of CHO and moderate total fat to help reduce SFA intake and because high-fat foods have a high-caloric content.

The 2000 recommendation on grain products, vegetables, and fruits does not specifically say that most Americans need to give greater emphasis to these products than they do now. The recommendation to aim for a healthy weight is followed by advice to be physically active each day. There is a national recognition that the population is too sedentary, and that both consumption (34) and food supply data indicate calories are up from a decade ago (14). Challenges remain, to translate the specific , lengthy, and complex information (Dietary Guidelines) into simple messages, and to develop strategies to help Americans achieve healthful eating patterns and daily physical activity.

In looking to the twenty-first century, another issue will present itself as a challenge for dietary guidance, again from the perspective of several disease conditions: the issue of dietary supplements. With an aging population, with an emerging science based on the importance of foods relatively higher in certain micronutrients, and with a population that seems already predisposed to the use of dietary supplements, the issue of such supplements will have to be more constructively engaged in any discussion of dietary guidance (35).

There are, of course, other components to nutrition policy beyond that of dietary guidance. Some examples of a few of the ways that public policy can better capture the convergence in perspectives for the benefit of Americans are shown in Table 9. The importance of the commitment to improve dietary patterns can be demonstrated by shaping the economic supports and incentives built into food assistance programs, aid to producer groups, determination to emphasize more healthful food and physical environments in schools, and support for sustained marketing of the agreed-upon principles. The current demographic and dietary trends transform these issues from "nice things to do" to that of social imperatives. Action is compelled, even in the face of uncertainty.

3.1. Clinical Implications

The role of the clinician (and other health-care providers) is to bring focus to the points of individual variation. Most policy processes are geared to the points of convergence, but the points of individual variation must also be addressed, and they will be increasingly prominent in the coming years, as the science unfolds. It ultimately falls to the clinician to aid people in the considerable challenge of sorting through what they perceive as conflicting advice, of developing strategies for applying general guidance to their particular living circumstances, and of identifying ways in which such guidance parts company with the character of their personal level of risk. Often, these are likely to be complex issues requiring more sophisticated information.

At this point, the community of health professionals is ill-equipped to respond appropriately to this obligation. More medical schools need what may be reasonably termed a clinical nutrition curriculum (*see* Chapter 23). The initiative of the National Institutes of Health to fund, in 1998, 10 awards at $150,000/yr for 5 yr, to be followed with a second group of awards in 1999, is much needed. The awards are intended to encourage the development or enhancement of medical school curricula, to increase opportunities for students, house staff, faculty, and practicing physicians to learn nutrition principles and clinical practice skills, with an emphasis on preventing cardiovascular disease, and to provide training modules for dissemination to other medical schools, as well as to other health care professional schools.

Physicians have lagged behind the general public in acknowledging the relationship between high blood cholesterol levels and risk of CHD. The solution to these shortfalls can only come with improvements in the nutritional component of educational programs for medical, nursing, and other health-care providers, changes in the structure of health service delivery to allow for competent dietary interventions, and introduction of economic incentives to ensure that those interventions are delivered. The fact that more than 75 million Americans are already enrolled in managed care settings, and that the number continues to grow exponentially, holds open the prospects for such changes, but only if a concerted and coordinated effort works to ensure that they occur *(36)*.

Futurists say that the years ahead will be dazzling. The results of advances in the research base could have major implications for the kinds of nutrition targets that will be set in the twenty-first century. As noted by Dr. W. Henry Sebrell, an early Director of the NIH *(1)*:

By many indications, this country's major needs in nutrition today are. . .: (1) control of obesity, (2) elucidation of the role of nutrition in the chronic diseases, (3) assessment of nutritional status as a step toward control of border-line deficiencies, (4) means for complete intravenous alimentation, and (5) additional knowledge regarding nutrition in the aged, under stress, and in convalescence.

The measure of success will be found in the extent to which the agenda will have changed 35 yr later.

REFERENCES

1. US Surgeon General. The Surgeon General's Report on Nutrition and Health. Washington, DC: US Department of Health and Human Services, 1998.
2. National Center for Health Statistics. Births and deaths: United States, 1996. Monthly Vital Statistics Report 1997; 46, Supplement 2.
3. McGinnis JM, Foege WH. Actual causes of death in the United States. JAMA 1993; 270:2207–2212.
4. U.S. Department of Health and Human Services. Healthy People 2010 Objectives: Draft for public comment. Office of Public Health and Science. September 15, 1998.
5. Hobbs FB, Damon BL. 65+ in the United States. U.S. Bureau of the Census. Current Population Reports; Special Studies. Washington, DC. 1996; No. 190: 23.
6. U.S. Department of Health and Human Services. Food and Drug Administration. "Food Labeling; Proposed Rules." Federal Register 1991; Vol. 56, No. 229, 60869-60873 November 27.
7. U.S. Department of Health and Human Services. Food and Drug Administration. "Food Labeling; Final Rules." Federal Register 1993; Vol. 58, No. 3, 2935-2941 January 6.
8. U.S. Department of Health and Human Services. Food and Drug Administration. "Folic Acid; Proposed Rules." Federal Register 1993; Vol. 58, No. 197, October 14.
9. Frazão E. High costs of poor eating patterns in the United States. In: America's Eating Habits. Changes and Consequences. Frazão E, ed. Food and Rural Economics Division. Economic Research Service. U.S. Department of Agriculture. Agriculture Information Bulletin No. 750. 1999; 5–32.
10. White House Conference. White House Conference on Food, Nutrition and Health, Final Report. Washington DC: U.S. Government Printing Office, 1970.
11. Levedahl JW, Oliveira V. Dietary Impact of food assistance programs. In: America's Eating Habits. Changes and Consequences. Frazão E, ed. Food and Rural Economics Division. Economic Research Service. U.S. Department of Agriculture. Agriculture Information Bulletin No. 750. 1999; 307–330.
12. Weiner J. Accelerating the trend toward healthy eating. Public and private efforts. In: Eating Habits. Changes and Consequences. Frazão E, ed. Food and Rural Economics Division. Economic Research Service. U.S. Department of Agriculture. Agriculture Information Bulletin No. 750. 1999; 385–401.
13. Tufts University Dialogue Conference on the Role of Fat-Modified Foods in Dietary Change. Nutr Rev 1997; 56:S1–S2.
14. Putnam J, Allhouse JE. Food Consumption, Prices, and Expenditures, 1970–97. Economic Research Service, USDA Statistical Bulletin No. 965. 1999.
15. United States Department of Agriculture. Nutrient Content of the U.S. Food Supply, 1909–1994. Home Economics Research Report No. 53, October, 1997.
16. New Product News. Food Institute Report, February 8, 1999.
17. Supermarket Business. September, 1998; 26.
18. U.S. Bureau of the Census. Statistical Abstract of the United States: 1998, 118th ed. Washington DC, 1998; 464.
19. Lin B, Guthrie J, Frazão E. Nutrient contribution of food away from home. In: America's Eating Habits. Changes and Consequences. Frazão E, ed. Food and Rural Economics Division. Economic Research Service. U.S. Department of Agriculture. Agriculture Information Bulletin No. 750. 1999; 213–242.
20. NHLBI Obesity Education Initiative Expert Panel on the Identification, Evaluation, and Treatment of Overweight and Obesity in Adults. Clinical Guidelines on the Identification, Evaluation, and Treatment of Overweight and Obesity in Adults. The Evidence Report. Obes Res 1998; 6(Suppl. 2):68S.
21. Kuczmarski RJ, Flegal KM, Campbell SM, Johnson CL. Increasing prevalence of overweight among US adults. The National Health and Nutrition Examination Surveys, 1960–1991. JAMA 1994; 272:205–211.
22. Heimbach JT. Cardiovascular disease and diet: the public view. Public Health Rep 1985; 100:5–12.
23. Guthrie JF, Derby BM, Levy AS. What people know and do not know about nutrition. In: America's Eating Habits. Changes Consequences, Frazao, E. ed. 1999; 243–280.
24. National Heart, Lung, and Blood Institute. Cholesterol awareness surveys [press conference]. Bethesda, MD: National Heart, Lung, and Blood Institute, December 4, 1995.
25. Cleeman JI, Lenfant C. The National Cholesterol Education Program. Progress and Prospects. JAMA 1998; 280:2099–2104.
26. Collins FS, Patrinos A, Jordan E, Chakravarti A, Gesteland R, Walters L. New goals for the U.S. Human Genome Project: 1998–2003. Science 1998; 282:682–689.

27. Pérusse L, Chagnon YC, Weisnagel J, Bouchard C. The human obesity gene map: the 1998 update. Obes Res 1999; 7:111–129.
28. Ohlrogge JB. Design of new plant products: engineering of fatty acid metabolism. Plant Physiol 1994; 104:821–826.
29. Budziszewski GJ, Croft KPC, Hildebrand DF. Use of biotechnology in modifying plant lipids. Lipids 1996; 31:557–569.
30. Knauf VC, Facciotti D. Genetic engineering of foods to reduce the risk of heart disease and cancer. In: Nutrition Biotechnology in Heart Disease and Cancer. Longnecker JB, et al., eds. New York: Plenum, 1995; pp. 221–228.
31. Reese DM. Fundamentals—Rudolf Virchow and modern medicine. West J Med 1998; 169:105–108.
32. Committee on Diet and Health. Food and Nutrition Board. Commission on Life Sciences. National Research Council. Diet and Health. Implications for Reducing Chronic Disease Risk. Washington, DC: National Academy Press, 1989.
33. Nutrition and Your Health: Dietary Guidelines for Americans, 5th ed. Home and Garden Bulletin No. 232. Washington, DC: U.S. Department of Agriculture and U.S. Department of Health and Human Services, 2000.
34. Ernst ND, Sempos CT, Briefel RR, Clark MB. Consistency between US dietary fat intake and serum total cholesterol concentrations: the National Health and Nutrition Examination Surveys. Am J Clin Nutr 1997; 66(Suppl. 4):965S–972S.
35. Commission on Dietary Supplement Labels. Commission on Dietary Supplement Labels Report to the President, Congress, and the Secretary of the Department of Health and Human Services. Washington, DC: U.S. Department of Health and Human Services, 1997.
36. HIAA and AHCPR join forces to help consumers choose and use managed care plans. www.ahcpr.gov/news/press/hia.htm, August 26, 1995.

II   CANCER

2

Vitamin Supplements and Cancer Risk
Epidemiologic Research and Recommendations

Ruth E. Patterson, Alan R. Kristal, and Marian L. Neuhouser

1. INTRODUCTION

Large numbers of Americans are taking vitamin and mineral supplements, despite the limited number of methodologically sound studies on whether supplement use affects disease risk. Recent randomized controlled trials of supplements have yielded some unexpected findings. β-carotene, which was believed to prevent cancer, was found to actually increase the incidence of lung cancer *(1,2)*. Selenium (Se), which was hypothesized to reduce risk of nonmelenomatous skin cancers, had no affect on skin cancer, but instead reduced the risk of a broad range of other cancers *(3)*. The widespread use of supplements can be viewed as a large, uncontrolled, natural experiment.

This chapter describes what is known about vitamin supplements and cancer risk, based on epidemiologic research. As an introduction, the chapter briefly reviews potential mechanisms whereby dietary supplements could prevent cancer, then also presents methodologic considerations important for understanding epidemiologic studies on supplement use and cancer risk. Most of this chapter is devoted to synthesizing results from studies that have provided data on supplement use and cancer risk, then discusses issues relevant to this research, with emphasis on problems in assessment of supplement use and potential confounding factors. Last, information is provided on new studies in this area and the authors give recommendations about the use of vitamin and mineral supplements to prevent cancer.

1.1. Hypothesized Mechanisms of Effect

There is extensive evidence that high consumption of plant foods is associated with lower risk of human cancers *(4–9)*. A comprehensive review of diet and cancer *(9)* concluded that current evidence demonstrates a protective effect of vegetable consumption, and, less definitively, fruit consumption, against almost all major cancers. The mechanisms underlying these associations are probably complex. There are a large number of compounds in plant foods that may influence the risk of cancer, including both micronutrients for normal metabolism and other bioactive compounds with unknown metabolic significance. Included among potential agents are a variety of vitamins (e.g., vitamins A, C, E, and folic acid), their precursors (e.g., β-carotene), and

From: *Primary and Secondary Preventive Nutrition*
Edited by: A. Bendich and R. J. Deckelbaum © Humana Press Inc., Totowa, NJ

minerals (e.g., calcium [Ca] and Se). Whether dietary supplements containing micro-nutrients found in plant foods would be effective chemopreventive agents is of considerable public health interest.

Laboratory studies have suggested many mechanisms whereby micronutrients commonly found in vitamin and mineral supplements could prevent, or promote, cancer. What follows is a very brief overview of some of the more plausible mechanisms. Most attention has focused on the antioxidant micronutrients: carotenoids, vitamins C and E, Se, and zinc (10–14). There are many potentially relevant functions for antioxidants, including protection of cell membranes and DNA from oxidative damage, scavenging and reduction of nitrites, and serving as co-factors for enzymes that protect against oxidative damage (7). However, these compounds may also, in certain conditions, have pro-oxidant effects (15). Vitamin A (i.e., retinol) plays a role in the differentiation of normal epithelial cells and the maintenance of intercellular communication through gap junctions, thus repressing the processes leading to abnormal cell replication (16). Vitamin C enhances immune response and connective tissue integrity (7). Inadequate folic acid may increase hypomethylation of DNA, with subsequent loss of the normal controls on gene expression (17). Iron may increase risk of cancer, because it enhances the growth of transformed cells, and acts as a pro-oxidant, thereby increasing carcinogenic DNA changes and general oxidative stress (18). Ca could reduce colon cancer (CC) risk by binding bile acids (19) and normalizing colorectal epithelial cell proliferation (20). Vitamin D may reduce risk of CC, because it controls the availability and intracellular functions of Ca (13). Se may block the clonal expansion of early malignant cells, perhaps by modulation of cell cycle proteins and apoptotic proteins (21). Improved understanding of cancer biology will be needed for identifying the metabolic processes that can be affected by vitamin and mineral supplementation.

1.2. Prevalence of Supplement Use in the United States

In the United States, consumption of vitamin and mineral supplements is widespread. Based on the 1988–1992 National Health and Nutrition Examination Survey (NHANES III), 35% of males and 44% of females reported taking a dietary supplement in the past month (22). The highest levels of use were seen in females aged 50 yr and older (52–55%), those with greater than high school education (50%), and people living in the West (48%). Supplement use in whites (43%) was considerably greater than in blacks and Mexican Americans (30%). Between 1987 and 1992, retail sales of vitamin and mineral supplements increased by 19% to approx $3.7 billion (23), indicating that there is a trend toward increased use of these products.

1.3. Objectives

The purpose of this chapter is to present human observational and experimental data on the use of vitamin supplements and cancer risk. To examine the role of supplement use, only studies have been included that presented findings on multivitamins or nutrients from supplements, separate from food. Studies on total intake of nutrients (diet plus supplements) are not presented, because it is not possible in such studies to separate effects of other bioactive compounds present in foods from those of the specific micronutrients of interest. Hereafter, the term "vitamin supplement" is meant to include both vitamin and mineral supplements, and the term "multivitamin" refers to a one-a-day type multivitamin with minerals.

Table 1
Vitamin and Mineral Supplement Use
Among 16,747 Participants in the Women's Health Initiative (WHI), 1995

Nutrient	Taking supplement containing nutrient (%)	Intake from supplements among supplement users (Median)	Intake from foods (Median)	Supplement intake as % of total intake among supplement users (Mean)	Supplement intake as % of total intake among all participants (Mean)
Retinol, mcg	43.5	2250	439	53.6	35.2
β-carotene, mcg	42.6	4500	3264	37.1	24.3
Vitamin C, mg	53.1	200	95	51.4	33.7
Vitamin E, mg	53.2	30	7	71.3	46.7
Folate, mcg	44.0	400	245	41.1	26.9
Calcium, mg	51.5	500	672	30.9	20.3
Iron, mg	37.0	18	13	33.4	21.9
Selenium, mcg	32.5	20	89	11.3	7.4

Adapted with permission from ref. 25.

2. BACKGROUND IMPORTANT IN INTERPRETING PUBLISHED STUDIES

2.1. Micronutrient Intakes from Foods and Supplements Differ Markedly

Vitamin and mineral supplements can provide a large proportion of total intakes of some micronutrients, and therefore the variability in total micronutrient intake attributable to supplements can overwhelm that from foods. For example, in a large study of women's health (24), supplement users obtained from 50–70% of their total retinol, vitamin C, and vitamin E from supplements, and the median dose from supplements was generally greater than that from foods (Table 1; 25). In addition, for many nutrients (such as vitamin E), the dose available from supplements (typically 200–1000 mg) is many times larger than can possibly be obtained from foods (about 8–10 mg) (26). Therefore, in many observational studies of cancer risk, the highest levels of intake of many micronutrients could only be obtained from supplements. It follows that some of the significant findings on vitamin or mineral intake were actually detecting an association between supplement use and cancer risk. However, because many studies do not present findings separately for nutrients from foods vs nutrients from supplements, the studies presented here are probably a subset of those that could address associations of supplements with cancer risk.

2.2. Effects of Micronutrients in Multivitamins Cannot Be Isolated

Findings from investigations that measure multivitamin use are a particular analytical challenge, because one cannot isolate the potential effect of the micronutrient of interest (e.g., vitamin A) from all the other vitamins and minerals in the supplement. To investigate micronutrients from supplements, study samples must have sufficient numbers of participants using single supplements (e.g., a capsule containing only vitamin E) to separate the effects of these micronutrients from multivitamin use. The authors suggest that findings on micronutrients that are seldom taken as single supplements (e.g., vitamin

A, folic acid, zinc) almost certainly reflect the use of multivitamins, and are thus confounded by other constituents. Therefore, here are presented only observational studies on multivitamins and the following micronutrients: vitamin C, vitamin E, and Ca. These micronutrients represent the most commonly taken single supplements (27), and therefore it is at least plausible that studies of these micronutrients had enough users to isolate their effect from that of multivitamins.

2.3. Issues of Study Design Related to Research on Vitamin Supplements

Three study designs used in epidemiologic research are described below, with additional comments on their strengths and weaknesses when used to study effects of supplements on cancer risk.

2.3.1. RANDOMIZED CONTROLLED TRIALS

In a randomized controlled trial (RCT), the investigators allocate the exposure (i.e., the supplement) at random. Participants are then followed over a period of time to assess the occurrence of a specified disease outcome. Assuming the sample is sufficiently large, the experimental design of an RCT provides a high degree of assurance about the validity of the results, far superior to that possible with any observational study. However, RCTs are too costly to conduct multiple trials for different types of cancers, nutrients, doses, combinations, or for long periods of time. In addition, in many trials, the participants are selected to be at high risk for the cancer of interest (e.g., smokers in studies of lung cancer [LC]) (1,2), limiting the generalizability of the findings. Finally, prevention trials cannot test an agent with known risk.

2.3.2. COHORT STUDIES

In cohort studies, the supplement use of a group of disease-free participants is measured. This group is then followed to assess the occurrence of multiple disease outcomes. Cohorts are attractive for studies of supplement use, because they can assess the effects of many types, doses, and combinations of supplements, with multiple cancers. Their primary limitation is that the exposure is self-selected, so that investigators must measure and control for factors (such as diet or exercise) likely to confound supplement–cancer associations. In addition, most long-standing cohort studies have inadequate statistical power to test associations of supplement use with cancer, because supplement use was relatively rare when these cohorts were established (27).

2.3.3. CASE–CONTROL STUDIES

In case–control studies, participants are selected based on whether they do (case) or do not (control) have cancer. The groups are then compared to see whether supplement use varies by disease status. Selection bias can occur if supplement users are more likely than nonusers to agree to be controls in a study. This bias is probable, because supplement users are more interested in health issues than nonusers (28), and therefore more likely to participate in a research study. Selection bias may, therefore, lead to finding a protective effect of a supplement, which may be erroneous. Recall bias can occur if individuals with cancer remember and report their use of supplements differently than controls, which can result in either an overestimation or underestimation of the association of supplement use with cancer risk.

3. REVIEW OF STUDIES
ON VITAMIN SUPPLEMENTS AND CANCER RISK

3.1. Methods

Below are summarized the published literature on vitamin supplements and cancer risk, organized by supplement type and by study design. Results are presented grouped by supplement type, because an evaluation of which vitamin supplements are associated with cancer at all sites is important for the development of public health recommendations for the prevention of cancer as a whole. Because "supplement(s)" is not a Medline subject heading, there is no straightforward way to identify relevant epidemiologic studies. The majority of the articles were found through a systematic survey of 18 major journals (see Appendix A) on nutrition, cancer, and epidemiology. The authors searched all articles on diet and cancer for findings on vitamin supplements, and conducted a bibliographic database search for randomized controlled trials, cohort studies, or case–control studies on diet (or nutrition) and neoplasms that contained the words "supplement," "supplements," or "supplementation" in the title or abstract.

This chapter is limited in several ways. Because few studies presented findings on vitamin supplements before 1985, the authors searched journals from 1980 onward (up to October, 1998). A paper was included only if there were at least 50 cancer end points (cases or deaths) in adults; studies of precancerous conditions (e.g., colon adenomas or leukoplakia) or treatment studies (e.g., prevention of cancer recurrence) were not reviewed.

When available, the authors present adjusted relative risks (and 95% confidence intervals [CI]) for higher vs lower levels of vitamin supplement use (i.e., dose). When relative risks and CIs were not provided, relative risks only are presented, relative risks from published tables are calculated, or a description of findings (e.g., no association) is provided.

Because the most tested agent in RCTs of supplements has been β-carotene, these findings are presented in a table (Table 2). β-carotene has only recently been available as a supplement to the general public, and therefore there are no observational studies on this compound. Because of the amount of attention given to an RCT of Se, these findings are described in detail. All data are presented on multivitamins and the other most common single supplements: vitamin C, vitamin E, and Ca. As noted, because other vitamins and minerals (e.g., vitamin A, folic acid, Se) are generally only obtained from multivitamin pills, results are not presented for those nutrients.

3.2. Randomized, Controlled Trials of β-Carotene

Table 2 gives results from the five randomized controlled trials that have examined either supplemental β-carotene alone or β-carotene combined with other supplemental nutrients (1,2,29–33). These trials were motivated by observational epidemiology, animal experiments, and mechanistic studies of carcinogenesis. There are strong and consistent findings of protective effects for fruit and vegetable consumption (primary dietary sources of carotenoids), total carotenoid intake, and serum carotenoid concentration on cancer incidence, particularly for cancer of the lung. However, not a single trial of β-carotene, either alone or combined with other agents, found protective effects for

Table 2
Randomized Controlled Trials of β-Carotene (or Combinations Containing β-Carotene) and Risk of Cancer

Study name (ref.)	Agent	End point(s)	Cases	Relative risk for supplementation
Skin Cancer Prevention Study (29,30)	50 mg β-carotene	Cancer mortality		
		All sites	82	0.8 (0.5–1.3)[a]
		Incidence		
		Nonmelanoma skin cancer	1952	1.0 (0.9–1.2)[a]
		Basal cell	651	1.0 (0.9–1.2)[a]
		Squamous cell	132	1.2 (0.9–1.7)[a]
Nutrition Intervention Trials in Linxian, China (31)	15 mg β-carotene, 50 mcg Se, and 30 mg AT	Cancer mortality		
		All sites	792	0.9 (0.8–1.0)
		Esophageal	360	1.0 (0.8–1.2)
		Stomach	331	0.8 (0.6–1.0)
		Cardia	253	0.8 (0.6–1.0)
		Noncardia	78	0.7 (0.5–1.1)
Nutrition Intervention Trials in Linxian, China (32)	High dose (2–3× the RDA) multivitamin with minerals and 15 mg β-carotene	Cancer mortality		
		All sites	176	1.0 (0.7–1.3)[a]
		Esophageal	82	0.8 (0.5–1.3)[a]
		Stomach	77	1.2 (0.9–1.9)[a]
		Incidence		
		All sites	448	1.0 (0.9–1.2)[a]
		Esophageal	251	0.9 (0.7–1.2)[a]
		Stomach	177	1.2 (0.9–1.6)[a]
The Alpha-Tocopherol, Beta-Carotene Study (1)	20 mg β-carotene	Cancer mortality		
		Lung	564	1.2 (ns)[b]
		Other	552	1.0 (ns)[b]

26

Table 2 (*continued*)

Physicians' Health Study (*33*)	50 mg β-carotene on alternate days	Incidence	
		Lung	876	1.2 (1.0–1.4)
		Four cancers	149–250	No associations
		Cancer mortality	
		All sites	766	1.0 (0.9–1.1)[a]
		Incidence	
		Nine cancers	50–1047	No associations
Beta Carotene and Retinol Efficacy Trial, or CARET (*2*)	30 mg β-carotene and 25,000 IU vitamin A	Cancer mortality	
		Lung cancer	254	1.5 (1.1–2.0)
		Incidence	
		Lung cancer	388	1.3 (1.0–1.6)
		Prostate cancer	300	No associations
		Other cancers	730	No associations

[a]Adjusted relative risk, see original studies for details.
[b]Nonsignificant.

27

any cancer, cancer mortality, or total mortality. In two studies of persons at high risk of LC, because of either smoking or asbestos exposure, β-carotene significantly increased LC incidence by 20 and 30% *(1,2)*. In one of these trials, β-carotene also significantly increased LC mortality and cardiovascular disease mortality *(2)*. In the single trial examining skin cancer, there was no effect on any type of skin cancer or cancer mortality, overall *(29,30)*. Two trials in China examined β-carotene combined with other micronutrients. In one trial focused on cancers of the upper digestive tract, supplementation of 15 mg β-carotene with Se and vitamin E resulted in a near statistically significant 20% reduction in mortality from stomach cancer *(31)*. In a trial of persons with esophageal dysplasia, supplementation with 15 mg β-carotene plus high-dose multivitamins with minerals had no effect on total, esophageal, or stomach cancer incidence or mortality *(32)*. The consistent negative findings from these clinical trials are perplexing, given the strong and consistent protective effects of dietary and serum carotenoids found in observational studies *(4–9,34–36)*. However, it is clear that high-dose β-carotene supplementation will not reduce LCs among smokers or among generally healthy populations.

The increased incidence of cancer among high-risk persons is difficult to understand, but consistency across these carefully designed and executed trials argues strongly against high-dose β-carotene supplementation.

3.3. Randomized, Controlled Trial of Se

A single randomized trial *(3)* has examined the association of Se supplementation with cancer incidence. This trial was designed to test whether Se supplementation would prevent recurrence of nonmelenomatous skin cancers among persons living in parts of the United States where soil Se levels are low. There were no associations of supplementation with skin cancer, but there were unexpected, large, and statistically significant results: a 50% reduction in cancer mortality, a 60% reduction in cancer incidence, and a 60% reduction in prostate cancer (PC) incidence *(3)*. Although these findings require careful replication, they do suggest that Se may be a dietary supplement effective against a number of cancers.

3.4. Multivitamins

Although multivitamins are the most commonly used dietary supplement, few studies have analyzed multivitamin use *per se*. Most studies have summed micronutrients from multivitamins plus single supplements, and reported results for single micronutrients only. Figure 1 shows results of 16 studies that have reported associations of multivitamin use with cancer incidence or mortality *(32,37–50)*. Only two studies have examined all cancer sites, and neither found statistically significant results *(32,37)*. The largest number of studies examined cancers of the upper digestive tract (oral cavity, pharynx, esophagus, and stomach). The single randomized, controlled trial found no associations with cancers of the upper digestive tract *(32)*. Four additional studies examined cancers of the oral cavity, esophagus, and pharynx *(38–40,50)*. One *(50)* found a statistically significant 70% increased risk for oral cancer, but, among the other studies, there were no significant associations or consistent trends. The two large studies of breast cancer (BC) were inconsistent: a cohort study *(41)* found a relative risk near zero, and a case–control study *(42)* found a statistically significant 30% increased risk. Both studies of CC found reduced risks *(43,44)*, although only one finding of a 50% decreased risk was statistically significant *(44)*. Both studies of cervical cancer found statistically significant 40 and

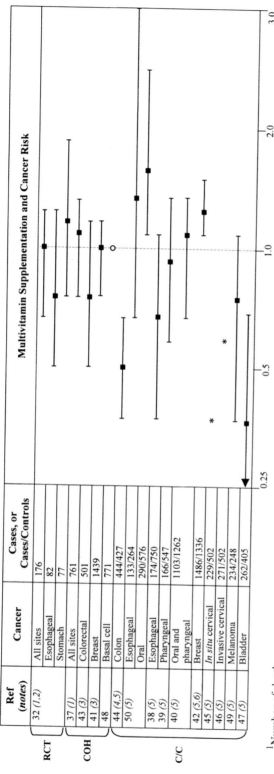

Multivitamin Supplementation and Cancer Risk

Ref (notes)	Cancer	Cases, or Cases/Controls
RCT		
32 (1,2)	All sites	176
	Esophageal	82
	Stomach	77
COH		
37 (1)	All sites	761
43 (3)	Colorectal	501
41 (3)	Breast	1439
48	Basal cell	771
C/C		
44 (4,5)	Colon	444/427
50 (5)	Esophageal	133/264
	Oral	290/576
38 (5)	Esophageal	174/750
39 (5)	Pharyngeal	166/547
40 (5)	Oral and pharyngeal	1103/1262
42 (5,6)	Breast	1486/1336
45 (5)	*In situ* cervical	229/502
46 (5)	Invasive cervical	271/502
49 (5)	Melanoma	234/248
47 (5)	Bladder	262/405

[1] Number of deaths.
[2] High dose multivitamins with minerals, including 15 mg beta-carotene.
[3] Adjusted relative risk.
[4] Average dose per year over a 10-year reference period.
[5] Adjusted odd ratio.
[6] Vitamins ABCDE and minerals. Other mixtures included ABCD with or without minerals, and ABCDE without minerals, and ABCDE with selenium only.
None of the other mixtures had statistically significant relative risks.

Fig. 1. Results of studies of multivitamin supplementation and cancer risk: Relative risks (RR) and odds ratios (ORs) with 95% CI, in which a point estimate < 1.0 indicates that multivitamins reduce risk of cancer, and a confidence interval (CI) that does not include zero indicates that the finding was statistically significant ($p < 0.05$). A "○" indicates that there was no statistically significant association, and the RR or OR was not presented in the original manuscript. A "*" indicates that there was a statistically significant association, but the CIs were not given in the original manuscript. An arrow indicates that the CI exceeds the scale. RCT = randomized controlled trial; COH = cohort; and C/C = case–control.

60% reduced risks *(45,46)*. The single study of bladder cancer found a statistically significant 39% reduced risk *(47)*.

Studies of multivitamins do not support a protective effect of multivitamins for cancers of the upper digestive tract (oral, pharyngeal, esophageal, and stomach) or breast. There is limited evidence for a protective effect for cancers of the colon, bladder, and cervix.

3.5. Vitamin C

Figure 2 shows results of the 24 studies that have reported associations of supplemental Vitamin C with cancer incidence or mortality *(31,37–41,44–48,50–62)*. Three studies examined all cancer sites combined, and none found either large or statistically significant effects *(31,37,51)*. The largest number of studies examined cancers of the upper digestive tract. The single randomized controlled trial *(31)* found no associations with cancers of the upper digestive tract. Of the five additional studies, two found statistically significant protective effects: a 50% reduced risk of pharyngeal *(39)* and 30% reduced risk of oral plus pharyngeal *(40)*. The remaining studies of upper digestive tract cancer found no statistically significant effects *(38,50,52)*. The five studies of BC found no statistically significant effects or consistent trends *(41,51,53–55)*. Of the three studies that examined LC, one found a statistically significant 60% reduced risk for men and a nonsignificant 40% increased risk for women *(56)*; results of other studies were inconsistent, and none were statistically significant *(51,57)*. Of the four studies that examined CC, one found a statistically significant 40% reduced risk *(44)*, two found nonstatistically significant reduced risks *(51,58)*, and one a reduced risk for women only *(59)*. Both studies of cervical cancer found statistically significantly reduced risks: 50% for *in situ* *(45)* and 30% for invasive *(46)*. Results from the four studies that examined bladder cancer were inconsistent: One study found a statistically significant 40% reduced risk for men only *(51)*; of the remaining studies, one found a nonsignificant 30% reduced risk *(60)*, one a 50% reduced risk *(47)*, and a third found a 50% reduced risk in women and a 20% increased risk in men *(61)*.

Studies of vitamin C do not support a protective effect for total cancers, BC, or LC. There is modest evidence for a protective effect for cancers of the upper digestive tract, cervix, bladder, and colon.

3.6. Vitamin E

Figure 3 shows results for the 22 studies that have reported associations of supplemental vitamin E with cancer incidence or mortality *(31,37,40,41,44–48,50–55,58,59,62–66)*. Only three studies report associations with all cancer sites combined; two found nonstatistically significant 20% *(31,51)* reductions in risk, and one found a nonstatistically significant 60% reduction in risk *(37)*. One of these studies was a randomized, controlled trial that combined vitamin E with β-carotene and Se, so that its result cannot be attributed to vitamin E alone *(31)*. None of the five studies of BC found statistically significant associations or consistent trends *(41,51,53–55)*. Of the three studies on LC, only the study among nonsmokers found a significant 50% reduced risk for both men and women *(64)*. The randomized trial designed specifically to test whether vitamin E could prevent LC in smokers found no effect *(1)*. However, an unexpected finding in this trial was a statistically significant 30% reduced risk for PC *(63)*. Ten studies examined upper digestive tract cancers. Of the two randomized controlled trials, the trial examining the vitamin E, Se, and β-carotene, combined, found a near statistically significant

20% reduction in stomach cancer *(31)*; the other trial of vitamin E alone found a nonstatistically significant 30% increased risk *(1)*. Of the three studies that examined oral cancer alone, or oral plus pharyngeal cancer, two found statistically significant protective effects, ranging from a 50 to 70% reduced risk *(40,65)*. The remaining studies of upper digestive tract cancers found nonstatistically significant protective effects *(50,52)*. Of the six studies that examined CC, two observational studies found statistically significant protective effects of 50 and 60% reduced risks *(44,58)*. The randomized controlled trial found a nonsignificant 20% reduced risk *(1)*, and the remaining observational studies found small reduced risks in women, but not men *(51,59,66)*.

Studies of vitamin E do not support an association with BC or smoking-related LCs. The single study of a protective effect for PC is important, but it is difficult to interpret this finding without evidence from other studies. There is modest evidence for associations of vitamin E with cancers of the upper digestive tract, and somewhat stronger evidence of an association with reduced risk of CC.

3.7. Calcium

Figure 4 gives results of the seven studies that have reported associations of Ca supplementation with cancer incidence *(44,62,67–71)*. Of the four studies that examined CC, one found a statistically significant reduced risk (the odds ratio [OR] was not reported) *(69)*, and two found nonstatistically significant 20 and 30% reduced risks *(44,68)*. The single report for endometrial cancer found a small, nonstatistically significant reduced risk *(62)*, and the single report for rectal cancer found a near statistically significant 24% reduced risk *(70)*. The single report on PC found a statistically significant and large (approx 300%) increased risk; however, the exceptionally wide CIs suggest that this finding be viewed with caution *(71)*.

Studies of Ca supplementation and cancer are very limited. There is modest evidence for a protective effect of Ca supplementation on CC, and perhaps rectal cancers.

4. DISCUSSION

Taken together, these results provide only modest support for an association of supplement use with cancer risk. Certainly the strongest findings are from the RCTs that indicate β-carotene can increase incidence of cancer in smokers, α-tocopherol (AT) (vitamin E) can reduce risk of PC, and Se may prevent a broad range of cancers. No supplements appear to be related to BC. Cancers of the gastrointestinal tract appear to be inversely associated with all the supplements examined here, with perhaps the most consistent associations seen between vitamin E and CC.

There are a number of methodologic problems in much of the epidemiologic research on supplement use. These limitations are important to consider before drawing conclusions from this review. Here are discussed three important issues: measurement error in assessment of supplement use, importance of a time-integrated measure, and supplement use as a marker for cancer-related behavior.

4.1. Measurement Error in Assessment of Supplement Use

Epidemiologic studies typically use personal interviews or self-administered questionnaires to obtain information on 3–5 general classes of multiple vitamins, and on single supplements, the dose of single supplements, and, sometimes, frequency and/or

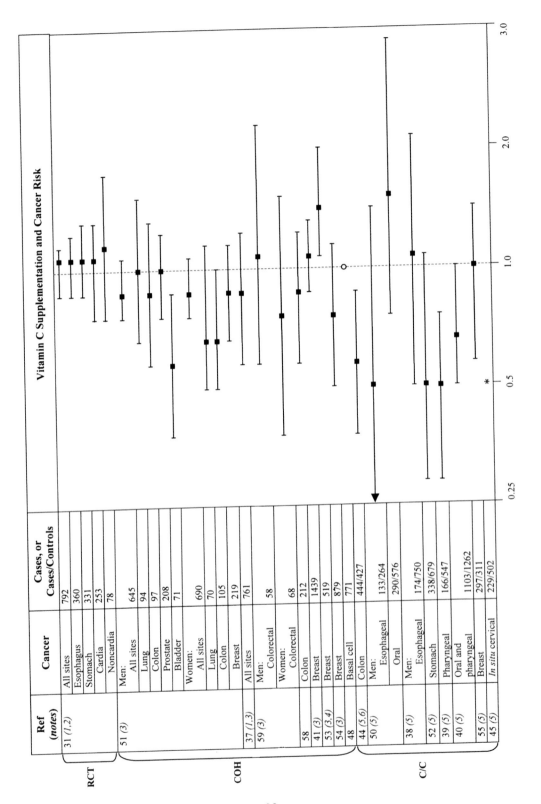

Vitamin C Supplementation and Cancer Risk

Ref (notes)	Cancer	Cases, or Cases/Controls	Vitamin C Supplementation and Cancer Risk
46 (5)	Invasive cervical	271/502	
62	Endometrial	103/236	
56 (5)	Men: Lung	230/597	
	Women: Lung	102/268	
57 (5)	Lung	839/772	
60 (5)	Bladder	323/392	
61 (5)	Men: Bladder		
	Women: Bladder	261/522	
47 (5,6)	Bladder	240/395	

C/C

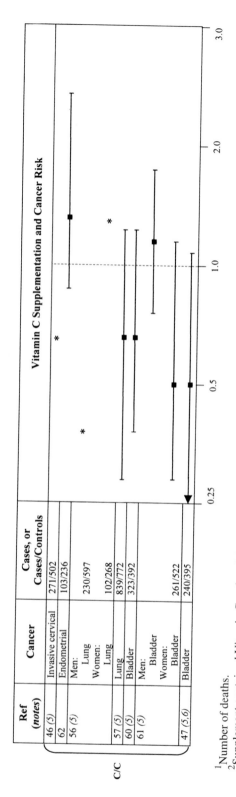

[1] Number of deaths.
[2] Supplement contained Vitamin C and molybdenum.
[3] Adjusted relative risk.
[4] Nestled case control analysis; odds ratio used to approximate relative risk.
[5] Adjusted odds ratio.
[6] Average dose per year over a 10 year reference period.

Fig. 2. Results of studies of vitamin C supplementation and cancer risk: RRs and ORs with 95% CI, in which a point estimate < 1.0 indicates that vitamin C reduces risk of cancer, and a CI that does not include zero indicates that the finding was statistically significant ($p < 0.05$). A "○" indicates that there was no statistically significant association, and the RR or OR was not presented in the original manuscript. A "*" indicates that there was a statistically significant association, but the CIs were not given in the original manuscript. First column gives types of study, in which RCT = randomized controlled trial, COH = cohort, and C/C = case–control.

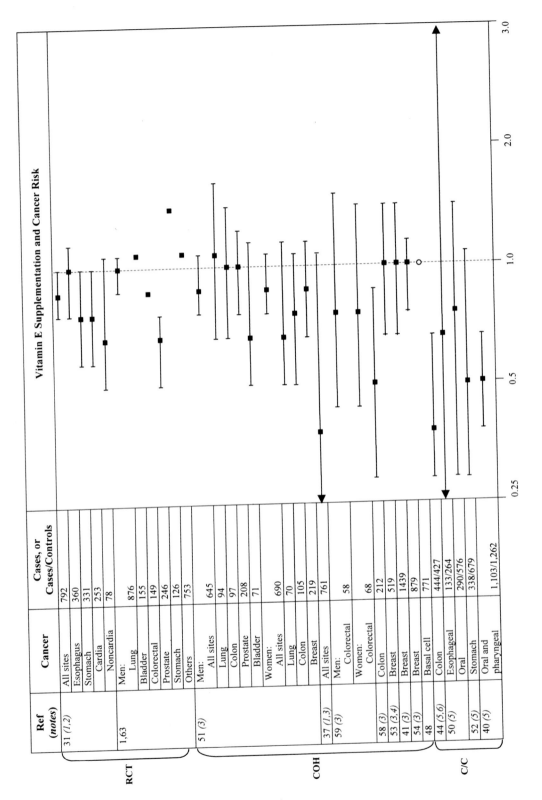

Vitamin E Supplementation and Cancer Risk

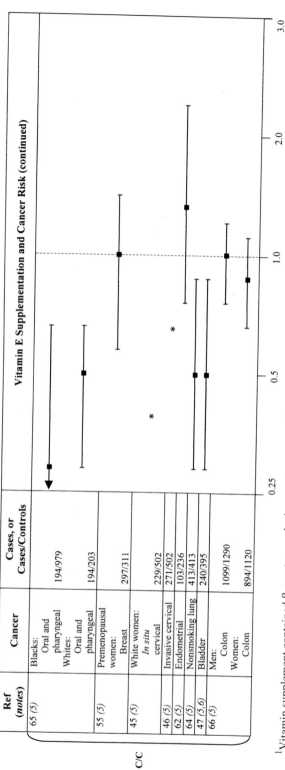

Vitamin E Supplementation and Cancer Risk (continued)

Ref (notes)	Cancer	Cases, or Cases/Controls
65 (5)	Blacks: Oral and pharyngeal	194/979
55 (5)	Whites: Oral and pharyngeal	194/203
55 (5)	Premenopausal women: Breast	297/311
45 (5)	White women: In situ cervical	229/502
46 (5)	Invasive cervical	271/502
62 (5)	Endometrial	103/236
64 (5)	Nonsmoking lung	413/413
47 (5,6)	Bladder	240/395
66 (5)	Men: Colon	1099/1290
	Women: Colon	894/1120

C/C

[1] Vitamin supplement contained β-carotene, selenium, and α-tocopherol.
[2] Number of deaths.
[3] Adjusted relative risks.
[4] Nested case-control analysis; odds ration used to approximate relative risk.
[5] Adjusted odds ratio.
[6] Average dose per year over 10-year reference period.

Fig. 3. Results of studies of vitamin E (AT) supplementation and cancer risk: Relative risk and odds ratios with 95% CI, in which a point estimate < 1.0 indicates that vitamin E reduces risk of cancer, and a CI that does not include zero indicates that the finding was statistically significant ($p < 0.05$). A "○" indicates that there was no statistically significant association, and the RR or OR was not presented in the original manuscript. A "■" indicates that there was no statistically significant association, and only the RR or OR is presented in the original manuscript, but not the CIs. A "*" indicates that there was a statistically significant association, but the CIs were not given in the original manuscript. First column gives types of study in which RCT = randomized controlled trial, COH = cohort, and C/C = case–control.

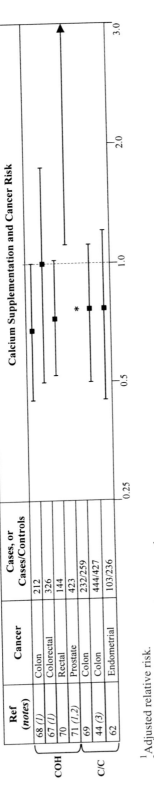

Calcium Supplementation and Cancer Risk

Ref (notes)	Cancer	Cases, or Cases/Controls
COH		
68 (1)	Colon	212
67 (1)	Colorectal	326
70	Rectal	144
71 (1,2)	Prostate	423
69	Colon	232/259
C/C		
44 (3)	Colon	444/427
62	Endometrial	103/236

[1] Adjusted relative risk.
[2] Relative risk based on metastatic cancer only.
[3] Adjusted odds ratio.

Fig. 4. Results of studies of Ca supplementation and cancer risk: RRs or ORs with 95% CI, in which a point estimate < 1.0 indicates that Ca was associated with reduced risk of cancer, and a CI that does not include zero indicates that the finding was statistically significant ($p < 0.05$). A "*" indicates that there was a statistically significant association, but the CIs were not given in the original manuscript. An arrow indicates that the point estimate and CI exceeds the scale. COH = cohort; C/C = case–control. There were no published randomized controlled trials of Ca supplementation and cancer incidence of mortality.

duration of use. However, until recently, scant attention has been paid to the validity of these types of instruments.

The authors conducted a validation study, comparing supplement data collected in a telephone interview and from a self-administered questionnaire with data derived from a detailed in-person interview and transcription of the labels of supplement bottles (i.e., a gold standard), among adult supplement users in Washington State ($n = 104$). Correlation coefficients, comparing average daily supplemental vitamin and mineral intake from the interview or questionnaire to the gold standard, ranged from 0.8 for vitamin C to 0.1 for iron *(72)*. These results suggest that commonly used epidemiologic methods of assessing supplement use may incorporate significant amounts of error in estimates of some nutrients. The effect of this type of nondifferential measurement error is to attenuate measures of association, which could obscure many significant associations of supplement use with cancer.

4.2. Importance of a Time-Integrated Measure of Supplement Use

Investigators studying diet and chronic diseases usually wish to measure an individual's long-term nutrient intake, because the induction and latent periods for these diseases are long *(4,5)*. However, many studies only asked participants about their current use of vitamin and mineral supplements, or only obtained information about supplement use at one point in time. Potential sources of variability in supplement use over time include changes in the type of multivitamin used, number of years the supplement was taken, formulations of multivitamins or dose of single supplements, and frequency of taking supplements.

The authors conducted a mailed survey to investigate the relationship between current and long-term (10-yr) supplement use ($n = 325$ adults) *(73)*. Estimates of current daily intakes for supplemental micronutrients were roughly twice that of average daily intake over the past 10 yr. Correlations between current intake and long-term intake from supplements alone were 0.77, 0.75, and 0.65 for vitamin C, E, and Ca, respectively *(73)*. This measurement error may also have contributed to many of the null associations in this review.

4.3. Supplement Use as Marker for Cancer-Related Behavior

Observational studies on supplement use can be seriously compromised by confounding, because supplement use is strongly related to other factors that affect cancer risk. Supplement users are more likely than nonusers to be female, Caucasian, better-educated, affluent, nonsmokers, light drinkers, and to consume diets lower in fat and higher in fiber and some micronutrients *(74–76)*. However, one set of potential confounding variables, only recently explored, are those specific to cancer risk: screening, use of potentially chemopreventive agents, and diet-related attitudes and behavior.

The authors used data from a random-digit-dial survey to monitor cancer risk behavior in adults in Washington State ($n = 1449$) *(28)*. Among women, supplement users were over twice as likely as nonusers to have had a sigmoidoscopy or a hemoccult, and 1.5× more likely to have had a mammogram. Among men, supplement users were about twice as likely to have had a prostate-specific antigen (PSA) test, or to regularly take aspirin. Supplement users were statistically significantly more likely to exercise regularly, eat four or more servings fruits and vegetables per day, follow a low-fat diet pattern, and believe in a connection between diet and cancer.

These relationships could confound studies of supplement use and cancer risk in complex ways. For example, male supplement users were more likely to have had a PSA test, which is associated with increased diagnosis of PC. Thus, supplement users could appear to have a higher incidence of PC. However, if early diagnosis of PC by PSA reduces mortality, supplement users could appear to have lower PC mortality. Health beliefs influence cancer risk through behavior such as diet and exercise. For example, in a previous prospective study, the authors found that belief in a connection between diet and cancer was a statistically significant predictor of changes to more healthful diets over time (77). In cohort studies, the increasing healthfulness of supplement users' diets and other health practices over time could result in a spurious positive association between supplement use and chronic disease.

In theory, control in analyses for demographics and health-related behavior adjusts for these confounding factors. However, absence of residual confounding cannot be assured, especially if important confounding factors are unknown, not assessed, or not included in the analyses.

4.4. Future Research

It is clear, from the above review and discussion, that there is not sufficient high-quality research on vitamin supplements and cancer risk from which to draw any firm conclusions. In particular, attention needs to be paid to obtaining measures of both dose and duration of use. However, there are several new initiatives that should result in considerable enhancement of the knowledge base regarding these compounds.

The National Cancer Institute recently funded a cohort study specifically designed to focus on dietary supplement use and cancer risk (E. White, personal communication). Investigators will assemble a cohort of 35,000 men and 40,000 women, recruited so that 75% have regularly used some type of dietary supplement (vitamins, minerals, or botanicals) over the last 10 yr. The cohort will be recruited by mail within the 13 counties of western Washington State, and cancer-related end points will be ascertained by periodic linkage to the western Washington Surveillance Epidemiology and End Results cancer registry.

A new randomized trial is being designed to test the individual and combined effects of AT and Se on PC risk (C. A. Coltman, Jr., personal communication). This trial is motivated, in part, by the secondary results from two RCTs, which suggested that supplementation with AT could reduce PC incidence (63), and Se could reduce incidence of several carcinomas (3). This trial is expected to begin recruitment in 2000.

In addition, there is reason to hope that the intriguing results of the β-carotene and Se RCTs will motivate epidemiologists to measure supplement use carefully, and to report findings on supplements separately from those on food.

5. RECOMMENDATIONS

As noted, increasing numbers of Americans are taking vitamin and mineral supplements. Because of these trends, health professionals are confronted regularly with questions regarding the efficacy of these compounds. It is no longer acceptable to simply state that these products do not work, or to claim ignorance regarding their efficacy.

Most supplement users have already decided that these compounds improve their health. In a small study on motivations and beliefs of supplement users ($n = 104$), the authors found that supplement users believed that multivitamins helped them feel better (41%), vitamin C prevents colds and/or flu (76%), and vitamin E and Ca prevent chronic disease (60–80%) *(78)*. Many participants felt that foods could not supply adequate amounts of certain nutrients, indicating that advice to eat a balanced diet would not reduce their motivation to take dietary supplements.

Given the large numbers of Americans taking supplements, it is important to formulate recommendations regarding their use, despite the inadequate research base. Recommendations for persons with rare disorders such as hemochromatosis, or with chronic diseases such as renal disease requiring hemodialysis, are complex, and require careful, informed, and individualized evaluation. For the general population, the authors feel the following recommendations regarding vitamin supplements and cancer risk are consistent with the literature, and are responsible.

- Results of randomized, controlled trials clearly indicate that cigarette smokers, or other individuals at high risk for LC, should not take β-carotene supplements. Healthy adults will receive no benefit from β-carotene supplementation.
- The authors believe it is premature to recommend Se supplementation. The evidence regarding Se and cancer is minimal: unexpected, secondary findings from a small trial of high-Se yeast tablets *(79)*. In addition, little is known about toxicity of the so-called food forms of Se vs inorganic forms of Se (selenate or selenite, the latter of which is relatively instable) *(80)*. If an individual chooses supplementation, the authors recommend use of an organic form, such as high-Se brewer's yeast, and a daily dose that does not exceed 200 mcg, a form and dose that appears to have been safe in the U.S. intervention trial *(3)*.
- A daily multivitamin and mineral pill is unlikely to be harmful, and may be beneficial.
- Vitamin C supplementation may reduce the risk of some cancers, particularly those of the GI tract and the bladder. Anecdotal evidence indicates that doses as high as 1 g/d are safe, and most recent research finds little or no evidence of toxicity at even higher levels *(81,82)*. Nonetheless, the authors suggest that doses not exceed 500 mg/d, based on two lines of evidence. First, there are pharmacokinetically determined limits on effects of oral vitamin C on plasma levels *(83)*; second, the long-term risks of very high levels of supplementation are unknown.
- Studies to date suggest that vitamin E supplementation may reduce risk of PC or CC. In addition, there is considerable evidence that vitamin E is protective against cardiovascular disease *(84,85)*. The toxicity of vitamin E is low and clinical trials indicate that large doses (200–800 mg/d) do not result in serious side effects in most adults *(86)*. The authors recommend doses ranging from 200 to 400 mg/d.
- There is some modest evidence that Ca supplements may reduce risk of CC. Given the much stronger evidence that this supplement can prevent osteoporosis *(87)*, use of Ca supplements in the range of 500–1000 mg/d may be prudent for many Americans.
- There is essentially no epidemiologic research on other vitamin (e.g., vitamin A, vitamin D, and the B vitamins) and mineral (e.g., chromium, copper, magnesium, iron, Zn) supplements and cancer, because most Americans obtain these supplementary micronutrients from a multivitamin. Because of the risk of toxicity, the authors do not recommend high-dose supplementation of vitamins A or D *(86,88)*. The B vitamins (including folic acid) are relatively nontoxic *(26)*, and therefore are low-risk supplements. Given the possibility that iron increases cancer risk *(18)*, the authors advise against large doses of this mineral for the purposes of preventing cancer. No recommendations are possible regarding other minerals.

Finally, Americans need a strong message that there are many nonnutritive compounds in foods, especially in fruits and vegetables, which probably play an important role in the prevention of cancer and other diseases *(4,5)*. Therefore, it should be emphasized that supplements are just that: food supplements, and not food replacements. Vitamin supplements cannot replace the benefits obtained from eating a diet high in fruit and vegetables, nor can they reverse the damage caused by a low-fiber, high-fat diet. It must be made clear to consumers that vitamin and minerals supplements do not, and cannot, compensate for a poor diet.

APPENDIX A: JOURNALS REVIEWED (1980–1998)

American Journal of Clinical Nutrition
American Journal of Epidemiology
American Journal of Public Health
Annals of Epidemiology
Cancer Causes and Control
Cancer Epidemiology, Biomarkers & Prevention
Cancer Research
Epidemiology
European Journal of Cancer Prevention
International Journal of Cancer
International Journal of Epidemiology
Journal of the American Medical Association
Journal of the National Cancer Institute
Journal of Nutrition
Lancet
New England Journal of Medicine
Nutrition and Cancer
Preventive Medicine

REFERENCES

1. The Alpha-Tocopherol Beta Carotene Cancer Prevention Study Group. The effect of vitamin E and beta carotene on the incidence of lung cancer and other cancers in male smokers. N Engl J Med 1994; 330:1029–1035.
2. Omenn GS, Goodman GE, Thornquist MD, et al. Effects of a combination of beta carotene and vitamin A on lung cancer and cardiovascular disease. N Engl J Med 1996; 334:1150–1155.
3. Clark LC, Combs GF Jr, Turnbull BW, et al. Effects of selenium supplementation for cancer prevention in patients with carcinoma of the skin. A randomized controlled trial. Nutritional Prevention of Cancer Study Group. JAMA 1996; 276:1957–1963.
4. Steinmetz K, Potter JD. A review of vegetables, fruit, and cancer. I: Epidemiology. Cancer Causes Control 1991; 2:325–357.
5. Steinmetz K, Potter JD. A review of vegetables, fruit, and cancer. II: Mechanisms. Cancer Causes Control 1991; 2:427–442.
6. Block G, Patterson BH, Subar AF. Fruit, vegetables, and cancer prevention: a review of the epidemiologic evidence. Nutr Cancer 1992; 18:1–29.
7. Steinmetz K, Potter JD. Vegetables, fruit and cancer prevention: a review. J Am Diet Assoc 1996; 96:1027–1039.
8. Verhoeven DTH, Goldbohm RA, Van Poppel G, et al. Epidemiological studies on brassica vegetables and cancer risk. Cancer Epidemiol Biomarkers Prev 1996; 5:733–748.
9. Willett WC, Trichopoulos D. Nutrition and cancer: a summary of the evidence. Cancer Causes Control 1996; 7:178–180.

10. Bertram JS, Dolonel LN, Meyskens FL. Rationale and strategies for chemoprevention of cancer in human. Cancer Res 1987; 47:3012–3031.
11. Moon TE, Micozzi MS. Nutrition and Cancer Prevention: Investigating the Role of Micronutrients. New York: Marcel Dekker, 1988.
12. Diplock AT. Antioxidant nutrients and disease prevention: an overview. Am J Clin Nutr 1991; 53(Suppl.):189–193.
13. Weisburger JH. Nutritional approach to cancer prevention with emphasis on vitamins, antioxidants, and carotenoids. Am J Clin Nutr 1992; 53(Suppl.):226S–2237S.
14. Willett WC. Micronutrients and cancer risk. Am J Clin Nutr 1994; 59(Suppl.):1162S–1165S.
15. Herbert V. Symposium: Prooxidant effects of antioxidant vitamins. J Nutr 1996; 126(Suppl.).
16. Hossian MZ, Wiliens LR, Mehta PP, et al. Enhancement of gap junctional communication by retinoids correlates with their ability to inhibit neoplastic transformation. Carcinogenesis 1989; 10:1743–1748.
17. Giovannucci E, Stampfer MJ, Colditz GA, et al. Folate, methionine, and alcohol intake and the risk of colorectal adenoma. J Natl Cancer Inst 1993; 85:875–884.
18. Bird Cl, Witte JS, Swendseid ME, et al. Plasma ferritin, iron intake, and the risk of colorectal polyps. Am J Epidemiol 1996; 144:34–41.
19. Alberts DS, Rittenbaugh C, Story JA, et al. Randomized, double-blinded, placebo-controlled study of effect of wheat bran fiber and calcium on fecal bile acids in patients with resected adenomatous colon polyps. J Natl Cancer Inst 1996; 88:81–92.
20. Bostick RM, Potter JD, Fosdick L, et al. Calcium and colorectal epithelial cell proliferation: a preliminary randomized, double-blinded, placebo-controlled clinical trial. J Natl Cancer Inst 1993; 85:132–141.
21. Ip C. Lessons from basic research in selenium and cancer prevention. J Nutr 1998; 128:1845–1854.
22. Ervin RB, Wright JD, Kennedy-Stephenson JJ. Use of dietary supplements in the United States, 1988–1994. Vital Health Stat; in press.
23. 1992 Overview of the Nutritional Supplement Market. Washington, DC: 1993.
24. Women's Health Initiative Study Group. Design of the Women's Health Initiative Clinical Trial and Observational Study. Cont Clin Trials 1998; 19:61–109.
25. Patterson RE, Kristal AR, Carter RA, et al. Measurement characteristics of the Women's Health Initiative food frequency questionnaire. Ann Epidemiol 1999; 9(3):178–187.
26. Subcommittee on the Tenth Edition of the RDAs. Recommended Dietary Allowances. Washington, DC: Food and Nutrition Board, Commission on Life Sciences, National Research Council, 1989.
27. Patterson RE, White E, Kristal AR, et al. Vitamin supplements and cancer risk: a review of the epidemiologic evidence. Cancer Causes Control 1997; 8:786–802.
28. Patterson RE, Neuhouser ML, White E, et al. Cancer-related behavior of vitamin supplement users. Cancer Epidemiol Biomarkers Prev 1998; 7:79–81.
29. Greenberg RE, Baron JA, Stukel TA, et al. A clinical trial of beta carotene to prevent basal-cell and squamous-cell cancers of the skin. N Engl J Med 1990; 323:789–795.
30. Greenberg ER, Baron JA, Karagas MR, et al. Mortality associated with low plasma concentration of beta carotene and the effect of oral supplementation. JAMA 1996; 275:699–703.
31. Blot WJ, Li JY, Taylor PR, et al. Nutrition intervention trials in Linxian, China: supplementation with specific vitamin/mineral combinations, cancer incidence, and disease-specific mortality in the general population. J Natl Cancer Inst 1993; 85:1483–1492.
32. Li J, Taylor PR, Li B, et al. Nutrition intervention trials in Linxian, China: multiple vitamin/mineral supplementation, cancer incidence, and disease-specific mortality among adults with esophageal dysplasia. J Natl Cancer Inst 1993; 85:1492–1498.
33. Hennekens CH, Buring JE, Manson JE, et al. Lack of effect of long-term supplementation with beta carotene on the incidence of malignant neoplasms and cardiovascular disease. N Engl J Med 1996; 334:1145–1149.
34. Ito Y, Sazuki S, Yakyu K, et al. Relationship between serum carotenoid levels and cancer death rates in the residents, living in a rural area of Hokkaido, Japan. J Epidemiol 1997; 7:1–8.
35. Comstock GW, Alberg AJ, Huang HY, et al. The risk of developing lung cancer associated with antioxidants in the blood: ascorbic acid, carotenoids, alpha-tocopherol, selenium, and total peroxyl radical absorbing capacity. Cancer Epidemiol Biomarkers Prev 1997; 6:907–916.
36. Dorgan JF, Sowell A, Swanson CA, et al. Relationships of serum carotenoids, retinol, alpha-tocopherol, and selenium with breast cancer risk: results from a prospective study in Columbia, Missouri (United States). Cancer Causes Control 1998; 9:89–97.

37. Losonczy KG, Harris TB, Havlik RJ. Vitamin E and vitamin C supplement use and risk of all-cause and coronary heart disease mortality in older persons: the Established Populations for Epidemiologic Studies of the Elderly. Am J Clin Nutr 1996; 64:190–196.

38. Brown LM, Swanson CA, Gridley G, et al. Adenocarcinoma of the esophagus: role of obesity and diet. J Natl Cancer Inst 1995; 87:104–109.

39. Rossing MA, Vaughan TL, McKnight B. Diet and pharyngeal cancer. Int J Cancer 1989; 44:593–597.

40. Gridley G, McLaughlin JK, Block G, et al. Vitamin supplement use and reduced risk of oral and pharyngeal cancer. Am J Epidemiol 1992; 135:1083–1092.

41. Hunter DF, Manson JE, Colditz GA, et al. A prospective study of the intake of vitamins C, E, and A and the risk of breast cancer. N Engl J Med 1993; 329:234–240.

42. Ewertz M, Gill C. Dietary factors and breast-cancer risk in Denmark. Int J Cancer 1990; 46:779–784.

43. Martinez ME, Giovannucci EL, Colditz GA, et al. Calcium, vitamin D, and the occurrence of colorectal cancer among women. J Natl Cancer Inst 1996; 88:1375–1382.

44. White E, Shannon JS, Patterson RE. Relationship between vitamin and calcium supplement use and colon cancer. Cancer Epidemiol Biomarkers Prev 1997; 6:769–774.

45. Ziegler RG, Jones CH, Brinton LA, et al. Diet and the risk of *in situ* cervical cancer among white women in the United States. Cancer Causes Control 1991; 2:17–29.

46. Ziegler RG, Brinton LA, Hamman RF, et al. Diet and the risk of invasive cervical cancer among white women in the United States. Am J Epidemiol 1990; 132:432–445.

47. Bruemmer B, White E, Vaughan TL, et al. Nutrient intake in relation to bladder cancer among middle-aged men and women. Am J Epidemiol 1996; 144:485–495.

48. Hunter DH, Colditz GA, Stampfer MJ, et al. Diet and risk of basal cell carcinoma of the skin in a prospective cohort of women. Ann Epidemiol 1992; 231–239.

49. Kirkpatrick CS, White E, Lee JAH. Case-control study of malignant melanoma in Washington State. II. Diet, alcohol, obesity. Am J Epidemiol 1994; 139:869–880.

50. Barone J, Tailoi E, Hebert JR, et al. Vitamin supplement use and risk for oral and esophageal cancer. Nutr Cancer 1992; 18:31–41.

51. Shibata A, Paganini-Hill A, Ross PK, et al. Intake of vegetables, fruits, beta-carotene, vitamin C and vitamin supplements and cancer incidence among the elderly: a prospective study. Br J Cancer 1992; 66:673–679.

52. Hansson L, Nyren O, Bergstrom R, et al. Nutrients and gastric cancer risk. A population-based case control study in Sweden. Int J Cancer 1994; 57:638–644.

53. Rohan TE, Howe GR, Friedenreich CM, et al. Dietary fiber, vitamins A, C, and E, and risk of breast cancer: a cohort study. Cancer Causes Control 1993; 4:29–37.

54. Kushi LJ, Fee RM, Sellers TA, et al. Intake of Vitamins A, C, E and postmenopausal breast cancer. Am J Epidemiol 1996; 144:165–174.

55. Freudenheim JL, Marshall JR, Vena JE, et al. Premenopausal breast cancer risk and intake of vegetables, fruits, and related nutrients. J Natl Cancer Inst 1996; 88:340–348.

56. Le Marchand L, Yoshizawa CN, Kolonel LN, et al. Vegetable consumption and lung cancer risk: a population-based case-control study in Hawaii. J Natl Cancer Inst 1989; 81:1158–1164.

57. Jain M, Burch JD, Howe GR, et al. Dietary factors and risk of lung cancer: results from a case-control study, Toronto, 1981–1985. Int J Cancer 1990; 86:33–38.

58. Bostick RM, Potter JC, McKenzie DR, et al. Reduced risk of colon cancer with high intake of vitamin E: the Iowa Women's Health Study. Cancer Res 1993; 53:4230–4237.

59. Wu HA, Paganini-Hill A, Ross RK, et al. Alcohol, physical activity and other risk factors for colorectal cancer: a prospective study. Br J Cancer 1987; 55:687–694.

60. Steineck G, Hagman U, Gerhardsson M, et al. Vitamin A supplements, fried foods, fat and urothelial cancer. A case-referent study in Stockholm in 1985–87. Int J Cancer 1990; 45:1006–1011.

61. Nomura AMY, Kolonel LN, Hankin JH, et al. Dietary factors in cancer of the lower urinary tract. Int J Cancer 1991; 48:199–205.

62. Barbone F, Austin H, Partridge EE. Diet and endometrial cancer: a case-control study. Am J Epidemiol 1993; 137:393–409.

63. Heinonen OP, Albanes D, Virtamo J, et al. Prostate cancer and supplementation with α-tocopherol and β-carotene: incidence and mortality in a controlled trial. J Natl Cancer Inst 1998; 90:440–446.

64. Mayne ST, Janerich DT, Greenwald P, et al. Dietary beta-carotene and lung cancer risk in U.S. nonsmokers. J Natl Cancer Inst 1994; 86:33–38.

65. Day GL, Blot WJ, Austin DF, et al. Racial differences in risk of oral and pharyngeal cancer: alcohol, tobacco, and other determinants. J Natl Cancer Inst 1993; 88:340–348.
66. Slattery ML, Edwares SL, Anderson K, et al. Vitamin E and colon cancer: Is there an association? Nutr Cancer 1998; 30:201–206.
67. Kampman E, Goldbohm RA, van den Brandt PA, et al. Fermented dairy products, calcium, and colorectal cancer in the Netherlands cohort study. Cancer Res 1994; 54:3186–3190.
68. Bostick RM, Potter JD, Sellers TA, et al. Relation of calcium, vitamin D, and dairy food intake to incidence of colon cancer among older women. Am J Epidemiol 1993; 137:1302–1317.
69. Kampman E, Verhoeven D, Sloots L. Vegetable and animal products as determinants of colon cancer risk in Dutch men and women. Cancer Causes Control 1995; 6:225–234.
70. Zheng W, Anderson KE, Kushi LH, et al. A prospective cohort study of intake of calcium, vitamin D, and other micronutrients in relation to incidence of rectal cancer among postmenopausal women. Cancer Epidemiol Biomark Prev 1998; 7:221–225.
71. Giovannucci E, Rimm EB, Wolk A, et al. Calcium and fructose intake in relation to risk of prostate cancer. Cancer Res 1998; 58:442–447.
72. Patterson RE, Kristal AR, Levy L, et al. Validity of methods used to assess vitamin and mineral supplement use. Am J Epidemiol 1998; 148:643–649.
73. Patterson RE, Neuhouser ML, White E, et al. Measurement error from assessing use of vitamin supplements at one point in time. Epidemiology 1998; 9:567–569.
74. Block G, Cox G, Madans J, et al. Vitamin supplement use, by demographic characteristics. Am J Epidemiol 1988; 127:297–309.
75. Subar AF, Block C. Use of vitamin and mineral supplements: demographics and amounts of nutrients consumed. Am J Epidemiol 1990; 132:1091–1101.
76. Slesinski MJ, Subar AF, Kahle LL. Dietary intake of fat, fiber and other nutrients is related to the use of vitamin and mineral supplements in the United States: the 1992 National Health Interview Survey. J Nutr 1996; 126:3001–3008.
77. Patterson RE, Kristal AR, White E. Do beliefs, knowledge, and perceived norms about diet and cancer predict dietary change? Am J Pub Health 1996; 86:1394–400.
78. Neuhouser ML, Patterson RE, Levy L. Motivations for using vitamin supplements. J Am Diet Assoc; in press.
79. Combs GFJ, Clark LC, Turnbull BW. Reduction of cancer risk with an oral supplement of selenium. Biomed Environ Sci 1997; 10:227–234.
80. Patterson BH, Levander OA. Naturally occurring selenium compounds in cancer chemoprevention trials: a workshop summary. Cancer Epidemiol Biomarkers Prev 1997; 6:63–69.
81. Diplock AT. Safety of antioxidant vitamins and beta-carotene. Am J Clin Nutr 1995; 62:1510S–1516S.
82. Johnston CS. Biomarkers for establishing a tolerable upper intake level for Vitamin C. Nutr Rev 1999; 57:771–777.
83. Blanchard J, Tozer TN, Rowland M. Pharmacokinetic perspectives in megadoses of ascorbic acid. Am J Clin Nutr 1997; 66:1165–1170.
84. Jha P, Flather M, Lonn E, et al. The antioxidant vitamins and cardiovascular disease: a critical review of epidemiologic and clinical trial data. Ann Intern Med 1995; 123:860–872.
85. Meydani M. Vitamin E. (Fat-soluble vitamins). Lancet 1995; 345:170–175.
86. Kaegi E. Unconventional therapies for cancer: 5. Vitamins A, C and E. Can Med Assoc J 1998; 158:1483–1488.
87. Nordin BE. Calcium and osteoporosis. Nutrition 1997; 13:664–686.
88. Marriott B. Vitamin D supplementation: a word of caution. Ann Intern Med 1997; 127:231–233.

3

Soy and Cancer Prevention

David B. Fournier, John W. Erdman, Jr.,
and Gary B. Gordon

1. INTRODUCTION

1999 marks the twentieth anniversary of the publication of the classic book entitled, *Soy Protein and Human Nutrition*, which reported the proceedings of a meeting in Keystone, CO, in 1978. The publication primarily addressed issues related to the quality of soy protein for infant and adult feeding *(1)*. One emerging issue was the hypocholesterolemic properties of soy protein, which has now become a mature field of study. There was a concern that a number of biologically active substances in soy products might result in adverse effects, including cancer. Trypsin inhibitors in soy were reported to increase pancreatic cancer in rats, and soy estrogens to depress food intake when fed at high levels *(2)*, but some of the antinutritional factors of concern two decades ago, such as trypsin inhibitors, phytic acid, saponins, and phytoestrogens, are now looked upon for potential health benefits.

2. SOY CONSUMPTION AND CANCER INCIDENCE

Over the past several years, an increasing body of evidence suggests that dietary consumption of fruits and vegetables may help to reduce the incidence of several chronic diseases. Soybeans, in particular, have been recognized as having a potential role in the prevention and treatment of cardiovascular disease, osteoporosis, kidney disease, and cancer. Overall, dietary factors contribute to approx one-third of potentially preventable cancers *(3)*. Conversely, diets high in animal fat and red meat are associated with an increased risk of cancer and other chronic diseases *(4,5)*. Evidence derived from epidemiological studies, although inconsistent, suggests that there may be an association between soy intake and a decreased risk of breast cancer (BC) *(6)*, prostate cancer (PC) *(7)*, stomach cancer *(8)*, colorectal cancer (CC) *(9)*, lung cancer (LC) *(10)*, and endometrial cancer *(11,12)*. However, potential pitfalls encountered by many of these studies have prevented conclusive results from being delineated. For example, some of these studies were not able to separate soy from other dietary variables, and had difficulty discerning between the different types and amounts of soy products being consumed. Further, there are also inherent difficulties in trying to relate specific dietary intakes to the development of cancer many years later.

Considerable research has identified several potential health benefits associated with increased soy consumption, and soybeans are also relatively efficient to produce.

From: *Primary and Secondary Preventive Nutrition*
Edited by: A. Bendich and R. J. Deckelbaum © Humana Press Inc., Totowa, NJ

According to one estimate, an acre of land devoted to soybean production can produce approx 25× the amount of protein as an acre of land devoted to beef production, and 10× the amount of protein as can be produced on an acre of land devoted to milk production (13). Thus, given increasing land and water constraints, soybeans may provide a relatively inexpensive source of high-quality protein to developing countries.

A wide variety of soybean preparations are typically consumed. Traditional soy foods, developed using oriental processing techniques, are generally classified as fermented or nonfermented. Popular Asian-style fermented soyfoods include tempeh, miso, natto, soy sauces, and fermented tofu and soymilk products (14). Nonfermented soy foods include fresh green soybeans, whole dry soybeans, soy nuts, soy sprouts, whole-fat soy flour, soy milk, tofu, okara, and yuba. More recently, soy protein products, including isolates, concentrates, and flour, have been developed. These products, consisting of 50–90% total protein, account for nearly 90% of all soybeans consumed by humans (15). Although nearly half of the world's soybeans are produced in the United States, people in the West consume relatively small amounts of soybeans. In general, people living in the United States and Western Europe eat between 1 and 3 g soyfoods/d; Asians typically consume an average of 20–80 g soy foods/d (16).

Like soy consumption patterns, cancer incidence rates, including those for BC, PC, and CC, vary substantially throughout the world. Typically, however, incidence rates for these cancers tend to be highest in the United States and in Western Europe, and lowest among native Japanese and Chinese peoples (17). Historically, people living in China and Japan have a 4–10-fold decreased risk of developing BC and PC, compared to people living in the West (18). In general, countries with high per capita daily intakes of soy foods have the lowest incidence rates of hormone-dependent cancers (Fig. 1). Moreover, the incidence of BC in Asians migrating to the West increases to levels similar to the native Caucasian population within two generations of migration, among those who assume a westernized diet (19). Conversely, migrants maintaining their traditional Asian diet do not have an increased risk of cancer (20). These observations suggest that variations in hormone-dependent cancer risk are caused by environmental, rather than genetic, factors.

3. POTENTIAL ANTICANCER SOY CONSTITUENTS

Several potential anticarcinogens have been identified in soybeans, including protease inhibitors (PI) (Bowman-Birk inhibitor [BBI] and Kunitz inhibitor), phytic acid, saponins, and isoflavones. Although each of these components have displayed anticarcinogenic activity in vitro, isoflavones have typically been considered the primary anticancer soy constituent. This review provides a brief overview of the in vitro actions of PIs, saponins, and phytic acid, but it focuses primarily on the anticancer data (epidemiology, in vitro, animal, and human) relevant to soybean isoflavones.

4. PIS, SAPONINS, AND PHYTIC ACID: POTENTIAL MECHANISMS OF ANTICARCINOGENIC ACTION

PIs are proteins with typical mol wt between 8000 and 10,000 Daltons. Two of the most extensively studied soy-derived PIs are the BBI and the soybean PI (Kunitz inhibitor). The BBI is a potent anticarcinogen, with activity resulting from the inhibition of both trypsin and chymotrypsin (21,22). Although the precise anticarcinogenic action of BBI

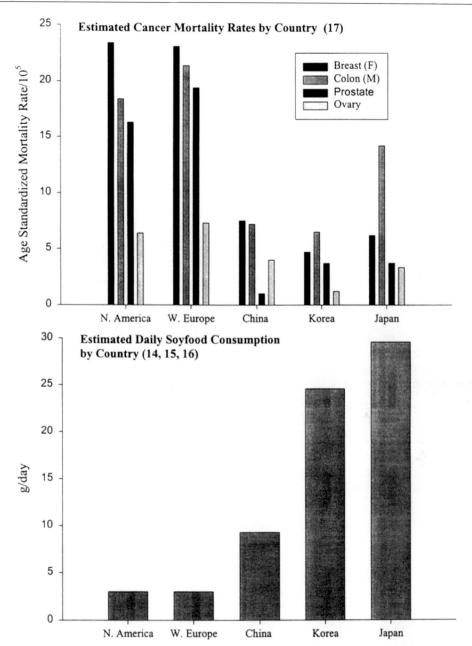

Fig. 1. Estimated cancer mortality rates and daily soyfood consumption by country.

is unknown, PIs have been suggested to suppress carcinogenesis via inhibition of specific oncogenes and proteases thought to be involved in the conversion of a cell from normal to malignant *(23)*.

Saponins are heat-stable glycosides composed of a lipid-soluble aglycone linked to one or more water-soluble sugar residues *(24,25)*. In vitro studies indicate that saponins may exert anticarcinogenic effects via various mechanisms, including selective toxicity toward cancer cells, immune modulation, and regulation of cell proliferation *(25)*. Soybeans and soy products contain approx 0.5 and 0.3–0.4% saponins, respectively *(26)*. Although saponins are reportedly toxic in some fish and cold-blooded animals *(27)*, most saponins, including those derived from soybeans, are not toxic to mammals *(28)*.

Phytic acid is a naturally occurring compound found in plants, cereals, and legumes, which appears primarily as a salt with monovalent and divalent cations (Ca^{2+}, Mg^{2+}, and K^+) *(29)*. In vitro anticarcinogenic properties of phytic acid include a suppressive effect on transition metal oxidant reactivity (decreasing radical generation) *(30)*, the inhibition of lipid peroxidation *(31)*, and as a second messenger involved in cellular proliferation and differentiation. Despite the anticarcinogenic properties exhibited by phytic acid, however, it has been shown to have an inhibitory effect on the bioavailability of several minerals, including calcium, iron, and zinc *(32)*. Consequently, the beneficial anticarcinogenic properties of phytic acid may need to be weighed against potential adverse effects on mineral bioavailability. Although a significant body of in vitro evidence suggests that soybean PIs, phytic acid, and saponins are anticarcinogenic, few studies have examined the specific actions of these components in animal models of cancer *(24,33,34)*.

5. ISOFLAVONE COMPONENT OF SOY AND SOY PRODUCTS

Isoflavones are a group of naturally occurring heterocyclic phenols found in soybeans and forage plants. Genistein (4',5,7-trihydroxyisoflavone) and daidzein (4',7-trihydroxy-isoflavone) are the principal isoflavones found in soybeans. Genistein is formed from biochanin A, and is metabolized to the estrogenically inactive *p*-ethyphenol; daidzein is formed from formononetom, and is metabolized, via intermediates, into equol and 0-desmethylangolensin *(35)*. Typically, genistein and daidzein occur in plants in their bound form as the glycosides, genistin and daidzin, respectively, and are biologically inactive. Metabolism of isoflavones in humans is thought to be facilitated by colonic bacteria, which remove the sugar moiety producing active compounds *(36)*. Several reports examining isoflavone pharmacokinetics suggest that the isoflavones, genistein and daidzein, are readily absorbed and excreted from the human body *(37–42)*. To date, isoflavones have been measured in human urine, plasma, feces, and breast milk, and preliminary studies indicate that urinary and plasma isoflavone levels are significantly increased during chronic soy intake, however, a large amount of interindividual variability may exist *(43)*. Pharmacokinetic calculations indicate that isoflavones ingested from soy-protein isolate may be bioavailable at levels as low as 9 mg/d, an amount equal to approx 1 oz of tofu *(41)*. Soy-based products, including soy milk, tofu, and soy flour, have total isoflavone concentrations in the range of 1.3–3.8 mg/g dry wt (0.2–2.3 mg/g wet wt); soybeans themselves contain genistein and daidzein levels up to 3 mg/g *(14)*. Soy-protein isolates typically contain between 100 and 150 mg total isoflavone per 100 g *(35)*.

5.1. Epidemiology: Intake and Cancer Risk

As indicated, numerous questionnaire-based studies have analyzed the relationship between total soy consumption and cancer risk. The data suggest that increased soy consumption may correlate with a decreased risk of hormone-dependent cancers, but the results are inconclusive, overall, and fail to point to the particular soy constituent(s) responsible for any beneficial effects seen. More recently, investigators have examined the relationship between cancer incidence and prior isoflavone intake, as measured through urine or serum concentrations. For example, Bundred et al. *(44)* compared serum phytoestrogen levels among healthy controls, women with BC treated more than 3 yr previously, and women presenting with BC. Serum phytoestrogens were measured using isotope dilution gas chromatography-mass spectrometry. Overall, the healthy control women had significantly higher serum levels of daidzein and genistein than either previously treated patients or new BC cases.

In a similar study, Ingram et al. *(45)* measured the association between urinary phytoestrogen excretion and subsequent cancer risk. Urine samples were collected from women with newly diagnosed early BC and analyzed for genistein, daidzein, equol, enterodiol, enterolactone, and matairesinol. Age-matched controls were randomly selected from the electoral role. After adjusting for other risk factors, high excretion of both equol and enterolactone was associated with a significant reduction in BC risk. These data corroborate previous observational studies reporting high phytoestrogen excretion among populations with low BC incidences *(46–48)*.

5.2. Potential Mechanisms of Anticarcinogenic Action

Isoflavones display a wide range of in vitro anticarcinogenic activity, including inhibition of protein tyrosine phosphorylation *(49–52)*, inhibition of DNA topoisomerases I and II and oncogenic transformation *(53)*, induction of differentiation in cancer cell lines *(54,55)*, inhibition of cell proliferation *(56,57)*, inhibition of tumor promoter-induced hydrogen peroxide formation *(58)*, induction of apoptosis *(59,60)*, and scavenging of exogenous hydrogen peroxide free radicals, and antipromotional effects *(61,62)*. Although the precise mechanism(s) by which isoflavones may protect against cancer have not yet been clearly defined, several hypotheses have emerged.

5.2.1. HORMONAL EFFECTS

One common theory holds that isoflavone phytoestrogens may reduce cancer risk by decreasing the promotional effects of high levels of endogenous estrogen *(63)*. Because genistein and daidzein have been shown to bind to estrogen receptors (ERs), these isoflavones have been implicated as antiestrogens through competition with endogenous estrogen for receptor binding. However, similar to the antiestrogen, tamoxifen, genistein exhibits paradoxical effects, either agonistic or antagonistic, depending on the species, tissue, and dose administered *(64–66)*. Moreover, studies showing that genistein inhibits cell proliferation similarly, in estrogen receptor (ER)-positive and ER-negative human cancer cell lines, suggests that at least some of the anticarcinogenic activity of isoflavones may be mediated through an ER-independent pathway *(67)*.

5.2.2. ANTIANGIOGENIC EFFECTS

A second line of research indicates that isoflavones may inhibit tumor growth through a reduction in invasion and angiogenesis. Angiogenesis, or the formation of new blood vessels, plays a critical role in the physiologic processes of menstrual cycle, embryonal development, and wound healing, and also contributes to the pathophysiology of a variety of diseases, including rheumatoid arthritis and malignant neoplasms *(68)*. Typically, avascular tumors do not grow beyond a diameter of 1–2 mm *(69)*; well-vascularized tumors can expand and metastasize. Although the exact mechanisms leading to angiogenesis are still unclear, the process is thought to be complex, involving the interaction between a tumor and normal endothelial cells (ECs), extracellular matrix proteins, and multiple stimulatory and inhibitory factors. Tumor cells release a variety of EC mitogens that stimulate angiogenesis, including basic fibroblast growth factor and vascular endothelial growth factor (VEGF). Other angiogenic stimulators include transforming growth factor α (TGF-α), TGF-β, and tumor necrosis factor α, among others.

Proliferation of ECs is accompanied by the degradation of extracellular matrix proteins and the migration of ECs, resulting in lumen formation and development of a new blood vessel *(70)*. Ultimately, the extent of angiogenesis is dependent on the balance between factors that induce or inhibit the formation of blood vessels. A relatively new paradigm in cancer research has been the search for exogenous compounds that modulate pathological angiogenesis. Fotsis et al. *(71)* recently studied the ability of various dietary compounds to inhibit angiogenesis. In that experiment, urine fractions from human subjects consuming a plant-based diet were examined for the presence of antiangiogenic compounds. One of the most potent of the fractions collected was found to contain isoflavonoids: Genistein was subsequently identified as the most effective inhibitor of vascular EC proliferation and in vitro angiogenesis.

More recently, genistein has been shown to exert multiple suppressive effects on breast carcinoma cells, including inhibition of invasion and downregulation of angiogenesis *(72)*. In that study, genistein inhibited invasion of MCF-7 and MDA-MB-231 BC cells, as characterized by downregulation of matrix metalloproteinase-9 and upregulation of tissue inhibitor of metalloproteinase-1. In the MDA-MB-231 zenograft model, genistein also inhibited angiogenesis by decreasing tumor blood vessel density and decreasing the levels of VEGF and TGF-β1.

6. ANIMAL MODELS

Isoflavones have also been examined in a variety of carcinogen-induced and genetic models of cancer, including those of the breast, colon, prostate, liver, and lung. In reports published prior to 1993, 17/26 indicated that soybeans exert some chemoprotective action, as measured through tumor number, incidence, latency, and metastasis *(73)*. However, because a variety of soy preparations were used in many of these studies, the particular action of individual soy components could not be evaluated. Through subsequent experimentation, isolated isoflavones and other soy constituents have been shown to inhibit tumor incidence and/or multiplicity in a wide variety of experimental models of cancer *(74)*.

7. ONGOING HUMAN TRIALS

Recently, the first randomized soy intervention trials, looking at cancer as the primary clinical endpoint, have been initiated. A double-blind, prospective study, seeking to determine if soy protein could reduce indicators of risk for CC, has recently been reported *(75)*. Seventy patients (41 males and 29 females) with previously confirmed adenomatous colon polyps or CC, were recruited. The subjects consumed either a soy or casein (control) supplement for 1 yr, each supplement providing 39–40 g protein. Four blood samples (two at baseline, 6 mo, and end) and eight colon mucosa biopsy samples (four at baseline, four at end) were obtained from each subject. Compliance was measured through bimonthly urinary isoflavone excretion. The biopsies from the sigmoid colon were evaluated for proliferating cellular nuclear antigen labeling index and proliferation zone analysis. The results demonstrate lowering of the proliferation capacity of colonic crypts in subjects consuming the soy supplement *(76)*.

Berrino et al. *(77)* conducted a randomized trial on 104 healthy postmenopausal women, aged 50–65 yr, at high risk of BC because of high serum testosterone levels. Fifty-two of the subjects were randomly assigned to follow a dietary modification, including foods rich in phytoestrogens, for 4.5 mo; another group consumed their usual diet. Compliance with the protocol was reportedly 98%. Fasting blood was collected at baseline and after 2 and 4.5 mo, and was analyzed for hormone levels. Serum testosterone decreased significantly in the diet group (–18.3%), compared to the control group (–7.0%, $p = 0.006$), and sex-hormone-binding globulin increased (–3.4% vs 4.1%, $p = 0.000$). Dietary intervention also significantly decreased total cholesterol, body wt, and waist circumference. Other hormonal assays are currently being performed, and have not yet been reported.

8. FUTURE DIRECTIONS

As the new century begins, we are convinced that soy protein is an excellent-quality protein for human feeding, and are also sure that soy protein will reduce the incidence of coronary heart disease, because soy is effective in the reduction of serum cholesterol. Regarding the second major killer of Americans, cancer, the effects of soy are not so clear. Epidemiological support exists for several cancers, including BC, PC, and CC. In addition, there is supporting cell culture and other in vitro and in vivo evidence, especially for the anticarcinogic actions of the isoflavones. These biologically active estrogens, once thought to be toxins, may play an anticarcinogic role in certain cell types. Researchers should be careful, however, with in vitro systems, to stay within physiologically relevant ranges of isoflavones. Future work should take advantage of the animal models for cancer and, when appropriate, utilize the human directly. Several pilot cancer trials are underway, and, based on the results of those trials, intervention trials may follow. In 10–20 yr, reviews on soy protein and human health may detail the anticancer benefits of soy.

9. RECOMMENDATIONS

It is prudent for health-conscious persons to include soy protein as part of their dietary selections throughout the week. Soy protein is a complete protein, with clear advantages for those who would like to reduce their intake of animal-based foods or those with elevated serum cholesterol. Soy foods are generally cholesterol-free, can be low in fat, but full-fat products provide a healthy fatty acid profile. Although it is not possible to suggest specific daily levels of soy product consumption, soy can be an important part of a balanced dietary approach to health.

There is strong epidemiological evidence for reduced incidence of several cancers in high soy-consuming populations. Because these populations ingest mostly foods derived from whole soybeans, and because the precise benefits of individual soy constituents have not yet been determined in humans, the authors suggest consumption of soy products that retain as much of the components of whole soy as practical. This is particularly true for the isoflavone fraction. As reviewed in this chapter, soy isoflavones exert a number of potential anticarcinogenic effects, in vitro. Results of ongoing animal and human trials should provide additional support for expanded recommendations regarding soy and cancer incidence.

REFERENCES

1. Wilcke HL, Hopkins DT, Waggle DH. Soy protein and human nutrition. New York: Academic, 1979.
2. Anderson RL, Rackis JJ, Tallent WH. Biological action of substances in soy products. In: Soy Protein and Human Nutrition. Wilke HL, Hopkins DT, Waggle, DH, eds., New York: Academic, 1979; 209–233.
3. Miller AB. Diet and cancer. A review. Acta Oncol 1990; 29:87–95.
4. Miller AB, Berrino F, Hill M, Pietinen P, Riboli E, Wahrendorf J. Diet in the aetiology of cancer: a review. Eur J Cancer 1994; 30A:207–220.
5. Goodman MT, Nomura AMY, Wilkens LR, Hankin J. The association of diet, obesity, and breast cancer in Hawaii. Cancer Epidemiol Biomarkers Prev 1992; 1:269–275.
6. Lee HP, Gourley L, Duffy SW, Esteve J, Lee J, Day NE. Dietary effects on breast-cancer risk in Singapore. Lancet 1991; 337:1197–1200.
7. Severson RK, Nomura AMY, Grove JS, Stemmermann GN. A prospective study of demographics, diet, and prostate cancer among men of Japanese ancestry in Hawaii. Cancer Res 1989; 49:1857–1860.
8. Hirayama T. Epidemiology of stomach cancer in Japan. Jpn J Clin Oncol 1984; 14:159–168.
9. Tajima K, Tominaga S. Dietary habits and gastro-intestinal cancers: a comparative case-control study of stomach and large intestine cancers in Nagoya, Japan. Jpn J Cancer Res 1985; 76:705–716.
10. Koo LC. Dietary habits and lung cancer risk among Chinese females in Hong Kong who never smoked. Nutr Cancer 1988; 11:155–172.
11. Goodman MT, Hankin JH, Wilkens LR, Lyu L-C, McDuffie K, Liu LQ, Kolonel LN. Diet, body size, physical activity, and the risk of endometrial cancer. Cancer Res 1997; 57:5077–5085.
12. Goodman MT, Hankin JH, Wilkens, Kolonel LN. Dietary phytoestrogens and the risk of endometrial cancer. Am J Clin Nutr 1998; 68(Suppl.):1524S–1530S.
13. Christiansen RP. Efficacious use of food resources in the United States. U.S.D.A. Technical Bulletin no. 963. Washington DC: U.S. Government Printing Office, 1948.
14. Golbitz P. Traditional soyfoods: processing and products. J Nutr 1995; 125:570S–572S.
15. Messina M, Messina V. Increasing use of soyfoods and their potential role in cancer prevention. J Am Diet Assoc 1991; 91:836–840.
16. Coward L, Barnes NC, Setchell KDR, Barnes S. Genistein, daidzein, and their β-glycoside conjugates: antitumor isoflavones in soybean foods from American and Asian diets. J Agriculture Food Chem 1993; 41:1961–1967.
17. Pisani P, Parkin DM, Ferlay J. Estimates of the worldwide mortality from eighteen major cancers in 1985. Implications for prevention and projections of future burden. Int J Cancer 1993; 55:891–903.
18. American Cancer Society. Facts and Figures. 1994. Atlanta, GA.
19. Parkin DM. Cancers of the breast, endometrium and ovary: geographic correlations. Eur J Cancer Clin Oncol 1989; 25:1917–1925.
20. Kolonel LN. Variability in diet and its relation to risk in ethnic and migrant groups. Basic Life Sci 1988; 43:129–135.
21. Kennedy AR, Szuhaj BF, Newberne PM, Billings PC. Preparation and production of a cancer chemopreventive agent, Bowman-Birk inhibitor concentrate. Nutr Cancer 1993; 19:281–302.
22. Billings PC, Newberne PM, Kennedy AR. Protease inhibitor suppression of colon and anal gland carcinogenesis induced by dimethylhydrazine. Carcinogenesis 1990; 11:1083–1086.
23. Kennedy AR. Anticarcinogenic activity of protease inhibitors. In: Protease Inhibitors as Cancer Chemopreventive Agents. Troll W, Kennedy AR, eds., New York: Plenum, 1993; 9–64.
24. Koratkar R, Rao AV. Effect of soya bean saponins on azoxymethane-induced preneoplastic lesions in the colon of mice. Nutr Cancer 1997; 27:206–209.
25. Rao AV, Sung MK. Saponins as anticarcinogens. J Nutr 1995; 125:717S–724S.
26. Anderson RL, Wolf WJ. Compositional changes in trypsin inhibitors, phytic acid, saponins and isoflavones related to soybean processing. J Nutr 1995; 125:581S–588S.
27. Oakenfull DG, Sidhu GS. Saponins. In: Toxicants of Plant Origin, Vol. 2. Cheeke P, ed., Boca Raton: CRC, 1989; pp. 98–99.
28. Oakenfull D, Sidhu GS. Could saponins be a useful treatment for hypercholesterolaemia? Eur J Clin Nutr 1990; 44:79–88.
29. Shamsuddin AM. Inositol phosphates have novel anticancer function. J Nutr 1997; 125:725S–732S.
30. Graf E, Eaton JW. Antioxidant functions of phytic acid. Free Radical Biol Med 1990; 8:61–69.
31. Graf E, Mahoney JR, Bryant RG, Eaton JW. Iron-catalyzed hydroxyl radical formation. Stringent requirement for free iron coordination site. J Biol Chem 1984; 259:3620–3624.

32. Wei H, Bowen R, Cai Q, Barnes S, Wang Y. Antioxidant and antipromotional effects of the soybean isoflavone genistein. Proc Soc Exp Biol Med 1995; 208:124–130.

33. Von Hofe E, Newberne PM, Kennedy AR. Inhibition of N-nitrosomethylbenzylamine-induced esophageal neoplasms by the Bowman-Birk protease inhibitor. Carcinogenesis 1991; 12:2147–2150.

34. Kennedy AR, Beazer-Barclay Y, Kinzler KW, Newberne PM. Suppression of carcinogenesis in the intestines of Min mice by the soybean-derived Bowman-Birk inhibitor. Cancer Res 1996; 56:679–682.

35. Knight DC, Eden JA. A review of the clinical effects of phytoestrogens. Obstet Gynecol 1996; 87:897–904.

36. Adlercreutz H, Hockerstedt K, Bannwart C, Bloigu S, Hamalainen E, Fotsis T, Ollus A. Effect of dietary components, including lignans and phytoestrogens, on enterohepatic circulation and liver metabolism of estrogens and on sex hormone binding globulin (SHBG). J Steroid Biochem 1987; 27:1135–1144.

37. Hutchins AM, Slavin JL, Lampe JW. Soybean feeding and urinary isoflavonoid phytoestrogen and lignan excretion in healthy men. J Nutr 1995; 125:802S.

38. Franke AA, Custer LJ, Cerna CM, Narala K. Rapid HPLC analysis of dietary phytoestrogens from legumes and from human urine. Proc Soc Exp Biol Med 1995; 208:18–26.

39. Franke AA, Custer LJ. High-performance liquid chromatographic assay of isoflavonoids and coumestrol from human urine. J Chromatogr B Biomed Appl 1994; 662:47–60.

40. Kelly GE, Nelson C, Waring MA, Joannou GE, Reeder AY. Metabolites of dietary (soya) isoflavones in human urine. Clin Chim Acta 1993; 223:9–22.

41. Karr SC, Lampe JW, Hutchins AM, Slavin JL. Urinary isoflavonoid excretion in humans is dose dependent at low to moderate levels of soy-protein consumption. Am J Clin Nutr 1997; 66:46–51.

42. Franke AA. Correspondence re: L-JW Lu et al.: a simplified method to quantify isoflavones in commercial soybean diets and human urine after legume consumption. Cancer Epidemiol Biomarkers Prev 1995; 4:497–503. Cancer Epidemiol Biomarkers Prev 1996; 5:407–408.

43. Lu LJ, Hokanson JA, Anderson KE, Marshall MV, Hu DM, Kinsky MP, Sadagopa Ramanujum VM. Urinary excretion of isoflavones in healthy subjects after soymilk consumption. Proc Annu Meet Am Assoc Cancer Res 1993; 34:A3314.

44. Bundred NJ, Harding C, McMichael Phillips D, Howell A, Morton M. Serum phytoestrogen concentrations in British women with breast cancer and controls. Am J Clin Nutr 1998; 68(Suppl.):1524S–1530S.

45. Ingram D, Sanders K, Kolybaba M, Lopez D. Case-control study of phyto-estrogens and breast cancer. Lancet 1997; 350:990–994.

46. Adlercreutz H, Fotsis T, Bannwart C, Wahala K, Makela T, Brunow G, Hase T. Determination of urinary lignans and phytoestrogen metabolites, potential antiestrogens and anticarcinogens, in urine of women on various habitual diets. J Steroid Biochem 1986; 25:791–797.

47. Adlercreutz H, Honjo H, Higashi A, Fotsis T, Hamalainen E, Hasegawa T, Okada H. Urinary excretion of lignans and isoflavonoid phytoestrogens in Japanese men and women consuming a traditional Japanese diet. Am J Clin Nutr 1991; 54:1093–1100.

48. Adlercreutz HC, Goldin BR, Gorbach SL, Hockerstedt KA, Watanabe S, Hamalainen EK, et al. Soybean phytoestrogen intake and cancer risk. J Nutr 1995; 125:757S–770S.

49. Makishima M, Honma Y, Hozumi M, Sampi K, Hattori M, Umezawa K, Motoyoshi K. Effects of inhibitors of protein tyrosine kinase activity and/or phosphatidylinositol turnover on differentiation of some human myelomonocytic leukemia cells. Leuk Res 1991; 15:701–708.

50. Carlo Stella C, Regazzi E, Garau D, Mangoni L, Rizzò MT, Bonati A, et al. Effect of the protein tyrosine kinase inhibitor genistein on normal and leukaemic haemopoietic progenitor cells. Br J Haematol 1996; 93:551–557.

51. Linassier C, Pierre M, Le Pecq J-B, Pierre J. Mechanisms of action in NIH-3T3 cells of genistein, an inhibitor of EGF receptor tyrosine kinase activity. Biochem Pharmacol 1990; 39:187–193.

52. Akiyama T, Ishida J, Nakagawa S, Ogawara H, Watanabe S, Itoh N, Shibuya M, Fukami Y. Genistein, a specific inhibitor of tyrosine-specific protein kinases. J Biol Chem 1987; 262:5592–5595.

53. Okura A, Arakawa H, Oka H, Yoshinari T, Monden Y. Effect of genistein on topoisomerase activity and on the growth of [Val 12]Ha-ras-transformed NIH 3T3 cells. Biochem Biophys Res Commun 1988; 157:183–189.

54. Kiguchi K, Constantinou AI, Huberman E. Genistein-induced cell differentiation and protein-linked DNA strand breakage in human melanoma cells. Cancer Commun 1990; 2:271–278.

55. Constantinou A, Huberman E. Genistein as an inducer of tumor cell differentiation: possible mechanisms of action. Proc Soc Exp Biol Med 1995; 208:109–115.

56. Okura A, Arakawa H, Oka H, Yoshihari T, Monden Y. Effect of genistein on topoisomerase activity and on the growth of [VAL 12]Ha-ras-transformed NIH 3t3 cells. Biochem Biophys Res Commun 157:183–189.

57. Bourquin LD, Bennink MR. Differential effects of genistein and daidzein on growth of human colon cancer cell lines. Am J Clin Nutr 1998; 68(Suppl.):1524S–1530S.
58. Hempstock J, Kavanagh JP, George NJR. Growth inhibition of human prostatic cell lines by phytoestrogens. Am J Clin Nutr 1998; 68(Suppl.):1524S–1530S.
59. McCabe MJ, Orrenius S. Genistein induces apoptosis in immature human thymocytes by inhibiting topoisomerase-II. Biochem Biophys Res Commun 1993; 194:944–950.
60. Spinozzi F, Pagiacci MC, Migliorati G, Moraca R, Grignani F, Riccardi C, Nicoletti I. The natural tyrosine kinase inhibitor genistein produces cell cycle arrest and apoptosis in jurkat T-leukemia cells. Leuk Res 1994; 18:431–439.
61. Wei H, Wei L, Frenkel K, Bowen R, Barnes S. Inhibition of tumor promoter-induced hydrogen peroxide formation in vitro and in vivo by genistein. Nutr Cancer 1993; 20:1–12.
62. Wei H, Bowen R, Cai Q, Barnes S, Wang Y. Antioxidant and antipromotional effects of the soybean isoflavone genistein. Proc Soc Exp Biol Med 1995; 208:124–130.
63. Lu L-JW, Lin S-N, Grady JJ, Nagamani M, Anderson KE. Altered kinetics and extent of urinary daidzein and genistein excretion in women during chronic soya exposure. Nutr Cancer 1996; 26:289–302.
64. Zava DT, Duwe G. Estrogenic and antiproliferative properties of genistein and other flavonoids in human breast cancer cells in vitro. Nutr Cancer 1997; 27:31–40.
65. Wang C, Kurzer MS. Phytoestrogen concentration determines effects on DNA synthesis in human breast cancer cells. Nutr Cancer 1997; 28:236–247.
66. Hsieh CY, Santell RC, Haslam SZ, Helferich WG. Estrogenic effects of genistein on growth of estrogen receptor-positive human breast cancer (MCF-7) cells in vitro and in vivo. Cancer Res 1998; 58:(17):3833–3838.
67. Shao Z-M, Alpaugh M, Fontana JA, Barskey SH. Genistein inhibits cell proliferation similarly in ER-positive and ER-negative human breast carcinoma cell lines characterized by p21$^{WAF/Cip1}$ induction, G$_2$/M arrest and apoptosis. J Cell Biochem 1998; 69:44–54.
68. Folkman J, Shing Y. Angiogenesis. J Biol Chem 1992; 267:10,931–10,934.
69. Folkman J, Cotran RS. Relation of vascular proliferation to tumor growth. Int Rev Exp Pathol 1976; 16:207–248.
70. Liotta L, Steeg PS, Stetler-Stevensen WG. Cancer metastasis and angiogenesis: an imbalance of positive and negative regulation. Cell 1991; 64:327–336.
71. Fotsis T, Pepper M, Adlercreutz H, Fleischmann G, Hase T, Montesano R, Schweigerer L. Genistein, a dietary-derived inhibitor of in vitro angiogenesis. Proc Natl Acad Sci USA 90:2690–2694.
72. Shao Z-M, Wu J, Shen Z-Z, Barsky SH. Genistein exerts multiple suppressive effects on human breast carcinoma cells. Cancer Res 1998; 58:4851–4857.
73. Messina MJ, Persky V, Setchell KD, Barnes S. Soy intake and cancer risk: a review of the in vitro and in vivo data. Nutr Cancer 1994; 21:113–131.
74. Fournier DB, Erdman J, Gordon GB. Soy, its components, and cancer prevention: a review of the in vitro, animal and human data. Cancer Epidemiol Biomarkers & Prev 1998; 7:1055–1065.
75. Bennink MR, Mayle JE, Bourquin LD, Thiagarajan D. Evaluation of soy protein in risk reduction for colon cancer and cardiovascular disease: preliminary results. Am J Clin Nutr 1998; 68(Suppl.):1529S.
76. Thiagarajan D, Bennink MR, Bourquin LD, Maple JE, Seymour EM, Mridvika M. Effects of soy protein consumption on colonic cell proliferation in humans. FASEB J 1999; 13:A370(Abstract).
77. Berrino F, Secreto G, Camerini E, Bellati C, Maffei F, Pala V, et al. A randomized trial to prevent hormonal patterns at high risk for breast cancer: the DIANA (Diet and Androgens) project. Am J Clin Nutr 1998; 68(Suppl.):1524S–1530S.

4

Micronutrients as Intermediate Biomarkers in Chemotherapy and Enhancement for Cancer Treatments

Wolfgang J. Issing

1. INTRODUCTION

After decades of rigorous investigation of countless cancer chemotherapy regimens, many cancers, including those of the lung and head and neck (HN), still remain beyond clinical ability to control. Despite therapeutic advances and intensive efforts in tobacco-cessation education and counseling, overall survival rates for patients with aerodigestive tract cancers have improved only marginally over the past 30 yr (1). Of all patients initially "cured" of early-stage head and neck cancer (HNC) 3–5%/yr will develop second primary tumors (2,3). Vikram (4) was able to show that the occurrence of second primaries was a serious threat to the survival rate of patients with HNC. After only 4 yr, the probability of developing a second primary is greater than the risk of recurrence of the initial malignancy.

The phenomenon of high risk of subsequent cancers has been explained by the concept of "field cancerization," which suggests that certain risk factors, such as smoking, result in diffuse changes in the entire lining of the upper aerodigestive tract (5,6). Thus, these mucous membranes as a whole are considered to be at high risk for subsequent neoplastic progression. The occurrence of multiple primary cancers, as well as premalignant lesions, in tissue exposed to carcinogenic substances, has great significance for the oncology of HN tumors. The oral cavity and hypopharynx are the most common sites of squamous cell carcinoma (SCC) of HN in the Western world.

Alcohol and tobacco seem to play a synergistic role in carcinogenesis in the oral cavity, hypopharynx, and esophagus. The risk of developing a carcinoma of the larynx increases directly proportional to the amount smoked. In the United States, 50 million people smoke cigarettes and 12 million chew tobacco. Worldwide, the corresponding figures are 1 billion and 600 million. Despite the large number of smokers in the United States, the estimated incidence of HNC in 1993 was only 32,000, and the estimated mortality was 8000 (7,8). Other examples of well-known site-specific carcinogens include dietary factors in Chinese nasopharyngeal carcinoma and wood dust exposure in nasal adenocarcinoma (9,10). Other factors, including vitamin A deficiency, cause epithelial metaplasia (11).

From: *Primary and Secondary Preventive Nutrition*
Edited by: A. Bendich and R. J. Deckelbaum © Humana Press Inc., Totowa, NJ

Leukoplakia, a white keratotic plaque in the oral cavity or in the larynx, which cannot be scraped off, may be a premalignant precursor of SCC, and is often tobacco-related and easily monitored. In addition to the chief cause, smoking, other risk factors, such as chemical fumes and dust, must be considered *(12)*. The rate of transformation of leukoplakia into invasive cancer is directly related to the degree of histologic abnormality. In the largest study with the longest follow-up in the United States (mean follow-up, 7.2 yr), the long-term transformation rate for all dysplastic lesions was 36%. Even though complete spontaneous remission has been reported, surgical removal is still considered the best therapy. However, many patients surgically treated for oral leukoplakia later develop local recurrences, new leukoplakias or even SCCs. Therefore, leukoplakia provides an ideal human model for aerodigestive tract carcinogenesis and the study of chemoprevention. Because of field carcinogenesis, results of trials in oral leukoplakia have important implications for cancers in other aerodigestive tract sites, including the lung *(13–20)*.

As a result of the knowledge about field cancerization and the increasing understanding of carcinogenesis as a process consisting of many small steps, clinical use of chemopreventive agents has increased in recent years. The goal of chemoprevention is to halt or reverse the progression of carcinogenesis, and thus avert the development of invasive tumors. Wide-scale epidemiological studies, such as the Physicians' Health Study (included 22,071 American physicians, who received β-carotene for 12 yr) and the Alpha-Tocopherol, Beta-Carotene Cancer Prevention (ATBC) Study, in which 29,000 male smokers from Finland were treated, showed that β-carotene exerted no positive influence on the development of malignancies *(21,22)*. In contrast, however, in a third study, vitamin A (retinyl palmitate [RP]) did indeed exhibit a positive effect in the prevention of second primary cancer in the head and neck region and in the lung. In an investigation by Hong et al. *(7)*, 28% in the placebo group, vs 6% in the verum group, developed a second primary cancer in the HN region ($p = 0.005$) *(7,23)*.

One of the most important oncologic developments in the last 10 yr is the elucidation of the molecular events within the cell that contribute to the process of carcinogenesis. The potential for using this expanding knowledge to reduce the morbidity and mortality caused by cancer continues to increase. Unfortunately, the application of this knowledge to clinical problems has not kept pace with the rapid advances in molecular biology of cancer. One new approach is to identify high-risk groups by means other than carcinogen exposure and family history. In order to accomplish this task, researchers have been looking more closely at the carcinogenic process. Genetic and cellular antigenic changes have been identified that may precede the histologic identification of a tumor cell. It is hoped that these intermediate end points can be used as surrogate end points for prevention trials, and ultimately have clinical use in identifying high-risk groups. One potential intermediate end point is the presence of retinoid acid receptors (RAR) in cells. Retinoic acid (RA), a metabolite of vitamin A, is essential for cell growth and differentiation, and also has antiproliferative effects. Topical and oral administration of RA has been shown to be effective in the treatment of basal cell carcinoma, bladder papilloma, and leukoplakia of the oral cavity and larynx *(24–26)*.

2. MOLECULAR BIOLOGY OF RARS

Retinoids are the best-studied chemopreventive agents. Recent major advances have been made toward understanding the retinoids' mechanisms of action. It is now apparent that the nuclear receptors for the retinoids belong to a common superfamily that also

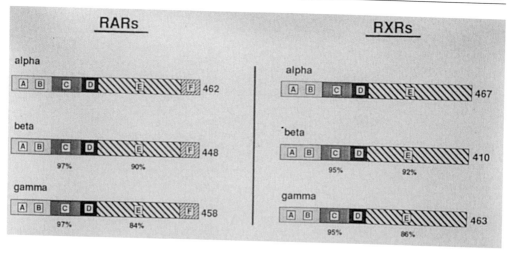

Fig. 1. Structure of RAR and RXR.

includes the steroid and thyroid receptors. As in steroid and thyroid hormone nuclear receptors, RARs consist of six distinct functional domains, designated A–F. Differences between the three receptor subtypes are found mostly in the A and F regions and in the middle part of the D region. The DNA-binding C region, the RA-binding E region, and the adjacent parts of the D region are highly conserved between receptors, and also between species (Fig. 1; 27). The two major classes of RARs, the RAR and RXR series, have α, β, and γ subtypes, and multiple isoforms (Fig. 2). These nuclear receptors are known to be influential factors that affect the transcription of target genes (e.g., the epidermal growth factor receptor) through binding to a specific RA response element (RARE), which in turn regulates cell differentiation and proliferation (28). RXRs act cooperatively with RARs through the formation of heterodimers, selectively enhancing the binding of RARs to RARE on target genes (29).

Explanation is multiple as to why vitamin A and natural metabolites, as well as synthetic derivatives, have positive effects on SCC in the HN region. Retinoids can exert effects at several points in the malignant transformation process. The multistep process of tumor genesis was recently described in a study discussing the most common genetic mutations (p53) in malignancies of the upper aerodigestive tract. It was shown that the initial malignancies expressed completely different mutations than the second primaries. This supports the theory of different clonal origins between initial and second cancers (30). Maxwell et al. (31) were able to prove that retinoids can regulate the expression level of p53 mRNA and proteins in certain in vitro systems.

An additional point of attack of retinoids is the re-establishment of normal cell differentiation and the ability to react to normal growth-control mechanisms. Two retinoid-related effects are an improvement in the gap junction communication and an increase in integrin expression (32). Thus, most important functions of retinoids are to influence the expression of certain genes, with the consequent modulation of gene differentiation to suppress the progression of premalignant lesions.

Retinoids bind to the nuclear receptors that in turn bind to the so-called response elements in the promoter region of certain genes. Investigations concerning the role of the individual receptors show that there are apparent differences in the biological func-

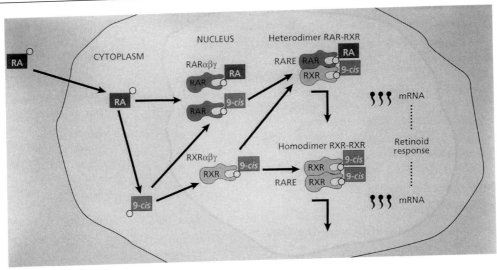

Fig. 2. Mechanism of action of vitamin A in the cell.

tions of the various receptors. For example, RARα plays an important role in acute promyelocytic leukemia, RARγ in malignant teratomas, and RARβ in the carcinogenesis of oral cancer *(33–35)*. The important role of RARβ in the carcinogenesis of the upper aerodigestive tract is supported by the presence of these cancers when this nuclear receptor is absent. RARβ has not been found in a large number of HN and lung cancers *(36,37)*. Additional evidence is found in the suppression of tumor genesis in lung carcinoma cell lines after transfection of RARβ *(38)*. Furthermore, the progressive loss of RARβ expression is associated with the progression of carcinogenesis in HN and lung carcinomas. The most significant evidence, however, is the absence of RARβ in approximately two-thirds of all premalignant lesions of the oral cavity, and the significant upregulation of the expression of RARβ after application of the retinoid, isotretinoin, and the resulting correlation between increased RARβ expression and clinical success. The author therefore believes that RARβ is the best indicator for the implementation of retinoids in chemoprevention, and at the same time represents an excellent biomarker *(38)*.

3. ROLE OF VITAMIN A IN CHEMOPREVENTION

The basic postulates of chemoprevention are as follows: Intervention with a chemopreventive agent will help prevent the field-wide appearance of invasive cancer; and carcinogenesis can be arrested or reversed in precancerous stages *(2,24)*.

Issing et al. used high-dose vitamin A retinyl Palmitate (RP) to treat leukoplakias of the larynx, especially in elderly patients who were considered at high risk for general anesthesia *(39)*. They observed a complete remission rate of 75% (15/20 patients), and a maintenance therapy of 150,000 IU/d was given in order to preserve the positive results (Fig. 3). Among the five patients with a partial response, three relapsed even under the treatment with RP within the first year of follow-up. Even though only 11/20 patients were histologically evaluated, it seems that all patients with severe dysplasia or carcinoma *in situ* did relapse more readily than patients with mild or moderate dysplasia. The median duration of treatment was 18 mo (range 12–24 mo). One of the chief advantages

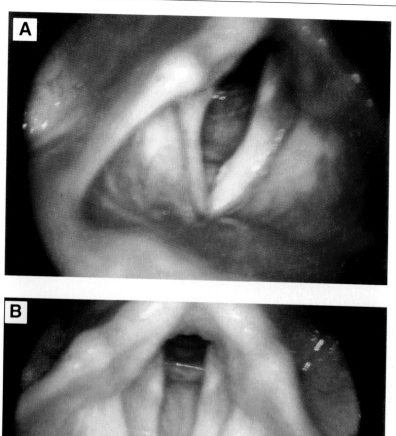

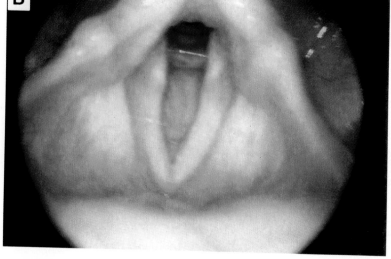

Fig. 3. (A and B) Typical example of a complete response of a larynx leukoplakia in an 80-yr-old man following 3-mo treatment.

of RP in patients with larynx leukoplakia was the avoidance of general anesthesia in elderly patients who were considered as high-risk patients for undergoing surgery *(26)*.

In general, therapeutic doses of vitamin A and other retinoids have been reported to cause severe side effects (skin dryness, cheilitis, hypertriglyceridemia, and conjunctivitis), and many patients are unable to continue the therapy *(16)*. In the author's trial, there were no severe toxic side effects seen, even at doses of up to 1,500,000 IU RP/d for 1 wk. Based on the experience gained in this investigation, the method of choice for the chemopreventive treatment of larynx leukoplakias appears to be the initial administration of relatively high doses of RP as induction therapy, followed by moderate doses during the maintenance phase, in order to keep recurrences low. Thus, the author's investigation

Table 1
Expression of RARs in Tumor Cell Lines

Number	Cell line	Tissue	RAR α	RAR β	RAR γ	RXRα
1	A 549	Lung	−	+	+	+
2	Ha 1182	Lung	+	+	+	+
3	Ha 146	Lung	−	−	+	+
4	Tera 2	Lung	−	+	+	+
5	H 128	Lung	−	−	+	+
6	A 427	Lung	−	−	+	+
7	SCC 4	SCCHN	+	+	+	−
8	SCC 9	SCCHN	−	+	+	+
9	SCC 15	SCCHN	−	+	+	+
10	SCC 25	SCCHN	−	−	+	+
11	Detroit	SCCHN	−	+	+	−
12	Hep 2	Larynx	−	−	+	+
13	FADU	Larynx	−	−	+	+
14		Placenta	+	+	+	+

+, present; −, not present.

showed that RP seems to be an effective chemopreventive agent in patients with recurring larynx leukoplakia or in patients who have an increased risk associated with undergoing surgery *(33)*.

4. MECHANISM OF ACTION OF VITAMIN A TREATMENT IN CHEMOPREVENTION

Currently, it is known that RARα, -β, and -γ can bind all-*trans* retinoic acid (ATRA), as well as 9-*cis* retinoic acid (9c-RA); the retinoid X receptors (RXRα, -β, -γ) can only bind 9c-RA *(40)*. With the help of a co-transfection assay (the RAR is co-transfected with a hormone response element and a reporter gene [luciferase]), the author was able to demonstrate the binding of RP to RARβ and RARγ at 25 and 24% of the binding sites, respectively, at 10 M. No binding to RARα could be observed (unpublished data).

Thus, in agreement with the current literature, it appears that RARβ and RARγ play a key role in interactions between vitamin A and its receptors *(41)*. The author screened a total of 13 cell lines and 29 tissue samples from SCC, as well as one malignant melanoma of HN for the expression of RARs α, β, γ and RXRα by polymerase chain reaction. Only RARγ was expressed 100% in tumor tissue, as well as in cell lines. RARβ showed 100% expression in tumor tissue; cell lines showed only a 54% expression. All other receptors were diminished in their expression (Tables 1–3). In positive controls of placenta and normal cheek mucosa, all receptors were constantly expressed. There was no significant difference in RAR/RXR expression, according to the various anatomic sites explored. There was also no significant correlation between RAR/RXR expression and tumor differentiation status.

Fanjul et al. *(42,43)* reported that selective retinoids stimulate certain RARs (mostly RARβ and RARγ), and therefore inhibit the activity of activator protein-1 (AP-1), a

Table 2
Expression of RARs in Tissue Specimens

Number	Tissue	RARα	RARβ	RARγ	RXRα	β-actin
1	Oropharynx	+	+	+	−	+
2	"	+	+	+		+
3	"	−	+	+	+	+
4	"	−	+	+	+	+
5	"	−	+	+	+	+
6	"	+	+	+	+	+
7	"	+	+	+	+	+
8	"	−	+	+	−	+
9	"	−	+	+	+	+
10	"	−	+	+	+	+
11	"	−	+	+	+	+
12	Hypophar	+	+	+	−	+
13	"	−	+	+	+	+
14	"	+	+	+	−	+
15	"	+	+	+	+	+
16	"	−	+	+	+	+
17	"	−	+	+	+	+
18	Larynx	+	+	+	−	+
19	"	+	+	+	−	+
20	"	−	+	+	+	+
21	"	−	+	+	+	+
22	Lymphnd	+	+	+	+	+
23	"	−	+	+	+	+
24	"	+	+	+	+	+
25	"	−	+	+	+	+
26	CUP	−	+	+	−	+
27	"	−	+	+	+	+
28	"	+	+	+	+	+
29	"	−	+	+	+	+
30	Melanoma	−	+	+	+	+

Cancer of unequal primary.

Table 3
RAR Expression in Cell Lines and Tissue

	Cell lines (%)	Tissue (%)
RARα	15	43
RARβ	54	100
RARγ	100	100
RXRα	85	77

product of both nuclear proto-oncogenes c-*jun* and c-*fos*, as well as various other related proteins that are usually responsible for cell proliferation. In this way, the retinoids could interfere with the abundant cell proliferation signals, either via RAR or through directly blocking the AP-1 *(42,43)*.

4.1. Clinical Implication of Assessment of Retinoid Receptor Status

Because changes in oncogene expression have been correlated with epithelial growth, transformation, and tumor progression, the effects of RA on oncogene expression has been explored by many groups. Lee et al. *(44)* described a RA-induced decrease of epidermal growth factor receptor (EGFR) mRNA expression in two cell lines established from SCCs of HN. Further analyses showed that the tyrosine kinase activity of EGFR was also suppressed. Because the kinase activity is considered to be essential for signal transduction, its inhibition by RA may be one mechanism by which tumor cell growth can be suppressed *(44)*. The same group demonstrated that RA can modify the structure of the EGFR by decreasing its glycosylation, and suggest that these changes may suppress the autophosphorylation activity of the receptor kinase *(45)*. Zheng et al. *(46)* proved that the EGFR promoter activity was negatively regulated by RA, in a dose-dependent manner, and this correlated highly with the decreased steady-state level of mRNA encoding RARγ. These data strongly suggest that the EGFR promoter is regulated by RARγ, which itself is under the control of RA *(46)*. Similar results were reported by Hudson et al. *(47)*, who found that the EGFR and *ERBB-2/HER-2* genes were inhibited by ligand-activated RARs. Dimitrovsky et al. *(48)* also reported the downregulation of transforming growth factor α (TGFα) and EGFR in human teratocarcinoma cells (NT2/D1) after stimulation with RA. These mechanisms of action studies at the molecular level provide a plausible explanation for the positive impact of RA on premalignant lesions, such as oral leukoplakia, as well as reduced incidence of second primary tumors in patients with HNC treated with retinoids. RA downregulates EGFR and TGF-α, and by doing so interrupts the autocrine loop often found in patients with unfavorable prognosis *(49,50)*.

Lotan et al. *(38)* recently described the expression of RARβ mRNA as selectively lost in premalignant oral lesions, and said that it could be restored after treatment with isotretinoin, and that this restoration was associated with a clinical response. There was no association between the expression of RARβ mRNA and age, smoking status, or use of alcohol. Because RARβ mRNA was detected in samples of normal tissue, but in only 40% of the samples of premalignant tissue, Lotan et al. suggest that the loss of RARβ mRNA is an early event in carcinogenesis. The ability of RA to induce the expression of RARβ mRNA supposes that RARβ is able to suppress the premalignant phenotype, and thus could be used as an intermediate marker in chemoprevention trials *(38)*. Gebert et al. *(37)* and Houle et al. *(51)* reported similar results about the expression of RARβ in lung carcinoma.

The development of surrogate end point biomarkers (SEBs) in cancer chemoprevention trials could change the approach to chemoprophylaxis. SEBs will probably include genes or gene products that are altered in neoplasia (dysplasia), and can be measured, e.g., by screening of high-risk groups, and are modulated by a chemopreventive agent. Molecular markers may enable more accurate selection of high-risk groups and chemopreventive agents, with higher efficiency and less side-effect potential *(52)*.

5. ROLE OF PROTEOLYTIC ENZYMES IN PREVENTION OF LOCAL RECURRENCES AND METASTASIS OF SCCHN

One of the most difficult problems in cancer research today remains the understanding of the causal relationship between cellular and molecular mechanisms and consequent malignant disease. Most patients do not die of their primary tumors: Death is often caused

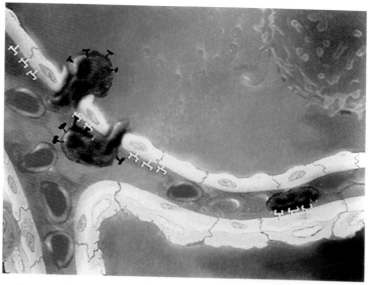

Fig. 4. By way of special adhesion molecules (black), such as vitronectin or CD44, the tumor cell is able to adhere to the inner wall of a vessel. The endothelial cell withdraws, and the tumor cell can penetrate deeper into the surrounding tissue (infiltration), and eventually develop into a metastasis. A macrophage of the tissue is seen in the upper right of the illustration.

by metastatic spread of the disease. It is therefore essential to detect malignancies as early as possible, in order to prevent the potential invasive growth of metastatic cells. A key problem in treatment and secondary prevention lies in understanding of the development of immune tolerance and metastasis.

In recent years, numerous molecular events have been identified as possible targets for effective oncological therapy. Unfortunately, experimental concepts have yet to produce satisfactory results in a clinical situation. This probably results from the heterogeneity of transformed cells and the dynamics of malignant processes.

There is no longer any doubt about the importance of dysregulation of various adhesion molecules in metastatic spread of disease (53,54). Research has shown that the overexpression of physiological and altered adhesion molecules (splice variants) increases potential migration for the tumor cells to new sites. In order for metastases to develop, cancer cells from the tumorous growth must pass into the circulatory system via the blood or lymph tracts. These cells then adhere to other sites within the organism, e.g., on the inner walls of vessels. From there, the tumor cells penetrate into surrounding tissues, multiply, and ultimately form a metastasis (Fig. 4). It has long been known that the overall adhesiveness of the blood and cells is increased during chronic and malignant diseases. The excessive production of the fibrin protein has been considered as a likely explanation for this phenomenon, and for the actual adhesion of cancer cells. Recently, evidence has been found that the metastasis of certain cancer cells also requires other agents. In order to adhere to the inner wall of vessels (endothelium), cancer cells use special agents, the so-called "adhesion molecules," which are found on cell surfaces. These cancer cells are only able to penetrate into the tissue (infiltration), grow, and eventually form metastases, after the malignant cells establish contact with an endothelial cell via these adhesion molecules. In the development of malignant melanoma, for

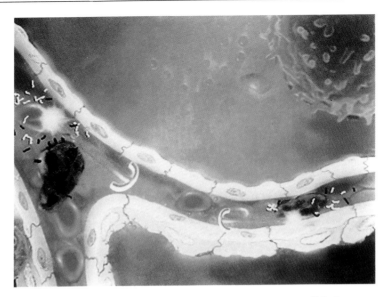

Fig. 5. Enzymes alter or hinder the development of the receptors responsible for metastasis. In this way, it is impossible for the tumor cell to bind to the vascular endothelium. The development of metastases is thereby hindered, or at least inhibited.

instance, the adhesion molecule, vitronectin, is of essential importance. Modern approaches in cancer therapy frequently target adhesion sites by using monoclonal antibodies (Abs) against cell surface molecules. For example, the use of Abs against CD44-receptor-positive cells prevents the dissemination of these malignant cells, and thus the growth of metastases.

The utilization of Abs presents two major disadvantages: first, the immune system of cancer patients eventually may produce neutralizing Abs, which in turn jeopardize the potential success of the treatment. Second, because the Abs are specific to each tumor, and must be developed in an individual basis, the costs of therapy are enormous, in many cases. Recently, there has been the development of enzyme therapies. Enzymes can possibly achieve a similar effect on adhesion molecules without the development of resistance, and at an acceptable price. Desser et al. *(55)* were able to show that enzymes hinder tumor cell adhesion by preventing the formation of vitronectin on the cell surfaces. The enzymes were thereby able to inhibit the development of metastases (Fig. 5). Similar relationships were also seen for metastasis of breast cancer and colon cancer. In these cancers, the cell-surface molecule, the CD44 receptor, is considered to be responsible for metastasis. After oral administration, approx 5% of the enzymes can be detected as enzymatically active molecules in plasma *(56)*. Other studies indicate that the percentage may be higher *(57,58)*. Potentially useful enzymes selectively split the CD44-receptor and other related cell-adhesion molecules. It is expected, therefore, that these enzymes can have a similar effect on malignant cells as anti-CD44 Abs.

5.1. Proteolytic Enzymes and Immune Function and Metastasis

Certain tumors spontaneously evoke an immune response by specific classes of T-cells (TH1 cells), and it appears that these tumors do not become malignant, because they are swiftly rejected. If the tumor is not destroyed, and is present, it is not expected that such tumors cause malignant growth in patients. Lehmann et al. (personal communication) studied an active cancer (glioblastoma), and were able to demonstrate a strong alternate immune response by TH2 cells to the tumor growth. However, with the application of enzymes (as described above), there was a reduction in CD44 expression, and a TH1 immune response replaced the TH2 response (Lehmann et al., personal communication). It remains to be clarified whether the splitting of the CD44 receptor on the cell surface, and the resultant reduced metastatic potential, involved the transformation of the TH2 response to a TH1 response.

Several research groups have studied the development of immune tolerance to tumors and the potential to reinitiate an antitumor response (59). Lehmann et al. (60) provide new information in an study about the TH1/TH2 immune response that was originally associated with autoimmune diseases. The recently developed test system allows detection of the reaction of individual immune cells (61). In general, the immune system reacts to autoantigens with the implementation of a mild TH2-response, in the absence of a definite danger signal. However, if a danger signal (i.e., accidental infection, strongly antigenic polypeptide) appears in the course of the immune reaction, the immune system reacts to the autoantigen with a strong TH1 response (cytotoxic T-cells, complement activation). Under normal conditions, this is a proper, protective response of the immune system. Unfortunately, this response can also result in inappropriate responses to auto (or self)-antigens, and can result in autoimmune disease. Lehmann et al. (60) have observed in vivo that malignant diseases show a TH1 response directed at the malignant cells. In the course of the disease, a switch to a massive TH2 response occurs, which suppresses the TH1 response, the consequence of which is that the individual's immune system acts to protect the tumor from destruction. An increased susceptibility to infections could be explained as a result. If it were possible to reduce the massive TH2 response, without suppressing the immune system as a whole, the application of an appropriate danger signal could then lead to the reinitiation of a TH1 response and, hopefully, tumor destruction.

In animal experiments, it has been possible to reduce the TH2 response, in autoimmune encephalitis, with the oral application of proteases (62). It is not yet clear whether this positive effect can be attributed to modulation of adhesion molecules or an alteration in signal transduction directly, via co-stimulating signals, or through T-cell-mediated cytokine regulation. Preliminary experiments suggest that the application of proteases could result in reduction of the massive TH2 response, so that reinitiation of a TH1 response may be possible.

Upon considering the current literature concerning the question of the role of proteases in the process of metastasis, it may at first seem inconsistent to suggest the addition of proteolytic enzymes to a cancer treatment regime. One hypothesis suggests that these proteases, which are taken in high concentrations, and are not bound to protease inhibitors, merely have a negligible effect. However, orally applied proteases are bound in large part to antiproteases, mostly to α-2-macroglobulin, following absorption. New data suggest that, in the region of immunologically active tissue, higher concentrations of α-2-macroglobulin-protease complexes are found. These complexes are assumed to have their own immune-stimulating and regulating influences on the local environment, and result in the production of various cytokines, especially TGF-β (55,63,64).

5.2. Proteolytic Enzymes as Adjuvants to Cancer Therapies

Proteolytic enzymes also seem to offer protection against the adverse effects of radio-therapy (RT), a method of treatment for certain types of cancer that has been quite successful. Radiotoxemia (radiation sickness), a feeling of malaise with a relatively long-term reduction in the endogenous immune-defensive powers, is a side effect that is seen most commonly following RT. In a large-scale clinical investigation performed by Beaufort et al. *(65)*, the concomitant application of enzymes, together with RT, was documented to provide substantial reductions in adverse effects. The patients were able to better tolerate the RT. The protective effect of proteolytic enzymes was specifically seen in the reduced symptoms of inflammation of the mucous membranes of the mouth following RT. The progress of radiogenic mucositis was clearly influenced positively through the use of enzyme therapy *(65)*. Sakalova et al. *(66)* observed a 50–60% decrease of the mortality risk in patients with multiple myeloma receiving optimized CT regimens and oral enzymes (Wobe-MugosE, Mucos Pharma, Geretsried, Germany). This compound recently received orphan drug status from the Food and Drug Administration for the treatment of multiple myeloma (O. Pecher, personal communication).

6. ANTIOXIDANTS

Epidemiologic studies show mostly an inverse relationship between cancer incidence and intake of specific foods high in antioxidant nutrients, such as β-carotene, selenium (Se), vitamin C (ascorbic acid), and vitamin E (α-tocopherol). β-carotene is one of the 600 carotenoids occurring in nature. Its major sources are green vegetables and colored fruits. One major mechanism of action for β-carotene is its antioxidant function, which involves the neutralization of free radicals. The source of free radicals can be photochemical reactions and oxidant stress, which are greatly increased by cigarette smoking. Free radicals and oxidants are able to damage RNA and DNA by reactions with guanine *(67)*. Another mechanism of action for β-carotene is its immunomodulatory effects, which were summarized by Bendich *(68)*.

The first results on human intervention studies on cancer prevention are now available. A combination of β-carotene, vitamin E, and Se reduced stomach cancer mortality in China (Linxian study) *(69)*. On the other hand, there are results available *(20,70,71)* indicating a lack of protection of β-carotene on lung cancer in smokers in Finland, and colorectal adenoma and second skin cancers in the United States. Similar observations were made for vitamin E, also a free-radical scavenger, because vitamin E was supplemented in the Finnish trial, as well.

Vitamin C, another free-radical scavenger, was associated with a lower incidence of stomach cancer, perhaps of reduced formation of carcinogenic N-nitroso compounds. Controlled clinical trials of high-dose vitamin C intake have failed to show any statistically significant survival advantage in patients with advanced cancer *(72)*. There are striking questions concerning vitamin C's role in cancer prevention, as well as progression. For instance, a minor effect was observed in patients with familial polyposis coli, with a significant decrease of polyps in a 9-mo follow-up, but a subsequent study showed no significant advantage for the vitamin C therapy *(73,74)* (*see* Chapter 2).

Data on Se, which may reduce cancer risk, are promising *(75)*. These data were derived from studies of single micronutrients or selected combinations of a few essential nutrients. Thus, researchers cannot rule out that other factors found in fruits and vegetables may be responsible for the protective effect of these dietary components, which have been consistently associated with reducing cancer risks.

7. FOLIC ACID

Although genetic alterations have been shown to play an important part in CC, it has been estimated that about 90% of CC in the United States can be associated with dietary factors and deficiencies. Recently, considerable interest has focused on folic acid, because low levels of the vitamin have been shown, in animal and epidemiological studies, to be associated with an increased risk of malignant transformation. Several clinical studies (76–78) have suggested an association between folate (FOL) deficiency and dysplasia in the cervical, bronchial, and colonic epithelium. Epidemiological studies conducted in people with ulcerative colitis, as well as in the general population, indicate a 30–50% reduction in colorectal neoplasia among those with higher folate status (78).

FOL is an essential factor for a number of critical metabolic pathways in the cell that involve the transfer of one carbon (methyl) groups. It is hypothesized that hypomethylation of DNA may be one mechanism of cancer initiation or progression. This mechanism can be stopped by adequate intake of folic acid. Folic acid is also a co-factor in the synthesis of S-adenosylmethionine (the principal methyl donor), and is exacerbated by alcohol, which is a FOL antagonist. It is in this manner that FOL may have an effect on DNA methylation at cytosine-guanine dinucleotides, an epigenetic modification of DNA that is observed in several human and experimental cancers. In particular, genome-wide and site-specific proto-oncogene DNA hypomethylation has been observed in early stages of colorectal carcinogenesis. Kim et al. (79) found an exon-specific DNA hypomethylation of the p53 tumor suppressor gene in rats that was induced by dimethylhydrazine. This is interesting, because the p53 tumor suppressor gene is implicated in over 70% of CCs, and the hypomethylation was effectively overcome by increasing levels of dietary FOL (79). However, in another study, Kim et al. (80) showed, in an animal model, that levels of dietary FOL beyond 4× the dietary requirement did not convey further benefit.

8. HIGH-DOSE MULTIVITAMINS

The belief that vitamins are essential nutrients for human life, and that they can affect serious diseases, has an ancient origin. There is evidence on an Egyptian papyrus that hemeralopia, a sight illness, was cured with the administration of liver. Now we know that the cause of this loss of vision was a lack of vitamin A. In the eighteenth century, cod liver oil was used for rachitism prophylaxis and therapy. About the same time, Lind showed the therapeutical power of fruit juice to cure scorbutus. According to the most recent studies, vitamins, multivitamins, and other essential nutrients are not only essential, but also play a major role in the concept of chemoprevention. For example, among Chinese at high risk for esophageal and gastric cancer, a 21% reduction in gastric cancer deaths, and a 9% reduction in total mortality, was observed among subjects receiving a combined treatment of β-carotene, vitamin E, and Se (81). The treatment prevented gastric cancer in nondysplastic, high-risk patients, but not in subjects with gastric dysplasia. Other studies (82) have examined the protective effect of vitamin C in animal models, because of its ability to inhibit nitrosamine formation. Giovannucci et al. (83) observed, in the Nurses' Health Study (88,756 women, from 1980 to 1994), a sharp

Table 4
Dietary Factors Examined for Potential Chemoprevention

Dietary factors	Cancer types	Ref.
Isotretinoin	Head and neck	Hong et al. 1990
Isotretinoin	Premalignant oral lesions	Lotan et al. 1995
Vitamin A	Lung	Pastorino et al. 1993
Retinyl palmitate	Larynx leukoplakia	Issing et al. 1996
All-*trans*-RA	Acute promyelocytic leukemia	Huang et al. 1988
13-*cis*-RA and α-tocopherol	Acute leukemia	Besa et al. 1990
Vitamin A, B$_6$, C, E, and zinc	Bladder	Lamm et al. 1994
β-carotene, vitamin E, Se	Stomach	Blot et al. 1993
Proteolytic enzymes	Multiple myeloma	Sakalova et al. 1998
Folic acid and vitamin A, C, D, E	Colorectal	Giovannucci et al. 1993
Folic acid	Bronchial metaplasia	Heimberger et al. 1987
Folic acid	Cervical	Kwasniewska et al. 1998

decline of new cases of CC (15 instead of 68 new cases per 10,000 women 55–69 yr of age) in women, after long-term use (15 yr) of multivitamins (vitamin A, C, D, E, and FOL). This may also explain the sharp reduction in CC incidence that occurred in white persons in the United States in the late 1980s. Approximately one-quarter of Americans began consuming an additional 400 µg folic acid daily from vitamin supplements or fortified breakfast cereals in 1973, when use of this amount of folic acid was first allowed *(83)*.

8.1. High-Dose Supplementation During CT

Lamm et al. *(84)* reported about a 40% decrease in tumor recurrence in patients with bladder carcinoma receiving megadose vitamins A, B$_6$, C, E, and zinc. They also observed that vitamin E decreased the toxic side effects of vitamin A *(84)*. Besa et al. *(85)* observed, in patients with myelodysplastic syndrome, a reduced rate (20–26%) of progression and transformation to acute leukemia, when patients were treated with 13-*cis*-RA or 13-*cis*-RA and α-tocopherol. They also reported an amelioration of the retinoid-related toxicities, including mucositis with α-tocopherol treatment *(85)*.

9. SUMMARY AND RECOMMENDATIONS

Vitamin A and its natural and synthetic metabolites appear to have the potential to modulate intermediate markers of HNC. Use of retinoids that can upregulate certain receptors has been associated with a reduced incidence of second primary tumors (Table 4). Regarding the use of nutrients as adjuncts to CT, the preliminary data are encouraging, and further research appears warranted. Greater emphasis should be placed on validating the clinical value of identifying intermediate markers of genetic changes associated with initiation and treatment of cancer. It seems that the use of high doses of RP may be effective in patients with recurring larynx leukoplakia, or in elderly patients with increased risk undergoing general anesthesia. Vitamin A (RP) showed a positive effect in the prevention of second primary cancers in HN and in the lung. Proteolytic enzymes seem to offer protection against adverse effects of RT, and also decreased mortality risk in patients with multiple myeloma. Folic acid is associated with significantly reduced incidence of CC. The data on antioxidant vitamins and prevention of cancer are not conclusive. However, the results are certainly in line with the advice that a diet rich in fruits and vegetables will help to reduce cancer risk.

ACKNOWLEDGMENTS

The author thanks Dr. Otto Pecher (Mucos Pharma) for Figs. 4 and 5. Also many thanks to Dr. Gail Wong, Ligand Pharmaceuticals, for the retinyl palmitate binding assays.

REFERENCES

1. Boring CC, Squires TS, Tong T. Cancer statistics, 1991. Cancer 1991; 41:19–36.
2. Lippman SM, Hong WK. Second malignant tumors in head and neck squamous cell carcinoma: the overshadowing threat for patients with early-stage disease. Int J Radiat Oncol Biol Phys 1989; 17:691–694.
3. Lippman SM, Hong WK. 13-cis-retinoic acid and cancer chemoprevention. J Natl Cancer Inst Monogr 1992; 13:111–115.
4. Vikram B. Changing patterns of failure in advanced head and neck cancer. Arch Otolaryngol 1984; 110:564–565.
5. Strong MS, Incze J, Vaughan CW. Field cancerization in the aerodigestive tract: its etiology, manifestation, and significance. J Otolaryngol 1984; 13:1–6.
6. Kelloff GJ, Boone CW, Steele VK, et al. Development of chemopreventive agents for lung and upper aerodigestive tract cancers. J Cell Biochem 1993; 17F(Suppl.):2–17.
7. Hong WK, Lippman SM, Itri LW, et al. Prevention of second primary tumors with isotretinoin in squamous cell carcinoma of the head and neck. N Engl J Med 1990; 323:795–801.
8. American Cancer Society. Cancer, Facts and Figures 1993. Atlanta, GA: American Cancer Society, 1993.
9. Maran AGD, Wilson JA, Gaze MN. The nature of the head and neck cancer. Eur Arch Otorhinolaryngol 1993; 250:127–132.
10. Acheson ED, Cowdell RH, Hadfield E, et al. Nasal cancer in wood workers in the furniture industry. BMJ 1968; 2:587–590.
11. de Vries N, Zandwijk N van, Pastorino U. The euroscan study. Br J Cancer 1991; 64:985–989.
12. Duchon J, Czinger J, Pupp L. Stimmbandpachydermien und das Rauchen. Z. Laryngol Rhinol 1972; 51:253–255.
13. Lippman SM, Batsakis JG, Toth BB, et al. Comparison of low-dose isotretinoin with beta carotene to prevent oral carcinogenesis. N Engl J Med 1993; 328:15–20.
14. Silverman S Jr, Gorsky M, Lozada F. Oral leukoplakia and malignant transformation: a follow-up study of 257 patients. Cancer 1984; 53:563–568.
15. Slaughter DP, Southwick HW, Smejkal W. Field cancerization in oral stratified squamous epithelium: clinical implications of multicentric origin. Cancer 1953; 6:963–968.
16. Lippman SM, Benner SE, Hong WK. Chemoprevention strategies in lung carcinogenesis. Chest 1993; 103:15S–19S.
17. Chiesa F, Tradati N, Marazza M, et al. Prevention of local relapses and new localisations of oral leukoplakias with the synthetic retinoid fenretinide (4-HPR). Preliminary results. Oral Oncol, Eur J Cancer 1992; 2:97–102.
18. Frame JW, Dasgupta AR, Dalton GA. Use of the carbon dioxide laser in the management of premalignant lesions of the oral mucosa. J Laryngol Otol 1984; 98:1251–1260.
19. Chiesa F, Sala L, Costa L, et al. Excision of oral leukoplakia by carbon dioxide laser on an out-patient basis: a useful procedure for prevention and early detection of oral carcinoma. Tumori 1986; 2:307–312.
20. Chu FWK, Silverman S Jr, Dedo HH. Carbon dioxide laser treatment of oral leukoplakia. Laryngoscope 1988; 98:125–130.
21. The Alpha-Tocopherol, Beta Carotene Cancer Prevention Study Group: The effect of vitamin E and beta carotene on the incidence of lung cancer and other cancers in male smokers. N Engl J Med 1994; 330:1029–1035.
22. Hennekens CH, Buring JE, Manson JE, et al. Lack of effect of long-term supplementation with beta carotene on the incidence of malignant neoplasms and cardiovascular disease. N Eng J Med 1996; 334:1145–1149.

23. Pastorino U, Infante M, Maioli M , Chiesa G, et al. Adjuvant treatment of stage I lung cancer with high-dose vitamin A. J Clin Oncol 1993; 11:1216–1222.
24. Sporn B. Approaches to prevention of epithelial cancer during the preneoplastic period. Cancer Res 1976; 36:2699–2702.
25. Benner SE, Hong WK, Lippman SM, et al. Intermediate biomarkers in upper aerodigestive tract and lung chemoprevention trials. J Cell Biochem 1992; 16G(Suppl.):33–38.
26. Issing WJ, Struck R, Naumann A. Long-term follow up of larynx leukoplakia under treatment with retinyl palmitate. Head Neck 1996; 18:560–565.
27. Leroy P, Krust A, Kastner P, Mendelsohn C, Zelent A, Chambon P. Retinoic acid receptors. In: Retinoids in Normal Development and Teratogenesis. Morriss-Kay GM, ed. Oxford: Oxford University Press, 1992; 7–25.
28. Smith MA, Parkinson DR, Cheson BD, et al. Retinoids in cancer therapy. J Clin Oncol 1992; 10:839–864.
29. Leid M, Kastner P, Lyons R, Nakshatri H, Saunders M, Zacharewski T, et al. Purification, cloning and RXR identity of the HeLa cell factor with which RAR or TR heterodimerizes to bind target sequences efficiently. Cell 1992; 68:377–395.
30. Chung KY, Mukhopadhyay T, Kim J, Casson A, Ro JY, Goepfert H, Hong WK, Roth JA. Discordant p53 gene mutations in primary head and neck cancers and corresponding second primary cancers of the upper aerodigestive tract. Cancer Res 1993; 53:1676–1683.
31. Maxwell SA, Mukhopadhyay T. Transient stabilization of p53 in non-small cell cultures arrested for growth by retinoic acid. Exp Cell Res 1994; 214:67–74.
32. Lotan R. Retinoids and squamous cell differentiation. In: Retinoids in Oncology. Hong WK, Lotan R, eds. New York: Marcel Dekker, 1993; 43–72.
33. Huang M, Ye Y, Cheng S, Chai J, Lu J, Zhoa L, Gu L, Wang Z. Use of all-trans-retinoic acid in the treatment of acute promyelocytic leukemia. Blood 1988; 72:567–572.
34. Moasser MM, Deblasio A, Dimitrowsky E. Response and resistance to retinoic acid are mediated through the retinoic acid nuclear receptor gamma in human teratocarcinomas. Oncogene 1994; 9: 833–840.
35. Zou CP, Clifford JL, Xu XC, Sacks PG, Chambon P, Hong WK, Lotan R. Modulation by retinoic acid (RA) of squamous cell differentiation, cellular RA-binding proteins, and nuclear RA receptors in human head and neck squamous cell carcinoma cell lines. Cancer Res 1994; 54:5479–5487.
36. Hu L, Crowe DL, Rheinwald JG, Chambon P, Gudas LJ. Abnormal expression of retinoic acid receptors and keratin 19 by human oral and epidermal squamous cell carcinoma cell lines. Cancer Res 1991; 51:3972–3981.
37. Gebert JF, Moghal N, Frangioni JV, Sugarbaker DJ, Neel BG. High frequency of retinoic acid receptor beta abnormalities in human lung cancer. Oncogene 1991; 6:1859–1868.
38. Lotan R, Xu X-C, Lippman SM, Ro JY, Lee JS, Lee JJ, Hong WK. Suppression of retinoic acid receptor-β in premalignant oral lesions and its upregulation by isotretinoin. N Engl J Med 1995; 332:1405–1410.
39. Issing WJ, Struck R, Naumann A, Kastenbauer E. A-Mulsin Hochkonzentrat, ein neues Therapiekonzept bei Larynxleukoplakien. Laryngo-Rhino-Otol 1996; 75:29–33.
40. Nakshatri H, Bouillet P, Bhat-Nakshatri P, et al. Isolation of retinoic acid-repressed genes from P19 embryonal carcinoma cells. Gene 1996; 174:79–84.
41. Issing WJ, Wustrow TPU. Expression of retinoic acid receptors in squamous cell carcinomas and their possible implication for chemoprevention. Anticancer Res 1996; 16:2373–2378.
42. Fanjul AN, Delia D, Pfahl MA, et al. 4-hydroxyphenyl retinamide is a highly selective activator of retinoid receptors. J Biol Chem 1996; 271:22,441–22,446.
43. Fanjul AN, Bouterfa H, Dawson M, et al. Potential role for retinoic acid receptor-β in the inhibition of breast cancer cells by selective retinoids and interferons. Cancer Res 1996; 56:1571–1577.
44. Lee JS, Kim JS, Blick M, Hong WK, Lotan R. Effects of retinoic acid on oncogene expression in a human head and neck squamous carcinoma cell line. In: Head and Neck Oncology Research. Wolf GT, Carey TE, eds. Berkeley: Kugler & Ghedini, 1987; 43–48.
45. Kim JS, Steck PA, Gallick GE, Lee JS, Blick M, Hong WK, Lotan R. Suppression by retinoic acid of epidermal growth factor receptor autophosphorylation and glycosylation in cultured human head and neck squamous carcinoma cells. J Natl Cancer Inst Monogr 1992; 13:101–110.
46. Zheng ZS, Polakowska R, Johnson A, Goldsmith LA. Transcriptional control of epidermal growth factor receptor by retinoic acid. Cell Growth Differ 1992; 3:225–232.
47. Hudson LG, Santon JB, Glass CK, Gill GN. Ligand-activated thyroid hormone and retinoic acid receptors inhibit growth factor receptor promoter expression. Cell 1990; 62:1165–1175.

48. Dimitrovsky E, Moy D, Miller WH, Li A, Masui H. Retinoic acid causes a decline in TGF-α expression, cloning efficiency, and tumorigenicity in a human embryonal cancer cell line. Oncogene Res 1990; 5:233–239.

49. Grandis JR, Tweardy DJ. TGF-α and EGFR in head and neck cancer. J Cell Biochem 1993; 17F:188–191.

50. Issing WJ, Liebich C, Wustrow TPU, Ullrich A. Coexpression of epidermal growth factor receptor and TGF-α and survival in upper aerodigestive tract cancer. Anticancer Res 1996; 16:283–288.

51. Houle B, Leduc F, Bradley WE. Implication of RARβ in epidermoid (squamous) lung cancer. Genes Chromosom Cancer 1991; 3:358–366.

52. Beenken SW, Huang P, Seller M, Peters G, Listinsky C, Stockard C, et al. Retinoid modulation of biomarkers in oral leukoplakia/dysplasia. J Cell Biochem 1994; 19:270–277.

53. Pantel K, Riethmüller G, Johnson JP, Izbicki JR, Passlick B, Angstwurm M, Schlimok G. Early metastasis of human solid tumours: expression of cell adhesion molecules. CIBA Found Symp 1995; 189:157–170.

54. Miyasaka M. Cancer metastasis and adhesion molecules. Clin Orthop 1995; 312:10–18.

55. Desser L, Rehberger A. Induction of tumor necrosis factor in human peripheral-blood mononuclear cells by proteolytic enzymes. Oncology 1990; 47:475.

56. Lamarre J, Wollenberg GK, Gonias SL, Hayes MA. Cytokine binding and clearance properties of proteinase-activated alpha 2-makroglobulin. Lab Invest 1991; 65:3–14.

57. Castell JV, Friedrich G, Kuhn CS, Poppe G. Intestinal absorption of undegraded proteins in men: presence of bromelain in plasma after oral intake. Am J Physiol 1997; 273:139–146.

58. Schiavo G, Benfenati F, Poulain B, et al. Tetanus and botulinum-B neurotoxins block neurotransmitter release by proteolytic cleavage of synaptobrevin. Nature 1992; 359:832–835.

59. Okada K, Yasumura S, Muller-Fleckenstein I, Fleckenstein B, Talib S, Koldovsky U, Whiteside, TL. Interactions between autologous CD4+ and CD8+ T lymphocytes and human squamous cell carcinoma of the head and neck. Cell Immunol 1997; 10:35–48.

60. Lehmann PV, Forsthuber T, Miller A, Ferzarz EE. Spreading of T-cell autoimmunity of cryptic determinants of an autoantigen. Nature 1992; 358:155–157.

61. Tary-Lehmann M, Saxon A, Lehmann PV. The human immune system in hu-PBL-SCID mice. Immunol. Today 1995; 529–533.

62. Lehmann PV. Immunmodulation by proteolytic enzymes. Nephrol Dial Transplant 1996; 11:953–955.

63. Wollenberg GK, Lamarre J, Rosendal S, et al. Binding of tumor necrosis factor alpha to activated forms of human plasma alpha 2-macroglobulin. Am J Pathol 1991; 138:265–272.

64. Webb DJ, Gonias SL, Atkins-Brady TL, Weaver AM. Proteinases are isoform-specific regulators of the binding of transforming growth factor beta to alpha 2-macroglobulin. Biochem J 1996; 320:551–555.

65. Beaufort F. Reduzierung von Strahlennebenwirkungen durch hydrolytische Enzyme. (Reduction in the adverse effects of radiation with hydrolytic enzymes.) Therapeutikon 1990; 10:577–580.

66. Sakalova A, Dedik L, Gazova S, Hanisch J, Schiess W. Survival analysis of an adjuvant therapy with oral enzymes in multiple myeloma patients. Br J Haematol 1998; 102:353.

67. Van Poppel G, Van den Berg H. Vitamins and cancer. Cancer Lett 1997; 114:195–202.

68. Bendich A. Carotenoids and the immune response. J Nutr 1989; 119:112–115.

69. Blot WJ, Li J, Taylor PR, et al. Nutrition intervention trials in Linxian China: supplementation with specific vitamin/mineral combinations, cancer incidence, and disease-specific mortality in the general population. J Natl Cancer Inst 1993; 85:1483–1492.

70. Greenberg ER, Baron JA, Tosteson TD, et al. A clinical trial of antioxidant vitamins to prevent colorectal adenoma. N Engl J Med 1994; 331:141–147.

71. Greenberg ER, Baron JA, Stukel TA, et al. A clinical trial of β-carotene to prevent basal-cell and squamous-cell cancers of the skin. N Engl J Med 1990; 323:789–795.

72. Moertel CG, Fleming TR, Creagen ET, Rubin J, O'Connell MJ, Ames MM. High-dose vitamin C versus placebo in the treatment of patients with advanced cancer who have had no prior chemotherapy. A randomized double-blind comparison. N Engl J Med 1985; 312:137.

73. Bussey HJ, DeCosse JJ, Deschner EE, Eyers AA, Lesser ML, Morson BC, et al. A randomized trial of ascorbic acid in polyposis coli. Cancer 1982; 50:1434.

74. DeCosse JJ, Miller HH, Lesser ML. Effect of wheat fiber and vitamins C and E on colorectal polyps in patients with familial adenomatous polyposis. J Natl Cancer Inst 1989; 81:1290.

75. Rogers AE, Longnecker MP. Biology of disease. Dietary and nutritional influences on cancer: a review of epidemiologic and experimental data. Lab Invest 1988; 59:729.

76. Heimburger DC, Krumdieck CL, Alexander B, Birch R, Dill SR, Bailey WC. Localized folic acid deficiency and bronchial metaplasia in smokers: hypothesis and preliminary report. Nutr Int 1987; 3:54–60.

77. Kwasniewska A, Tukendorf A, Semczuk M. Folate deficiency and cervical intraepithelial neoplasia. Eur J Gynaec Oncol 1997; 6:526–530.

78. Giovannucci E, Stampfer MJ, Colditz GA, Rimm EB, Trichopoulos D, Rosner BA. Folate, methionine, and alcohol intake and risk of colorectal adenoma. J Natl Cancer Inst 1993; 85:875–883.

79. Kim Y-I, Pogribny IP, Salomon RN, Choi SW, Smith DE, James SJ, Mason JB. Exon-specific DNA hypomethylation of the p53 gene of rat colon induced by dimethylhydrazine. Am J Pathol 1996; 149:1129–1137.

80. Kim Y-I, Salomon RN, Graeme-Cook F, Choi S-W, Smith DE, Dallal GE, Mason JB. Dietary folate protects against the development of macroscopic colonic neoplasia in a dose responsive manner in rats. Gut 1996; 39:732–740.

81. Grio R, Piacentino R, Marchino GL, Navone R. Antineoblastic activity of antioxidant vitamins: the role of folic acid in the prevention of cervical dysplasia. Panminerva Med 1993; 35:193–196.

82. Giacosa A, Filiberti R, Hill MJ, Faivre J. Vitamins and cancer chemoprevention. Eur J Cancer Prev 1997; 6:47–54.

83. Giovannucci E, Stampfer MJ, Colditz GA, Hunter DJ, Fuchs C, Rosner BA, Speizer FE, Willet WC. Multivitamin use, folate, and colon cancer in women in the Nurses' Health Study. Ann Intern Med 1998; 129:517–524.

84. Lamm DL, Riggs DR, Shriver JS, VanGilder PF, Rach JF, DeHaven JI. Megadose vitamins in bladder cancer: a double-blind clinical trial. J Urol 1994; 151:21–26.

85. Besa EC, Abrahm JL, Bartholomew MJ, Hyzinski M, Nowell PC. Treatment with 13-cis-retinoic acid in transfusion-dependent patients with myelodysplastic syndrome and decreased toxicity with addition of alpha-tocopherol. Am J Med 1990; 89:739–747.

III Cardiovascular/Renal Disease, Diabetes, and Obesity

5

Health Effects of *Trans* Fatty Acids

Susanne H. F. Vermunt and Ronald P. Mensink

1. INTRODUCTION

Trans fatty acids (TFAs) differ from their *cis* counterparts in the *trans* configuration of at least one double bond. This means that both carbon (C) atoms adjacent to the double bond are located at its opposite sides. The position of the double bond in the C-chain can be counted from the carboxyl-end (-COOH) of the molecule, which is symbolized as 'Δ', or from the methyl end (-CH$_3$), which is symbolized as "n minus." Thus, "n-3" means that the double bond is located at the third C atom from the methyl end. Chain elongation and desaturation always occur at the C-end of the FA molecule. Consequently, the position of the first double bond at the methyl end will not change during conversion reactions. Figure 1 shows α-linolenic acid (ALA) (C18:3n-3), which belongs to the n-3 family, and one of its *trans* isomers, C18:3n-3 Δ9c,12c,15tr. These two molecules are geometrical isomers.

TFAs can be formed from dietary (poly)unsaturated fatty acids (PUFAs) by bacteria in the first stomach (rumen) of ruminant animals, and by industrial hydrogenation and deodorization. During industrial hydrogenation, the chemical, physical, and sensory characteristics of the vegetable oil change, in order to make the oil suitable for food. The *cis* double bonds of PUFAs, in particular, are saturated (hydrogenated) by adding hydrogen to the oil. When all double bonds are hydrogenated, a saturated fatty acid (SFA) is formed. However, the *cis* configuration may also isomerize without net uptake of hydrogen. Consequently, *trans* double bonds are formed. Furthermore, the double bonds can migrate along the molecule, so that positional isomers will be formed. In this way, many different molecules can be formed from linoleic acid (LA) (Fig. 2). *Trans* monounsaturated fatty acids (MUFAs), in particular, are formed by hydrogenation.

Deodorization is the last step in the refining process, during which oils are prepared for use as an ingredient in margarine, shortening, cooking oil, and so on. *Trans* PUFAs can be easily formed by deodorization of oil *(1,2)*. Finally, *trans* PUFAs can be formed during heat or frying treatments *(3)*.

This chapter focuses on the effects of TFAs on various risk parameters for coronary heart disease (CHD), including lipids and lipoproteins (Lps), low-density lipoprotein (LDL) oxidation and hemostasis, and on cancer. Furthermore, the metabolism of TFAs and their effects on the desaturation and elongation of other FAs is discussed.

2. TFAs in Foods

TFA intake of the U.S. population has been estimated using availability or disappearance data, food frequency questionnaires, analysis of self-selected diets, duplicate diet

From: *Primary and Secondary Preventive Nutrition*
Edited by: A. Bendich and R. J. Deckelbaum © Humana Press Inc., Totowa, NJ

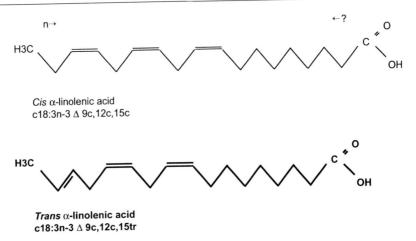

Cis α-linolenic acid
c18:3n-3 Δ 9c,12c,15c

Trans α-linolenic acid
c18:3n-3 Δ 9c,12c,15tr

Fig. 1. Chemical structure of all-*cis* C18:3n-3 and 9-*cis*,12-*cis*,15-*trans* C18:3n-3 (C18:3n-3 Δ9c,12c,15tr).

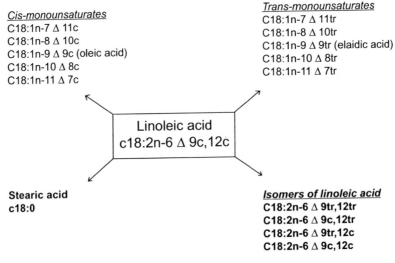

Cis-monounsaturates
C18:1n-7 Δ 11c
C18:1n-8 Δ 10c
C18:1n-9 Δ 9c (oleic acid)
C18:1n-10 Δ 8c
C18:1n-11 Δ 7c

Trans-monounsaturates
C18:1n-7 Δ 11tr
C18:1n-8 Δ 10tr
C18:1n-9 Δ 9tr (elaidic acid)
C18:1n-10 Δ 8tr
C18:1n-11 Δ 7tr

Linoleic acid
c18:2n-6 Δ 9c,12c

Stearic acid
c18:0

Isomers of linoleic acid
C18:2n-6 Δ 9tr,12tr
C18:2n-6 Δ 9c,12tr
C18:2n-6 Δ 9tr,12c
C18:2n-6 Δ 9c,12c

Fig. 2. Potential conversions of LA into its positional and geometrical isomers.

analysis, and/or adipose tissue composition data. The most recent estimate of the daily total TFA intake in the United States is 2.6% energy or 7.4% total fat intake for the total population aged 3 yr and older *(4)*. Estimates ranged from 2.6 to 2.8% and from 7.1 to 7.9%, respectively, across different age and gender groups. Values were based on results of the 1989–1991 Continuing Survey of Food Intakes by Individuals of the U.S. Department of Agriculture (USDA), and the TFA contents of specific foods calculated from a database compiled by the USDA. In Europe, the daily total TFA intake varied between 0.5% energy in Italy to 2.0% energy in Iceland *(5)*. These data were based on analysis of food samples and food consumption survey data, which were collected in 1995–1996 in 14 European countries.

Trans MUFAs contribute about 85% of total TFAs *(4)*. *Trans* monounsaturates from milk and meat fat are produced by bacteria in the rumen of animals. The major *trans*

Table 1
Per Capita Consumption of TFAs from Primary Food Sources

Food source	TFAs (g/d)	Total FAs (g/d)
Fried foods	0.8	3.9
Margarine, stick	0.5	1.7
Bread, commercial	0.3	4.0
Cakes and related baked goods	0.3	2.9
Savory snacks	0.3	2.3
Margarine, soft and spreads	0.2	1.2
Cookies	0.2	1.2
Milk	0.2	5.5
Butter	0.1	1.3
Crackers	0.1	0.5
Household shortenings	0.1	0.4
Ground beef	0.1	3.4

Values were based on results of the 1989–1991 CSFII of the USDA, and the TFA composition data was adapted from Nutrient Data Bank Bulletin Board (USDA). Reproduced with permission from ref. 6.

isomer in fat from ruminants is vaccenic acid (C18:1 Δ11tr), although *trans* double bonds at the Δ5–Δ16 positions are also present. Nonruminants that are fed diets containing *trans* C18:1 also have *trans* C18:1 isomers in their tissues.

More important sources of *trans* MUFAs, however, are partially hydrogenated vegetable oils and products made from these oils. Fried foods and stick margarine are the major contributors to the TFA intake in the United States, as shown in Table 1. Most *trans* double bonds are at the Δ10, Δ9, or Δ8 position.

Trans PUFAs are mostly formed during the deodorization process. In U.S. vegetable oils, the degree of isomerization of LA and ALA range from 0.3 to 3.3% and from 6.6 to 37.1%, respectively *(7)*. Most *trans* PUFAs are mono-*trans* isomers of LA and ALA, but only a few di-*trans* isomers are detected. Finally, *trans* PUFAs are formed during heat treatment of vegetable oils, such as during deep-frying processes *(3)*. Again, most *trans* isomers are mono-*trans* isomers.

3. METABOLISM

3.1. Digestion, Absorption and Incorporation into Blood Lipids

TFAs in margarines and dairy fats are incorporated in triacylglycerols (TGs); in meat, TFAs are found in phospholipids (PLs). Figure 3 shows the metabolic pathways of TFAs after dietary intake. After ingestion, TGs are split by pancreatic lipase into free fatty acids (FFAs) and sn2-monoglycerides. Small portions remain as diglycerides. PLs are split by pancreatic phospholipases, which remove the FA from the sn1 or sn2 position of the PL. Consequently, lysophospholipids and FFAs are formed. The digestion of *trans* MUFAs does not differ from that of their *cis*-isomers *(8)*.

After ingestion, FAs are absorbed by the enterocyte, after formation of micelles. Absorption of oleic acid (OA) and its positional and geometrical isomers is comparable *(9–12)*. In the enterocyte, FFAs, sn2-monoglycerides, and diglycerides may be re-esterified to TGs, cholesteryl esters, and PLs. The incorporation of positional and geometrical

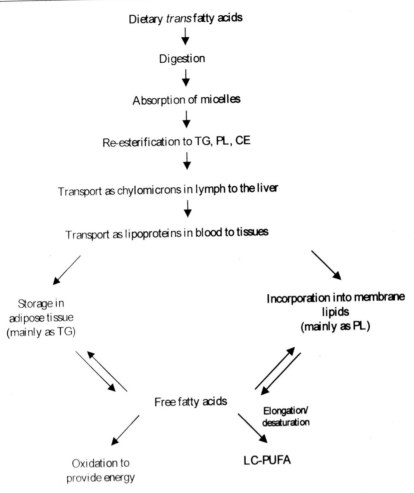

Fig. 3. Simplified scheme of TFA metabolism in humans. TG, triacylglycerols; PL, phospholipids; CE, cholesteryl esters; LCPUFA, long chain polyunsaturated FAs.

isomers of C18:1 Δ9c in TGs, cholesteryl esters, and PLs may differ from that of C18:1 Δ9c *(12).* After re-esterification, lipids may be taken up by chylomicrons, which transport the FAs through the lymph to the liver. Then, TFAs are transported by Lps through the blood stream. The incorporation of *trans* isomers of C18:1 Δ9 into very low density lipoproteins (VLDLs), LDL, and high density lipoproteins (HDLs) is lower than that of C18:1 Δ9c *(10–12).*

TFAs may also be incorporated into tissue PLs, stored in adipose tissue, desaturated and elongated into longer-chain polyunsaturated fatty acids (LCPUFAs), or oxidized via β-oxidation and peroxisomal systems.

3.2. Tissue Levels

In the human body, TFAs are found in TGs, mostly at positions 1 and 3. The TFA content of adipose tissue for U.S. subjects is about 4% of total FAs *(13).* Approximately 70% of TFAs are C18:1 isomers, which have their double bonds on the Δ8, 9, 10, 11, 12, or 13 position. *Trans* C16:1 isomers, which originate mostly from dairy fat, are also found in adipose tissue. About 20% of the *trans* isomers in adipose tissue are *trans* C18:2 isomers. Both mono-*trans* (Δ9c,12t and Δ9t,12c) and di-*trans* (Δ9t,12t) C18:2 isomers, and several *trans* C18:3 isomers, have been detected in adipose tissue.

TFAs in other tissues than adipose tissue are incorporated mostly into PLs predominantly at position 1. *Trans* C18:1 and C18:2 FAs have been found in human kidney, brain, heart, liver, aorta, jejunum, and human milk *(14,15)*; *trans* C18:3 has been detected in platelets and human milk *(16,17)*.

3.3. Desaturation and Elongation

Human liver microsomal complexes contain three different desaturation enzymes: Δ9, Δ6, and Δ5 desaturases, which insert double bonds at the Δ9, Δ6, or Δ5 position of the FA molecule, respectively. Furthermore, FAs can be elongated by addition of a two-C unit to the FAs. In this way, stearic acid, LA, and ALA are converted into their longer-chain metabolites (Fig. 4), which play an important role in many physiological processes *(18)*.

TFAs are desaturated by the same enzymes as *cis* FAs. Except for Δ8, Δ9, and Δ10 *trans* isomers, C18:1 positional isomers are good substrates for Δ9 desaturase *(19)*. Consequently, *cis,trans*, and *trans,cis* FAs can be formed. Some *trans* isomers of C18:1 are also substrates for Δ6 and Δ5 desaturase *(20)*. In addition, C18:1 *trans* isomers can be elongated into C20 and C22 FAs.

Trans LA may be converted into *trans* isomers of arachidonic acid (AA) (C20:4n-6); however, this may occur at a lower rate than all-*cis* C18:2 *(21)*. *Trans* isomers of ALA can be converted into *trans* isomers of docosahexaenoic acid (DHA; C22:6n-3) *(22,23)*. Observations, however, are mostly based on animal and in vitro studies, and may be different for the in vivo situation in humans.

3.4. Oxidation

Only a few human studies have been carried out to examine the effects of TFAs on FA oxidation. So far, it is only known that whole-body oxidation, measured with ^{13}C-labeled FAs, and oxidation rates by human heart homogenates, were equal between the TFA elaidic acid and the non-TFA with equivalent chain-length OA *(24,25)*.

3.5. Influence of TFAs on Desaturation and Elongation

Because TFAs and *cis* FAs can be converted by the same desaturase and elongase enzymes, competition between FAs exists. Both the *cis* and *trans* monoenoic positional isomers have been reported to inhibit the conversion of LA into AA in cultured glioma cells *(26)*. Furthermore, in human skin fibroblasts, C18:1 Δ9tr increased Δ9 desaturation of stearic acid; C18:1 Δ11tr and C18:2 Δ9tr,12tr had no effect *(27)*. In addition, C18:1 Δ9tr and C18:2 Δ9tr,12tr inhibited Δ6 desaturation. However, because levels of *cis* n-3 and n-6 FAs in human tissues are much higher than levels of TFAs, these FAs are physiologically more important competitive inhibitors for the conversion of LA into AA and ALA into DHA, compared to *trans* isomers.

4. EFFECTS OF *TRANS* MUFAS ON SERUM LIPIDS AND LPS

4.1. Total Cholesterol and LDL and HDL Cholesterol

The effect of dietary *trans* MUFAs on serum cholesterol concentrations has been investigated since the early 1960s *(17)*. Most studies have found increased serum total

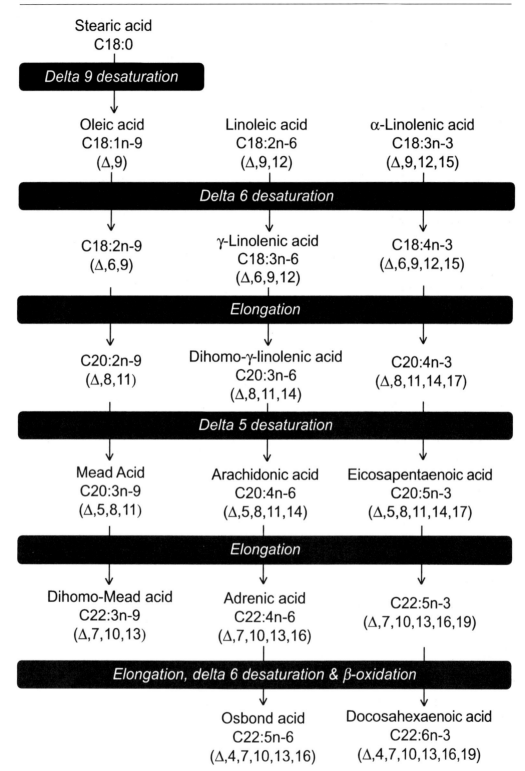

Fig. 4. Desaturation and elongation of FAs.

cholesterol levels in humans consuming partially hydrogenated vegetable oil. Results, however, were not uniform (28). In addition, these earlier studies did not examine the relationship between dietary *trans* MUFAs and the distribution of cholesterol among Lps. The first controlled intervention trial in which the effects of *trans* MUFA intake on serum LDL cholesterol (LDL-C) and HDL cholesterol (HDL-C) were examined, was reported in 1990 by Mensink and Katan (29). Twenty-five men and 34 women were fed a diet high in OA, high in *trans* isomers of OA, or high in a mixture of the SFAs, lauric and palmitic acid. Each diet was fed for 3 wk. The level of *trans* C18:1 in the *trans* diet was 11% of total energy. Results showed that *trans* C18:1 significantly raised total and LDL-C levels by 0.26 mmol/L and 0.37 mmol/L, respectively, and lowered HDL-C levels by 0.17 mmol/L, compared to OA. Later studies (30–34) investigated effects of lower intakes of TFAs (Table 2). The general conclusion is that TFAs and SFAs have similar effects on LDL-C, but increase LDL-C, compared to MUFAs and PUFAs. Also, TFAs lower HDL-C, compared to the other major categories of FAs. Because of differences in TFA intake, intakes of other dietary FAs and experimental designs, results of studies are difficult to compare. Therefore, results of five studies have been combined, and effects of TFAs on Lps were compared with those of OA (28). It is suggested that each additional percent of dietary energy as *trans* MUFAs, at the expense of OA, results in an increase in LDL-C levels of 0.040 mmol/L, and a decrease in HDL-C levels of 0.013 mmol/L (Fig. 5; 28). Such changes in LDL- and HDL-C are associated with an increased risk for CHD.

4.2. Lipoprotein(a)

Lipoprotein(a) (Lp[a]) is a LDL molecule with an extra glycoprotein (apoprotein [a]), attached through a disulfide link. High levels of Lp(a) increase the risk for CHD (35). Therefore, effects of *trans* MUFAs on Lp(a) have been investigated in several intervention studies. Nestel et al. (36) found that Lp(a) levels were significantly higher on a *trans* diet, compared to palmitic acid, but not compared to OA. Mensink et al. (37) reported significantly higher Lp(a) levels on TFAs, compared to SFAs, OA, stearic acid, and LA. Lichtenstein et al. (38) did not find an increase in Lp(a) concentrations; Almendingen et al. (30) found increased Lp(a) levels when butter was exchanged for partially hydrogenated soybean oil or fish oil. Aro et al. (31) observed increased Lp(a) levels on a TFA diet, compared to a dairy-fat-based diet. Most studies showed that *trans* MUFAs may raise Lp(a) levels, particularly in subjects who already have high Lp(a) levels (37).

4.3. Triacylglycerols

An elevated fasting TG level is also a risk marker for CHD (39). Katan et al. (28) summarized studies concerning the *trans* MUFA effect on fasting TG levels. It was calculated that each additional percent of energy as *trans* MUFAs, at the expense of OA, increases TG levels by 0.013 mmol/L (27).

4.4. Conclusion

Trans MUFAs raise serum LDL-C, Lp(a), and TG levels; HDL-C levels are lowered. The effects of *trans* PUFAs on serum lipids and Lps are not yet known.

4.5. Mechanism

Although a number of studies have shown that dietary TFAs affect serum LDL- and HDL-C levels, the underlying mechanisms for these effects are still not understood. It has

Table 2
Effects of TFAs on Serum LDL- and HDL-C Levels[a]

Ref.	Year	No. subjects Men	No. subjects Women	Design	Days of test period	Test diet[b]	FA content of test diet (% of daily energy intake)[b] S	M	P	T	Diet effects (mmol/L) HDL	LDL
Almendingen et al. (30)	1995	31		c	21	I	15.7	8.1	5.9	0.9	1.05	3.81
						II	10.5	9.2	6.5	8.5	1.05	3.58[d]
						III	10.8	5.7	7.0	8.0	0.98[d,e]	3.94[e]
Aro et al. (31)	1997	29	29	f	35	C	13.8	12.2	3.4	0.8		
						I	15.0	12.2	3.5	0.4	1.42	2.89
						II	7.1	21.2	2.9	8.7	1.36[d,g]	3.06[d,g]
Müller et al. (32)	1998		27	c	17	I	11.2	11.8	5.7	0.1	1.47	2.90
						II	3.8	10.6	5.5	7.0	1.32[d]	2.88
						III	6.1	11.7	10.2	0.2	1.43[e]	2.61[d,e]
Judd et al. (33)	1998	23	23	c	35	I	11.2	10.8	7.2	2.7	1.27	3.44
						II	7.9	11.2	9.0	3.9	1.24	3.27[d]
						III	8.3	10.4	10.8	2.4	1.24	3.21[d,e]
Lichtenstein et al. (34)	1999	18	18	c	35	I	16.7	8.1	2.4	1.3	1.16	4.58
						II	7.3	8.1	12.5	0.6	1.11	3.98[d]
						III	8.6	8.1	13.5	0.9	1.11	4.01[d]
						IV	8.4	8.0	11.1	3.3	1.11	4.11[d]
						V	8.6	9.9	8.1	4.2	1.11	4.24[d,e]
						VI	8.5	8.5	6.3	6.7	1.09[d]	4.34[d,e,h]

[a]Only studies with a thorough control of food intake, with dietary FAs being the sole variable, and designs that eliminated the effect of nonspecific drifts of the outcome variables with time, were selected.
[b]C, control diet; S, saturated FAs; M, MUFAs; P, PUFAs; T, TFAs.
[c]Crossover or Latin square design.
[d]For comparison with I.
[e]For comparison with II.
[f]Parallel design.
[g]Corrected for differences in lipid values between groups when on the control diets.
[h]For comparison with III.

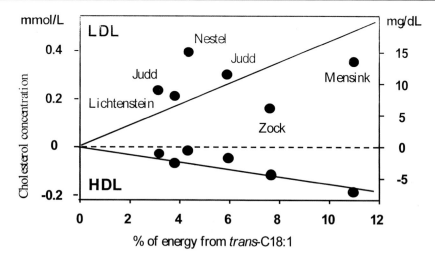

Fig. 5. Effects of exchanging OA for *trans* MUFAs on LDL- and HDL-C levels. Data are derived from six previous studies. Regression coefficients are 0.040 mmol/L for LDL and –0.013 mmol/L for HDL-C, which represent the predicted changes in serum LDL- and HDL-C levels, if 1% of daily energy intake from OA is replaced by *trans* MUFAs *(28)*.

been hypothesized that cholesteryl ester transfer protein (CETP) is involved. CETP transfers cholesteryl esters from HDL to the apolipoprotein B-containing Lps LDL and VLDL, in exchange for TG. Indeed, an increased CETP activity has been found in volunteers who consumed a TFA-enriched diet *(40,41)*, and after addition of TFAs to human plasma in vitro *(42)*. However, other studies *(31,43)* did not confirm these results.

Lecithin cholesterol acyltransferase (LCAT) has also been suggested to be involved. LCAT, which is bound to HDL, esterifies free cholesterol from tissues by the transfer of an acyl group from phosphatidyl-choline (PC). Because a significant part of the dietary TFAs is incorporated into PC *(12)*, a few studies have investigated the effect of TFAs on LCAT. Subbaiah et al. *(44)* reported a decrease of LCAT activity on TFAs. Tol et al. *(41)*, however, did not demonstrate an effect of TFAs on LCAT activity.

In the liver, FAs from chylomicrons are esterified to free cholesterol by acyl-CoA:cholesterol acyl transferase (ACAT). The affinity of ACAT differs for different FAs. A low affinity of the enzyme for a particular FA may result in an increase of free cholesterol in the liver. This causes a decrease of the LDL receptor activity. Since the LDL receptor is involved in the uptake of LDL from plasma, a decreased LDL receptor activity may result in higher LDL concentrations in plasma. Thus, through this pathway, dietary FAs may influence the plasma LDL-C concentration. In a hamster study by Woollett et al. *(45)*, *trans* C18:1 decreased the cholesteryl ester concentration in the liver, relative to OA. This could suggest that the affinity of ACAT is lower for *trans* C18:1, compared to OA, which may result in higher free cholesterol levels in the liver. In addition, the plasma LDL-C concentration was increased, and the LDL receptor activity was decreased on *trans* C18:1. Possibly, *trans* C18:1 affects plasma LDL-C via the pathway described above. This mechanism, however, has not been investigated in humans. Finally, *de novo* cholesterol synthesis did not differ between a high *trans*-hydrogenated corn oil-rich diet and an unhydrogenated corn oil-rich diet low in TFAs in healthy volunteers *(46)*.

5. EFFECTS OF TFAS ON OTHER RISK FACTORS FOR CHD

5.1. LDL Oxidation

Free radicals may initiate oxidation of PUFAs in the LDL particle, which eventually may lead to formation of an atherosclerotic plaque. The FA composition of the LDL particle is a reflection of the FA composition of the diet. Consequently, increased dietary TFA intake leads to higher proportions of TFAs in the LDL particle. Whether this influences the susceptibility for LDL to oxidation has been investigated in several intervention trials. However, no effect on in vitro LDL oxidation was found after consumption of *trans* MUFAs, compared to OA or palmitic acid *(36)*, of hydrogenated, compared to unhydrogenated, corn oil *(46)*, or of partially hydrogenated fish oil or partially hydrogenated soybean oil, compared to butter fat *(47)*. Therefore, it appears that, at least in vitro, TFAs do not have a major impact on LDL oxidizability.

5.2. Hemostasis

Human studies investigating the effects of TFAs on platelet aggregation, coagulation, and fibrinolysis are limited. Almendingen et al. *(48)* have found that a diet enriched in partially hydrogenated soybean oil increased concentrations of plasminogen activator inhibitor type 1 (PAI-1) antigen and PAI-1 activity, compared with a diet high in partially hydrogenated fish oil or butter fat. This indicates an inhibition of the fibrinolytic pathway. Fibrinogen levels were increased on butter, compared to partially hydrogenated fish oil; levels of factor VII were not affected by the diets. It was therefore concluded that partially hydrogenated fish oil had the most favorable hemostatic effects; partially hydrogenated soybean oil had the worst. Mutanen and Aro *(49)* did not see differences in concentrations of fibrinogen, factor VII coagulation activity, tissue type plasminogen activity, and PAI-1 activity between dietary TFAs from partially hydrogenated vegetable oil and stearic acid, in healthy subjects. However, collagen-induced platelet aggregation was significantly decreased on TFAs, compared to stearic acid *(50)*. No effects of TFAs were found on in vitro tromboxane B_2 production, adenosine diphosphate-induced aggregation, and production of endothelial prostacyclin *(50)*.

Few studies have investigated the effects of *trans* PUFAs on human platelet aggregation. Collagen-induced platelet aggregation was less inhibited on *trans* isomers of the LCPUFAs from fish, eicosapentaenoic acid (EPA) and DHA, compared to their *cis* isomers, when these FAs were incorporated into platelets *(16)*. O'Keefe et al. *(51)* has also shown this for EPA in AA-induced platelet aggregation, but not for DHA.

The effects of TFAs on aggregation, coagulation, and fibrinolysis have hardly been investigated. At present, however, it does not seem that TFAs have significant effects on hemostasis.

6. EPIDEMIOLOGICAL STUDIES

Various approaches have been used in epidemiological studies to examine the relationship between the intake of TFAs and the risk for CHD. Because high serum LDL-C levels are negatively associated with CHD, and high levels of HDL-C are thought to be antiatherogenic, some epidemiological studies have focused on the relation between the proportion of TFAs in tissues, which reflects dietary intakes, or the dietary TFA intake and the lipid profile *(52,54)*. In the cross-sectional study by Hudgins et al. *(52)*, no significant correlations between total TFAs in adipose tissue and plasma HDL-C, total to HDL and LDL to HDL-C ratios, and TG were observed in Caucasian men. On the contrary, in another cross-sectional study, the energy-adjusted TFA intake (3.4 ± 1.2 g/d, mean ± SD) was positively related to serum LDL-C, and to total: HDL and LDL:HDL-C ratios, and inversely related to HDL-C *(53)*. In the case–control study of Siguel and Lerman *(54)*, the relationships between plasma TFAs and lipid profile, and between plasma TFAs and risk for CHD, were investigated. It was shown that *trans*-16:1 was positively related to plasma total and LDL-C, TG, and risk for CHD, and negatively related to HDL-C and the HDL:total cholesterol ratio. Altogether, these studies confirm the dietary intervention studies, that TFAs have a negative impact on the lipid profile *(29–34,36,37)*. Most of these studies, however, did not address the question of whether high intakes of TFAs are related to the risk for CHD.

In case–control studies, the proportion of TFAs in tissues or the dietary TFA intake of case subjects, e.g., subjects with CHD, has been compared with that of control subjects, e.g., subjects without CHD *(14,55,61)*. Some studies suggested higher *trans*-C16:1 *(55,56)* or total TFA intakes *(61)* in cases, compared to controls; other studies have not found any effects of TFAs on CHD risk *(14,57,58,60,62)*. One study even showed that the proportion of *trans*-18:1 in adipose tissue was negatively associated with the risk for CHD *(59)*. Case–control studies, however, have the disadvantage that they are sensitive to information bias, selection bias, and confounding.

Prospective cohort studies suffer from fewer of the disadvantages attributed to case–control studies. Four cohort studies have examined the relationship between TFA intake and the risk for CHD. In the Nurses' Health Study, the relative risk (RR) of CHD was 1.27 (95% confidence interval [CI], 1.03–1.56) for the highest quintile of TFA intake (mean intake of 2.9% energy), relative to the lowest (mean intake of 1.3% energy), after adjustment for age and other CHD risk factors *(63)*. This means that women who consume 2.9% energy as TFAs per day have a 27% higher risk for CHD, compared to women with a TFA intake of 1.3% energy. Pietinen et al. *(64)* found, in the Finnish α-Tocopherol, β-Carotene Cancer Prevention Study, a positive association between TFA intake and risk of coronary death, after adjustment for age, supplementation group, and several coronary risk factors. The RR for CHD was 1.39 (95% CI, 1.09–1.78) for the highest quintile of TFA intake (median intake of 5.6 g/d), compared to the lowest (median intake of 1.3 g/d). In addition, in the Health Professionals Follow-up Study, subjects in the highest quintile of *trans* intake (median intake of 4.3 g/d) had a 78% (RR of 1.78; 95% CI, 1.11–1.84) higher risk on fatal CHD, compared to subjects in the lowest quintile of *trans* intake (median intake of 1.5 g/d), after controlling for age and several coronary risk factors *(65)*. Multivariate RRs of these three cohort studies are summarized in Fig. 6, which shows that multivariate RRs increase with TFA intakes. Finally, Kromhout et al. *(66)* have reported that TFA intake was positively related to 25-yr mortality from CHD in the Seven Countries Study.

Results from case–control studies are inconsistent. In the cohort studies, results are more uniform: A high intake of TFAs was associated with an increased risk of CHD. Therefore, based on the results of the cohort studies, it seems advisable to avoid high intakes of TFAs.

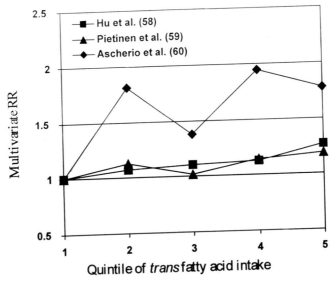

Fig. 6. Multivariate relative risk of CHD according to the quintiles of TFA intake of three cohort studies: the Nurses Health study of Hu et al. *(63)*; the α-Tocopherol, β-Carotene Cancer Prevention Study of Pietinen et al. *(64)*; and the Health Professionals Follow-up Study of Ascherio et al. *(65)*.

7. CANCER

The association between fat intake and carcinogenesis has been investigated in many animal and human studies. Only a few human studies, however, have focused on TFAs and cancer, particularly the risk for breast cancer (BC). Holmes et al. *(67)* found, in the Nurses' Healthy Study (a large cohort study), a RR on BC of 0.92 (95% CI, 0.86–0.98), when the TFA intake would increase with 1% of energy.

Three case–control studies have related the TFA content of adipose tissue to cancer risk. In the European Community Multicenter Study on Antioxidants, Myocardial Infarction, and Cancer of the Breast (EURAMIC) study *(68)*, the TFA content of subcutaneous adipose tissue was positively associated with risk for BC *(68)*. On the contrary, in women with BC, the TFA content in adipose tissue was negatively associated with having BC, as well as cancer in lymph nodes *(69)*. Finally, London et al. *(70)* did not find an association between the TFA content of subcutaneous adipose tissue and BC risk.

Human studies investigating the relationship between TFAs and other classes of cancers are scarce. In the EURAMIC study *(71)*, significant correlations were found between TFAs in adipose tissue and incidence of colon cancer. No association was found with prostate cancer *(71)*. There is not a consistent relationship from human studies between the intake and/or tissue levels of *trans* MUFAs and cancer risk.

8. CONCLUSIONS AND RECOMMENDATIONS

The digestion and absorption of *trans* MUFAs are comparable with those of their *cis* isomers. However, incorporation of various *trans* monoenoic isomers into lipid classes and Lps appears to be lower than that of the *cis* isomers. Furthermore, both *trans* MUFAs and PUFAs can be desaturated and elongated into longer-chain metabolites. However, conversion of *trans* LA may be less than that of LA. *Trans* MUFAs inhibit the conversion of LA; conversion of stearic acid may increase. The oxidation seems to be similar. These processes, however, have been investigated mostly in animal and in vitro studies. More human in vivo studies are therefore necessary.

Most studies on the effects of TFAs on health have focused on *trans* MUFAs, and effects of *trans* PUFAs are hardly known. *Trans* MUFAs increase serum LDL-C, TGs, and Lp(a) concentrations, and decrease serum HDL-C, compared with OA. The underlying mechanisms for these effects are not exactly known. Furthermore, *trans* MUFAs seem to have no major impact on LDL oxidizability, platelet aggregation, coagulation, and fibrinolysis. Several prospective epidemiological studies have shown a positive association between TFAs and the risk for CHD, but not with cancer risk. Therefore, a limitation of the TFA intake, as recommended by the American Heart Association, is justified *(71)*.

REFERENCES

1. Ackman R, Hooper S, Hooper D. Linolenic acid artifacts from the deodorization of oils. J Am Oil Chem Soc 1974; 51:42–49.
2. Wolff R. Further studies on artificial geometrical isomers of α-linolenic acid in edible linolenic acid-containing oils. J Am Oil Chem Soc 1993; 70:219–224.
3. Grandgirard A, Sébédio J, Fleury J. Geometrical isomerization of linolenic acid during heat treatment of vegetable oils. J Am Oil Chem Soc 1984; 61:1563–1568.
4. Allison D, Egan S, Barraj L, Caughman C, Infante M, Heimbach J. Estimated intakes of *trans* fatty and other fatty acids in the US population. J Am Diet Assoc 1999; 99:166–174.
5. Hulshof K, Van Erp-Baart M, Anttolainen M, et al. Intake of fatty acids in Western Europe with emphasis on *trans* fatty acids: the TRANSFAIR study. Eur J Clin Nutr 1999; 53:143–157.
6. Position paper on transfatty acid. ASCN/AIN Task force on transfatty acid. American Society for Clinical Nutrition and American Institute of Nutrition. Am J Clin Nutr 1996;63:663–670.
7. O'Keefe S, Gaskins-Wright S, Wiley V, Chen Chen I. Levels of *trans* geometrical isomers of essential fatty acids in some unhydrogenated U.S. vegetable oils. J Food Lipids 1994; 1:165–176.
8. Emken E. Do *trans* acids have adverse health consequences? In: Health Effects of Dietary Fatty Acids. Nelson G, ed. Champaign, IL: American Oil Chemists Society, 1991; 245–260.
9. Emken E, Dutton H, Rohwedder W, Rakoff H, Adlof R. Distribution of deuterium-labeled *cis* and *trans*-12-octadecemoic acids in human plasma and lipoprotein lipids. Lipids 1980; 15:864–871.
10. Emken E, Adlof R, Rohwedder W, Gulley R. Incorporation of deuterium-labeled *trans*- and *cis*-13-octadecenic acids in human plasma lipids. J Lipid Res 1983; 24:34–46.
11. Emken E, Rohwedder W, Adlof R, DeJarlais W, Gulley R. Absorption and distribution of deuterium-labeled *trans*- and *cis*-11-octadecenoic acid in human plasma and lipoprotein lipids. Lipids 1986; 21: 589–595.
12. Emken E, Adlof R, Rohwedder W, Gulley R. Incorporation of *trans*-8- and *cis*-8-octadecenoic acid isomers in human plasma and lipoprotein lipids. Lipids 1989; 24:61–69.
13. Kris-Etherton P, ed. *Trans* fatty acids and coronary heart disease risk. Am J Clin Nutr 1995; 62: 655S–708S.
14. Heckers H, Korner M, Tuschen T, Melcher F. Occurrence of individual *trans*-isomeric fatty acids in human myocardium, jejunum and aorta in relation to different degrees of atherosclerosis. Atherosclerosis 1977; 28:389–398.
15. Adlof R, Emken E. Distribution of hexadecenoic, octadecenoic and octadecadienoic acid isomers in human tissue lipids. Lipids 1986; 21:543–547.
16. Chardigny J, Sébédio J, Juanéda P, Vatèle J, Grandgirard A. Occurrence of n-3 *trans* polyunsaturated fatty acids in human platelets. Nutr Res 1993; 13:1105–1111.
17. Chardigny J, Wolff R, Mager E, Sébédio J, Martine L, Juanéda P. *Trans* mono- and polyunsaturated fatty acids in human milk. Eur J Clin Nutr 1995; 49:523–531.
18. Kinsella J. α-Linolenic acid: functions and effects on linoleic acid metabolism and eicosanoid-mediated reactions. In: Advances in Food and Nutrition Research. Kinsella J, ed. San Diego: Academic, 1991; 1–184.
19. Mahfouz M, Valicenti A, Holman R. Desaturation of isomeric trans-octadecenoic acids by rat liver microsomes. Biochim Biophys Acta 1980; 618:1–12.

20. Pollard M, Gunstone F, James A, Morris L. Desaturation of positional and geometric isomers of monoenoic fatty acids by microsomal preparations from rat liver. Lipids 1980; 15:306–314.

21. Beyers E, Emken E. Metabolites of *cis,trans*, and *trans,cis* isomers of linoleic acid in mice and incorporation into tissue lipids. Biochim Biophys Acta 1991; 1082:275–284.

22. Grandgirard A, Piconneaux A, Sébédio J, O'Keefe S, Semon E, Quere Le J. Occurrence of geometrical isomers of eicosapentaenoic and docosahexaenoic acids in liver lipids of rats fed heated linseed oil. Lipids 1989; 24:799–804.

23. Grandgirard A, Bourre J, Julliard F, et al. Incorporation of *trans* long-chain n-3 polyunsaturated fatty acids in rat brain structures and retina. Lipids 1994; 29:251–258.

24. Delany J, Bray G. Differential oxidation of various fatty acids. Obes Res 1993; 1:41S (Abstract).

25. Lanser A, Emken E, Ohlrogge J. Oxidation of oleic and elaidic acids in rat and human heart homogenates. Biochim Biophys Acta 1986; 875:510–515.

26. Cook H, Emken E. Geometric and positional fatty acid isomers interact differently with desaturation and elongation of linoleic and linolenic acids in cultured glioma cells. Biochem Cell Biol 1990; 68:653–660.

27. Rosenthal M, Whitehurst M. Selective effects of isomeric *cis* and *trans* fatty acids on fatty acyl Δ9 and Δ6 desaturation by human skin fibroblasts. Biochim Biophys Acta 1983; 753:450–459.

28. Katan M, Mensink R, Zock P. *Trans* fatty acids and their effects on lipoproteins in humans. Ann Rev Nutr 1995; 15:473–493.

29. Mensink R, Katan M. Effect of dietary *trans* fatty acids on high-density and low-density lipoprotein cholesterol levels in healthy subjects. N Engl J Med 1990; 323:439–445.

30. Almendingen K, Jordal O, Kierulf P, Sandstad B, Pedersen J. Effects of partially hydrogenated fish oil, partially hydrogenated soybean oil, and butter on serum lipoproteins and Lp(a) in men. J Lipid Res 1995; 36:1370–1384.

31. Aro A, Jauhiainen M, Partanen R, Salminen I, Mutanen M. Stearic acid, *trans* fatty acids, and dairy fat: effects on serum and lipoprotein lipids, apolipoproteins, lipoprotein(a), and lipid transfer proteins in healthy subjects. Am J Clin Nutr 1997; 65:1419–1426.

32. Müller H, Jordal O, Kierulf P, Kirkhus B, Pedersen J. Replacement of partially hydrogenated soybean oil by palm oil in margarine without unfavorable effects on serum lipoproteins. Lipids 1998; 33:879–887.

33. Judd J, Baer D, Clevidence B, et al. Effects of margarine compared with those of butter on blood lipid profiles related to cardiovascular disease risk factors in normolipemic adults fed controlled diets. Am J Clin Nutr 1998; 68:768–77.

34. Lichtenstein A, Ausman L, Jalbert M, Schaefer E. Effects of different forms of dietary hydrogenated fats on serum lipoprotein cholesterol levels. N Engl J Med 1999; 340:1933–1940.

35. Sandkamp M, Funke H, Schulte H, Kohler E, Assmann G. Lipoprotein(a) is an independent risk factor for myocardial infarction at a young age. Clin Chem 1990; 36:20–23.

36. Nestel P, Noakes M, Belling B, et al. Plasma lipoprotein lipid and Lp(a) changes with substitution of elaidic acid for oleic acid in the diet. J Lipid Res 1992; 33:1029–1036.

37. Mensink R, Zock P, Katan M, Hornstra G. Effect of dietary *cis* and *trans* fatty acids on serum lipoprotein(a) levels in humans. J Lipid Res 1992; 33:1493–1501.

38. Lichtenstein A, Ausman L, Carrasco W, Jenner J, Ordovas J, Schaefer E. Hydrogenation impairs the hypolipidemic effect of corn oil in humans. Arterioscl Thromb 1993; 13:154–161.

39. Austin M. Plasma triglyceride and coronary heart disease. Arterioscl Thromb 1991; 11:2–14.

40. Abbey M, Nestel P. Plasma cholesteryl ester transfer protein activity is increased when *trans*-elaidic acid is substituted for *cis*-oleic acid in the diet. Atherosclerosis 1994; 106:99–107.

41. Van Tol A, Zock P, Van Gent T, Scheek L, Katan M. Dietary *trans* fatty acids increase serum cholesteryl ester transfer protein activity in man. Atherosclerosis 1995; 115:129–134.

42. Lagrost L. Differential effects of *cis* and *trans* fatty acid isomers, oleic and elaidic acids, on the cholesteryl ester transfer protein activity. Biochim Biophys Acta 1992; 1124:159–162.

43. Nishida H, Arai H, Nishida T. Cholesterol ester transfer mediated by lipid transfer protein as influenced by changes in the charge characteristics of plasma lipoproteins. J Biol Chem 1993; 268:16,352–16,360.

44. Subbaiah P, Subramanian V, Liu M. *Trans* unsaturated fatty acids inhibit lecithin: cholesterol acyltransferase and alter its positional specificity. J Lipid Res 1998; 39:1438–1447.

45. Woollett L, Daumerie C, Dietschy J. *Trans*-9-octadecenoic acid is biologically neutral and does not regulate the low density lipoprotein receptor as the *cis* isomer does in the hamster. J Lipid Res 1994; 35:1661–1673.

46. Cuchel M, Schwab U, Jones P, et al. Impact of hydrogenated fat consumption on endogenous cholesterol synthesis and susceptibility of low-density lipoprotein to oxidation in moderately hypercholesterolemic individuals. Metabolism 1996; 45:241–247.

47. Halvorsen B, Almendingen K, Nenseter M, Pedersen J, Christiansen E. Effects of partially hydrogenated fish oil, partially hydrogenated soybean oil and butter on the susceptibility of low density lipoprotein to oxidative modification in men. Eur J Clin Nutr 1996; 50:364–370.

48. Almendingen K, Seljeflot I, Sandstad B, Pedersen J. Effects of partially hydrogenated fish oil partially hydrogenated soybean oil and butter on hemostatic variables in men. Arterioscl Thromb Vascular Biol 1996; 16:375–380.

49. Mutanen M, Aro A. Coagulation and fibrinolysis factors in healthy subjects consuming high stearic or *trans* fatty acid diets. Thrombosis Haemostasis 1997; 77:99–104.

50. Turpeinen A, Wubert J, Aro A, Lorenz R, Mutanen M. Similar effects of diets rich in stearic acid or *trans*-fatty acids on platelet function and endothelial prostacyclin production in humans. Arterioscl Thromb Vascular Biol 1998; 18:316–322.

51. O'Keefe S, Lagarde M, Grandgirard A, Sébédio J. *Trans* n-3 eicosapentaenoic and docosahexaenoic acid isomers exhibit different inhibitory effects on arachidonic acid metabolism in human platelets compared to the respective *cis* fatty acids. J Lipid Res 1990; 31:1241–1246.

52. Hudgins L, Hirsch J, Emken E. Correlation of isomeric fatty acids in human adipose tissue with clinical risk factors for cardiovascular disease. Am J Clin Nutr 1991; 53:474–482.

53. Troisi R, Willett W, Weiss S. *Trans*-fatty acid intake in relation to serum lipid concentrations in adult men. Am J Clin Nutr 1992; 56:1019–1024.

54. Siguel E, Lerman R. *Trans*-fatty acid patterns in patients with angiographically documented coronary artery disease. Am J Cardiol 1993; 71:916–920.

55. Thomas L, Winter J, Scott R. Concentration of 18:1 and 16:1 *trans* unsaturated fatty acids in the adipose body tissue of decedents dying of ischaemic heart disease compared with controls: analysis by gas liquid chromatography. J Epidemiol Community Health 1983; 37:16–21.

56. Thomas L, Winter J. Ischaemic heart disease and consumption of hydrogenated marine oils. Human Nutr Food Sci Nutr 1987; 41F:153–165.

57. Thomas L, Olpin S, Scott R, Wilkins M. Coronary heart disease and the composition of adipose tissue taken at biopsy. Human Nutr Food Sci Nutr 1987; 41F:167–172.

58. Aro A, Kardinaal A, Salminen I, et al. Adipose tissue isomeric *trans* fatty acids and risk of myocardial infarction in nine countries: the EURAMIC study. Lancet 1995; 345:273–278.

59. Roberts T, Wood D, Riemersma R, Gallagher P, Lampe F. *Trans* isomers of oleic and linoleic acids in adipose tissue and sudden cardiac death. Lancet 1995; 345:278–282.

60. Van de Vijver L, Van Poppel G, Van Houwelingen A, Kruyssen D, Hornstra G. *Trans* unsaturated fatty acids in plasma phospholipids and coronary heart disease: a case-control study. Atherosclerosis 1996; 126:155–161.

61. Ascherio A, Hennekens C, Buring J, Master C, Stampfer M, Willett W. *Trans*-fatty acids intake and risk of myocardial infarction. Circulation 1994; 89:94–101.

62. Tzonou A, Kalandidi A, Trichopoulou A, et al. Diet and coronary heart disease: a case-control study in Athens, Greece. Epidemiology 1993; 4:511–516.

63. Hu F, Stampfer M, Manson J, et al. Dietary fat intake and the risk of coronary heart disease in women. N Engl J Med 1997; 337:1491–1499.

64. Pietinen P, Ascherio A, Korhonen P, et al. Intake of fatty acids and risk of coronary heart disease in a cohort of Finnish men. Am J Epidemiol 1997; 145:876–887.

65. Ascherio A, Rimm E, Giovannucci E, Spiegelman D, Stampfer M, Willett W. Dietary fat and risk of coronary heart disease in men: cohort follow up study in the United States. Br Med J 1996; 313:84–90.

66. Kromhout D, Menotti A, Bloemberg B, et al. Dietary saturated and *trans* fatty acids and cholesterol and 25-year mortality from coronary heart disease: The Seven Countries Study. Prev Med 1995; 24:308–315.

67. Holmes M, Hunter D, Colditz G, et al. Association of dietary intake of fat and fatty acids with risk of breast cancer. JAMA 1999; 281:914–920.

68. Kohlmeier L, Simonsen N, Van het Veer P, et al. Adipose tissue *trans* fatty acids and breast cancer in the European community multicenter study on antioxidant, myocardial infarction, and breast cancer. Cancer Epidemiol Biomarkers Prev 1997; 6:705–710.

69. Petrek J, Hudgins L, Ho M, Bajorunas D, Hirsch J. Fatty acid composition of adipose tissue and indication of dietary fatty acids, and breast cancer prognosis. J Clin Oncol 1997; 15:1377–1384.

70. London S, Sacks F, Stampfer M, et al. Fatty acid composition of the subcutaneous adipose tissue and risk of proliferative benign breast disease and breast cancer. J Natl Cancer Inst 1993; 85:785–793.

71. Bakker N, Van het Veer P, Zock P, EURAMIC group. Adipose fatty acids and cancers of the breast, prostate and colon: an ecological study. Int J Cancer 1997; 72:587–591.

72. Krauss R, Deckelbaum R, Ernst N, et al. Dietary guidelines for healthy American adults. Circulation 1996; 94:1795–1800.

6

Antioxidant Vitamins and Atherosclerosis

Howard N. Hodis, Wendy J. Mack, and Alex Sevanian

1. INTRODUCTION

A large body of laboratory evidence suggests that the early stages of atherosclerosis (Athsc) are comprised of a series of oxidative processes *(1)*. Animal studies suggest that oxidative damage may be involved with atherogenic-promoting processes, such as endothelial damage *(2)*, and that antioxidants reduce oxidative damage and Athsc lesions *(3,4)*. As such, a large body of basic science research and animal studies support the antiatherogenic hypothesis of antioxidants. Although information concerning antioxidants and human Athsc is accumulating, the relevance of this hypothesis to Athsc prevention in humans remains unproven.

Studies in humans indicate an association between blood measures of oxidative processes and Athsc *(5)*. These data are paralleled by observational studies, including arterial imaging studies *(6,7)* that have demonstrated an inverse association between use of antioxidant vitamin supplements and cardiovascular disease (CVD). Data from randomized clinical trials have been less consistent, and the safety of certain antioxidant supplementations has been questioned in some studies *(8–13)*. The purpose of this chapter is to review evidence from observational studies, randomized clinical trials, and Athsc arterial-imaging studies for an antiatherogenic effect of antioxidant vitamins in humans.

2. FREE RADICALS, OXIDATION, ANTIOXIDANTS, AND ATHSC

Oxidative processes that evoke early atherogenesis parallel mechanisms described for lipid and protein oxidation by free radical species. Relative to free-radical-mediated injury to cell and tissues, certain antioxidants provide significant scavenging and protective effects. It has been suggested that oxidative damage to tissues is the outcome of an imbalance between free-radical species formation and elimination. Accordingly, emphasis has been placed on antioxidant interventions. Different categories of antioxidant defenses have been described, and are subdivided into nonenzymatic and enzymatic antioxidants *(14)*. A detailed overview of free-radical mechanisms that are relevant to the modification of lipoproteins (Lps) and injury to vascular tissues has recently been published *(15)*.

Lipid peroxidation, a free-radical-related process, underlies many of the proinflammatory and vascular cell changes associated with atherogenesis. Mechanisms to prevent

From: *Primary and Secondary Preventive Nutrition*
Edited by: A. Bendich and R. J. Deckelbaum © Humana Press Inc., Totowa, NJ

lipid peroxidation have been the focus of antioxidant research. Free-radical-related mechanisms initiating lipid peroxidation in tissues and Lps involve a host of reactive oxygen species (ROS), including superoxide anion radicals (O_2^-) and H_2O_2, both formed metabolically and by redox cycling of many compounds (16). Metabolic sources for ROS include enzymes of the mitochondrial respiratory chain (17), the cytochrome P-450 enzyme family (18), and lipoxygenases (19). The reactivity of ROS and rate of lipid peroxidation is facilitated by certain transition metals probably complexed to proteins, because free transition metals do not exist in normal tissues at catalytic levels sufficient for ROS production rates needed to induce cellular lipid peroxidation. Iron or copper bound to protein serve as effective catalysts, especially with saturation of protein-binding sites (20). This has been described for ceruloplasmin, which has been implicated in the oxidation of serum Lps (21). Plausible mechanisms for initiating lipid peroxidation may also involve heme proteins, known to be converted to potent oxidants (22).

Certain steps of arterial wall cellular metabolism that lead to atheroma formation can be modulated by low density lipoprotein (LDL)-derived oxidation products. The type and proportion of oxidation products are dependent on the radical-generating system. Cu^{2+}-mediated oxidation is a common in vitro system used to investigate the role of LDL components during lipid peroxidation. It has also been used to determine LDL oxidative susceptibility in healthy subjects, and in patients with circumstances associated with oxidative stress, such as myocardial infarction (MI). Measurements are often based on the inhibition period of oxidation (lag time), typically using 5–10 µmol Cu^{2+}/LDL. The susceptibility of LDL to oxidation is dependent on the composition of LDL, i.e., on its antioxidant, lipid hydroperoxide, and fatty acid content (23). Cu^{2+}-oxidized LDL (Ox-LDL) shares similar properties to LDL isolated from arterial lesions (23).

Oxidation of Lps, particularly LDL, forms a heterogeneous group of unsaturated carbonyls that react with the lysine ε-amino groups of apolipoprotein B (apoB), thus reducing the proportion of positively charged amino acids (24). LDL accordingly acquires a progressively negative net charge, and is taken up by a receptor that binds negatively charged apoB, scavenger receptor-A1 (25). A continuum of increasingly Ox-LDL can be formed, based on the duration and/or severity of oxidation. A threshold for oxidative modification of LDL apoprotein has been proposed, on the basis of the number of covalently modified lysine groups (26), and by modifications at other domains of the apoprotein (27). Progressive modifications along important domains of apoB, particularly at the ligand epitopes for cell LDL receptors, reduce its capacity for assimilation by receptor-mediated endocytosis (27). Ox-LDL can exist as both soluble and insoluble (aggregate) particles when LDL is oxidized with Cu^{+2} to varying degrees (28).

Lipid hydroperoxides formed in Lps react with apoproteins via two mechanisms: by decomposition to reactive carbonyls; or by addition of the peroxy radical to free amino groups, including those found in phosphatidylethanolamine (29). A reaction of the hydroperoxide with protein has been proposed to involve release of O_2^-, which may participate in further ROS-mediated oxidation reactions. This second mechanism may account for more fluorescent products after LDL oxidation than are found by reactions with aldehydic products. This reaction may take place in parallel with formation of Schiff bases, which are common reaction products of reactive carbonyls. The spectrum for the fluorescent products for reactions, via either mechanisms 1 or 2, resembles the spectrum obtained for Ox-LDL isolated from Athsc tissues or LDL subjected to a variety of oxidation reactions. This suggests that similar reactions may occur during the oxidation of Lps in vivo.

Oxidized Lps are known to be cytotoxic to vascular cells *(30)*, with toxicity attributable to the lipid components *(31)*. The cytotoxic effects appear to result from a free-radical-mediated oxidation process induced in cells upon exposure to Ox-LDL, since toxicity is mostly prevented by antioxidant pretreatments *(32)*. Receptor-mediated delivery of the oxidized Lps provides a targeted means for delivering oxidized lipids and their decomposition products to intracellular sites, resulting in the signaling and expression of stress–response genes, cytokines, and adhesion molecules. Ox-LDL is chemotactic to monocytes, and inhibits macrophage motility, which are effects also attributable to the lipid components *(33,34)*. Further evidence that these effects result from oxidized lipids comes from studies *(35)* showing that lipid loading and binding to collagen are inhibited by antioxidants. Studies using the antioxidants, probucol and butylated hydroxytoluene, offer compelling but indirect evidence for LDL oxidation as an important factor contributing to atherogenesis *(3,4)*. In Athsc animal studies *(3,4)*, these agents have been shown to slow the development of Athsc. These events may be evoked, either directly or indirectly, through the presence of lipid peroxidation products, and, in a concerted manner, facilitate the development of an Athsc lesion. The ability to induce the expression of cytokine genes, along with a series of other acute response proteins in vascular cells, is shared by both Ox-LDL and fatty acid hydroperoxides. Treatment of endothelial cells with either oxidant results in augmented expression of cytokine-mediated formation of adhesion molecules (vascular cell adhesion molecule and intercellular adhesion molecule) *(36)*. Inhibition of these responses by antioxidants is taken as evidence that the effects occur through cellular oxidant stress involving redox-sensitive transcriptional or posttranscriptional factors *(37)*. Similarly, the induction of factors, such as monocyte chemotactic peptide, is evoked by Ox-LDL and lipid peroxidation products through oxidant-sensitive transcriptional factors *(37)*. In this respect, it has been shown that vitamin E, and specifically R,R,R-α-tocopherol, may have a modulatory role on signal transduction events associated with the regulation of smooth muscle cell proliferation. The effect appears to be unrelated to its direct antioxidant activity, i.e., inhibition of lipid peroxidation and free-radical generation, although an indirect action related to modulating the cellular redox state is plausible. It is proposed *(38)* that protein kinase C-α (PKCα) inhibition by AT is linked to the activation of a protein phosphatase, which in turn dephosphorylates PKCα and inhibits its activity. This mechanism of action may not only influence the signaling events regulating smooth muscle cell proliferation, but may also inhibit formation of early Athsc lesions, as demonstrated recently in rabbits in which vitamin E prevented cholesterol-induced Athsc lesions and the induction of PKC activity *(39)*. In each of these cases, the oxidant-sensitive/antioxidant-inhibitable mechanism involves activation of transcription factors that signal cell proliferation, chemotaxis, and adhesion of inflammatory cells at vascular loci where Athsc lesions are prone to develop. The extent to which specific antioxidants are able to modulate these responses is presently under investigation.

3. OBSERVATIONAL EVIDENCE FOR ANTIATHEROGENIC EFFECT OF ANTIOXIDANTS

3.1. Ecologic Studies

Several early ecologic studies, reporting an inverse correlation between consumption of vitamin-containing foods and CVD, suggest a possible role of dietary antioxidants in the prevention of Athsc. In Scotland and England, fresh fruit and vegetable consumption was inversely associated with CVD mortality *(40,41)*. Vitamin C from fresh fruit and vegetable consumption was inversely related with coronary heart disease (CHD) mortality *(40,41)*. Data from the U.S. Department of Agriculture, and vital statistics from 1964 to 1978, indicated an inverse correlation between fruit and vegetable consumption and CVD mortality, which was especially true for foods rich in vitamin C *(42)*. A similar correlation was observed between increased ascorbate production and reduction in CHD mortality in the United States between 1958 and 1978 *(43)*. Although these represent important observations, results from these ecologic studies are limited, since they are susceptible to large interpretative biases from the inability to link CVD risk with food consumption in specific individuals. Further, these studies were not adjusted for concomitant CVD risk factors.

3.2. Epidemiologic Studies

3.2.1. VITAMIN E DIETARY AND SUPPLEMENTARY INTAKE

Five large-scale prospective cohort studies *(44–48)* have investigated the relationship between vitamin E intake and CVD (Table 1). Although only one of these studies *(46)* found decreased CHD risk associated with dietary intake of vitamin E, three of these studies found that supplementary vitamin E intake was significantly associated with lower CHD risk in the elderly *(48)*, middle-aged women *(44)*, and men *(45)*. The Nurses' Health Study was the largest of these studies, with 87,245 female nurses initially free of CVD, 34–59 yr old, who completed dietary questionnaires that assessed daily dietary and supplementary antioxidant vitamin intake *(44)*. During follow-up of 8 yr, 552 cases of CHD were documented, including 437 nonfatal MIs and 115 coronary deaths. Compared with women in the lowest quintile of vitamin E intake (<3.5 IU/d), those in the top quintile (>21.5 IU/d) had a relative risk (RR) of CHD of 0.66 (95% confidence interval [CI], 0.50–0.87, $p < 0.001$), after adjustment for age, smoking, and a variety of additional CVD risk factors. Benefit was attributable primarily to supplementary vitamin E intake, because dietary sources were not associated with significant reductions in CHD. Users of supplementary vitamin E for <2 yr had no significant reduction in CHD risk, RR 0.86 (95% CI, 0.52–1.43). However, use of supplementary vitamin E for ≥2 yr was associated with a significant reduction in CHD risk, after adjustment for CVD risk factors and other antioxidant vitamins, RR 0.59 (95% CI, 0.38–0.91). Women taking at least 100 IU/d specific vitamin E supplements (i.e., not multivitamins) had a RR of CHD of 0.57 (95% CI, 0.41–0.78), compared with nonusers. There was no trend toward a greater decrease in CHD risk with increasing daily intake of supplementary vitamin E, RR 0.56 (95% CI, 0.21–1.51) for intake of 100–250 IU/d; 0.56 (95% CI, 0.33–0.96) for intake of 300–500 IU/d; and 0.58 (95% CI, 0.24–1.42) for intake of ≥600 IU/d.

In the Health Professionals Follow-up Study, 39,910 male health professionals, 40–75 yr of age, and initially free of CVD, completed dietary questionnaires that assessed daily dietary and supplementary antioxidant vitamin intake *(45)*. During 4 yr of follow-up, 667 cases of CHD were documented, including 360 coronary artery (CA) bypass grafts or percutaneous transluminal coronary angioplasties, 201 nonfatal MI, and 106 fatal MI. Compared with men in the lowest quintile of vitamin E intake (median intake = 6.4 IU/d), those in the top quintile (median intake = 419 IU/d) had a RR of CHD of 0.64 (95% CI, 0.49–0.83, $p < 0.003$), after adjustment for age, smoking, body mass index, hypertension, and additional CVD risk factors, and a RR of CHD of 0.60 (95% CI, 0.44–

Table 1
Epidemiological Studies of Dietary and Supplementary Vitamin Intake

---

Vitamin E
    Nurses' Health Study
    Health Professionals Follow-Up Study
    Iowa Women's Health Study
    Finnish Mobile Clinic Study
    Established Populations for Epidemiologic Studies of the Elderly
Vitamin C
    Nurses' Health Study
    Health Professionals Follow-Up Study
    Iowa Women's Health Study
    Finnish Mobile Clinic Study
    Established Populations for Epidemiologic Studies of the Elderly
    Alameda County Study
    Western Electric Study
    Swedish Women's Study
    British Department of Health and Social Security Nutritional Survey
    First National Health and Nutrition Examination Survey Epidemiologic Follow-Up Study
β-carotene
    Nurses' Health Study
    Health Professionals Follow-Up Study
    Iowa Women's Health Study
    Finnish Mobile Clinic Study
    Western Electric Study
    Massachusetts Health Care Panel Study

0.81, $p < 0.01$), with further adjustments for vitamin C and carotene intake. Benefit was attributable primarily to supplementary vitamin E intake, since dietary sources were not associated with significant reductions in CHD. For men consuming ≥60 IU/d vitamin E, the RR of CHD was 0.64 (95% CI, 0.49–0.83), compared with those consuming <7.5 IU/d. Maximal reduction in risk was seen with an intake of 100–249 IU/d vitamin E, with no further decrease in risk at higher intakes. Men taking at least 100 IU/d vitamin E supplements for ≥2 yr had a RR of CHD of 0.63 (95% CI, 0.47–0.84), compared with nonusers, after controlling for multivitamin use. Men taking at least 100 IU/d of specific vitamin E supplements (i.e., not multivitamins) had a RR of CHD of 0.75 (95% CI, 0.61–0.93), compared with nonusers.

The Iowa Women's Health Study followed 34,486 postmenopausal women for up to 7 yr (46). The women, 55–69 yr of age and initially free of CVD, completed questionnaires that assessed daily dietary and supplementary antioxidant vitamin intake. During follow-up, 242 women died of CHD. In the overall cohort, vitamin E intake from food and supplements was not associated with a lower risk of CHD death, RR of 0.96 (95% CI, 0.62–1.51, $p = 0.27$). However, vitamin E intake from food was inversely associated with CHD death among the subgroup of 21,809 women who did not consume vitamin supplements. Compared with women in the lowest quintile of vitamin E intake (≤4.91 IU/d), those in the top quintile (≥9.64 IU/d) had a RR for CHD death of 0.38 (95% CI, 0.18–0.80, $p < 0.004$), after adjustment for age, total energy intake, and a variety of additional CVD risk factors. Unlike the Nurses' Health Study (44) and the Health Professionals Follow-up Study (45), supplementary intake of vitamin E was not associated with lower CHD risk. Intake of foods rich in vitamin E, such as margarine, nuts and seeds, and mayonnaise or creamy salad dressings, were each inversely associated with a lower risk for CHD death.

The Finnish Mobile Clinic Study was conducted in 5133 Finnish men and women, 30–69 yr of age, who were initially free of CVD (47). Daily dietary and supplementary antioxidant vitamin intake was assessed with questionnaires at baseline. During the mean 14-yr follow-up period, there were 186 CHD deaths in men and 58 CHD deaths in women. In the 2748 men, those in the highest vs lowest tertile of vitamin E intake had a RR for CHD death of 0.68 (95% CI, 0.42–1.11, p-value for trend = 0.01), after adjustment for CVD risk factors. In the 2385 women, those in the highest vs lowest tertile of vitamin E intake had a RR for CHD death of 0.35 (95% CI, 0.14–0.88, p-value for trend <0.01), after adjustment for CVD risk factors. Individuals who died of CHD consumed more dairy products and less vegetables, fruits, and margarine than did the survivors. The adjusted RR for CHD mortality, among the 3% of men and women who used supplements containing vitamin E or vitamin C vs those individuals who did not use supplements, was 0.55 (95% CI, 0.18–1.73).

The Established Populations for Epidemiologic Studies of the Elderly was a prospective study designed to determine the effect of vitamin E and vitamin C supplement intake (not part of a multivitamin) on CHD mortality in 11,178 men and women aged 67–105 yr (48). During the 6 to 9 yr of follow-up, there were 3490 deaths, including 1101 CHD deaths. Vitamin E supplement intake was associated with a RR for CHD mortality of 0.59 (95% CI, 0.37–0.93), as well as a RR for all-cause mortality of 0.73 (95% CI, 0.58–0.91), after adjustment for CVD risk factors. However, the dosages of the vitamin supplements and consistency of their use were not assessed.

3.2.2. Vitamin C Dietary and Supplementary Intake

Ten large-scale prospective cohort studies (45–54) have examined the relationship between vitamin C intake and CVD (Table 1). The results from these studies have been less consistent than those for vitamin E, and the majority of the studies do not support a relationship between vitamin C intake and CVD protection. Eight of these studies (45–52) have found no CVD risk reduction from vitamin C intake. After adjustment for other vitamin and multivitamin intake, both the Nurses' Health Study (49) and the Health Professionals Follow-up Study (45) showed no additional CVD benefit from vitamin C intake. In fact, in the Health Professionals Follow-up Study, men in the top quintile of vitamin C intake (median intake = 1162 mg/d) vs the lowest quintile (median intake = 92 mg/d) had a nonsignificantly increased risk for CHD (RR = 1.25, 95% CI, 0.68–1.16) (45). In addition, in the Iowa Women's Health Study, women in the top quintile of vitamin C intake (≥196.3 mg/d) vs the lowest quintile (≤87.3 mg/d) also had a nonsignificant increased risk for CHD mortality (RR = 1.43, 95% CI, 0.75–2.70) (46).

In the Finnish Mobile Clinic Study, women in the highest vs lowest tertile of vitamin C intake had a RR of CHD death of 0.49 (95% CI, 0.24–0.98, p = 0.06), after adjustment for CVD risk factors; men had a RR of 1.00 (95% CI, 0.68–1.45, p = 0.94) (47). In the Established Populations for Epidemiologic Studies of the Elderly, vitamin C supplement vs no supplement intake was associated with a RR of CHD mortality of 0.99 (95% CI, 0.74–1.33), after adjustment for CVD risk factors (48).

In the Alameda County Study, 3119 men and women, 16 yr of age and older, were followed for up to 10 yr (50). The subjects completed dietary questionnaires that assessed daily dietary and supplementary antioxidant vitamin intake. During follow-up, 276 deaths occurred. There were no significant relationships between vitamin C intake above and below 250 mg/d in mortality from cancer, CVD, or total mortality.

In the Western Electric Study, 1556 men, 40–55 yr old, were followed for 24 yr (51). Although there was a 0.75 (95% CI, 0.52–1.07) RR of CHD death in the highest tertile of vitamin C intake (>112 mg/d) vs the lowest tertile (<83 mg/d), this was not statistically significant. In a 12-yr follow-up study of 1462 Swedish women, 38–60 yr old, vitamin C intake, estimated from 24-h dietary recalls, was not associated with CVD mortality, MI, or stroke, after controlling for CV risk factors (52).

In the British Department of Health and Social Security Nutritional Survey, 730 British men and women, 65 yr and older, were followed for up to 20 yr (53). The subjects were initially free of CVD, and completed 7-d dietary records. During follow-up, there were 124 deaths from stroke and 182 deaths from CHD. Compared with subjects in the lowest tertile of vitamin C intake (≤27.9 mg/d), those in the top tertile (>44.9 mg/d) had a RR of death from stroke of 0.50 (95% CI, 0.30–0.80, $p < 0.003$), after adjustment for age, sex, and CVD risk factors. In contrast to the stroke results, there was no significant association between vitamin C intake and CHD mortality (RR = 0.8 [95% CI, 0.6–1.2]).

The First National Health and Nutrition Examination Survey Epidemiologic Follow-up Study was the only large-scale prospective cohort study to find a significant CVD benefit from vitamin C intake (54). This study involved a median follow-up of 10 yr in 11,348 men and women, 15–74 yr old. In the cohort of 4479 men, there were 1069 verified deaths, and, in the 6869 women, there were 740 verified deaths. Men who had a dietary intake of vitamin C of 50 mg/d or more, and who consumed vitamin C supplements on a regular basis, had a CVD standardized mortality ratio of 0.58 (95% CI, 0.41–0.78). Women with the same vitamin C intake had a CVD standardized mortality ratio of 0.66 (95% CI, 0.53–0.82). The average vitamin C supplement intake among users was 800 mg/d. The inverse association between vitamin C intake and CVD mortality appeared to be explained by supplementary intake, since vitamin C dietary intake was not significantly associated with reduced CVD mortality. Caution in the interpretation of these results is warranted, however, because the use of other vitamin supplements or multivitamins was not considered in the data analyses.

3.2.3. β-CAROTENE DIETARY AND SUPPLEMENTARY INTAKE

Six large-scale prospective cohort studies (45–47,51,55,56) have investigated the relationship between β-carotene intake and CVD (Table 1). As in the case with vitamin C, the reported relationships between β-carotene intake and CVD have been inconsistent. Of the six reported prospective cohort studies, only two have shown a statistically significant inverse relationship between β-carotene intake and CVD (45,55). Although women in the highest vs lowest quintile of β-carotene intake had a RR of 0.78 (95% CI, 0.59–1.03) for CHD risk in the Nurses' Health Study (56), this did not reach statistical significance after adjustment for age, smoking, and other CHD risk factors. In the Iowa Women's Health Study, no association was found between CHD mortality and vitamin A, retinol, or carotenoids from dietary or supplement intake alone, or from dietary and supplement intake combined (46). In the Finnish Mobile Clinic Study, women in the highest vs lowest tertile of β-carotene intake had a RR of CHD death of 0.62 (95% CI, 0.30–1.29, $p = 0.60$), after adjustment for CVD risk factors; men had a RR of 1.02 (95% CI, 0.70–1.48, $p = 0.36$) (47). Although there was a 0.79 (95% CI, 0.60–1.04) RR for CHD death in middle-aged men in the highest (>15.9 mg/d) vs the lowest tertile (<2.9 mg/d) of β-carotene intake in the Western Electric Study, this did not reach statistical significance *(51)*.

In the Health Professionals Follow-up Study, men in the top quintile of carotene intake (dietary and supplementary median intake = 19,034 IU/d) vs the lowest quintile (median intake = 3969 IU/d) had a lower risk for CHD (RR = 0.71 [95% CI, 0.53–0.86] $p = 0.03$) *(45)*. Although this inverse relationship between carotene intake and CHD risk was not found among those men who had never smoked (RR = 1.09 [95% CI, 0.66–1.79] $p = 0.64$), an inverse association was apparent among current smokers (RR = 0.30 [95% CI, 0.11– 0.82] $p = 0.02$) and former smokers (RR = 0.60 [95% CI, 0.38–0.94] $p = 0.04$).

The Massachusetts Health Care Panel Study examined the association between consumption of carotene-containing fruits and vegetables and CVD mortality in a prospective cohort of 1299 Massachusetts residents 66 yr old and older, initially free of CVD *(55)*. During 4.75 yr follow-up, 161 cases of CVD mortality were documented, including 48 confirmed fatal MI. Compared with men and women in the lowest quartile of carotene-containing fruit and vegetable consumption (<0.8 servings/d), those in the top quartile (≥2.05 servings/d) had a RR of CVD death of 0.59 (95% CI, 0.37–0.94, $p = 0.014$), after adjustment for age, smoking, cholesterol intake, alcohol consumption, and additional CVD risk factors, and a RR of 0.27 (95% CI, 0.10–0.74, $p = 0.005$) for fatal MI.

3.3. Studies Measuring Serum Antioxidant Concentrations

In general, studies examining the relationship between serum antioxidant concentrations and CVD have been inconclusive *(57–74)*. Specifically, studies examining the relationship between serum β-carotene, vitamin A, and vitamin C concentrations and CVD have been as inconsistent as the observational studies examining CVD and dietary and supplementary intake of these antioxidant vitamins. Also, studies examining the relationship between serum vitamin E concentrations and CVD have not consistently confirmed the observational studies examining dietary and supplementary intake of vitamin E and CVD.

3.3.1. Cross-Sectional Studies

In the cross-sectional World Health Organization/Multinational Monitoring Project of Trends and Determinants of Cardiovascular Disease Study (WHO/MONICA), multiple groups of approx 100 healthy men, aged 40–49 yr, from 16 different worldwide regions differing sixfold in age-standardized CHD mortality, were compared regarding plasma levels of vitamin A, C, E, and carotene *(57,58)*. Independent of lipid levels, the plasma vitamin E concentration was the strongest inverse predictive factor for cross-cultural CHD mortality rates. This study also indicated that the RR, because of a low vitamin E plasma level, may have a greater importance for CHD mortality than classical risk factors, such as a higher total cholesterol or blood pressure. Across all 16 regions, where LDL-cholesterol (LDL-C) levels ranged from 3.36 mmol/L (130 mg/dL) to 4.91 mmol/L (190 mg/dL), moderate associations between CHD mortality rates and plasma cholesterol ($r^2 = 0.29$, $p = 0.03$) and diastolic blood pressure (BP) ($r^2 = 0.25$, $p = 0.05$) were found; a considerably stronger inverse association was found for lipid-standardized vitamin E plasma levels ($r^2 = 0.62$, $p = 0.0003$). Lipid-standardized vitamin A ($r^2 = 0.24$, $p = 0.05$), vitamin C ($r^2 = 0.11$, $p = 0.22$), and carotene ($r^2 = 0.04$, $p = 0.48$) plasma levels showed weaker associations with CHD mortality rates. Among 12 regions with common plasma LDL-C levels, ranging from 3.88 mmol/L (150 mg/dL) to 4.40 mmol/L (170 mg/dL), absolute levels of vitamin E ($r^2 = 0.63$, $p = 0.002$) and lipid-standardized vitamin E ($r^2 = 0.73$, $p = 0.0004$) showed strong inverse correlations with CHD mortality rates. Additionally, vitamin C plasma levels showed a moderately strong, statistically significant inverse correlation with CHD mortality rates among the 12 regions ($r^2 = 0.41$, $p = 0.03$). Lipid-standardized vitamin A ($r^2 = 0.16$, $p = 0.19$) and carotene ($r^2 = 0.21$, $p = 0.14$) plasma levels showed no association with CHD mortality rates among the 12 regions. In regions with low and medium CHD risk (Italy, Switzerland, and Northern Ireland), average vitamin E plasma levels, among healthy middle-aged males, were 26–28 µmol/L; in regions with highest CHD risk (Finland and Scotland), vitamin E plasma levels were 20–21.5 µmol/L *(58)*. On average, vitamin E plasma levels were about 25% lower ($p < 0.01$) in regions with high CHD risk vs regions of low-to-medium risk, and there was only a small overlap in the distributions of vitamin E plasma levels. This indicates that there may be a threshold of CHD risk from vitamin E plasma levels below 25–30 µmol/L *(58)*. A similar threshold for CHD risk may be operational for vitamin C plasma levels below 23–51 µmol/L *(58)*. In a smaller cross-sectional survey *(59)* of four European regions, the evidence did not support the hypothesis that plasma antioxidant concentrations explain regional differences in CHD mortality.

In a cross-sectional survey *(60)* of 595 individuals, 50–84 yr old, conducted in an urban population of India, a significant inverse association between plasma vitamin A, vitamin C, vitamin E, and β-carotene levels and prevalence of coronary artery disease (CAD) (defined as presence of angina or diagnosis of MI) was found. The vitamin A and E levels remained inversely related to CAD, after adjustment for other CVD risk factors. The adjusted odds ratio for CAD, between the lowest and highest quintiles of plasma vitamin levels in 523 subjects without CAD and 72 subjects with CAD, was only significant for plasma vitamin E levels, 2.53 (95% CI, 1.11–5.31); lowest quintile <11.8 µmol/L, highest quintile >19.2 µmol/L.

The relation between serum ascorbic acid level and the prevalence of CVD was analyzed from 6624 U.S. men and women, 40–74 yr of age, enrolled in the National Health and Nutrition Examination Survey *(61)*. Compared with subjects in the lowest (≤0.4 mg/dL) vs highest (≥1.1 mg/dL) tertile of serum vitamin C concentrations, there was a 27% (95% CI, 10–41%) decreased prevalence of CHD and a 26% (95% CI, 3–44%) decreased prevalence of stroke, after adjustment for CVD risk factors obtained from demographic and historical information. Other CVD risk factors, such as plasma cholesterol levels and other serum antioxidant levels, were not controlled for in the analyses. In addition, misclassification of CVD may have occurred, since this diagnosis was self-reported.

3.3.2. CASE–CONTROL STUDIES

Case–control and prospective cohort studies have yielded mixed results, and, in general, have not confirmed the inverse relationship between serum vitamin antioxidant levels and CVD found in cross-sectional/ecologic studies. Three nested case–control studies, conducted within large prospective cohort studies, have been reported *(62–64)*. In two of these studies, no association between serum vitamin E or vitamin A concentrations and subsequent CVD mortality was found *(62,63)*. However, in the nested case–control studies from the Netherlands *(62)* and eastern Finland *(63)*, blood samples were collected at baseline, and vitamin assays were determined 7–10 yr after sampling. Blood samples were frozen at $-20°C$, a temperature at which antioxidant vitamins are unstable and undergo degradation. Thus, it is probable that the measured vitamin E levels were inaccurate. In the nested case–control study from Washington County, MD, blood samples were properly frozen at $-70°C$, and analyzed for vitamin levels 16 yr after collection (64). Although no overall association between serum R,R,R-α-tocopherol levels and risk for MI was found, a protective association was suggested with higher serum levels of AT among individuals with serum cholesterol levels ≥6.21 mmol/L (≥240 mg/dL). In addition, an increasing risk for MI was found with decreasing serum β-carotene concentrations ($p = 0.02$), with a similar trend found with decreasing levels of lutein ($p = 0.09$). However, the excess risk for MI associated with low serum carotenoid concentrations was limited to current smokers.

In a case–control study of 110 cases of angina pectoris (AP) and 394 controls, selected from a sample of 6000 men, aged 35–54 yr, a significant inverse association between vitamin E plasma levels and AP was found (65). Vitamin E levels remained independently and inversely associated with the risk of AP, after adjustment for age, smoking, BP, lipids, and weight. The adjusted odds ratio for AP between the lowest vs highest quintiles of vitamin E plasma levels was 2.68 (95% CI, 1.07–6.70, $p = 0.02$). Adjusted plasma levels of vitamin C, vitamin A, and carotene were inversely, but not significantly, associated with AP. Several double-blind randomized controlled trials examining the effect of vitamin E administration on AP have yielded mixed results (75–77).

3.3.3. PROSPECTIVE COHORT STUDIES

At least three prospective cohort studies (66–68) have reported the relationship between serum vitamin E, vitamin C, and β-carotene concentrations and CVD risk. The Basel Prospective Study examined the relationship between baseline serum vitamin C, vitamin E, and β-carotene concentrations and subsequent CVD mortality in 2974 male Swiss pharmaceutical company employees, aged 41–59 yr, initially without CVD (66). During 12 yr of follow-up, 553 men died, including 132 from ischemic heart disease (IHD) and 31 from stroke. Compared with men in the highest quartile of serum carotene (β-carotene plus α-carotene) concentration, those in the lowest quartile (<0.23 μmol/L) had a RR of CVD mortality of 1.53 (95% CI, 1.07–2.20, $p < 0.024$), after adjustment for age, smoking, BP, and cholesterol. Compared with men in the highest quartile of serum vitamin C concentration, those in the lowest quartile (<22.7 μmol/L) had a RR of CVD mortality of 1.25 (95% CI, 0.77–2.01, $p = 0.38$). Separately, low serum concentrations of carotene and vitamin C were not associated with death from stroke, RR of 2.07 (95% CI, 0.78–5.46, $p = 0.14$) and 1.28 (95% CI, 0.40–4.09, $p = 0.34$), respectively. However, the risk of death from stroke was significantly increased in subjects who were in both the lowest quartile of carotene (<0.23 μmol/L) and vitamin C (<22.7 μmol/L) plasma levels, relative to those in the highest quartile of both carotene and vitamin C, RR of 4.17 (95% CI, 1.68–10.33, $p = 0.002$). There was no association between CVD mortality and serum vitamin E concentrations. This latter finding may result from the fact that the median serum vitamin E concentration in the cohort was 35 μmol/L, and, as such, all of the serum vitamin E concentration quartiles were above the presumed threshold for CHD risk of 25–30 μmol/L, as suggested by the WHO/MONICA cross-sectional study (58). This also may have been true for the vitamin A levels.

The relationship between serum carotenoid concentration and subsequent CHD events (nonfatal MI and CHD death) was prospectively assessed in 1899 hyperlipidemic men assigned to the placebo arm of the Lipid Research Clinics Coronary Primary Prevention Trial (67). A total of 1883 men, aged 40–59 yr, had data for serum carotenoid levels and smoking status. After 13 yr follow-up, men in the highest quartile of serum β-carotene concentration (>3.16 µmol/L) had a RR for CHD events of 0.64 (95% CI, 0.44–0.92, $p = 0.01$), compared with those in the lowest quartile (<2.33 µmol/L), after adjustment for age, smoking, high-density cholesterol, low-density cholesterol, and other known CHD risk factors. This finding was stronger among the 441 men who never smoked, in whom the RR was 0.28 (95% CI, 0.11–0.73, p-value for trend = 0.06). For the 679 current smokers, the RR was 0.78 (95% CI, 0.44–1.34, p-value for trend = 0.04).

The relationship between serum vitamin C concentration and subsequent MI was prospectively assessed in 1605 randomly selected men with an average age of 54 yr initially free of CVD, in eastern Finland (68). After up to 8.75 yr follow-up, there were 70 fatal or nonfatal MIs. Compared with men in the highest quintile of plasma vitamin C concentration (>64.8 µmol/L), men in the lowest quintile (<11.4 µmol/L) had a RR of fatal or nonfatal MI of 4.03 (95% CI, 1.74–9.36, $p = 0.001$), after adjustment for age, season, and examination year. However, after adjustment for a variety of CVD risk factors, the RR was substantially diminished to 2.08 (95% CI, 0.82–5.30), and was no longer statistically significant.

Taken together, the studies relating serum antioxidant vitamin concentrations with CVD have been inconsistent and inconclusive. These studies further complicate the inconsistencies seen with the vitamin C and carotene dietary-intake studies, and have in general failed to confirm the apparent protective effect of high dietary and supplementary intake of vitamin E.

3.4. Arterial Imaging Studies

3.4.1. ANGIOGRAPHIC STUDIES

In contrast to the relatively large number of epidemiological studies examining the association between antioxidant vitamin intake and CVD, antioxidant relationships with Athsc, through direct arterial visualization, have been studied infrequently. Leukocyte ascorbic acid levels were significantly lower in patients with angiographically proven CAD than in patients without CAD (69). Vitamin E plasma levels were equal between patients with and without angiographically proven CAD, but plasma levels were ≥30 µmol/L in both groups (70). In another study, plasma total R,R,R-α-tocopherol levels were not different between patients with and without angiographically proven CAD; LDL R,R,R-α-tocopherol levels were unexpectedly significantly higher in patients with angiographically proven CAD (71). These studies are difficult to interpret, because no details of angiographic results were provided, and the classification systems used for categorizing patients with and without angiographically proven CAD were too imprecise to determine associations with risk factors. Additionally, the plasma antioxidant levels measured after diagnosis may have reflected lifestyle changes.

The first data relating antioxidant vitamin intake with progression of Athsc came from the Cholesterol Lowering Atherosclerosis Study (CLAS) (6,7). A randomized, placebo-controlled, serial arterial imaging clinical trial, CLAS was designed to determine whether drug reduction of LDL-C would reduce the progression of Athsc in the coronary (78,79), carotid (80,81), and femoral (82) arteries, as determined from serial angiographic and ultrasonographic measurements of change in Athsc (83). Ancillary analyses of dietary and supplementary antioxidant vitamin intake used a large database derived from 7-d food records collected on the 188 CLAS subjects every 2 mo *(83)*. The association between self-selected dietary and supplementary antioxidant vitamin intake and progression of CAD was derived from analysis of the serial quantitative coronary angiographic data from CLAS *(6)*. Overall, subjects with supplementary vitamin E intake ≥100 IU/d demonstrated less CA lesion progression (average per-subject change in percent diameter stenosis [%S]) than did subjects with supplementary vitamin E intake <100 IU/d for all lesions (–0.8 vs 2.0% S, $p < 0.04$) and for mild/moderate lesions <50% S (–0.6 vs 3.1% S, $p < 0.02$). In the drug group in which LDL-C was reduced to less than 2.59 mmol/L (100 mg/dL) with colestipol/niacin therapy, benefit of supplementary vitamin E intake was found for all lesions (–3.4 vs 1.1% S, $p < 0.03$) and mild/moderate lesions (–3.2 vs 2.2% S, $p < 0.02$). Although placebo subjects with supplementary vitamin E intake ≥100 IU/d demonstrated less CA lesion progression than did placebo subjects with supplementary vitamin E intake <100 IU/d for all lesions (1.7 vs 2.9% S) and mild/moderate lesions (1.8 vs 4.0% S), these differences were not significant. Dietary vitamin E intake was inversely, but nonsignificantly, associated with progression of CAD. No benefit was found for intake of dietary or supplementary intake of vitamin C. Since CAD progression (specifically, progression of lesions <50% S) is linked to the risk of clinical coronary events *(84)*, CLAS results present a plausible explanation for reduced CHD events seen with supplementary vitamin E intake in other studies.

Angiographic studies examining the effects of supplementary antioxidant vitamins for preventing restenosis after CA angioplasty have been less successful. In a double-blind, placebo-controlled trial, 115 subjects, with an average age of 54 yr, were randomized to either 400 IU AT 3×/d or placebo 48 h after angioplasty *(85)*. Four months after therapy, 36% of subjects who received R,R,R-α-tocopherol had restenosis vs 48% of subjects who had received placebo ($p = 0.06$).

In the Multivitamins and Probucol (MVP) trial *(86)*, 317 subjects, with a mean age of 60 yr, were randomly assigned to one of four treatments: probucol (500 mg), multivitamins (700 IU vitamin E, 500 mg vitamin C, and 30,000 IU β-carotene), both probucol and multivitamins, or placebo. Subjects were assigned the agents twice daily 4 wk before and 6 mo after angioplasty, as well as given an extra 1000 mg probucol, 2000 IU vitamin E, both probucol and vitamin E, or placebo 12 h prior to the angioplasty, according to their treatment assignments. Six months after angioplasty, the mean ± SD reduction in luminal diameter was 0.12 ± 0.41 mm in the probucol-treated group, 0.22 ± 0.46 mm in the combined probucol–multivitamin group, 0.33 ± 0.51 mm in the multivitamin group, and 0.38 ± 0.50 mm in the placebo-treated group. For those subjects receiving probucol vs those not receiving probucol, these results were significant ($p = 0.006$); for those subjects receiving vitamins vs those not receiving vitamins, these results were not significant ($p = 0.70$). Restenosis occurred in 25.0% of the probucol-treated subjects, 35.9% of the combined probucol–multivitamin-treated subjects, 42.2% of the multivitamin-treated subjects, and 42.9% of the placebo-treated subjects. For those subjects receiving probucol vs those not receiving probucol, these results were significant ($p = 0.004$); for those subjects receiving vitamins vs those not receiving vitamins, these results were not significant ($p = 0.49$). It is not clear why probucol (a potent antioxidant) prevented restenosis; multivitamin antioxidants, either alone or in combination with probucol, did not, but results similar to those with MVP have been reported from the Probucol Angioplasty Restenosis Trial, another trial of probucol vs placebo *(87)*.

3.4.2. B-Mode Ultrasound Studies

High-resolution, B-mode ultrasound measurement of arterial wall intima-media thickness (IMT) determines the extent and progression of subclinical Athsc in its earliest stages, and can be used to determine Athsc relationships in asymptomatic individuals (88–91). Further, since antioxidants are hypothesized to effect Athsc at its earliest stages, carotid wall measurements are ideal for determining associations with the earliest clinical stages of Athsc. Several reports have investigated the association between carotid artery IMT and antioxidant vitamin intake and their plasma levels.

In the largest cross-sectional arterial imaging study (92), average carotid artery IMT was determined by quintile of R,R,R-α-tocopherol, ascorbic acid, and carotene dietary intake in 6318 women and 4989 men, aged 45–65 yr, without clinical evidence of Athsc. Vitamin intake was adjusted for age, race, body mass index, LDL-C, HDL-C, smoking, plasma glucose, BP, and caloric intake. Among women and men <55 yr old, there was no association between dietary intake of any of the antioxidant vitamins and carotid wall thickness. Among women ≥55 yr of age, those consuming more dietary vitamin C or AT had less carotid wall-thickening (p-value for trend across quintiles of vitamin intake were 0.019 and 0.033, respectively). Among men ≥55 yr of age, those consuming more dietary vitamin C had less carotid wall-thickening (p-value for trend across quintiles was 0.035). No significant associations were found between antioxidant vitamin supplement intake and carotid wall thickness. Serum vitamin antioxidant levels from 231 cases (defined as subjects exceeding the 90th percentile for carotid IMT) and 231 controls (defined as subjects below the 75th percentile for carotid IMT) were examined from the same cohort (72). Cases with a thicker carotid artery IMT had significantly lower levels of the specific carotenoids, β-cryptoxanthin and lutein plus zeaxanthin. However, after adjustment for other CVD risk factors, this association became nonsignificant. Serum levels of retinol and AT were nonsignificantly higher among case than control subjects.

In another large cross-sectional arterial imaging study, carotid artery IMT was determined by quartile of erythrocyte vitamin E and plasma carotenoid levels in 1187 men and women, 59–71 yr old, initially without CVD (73). After adjustment for CVD risk factors, erythrocyte vitamin E levels were inversely and significantly associated with carotid artery IMT in men and women; plasma carotenoid levels were not associated with carotid IMT in either sex.

The relationship of vitamin E and β-carotene plasma levels with the 12-mo progression of carotid IMT in 216 men free of CVD, with serum LDL-C levels >4.01 mmol/L (>155 mg/dL), was examined in a longitudinal study (74). After adjusting for age, LDL-C level, systolic BP, smoking, and other variables, there was an inverse correlation between progression of carotid artery IMT and vitamin E plasma levels (p = 0.018), as well as with β-carotene levels (p = 0.012). The adjusted mean 12-mo carotid IMT increase was 78% (p = 0.045) greater in the lowest (≤22.5 μmol/L) vs the highest (≥32.7 μmol/L) quartile of vitamin E plasma levels, and 92% greater (p = 0.028) in the lowest (≤0.27 μmol/L) vs the highest (≥0.64 μmol/L) quartile of β-carotene plasma levels.

Evidence demonstrating a beneficial effect of supplementary vitamin E intake on progression of early Athsc was obtained from analysis of the CLAS carotid artery IMT data (7). Subjects in the CLAS placebo group who ingested >100 IU/d supplemental vitamin E demonstrated less progression of carotid IMT over a 2-yr period than those who ingested <100 IU/d (0.008 vs 0.023 mm/yr, $p = 0.02$). These data indicate that supplemental vitamin E intake may have a beneficial effect on reducing the progression of early preintrusive Athsc. The lack of effect of supplemental vitamin E intake on the progression of carotid IMT in the drug group most likely reflects a dominating effect of lipid-lowering on the progression of early Athsc. When examined independently of supplementary vitamin intake, dietary vitamin E and C intake had no beneficial effect on the progression of carotid IMT. Supplementary vitamin C intake had no beneficial effect on the progression of carotid IMT.

4. COMPLETED μNDOMIZED CONTROLLED TRIALS

Although the conclusions from epidemiological studies, concerning the CVD protective effects of antioxidant vitamins, have been mixed, there was enough consistency in the data, and potential benefit in reducing disease risk, to warrant clinical trials. Epidemiological studies are unable to completely control for confounding variables that could affect disease outcome. It is not possible to conclusively determine whether the association of CVD with dietary assessment or serum measurements of antioxidant vitamins represent a true association, or are confounded by other dietary or lifestyle practices, which themselves are protective. Additionally, the protective effects seen in these studies may be a result of other components of the foods or a combination of antioxidants or these other food components. The epidemiological data examining the relationship between antioxidant vitamin intake and CVD are limited in providing definitive answers about whether antioxidant vitamins are protective for CVD. Unbiased estimates of the efficacy of antioxidant vitamins as therapeutic or preventive agents can only be obtained from randomized controlled trials.

To date, seven randomized controlled trials of antioxidant vitamins examining CVD events have been published (8–13,93,94; Table 2). Of these, six (9,11–13,93,94) were specifically designed to determine whether antioxidant vitamins were effective in preventing cancer, not CVD. The only randomized controlled trial specifically designed to study CVD outcome (8) was conducted in individuals with established CAD (see below). The other trials were conducted predominantly in asymptomatic individuals. The results of these trials have not been consistent.

4.1. Vitamin E

The Alpha-Tocopherol Beta-Carotene Cancer Prevention Study (ATBC) was a randomized, double-blind, placebo-controlled, primary prevention trial designed to determine whether daily R,R,R-α-tocopherol (AT), β-carotene, or both, would reduce the incidence of lung and other cancers (9). A total of 29,133 male Finnish smokers, 50–69 yr of age, were randomized in a 2×2 factorial design to AT (50 mg/d) alone, β-carotene (20 mg/d) alone, both AT and β-carotene, or placebo. After a median follow-up of 6.1 yr of randomized treatment, there was no overall benefit of either supplement on CVD. Relative to the individuals who did not receive AT, those assigned to AT experienced a –16% (95% CI, –41–19%) nonsignificant reduction in death from ischemic stroke, but a statistically significant 50% (95% CI, 2–120%) increase in death from hemorrhagic stroke. Individuals assigned to AT had a –5% (95% CI, –15–6%) nonsignificant reduction in death from IHD, but a 2% (95% CI, –5–9%) nonsignificantly higher overall mortality, compared to those individuals who did not receive AT. Regarding the primary trial end point, the β-carotene group experienced a statistically significant 18% (95% CI,

Table 2

Completed Randomized Controlled Trials of Supplementary Vitamin Intake

Vitamin E
   Alpha-Tocopherol Beta-Carotene Cancer Prevention Study
   Linxian study
   Cambridge Heart Antioxidant Study
Vitamin C
   Linxian study
β-carotene
   Alpha-Tocopherol Beta-Carotene Cancer Prevention Study
   Linxian study
   Beta-Carotene and Retinol Efficacy Trial
   Skin Cancer Prevention Study
   Physicians' Health Study

3–36%, $p = 0.01$) increase in the incidence of lung cancer (LC), relative to the placebo group. Subjects receiving AT had a statistically significant –34% (95% CI, –49 to –15%) lower incidence of prostate cancer than control subjects; those receiving β-carotene had a 23% (95% CI, –4–58%) nonsignificantly greater incidence of prostate cancer than control subjects. Those receiving AT also had a nonsignificantly increased incidence of bladder and stomach cancer. The incidence of LC was unaffected by AT supplementation.

In an ATBC substudy, the first major coronary event after randomization was determined in 1862 men who had a previous MI *(10)*. In this substudy, 424 nonfatal MI and fatal CHD cases occurred during follow-up. Relative to subjects who received placebo (438 subjects), those assigned to the AT group (466 subjects) experienced a –38% (95% CI, –59 to –4%) significant reduction in nonfatal MI. However, there was a 33% (95% CI, –14–105%) nonsignificant increase in fatal CHD cases in the AT group. All events combined, nonfatal MI and fatal CHD, were nonsignificantly reduced –10% (95% CI, –33–22%) in subjects assigned to the AT group. Subjects assigned to the AT + β-carotene group experienced a 58% (95% CI, 5–140%) significant increase in death from CHD, relative to the placebo group. All events combined, nonfatal MI and fatal CHD, were nonsignificantly increased 14% (95% CI, –13–51%) in the AT + β-carotene group. Nonfatal MI was nonsignificantly reduced –14% (95% CI, –42–26%) in the AT + β-carotene group.

The Linxian study was a randomized, double-blind, placebo-controlled, primary prevention trial designed to determine whether daily intake of four combinations of nine individual vitamin–mineral supplements (2×4 factorial design) would reduce overall or cancer mortality or incidence of cancer *(93)*. Subjects 40–69 yr of age were recruited from four Linxian (Chinese) communities, and 29,584 individuals were randomized to placebo or retinol (5000 IU) and zinc (22.5 mg); riboflavin (3.2 mg) and niacin (40 mg); vitamin C (120 mg) and molybdenum (30 µg); and vitamin E (30 mg), β-carotene (15 mg), and selenium (Se) (50 µg). Linxian Provence was chosen because inhabitants of this area have one of the highest esophageal/gastric cancer rates in the world, as well as a low intake of several micronutrients. After a follow-up of 5.25 yr of randomized treatment, total mortality was significantly reduced, RR = –9% (95% CI, –16 to –1%, $p = 0.03$) among those randomized to the vitamin E, β-carotene, Se supplementation group. This reduction mostly resulted from lower cancer mortality, especially stomach cancer. There was also a nonsignificant reduction in cerebrovascular mortality, RR = −10% (95% CI, −24–7%). Because vitamin E, β-carotene, and Se were used in combination, it was not possible to determine which supplement or supplements contributed to the lower mortality rates. The other three combination regimens of retinol and zinc, riboflavin and niacin, and vitamin C and molybdenum had no significant effects on mortality rates. The relevance of these results to Western populations is unclear.

The Cambridge Heart antioxidant Study (CHAOS) was a randomized, double-blind, placebo-controlled, secondary prevention trial designed to determine whether AT would reduce CVD risk *(8)*. The primary trial outcomes were a combined end point of CVD death and nonfatal MI, and nonfatal MI alone. A total of 2002 subjects with angiographically proven CAD were randomized to AT (1035 subjects) and placebo (967 subjects). The first 546 subjects assigned to the AT group received 800 IU/d; the remainder received 400 IU/d. After a median follow-up of 510 d, subjects assigned to the AT group experienced a −47% (95% CI, −66 to −17%, $p = 0.005$) significant reduction in the CVD death and nonfatal MI combined end point. The beneficial effect on the composite end point resulted from a −77% (95% CI, −89 to −53%, $p = 0.005$) significant reduction in the risk for nonfatal MI. However, there was an 18% (95% CI, −38–127%) nonsignificant increase in CVD death in the AT group. In addition, total mortality was nonsignificantly greater in the AT group than in the placebo group (3.5 vs 2.7%, $p = 0.31$). The pattern of a significant reduction in nonfatal MI and a nonsignificant increase in CVD death in CHAOS is similar to the results from the ATBC substudy, and remains unexplained *(10)*.

4.2. Vitamin C

In the Linxian study, there was no significant effect on mortality rates in the vitamin C plus molybdenum supplement group *(93)*. In a smaller separate study of 538 subjects, 52–97 yr old, there was no reduction in total mortality at 6 mo in those individuals randomized to 200 mg/d vitamin C vs placebo *(94)*.

4.3. β-Carotene

In the ATBC study, subjects randomized to β-carotene experienced an 8% (95% CI, 1–16%) significant increase in total mortality and a 12% (95% CI, 1–25%) significant increase in death from IHD compared to those who did not receive β-carotene *(9)*. In addition, relative to those individuals who did not receive β-carotene, those assigned to β-carotene experienced a 23% (95% CI, −14–76%) nonsignificant increase in death from ischemic stroke and a 17% (95% CI, −20–70%) nonsignificant increase in death from hemorrhagic stroke. In addition to apparently increasing all of the CV mortality end points, β-carotene also significantly increased the incidence of LC, as well as nonsignificantly increased prostate, colon and rectal, and stomach cancer.

In the ATBC substudy *(10)*, compared to subjects who received placebo (438 subjects), those assigned to the β-carotene group (461 subjects) experienced a 75% (95% CI, 16–164%) significant increase in death from CHD. All events combined, nonfatal MI and fatal CHD, were nonsignificantly increased 11% (95% CI, −16–48%) in subjects assigned to the β-carotene group. In the β-carotene group, nonfatal MI was nonsignificantly reduced −33% (95% CI, −56–2%), relative to the placebo group.

In the Linxian study, β-carotene supplementation was used in combination with vitamin E and Se *(93)*. The results of this combination of supplements on total mortality, CVD mortality, and cancer are summarized in Subheading 4.1.

The Beta-Carotene and Retinol Efficacy Trial (CARET) was a randomized, double-blind, placebo-controlled, primary prevention trial designed to determine whether daily treatment with a combined supplement containing β-carotene and vitamin A would reduce the incidence of LC, the primary trial end point (11). A total of 18,314 men and women, 45–74 yr of age, with a high risk for LC from asbestos and/or smoking exposure, were randomized to placebo or a combined supplement of β-carotene (30 mg/d) and vitamin A (25,000 IU/d) in the form of retinyl palmitate. After a mean follow-up of 4 yr of randomized treatment, CARET was terminated early, because of a 28% (95% CI, 4–57%, $p = 0.02$) significantly increased risk for LC in the combined supplement group, compared with the placebo group. In the combined supplement group, overall mortality was significantly increased 17% (95% CI, 3–33%, $p = 0.02$), and death from CVD was nonsignificantly increased 26% (95% CI, –1–61%), compared with the placebo group.

The Skin Cancer Prevention Study (SCPS) was a randomized, double-blind, placebo-controlled, secondary prevention trial designed to determine the effect of daily β-carotene supplementation on all-cause mortality and mortality from CVD and cancer, in subjects with at least one biopsy-proven basal cell or squamous cell skin cancer (12). A total of 1188 men and 532 women, with a mean age of 63 yr, were randomized to placebo or β-carotene (50 mg/d) supplementation. After a median follow-up of 4.3 yr of randomized treatment, subjects randomized to β-carotene supplementation showed a 3% (95% CI, –18–30%) nonsignificant increase in all-cause mortality and a 16% (95% CI, –18–64%) nonsignificant increase in CVD mortality, compared with the placebo group. In subgroup analyses, there was no evidence of a protective effect of β-carotene supplementation on mortality in subjects with initial plasma β-carotene levels below the median concentration or among subjects classified by smoking history.

The Physicians' Health Study (PHS) was a randomized, double-blind, placebo-controlled, primary prevention trial designed to test whether aspirin and β-carotene supplementation could prevent cancer and CVD (13). Using a 2 × 2 factorial design, 22,071 U.S. male physicians, 40–84 yr old, without a history of cancer (except nonmelanomatous skin cancer) and CVD, were randomized to aspirin (325 mg/d) plus β-carotene placebo, β-carotene (50 mg every other day) plus aspirin placebo, both active agents, or both placebos. At the beginning of the study, 11% of the subjects were current smokers and 39% were former smokers. The aspirin portion of the study was terminated early, because of a 44% statistically significant ($p < 0.001$) reduction in risk for a first MI (95). After a mean follow-up of 12 yr of randomized treatment, subjects randomized to β-carotene supplementation showed no statistically significant overall benefit or harm with respect to cancer, CV events, CVD mortality, or total mortality (13). However, there were certain trends consistent with the ATBC (9,10), CARET (11), and SCPS (12) studies in the current smokers who were randomized to β-carotene supplementation. Current smokers randomized to β-carotene supplementation had an 8% (95% CI, –20–48%) greater relative risk for MI, 18% (95% CI, –17–67%) greater RR for stroke, 15% (95% CI, –7–43%) greater RR for CV events (nonfatal MI, nonfatal stroke, and CVD deaths), 13% (95% CI, –20–61%) greater RR for CVD mortality, and 5% (95% CI, –14–29%) greater RR for death from all causes, compared with placebo subjects; all RRs were nonsignificant (13).

5. SUMMARY OF ANTIOXIDANT VITAMIN SUPPLEMENTATION RANDOMIZED CLINICAL TRIALS

The results of randomized clinical trials that have evaluated the effect of AT supplementation on CVD events are mixed and somewhat troubling. In ATBC, there was no overall benefit of AT supplementation on CVD. In fact, subjects who received AT had a significantly increased risk of death from hemorrhagic stroke *(9)*. In CHAOS, although there was a reduction in risk for nonfatal MI, there was a nonsignificant increased risk for both CVD death and total mortality *(8)*. Similar to the CHAOS study, the ATBC substudy *(10)* showed the same pattern of a significant reduction in nonfatal MI, but a nonsignificant increase in CVD death.

In the two randomized controlled trials that have studied vitamin C *(93,94)*, there is no evidence that vitamin C is effective in reducing CVD or mortality. No adverse effects were observed.

The results of the ATBC *(9,10)*, Linxian *(93)*, CARET *(11)*, SCPS *(12)*, and PHS *(13)* studies provide no support for a beneficial effect of β-carotene in the prevention of CVD, in contradistinction to the beneficial effects inferred from observational studies. In fact, taken together, the results of these trials are troubling, because subjects, particularly smokers, randomized to the β-carotene supplementation groups, had increased rates of cancer, CV events, CVD death, and overall mortality. These trials indicate that β-carotene is not the primary component responsible for the lower risks of cancer and CVD death associated with the high intakes of fruits and vegetables. Although one could argue that β-carotene should still be tested in other populations, there is little support for efficacy, and good reason for concern for the safety of supplemental β-carotene for the prevention of cancer and CVD in certain populations, such as smokers.

Other than CHAOS, all of the randomized controlled trials thus far published were primarily designed for cancer outcomes. Therefore, these studies were not specifically designed to determine differences in CVD outcomes. CHAOS was the first published randomized controlled trial designed to determine the effect of antioxidant vitamin supplementation on CVD as a primary outcome. Unlike the majority of epidemiological studies that were carried out in individuals without clinical evidence of CVD, CHAOS was conducted in individuals with established CVD. By the time Athsc is well established, it is possible that antioxidant supplementation may be ineffective in reducing clinical coronary events. Animal studies have predominantly demonstrated antioxidants to be effective in preventing Athsc, usually at its earliest stages. There are very little data indicating that antioxidant vitamin supplementation may be effective therapeutically in treating Athsc, once it is established. Epidemiological studies probably reflect lifestyle behaviors, such as high dietary and supplementary intake of vitamins over many years, perhaps even during the early formative years of Athsc development. In contrast, the randomized controlled trials have investigated vitamin intervention for a limited period of time. The differential results of these studies suggest that antioxidant vitamins may have different effects on preventing Athsc, reducing the progression of Athsc, or effecting the rupture of Athsc plaques. Before final conclusions are reached regarding the effects of antioxidant vitamin supplements on CVD, the limitations of these randomized trials need to be realized, and the results of on-going trials published.

6. ONGOING RANDOMIZED CONTROLLED TRIALS

Several ongoing randomized clinical trials are underway, evaluating the effects of vitamin E, vitamin C, and β-carotene, either alone or in combination, on a variety of CVD end points, as well as on total mortality *(96–101*; Table 3). These studies are testing antioxidant vitamin supplementation in both primary and secondary prevention of CVD

Table 3
Ongoing Randomized, Double-Blind, Placebo-Controlled Trials Testing Antioxidants Alone or in Combination with Other Agents in the Primary and Secondary Prevention of CVD

Trial	Cohort	Agent and dosage	Primary end point
Primary prevention			
PHS	22,000 U.S. males	Vitamin E (400 IU qod[a]) + Vitamin C (500 mg/d) + β-carotene (50 mg qod) + Multivitamin (standard dose) (factorial design)	MI, stroke, and CVD mortality
WHS	40,000 U.S. women	Vitamin E (600 IU qod) + aspirin (100 mg qod)	MI, stroke, and CVD mortality
SU.VI.MAX	15,000 French men and women	Vitamin E (30 IU/d) + β-carotene (6 mg/d) + vitamin C (120 mg/d) + Se (100 µg/d) + zinc (20 mg/d)	MI, stroke, and CVD mortality
Secondary prevention			
HPS[b]	20,000 UK men and women	Vitamin E (600 IU/d) + β-carotene (20 mg/d) + vitamin C (250 mg/d) + simvastatin	MI, stroke, and CVD mortality
HOPE[b]	9500 Canadian men and women	Vitamin E (400 IU/d), ramipril (factorial design)	MI, stroke, and CVD mortality
WACS[c]	8000 U.S. women	Vitamin E (600 IU qod), β-carotene (50 mg qod[d]), vitamin C (500 mg qod), (factorial design)	MI, stroke, CA revascularization and CVD mortality
GISSI[e]	11,000 Italian men and women with recent MI (<3 mo)	Vitamin E (300 IU/d)	Total mortality
Arterial imaging			
VEAPS	353 healthy men and women	Vitamin E (400 IU/d)	Progression of carotid artery IMT by B-mode ultrasound
SECURE	700 men and women with CVD	Vitamin E (400 IU/d) + ramipril	Progression of carotid artery lesions on B-mode ultrasound

(continued)

Table 3 (*continued*)

Trial	Cohort	Agent and dosage	Primary end point
Arterial imaging			
WAVE	400 postmenopausal women with CAD	Vitamin E (400 IU BID[f]), vitamin C (500 mg BID) HRT (Premarin in hysterectomized women; Prempro in nonhysterectomized women) (factorial design)	Progression of CAD by quantitative coronary angiography
HATS	160 men and women with CAD and low HDL-C	Vitamin E (400 IU BID), vitamin C (500 mg BID), β-carotene (12.5 mg BID), Se (50 μg BID), nicotinic acid (factorial design)	Progression of CAD by quantitative coronary angiography
FATS	60 men with CAD	Vitamin E (400 IU BID) + vitamin C (500 mg BID) + β-carotene (12.5 mg BID) + Se (50 μg BID) + triple lipid-lowering medication	Progression of CAD by quantitative coronary angiography
SMARTFED	150 men and women with diabetes and dyslipidemia	Vitamin E (400 IU/d)	Progression of CAD by quantitative coronary angiography
MCBIT	600 men and women with CA bypass surgery	Vitamin E (800 IU/d) + lovastatin (±LDL-pheresis)	Progression of CAD by quantitative coronary angiography

[a] qod = every other day.
[b] Prior CVD or diabetes mellitus.
[c] Prior CVD or three or more coronary risk factors.
[d] β-carotene was replaced with folate.
[e] Unblinded trial.
[f] BID = two times each day.

PHS = Physicians' Health Study; WHS = Women's Health Study; SU.VI.MAX = Supplementation en Vitamines et Mineraux Antioxidants trial; HPS = Heart Protection Study; HOPE = Heart Outcomes Prevention Evaluation; WACS = Women's Antioxidant Cardiovascular Study; GISSI = Gruppo Italiano per lo Studio della Sopravvivenza nell'Infarto Miocardico Acuto; VEAPS = Vitamin E Atherosclerosis Prevention Study; SECURE = Study to Evaluate Carotid Ultrasound Changes in Patients Treated with Ramipril and Vitamin E; WAVE = Women's Antioxidant Vitamin Estrogen Trial; HATS = HDL Atherosclerosis Treatment Study; FATS = Familial Atherosclerosis Treatment Study—Long-Term Follow-Up; SMARTFED = St. Michael's Atherosclerosis Regression Trial with Fenofibrate and Vitamin E in Diabetics; MCBIT = Munich Coronary Bypass Intervention Trial.

events, in sample sizes varying from 10,000 to 40,000 subjects. Several of the ongoing randomized clinical trials are arterial imaging trials, using ultrasonographic and angiographic techniques designed to determine the effects of antioxidant vitamin supplements on the progression of Athsc, both in its early (subclinical) and later stages of development, respectively.

7. RECOMMENDATIONS

Although observational data suggest that antioxidant vitamins may reduce CVD risk, and basic research provides plausible mechanisms for such an effect, these data have not been substantiated by completed randomized clinical trials. Additionally, results of the completed randomized trials raise a level of concern for the safety of certain antioxidant vitamin supplementation. In the final analysis, current data do not support the use of antioxidant vitamin supplements for the prevention or treatment of CVD *(102)*. Guidelines for the use of antioxidant vitamin supplements for the prevention or treatment of CVD will have to await the results of ongoing randomized clinical trials, which will provide a large amount of information concerning the efficacy and safety of antioxidant vitamin supplementation. Regardless of the results of these trials, however, consumption of fruits and vegetables high in antioxidant vitamins appears to be an important component of a healthy dietary intake.

REFERENCES

1. Steinberg D, Parthasarathy S, Carew TE, Khoo JD, Witztum JL. Beyond cholesterol: modifications of low density lipoproteins that increase its atherogenicity. N Engl J Med 1989; 320:915–924.
2. Rong JX, Rangaswamy S, Shen L, Dave R, Chang YH, Peterson H, et al. Arterial injury by cholesterol oxidation products causes endothelial dysfunction and arterial wall cholesterol accumulation. Arterioscl Thromb Vasc Biol 1998; 18:1885–1894.
3. Bjorkhem I, Henriksson-Freyschuss A, Breuer O, Diczfalusy U, Berglund L, Henriksson P. The antioxidant butylated hydroxytoluene protects against atherosclerosis. Arterioscl Thromb 1991; 11:15–22.
4. Hodis HN, Chauhan A, Hashimoto S, Crawford DW, Sevanian A. Probucol reduces plasma and aortic wall oxysterol levels in cholesterol fed rabbits independently of its plasma cholesterol lowering effect. Atherosclerosis 1992; 96:125–134.
5. Stringer MD, Görög PG, Freeman A, Kakkar VV. Lipid peroxides and atherosclerosis. Br Med J 1989; 298:281–284.
6. Hodis HN, Mack WJ, LaBree L, Cashin-Hemphill L, Sevanian A, Johnson R, Azen SP. Serial coronary angiographic evidence that antioxidant vitamin intake reduces progression of coronary artery atherosclerosis. JAMA 1995; 273:1849–1854.
7. Azen SP, Qian D, Mack WJ, Sevanian A, Selzer RH, Liu CR, Liu CH, Hodis HN. Effect of supplementary antioxidant vitamin intake on carotid arterial wall intima-media thickness in a controlled clinical trial of cholesterol lowering. Circulation 1996; 94:2369–2372.
8. Stephens NG, Parsons A, Schofield PM, Kelly F, Cheeseman K, Mitchinson MJ, Brown MJ. Randomised controlled trial of vitamin E in patients with coronary disease: Cambridge Heart Antioxidant Study (CHAOS). Lancet 1996; 347:781–786.
9. The Alpha-Tocopherol, Beta Carotene Cancer Prevention Study Group. The effect of vitamin E and beta carotene on the incidence of lung cancer and other cancers in male smokers. N Engl J Med 1994; 330:1029–1035.
10. Rapola J, Virtamo J, Ripatti S, Huttunen JK, Albanes D, Taylor PR, Heinonen OP. Randomised trial of α-tocopherol and β-carotene supplements on incidence of major coronary events in men with previous myocardial infarction. Lancet 1997; 349:1715–1720.
11. Omenn GS, Goodman GE, Thornquist MD, Balmes J, Cullen MR, Glass A, et al. Effects of a combination of beta carotene and vitamin A on lung cancer and cardiovascular disease. N Engl J Med 1996; 334:1150–1155.

12. Greenberg ER, Baron JA, Karagas MR, Stukel TA, Nierenberg DW, Stevens MM, Mandel JS, Haile RW. Mortality associated with low plasma concentration of beta carotene and the effect of oral supplementation. JAMA 1996; 275:699–703.

13. Hennekens CH, Buring JE, Manson JE, Stampfer M, Rosner B, Cook NR, et al. Lack of effect of long-term supplementation with beta carotene on the incidence of malignant neoplasms and cardiovascular disease. N Engl J Med 1996; 334:1145–1149.

14. Davies KJA, Weise AG, Sevanian A, Kim E. Repair systems in oxidative stress. In: Molecular Biology of Aging, UCLA Symposium on Molecular and Cellular Biology. New York: Alan R. Liss, 1990; 123–141.

15. Sevanian A, Hodis HN. Antioxidants and atherosclerosis: an overview. BioFactors 1997; 6:385–390.

16. Brunmark A, Cadenas E. Redox and addition chemistry of quinoid compounds and its biological implications. Free Rad Biol Med 1989; 7:435–477.

17. Boveris A, Cadenas E. Production of superoxide radicals and hydrogen peroxide in mitochondria. In: Superoxide Dismutase, Vol. II. Oberley LW, ed., Boca Raton: CRC, 1982; 16–28.

18. Sevanian A, Nordenbrand K, Kim E, Ernster L, Hochstein P. Microsomal lipid peroxidation: the role of NADPH-cytochrome P-450 reductase and cytochrome P-450. Free Rad Biol Med 1990; 8:145–152.

19. Schewe T, Kuhn H. Do 15-lipoxygenases have a common biological role? Trends Biochem Sci 1991; 16:369–373.

20. de Silva DM, Aust SD. Ferritin and ceruloplasmin in oxidative damage: review and recent findings. Can J Physiol Pharmacol 1993; 71:84,322–84,705.

21. Ehrenwald E, Chisholm GM, Fox PL. Intact human ceruloplasmin oxidatively modifies low density lipoprotein. J Clin Invest 1994; 93:1493–1501.

22. Patel RP, Svistunenko DA, Darley-Usmar VM, Symons MCR, Wilson MT. Redox cycling of human methaemoglobin by H_2O_2 yields persistent ferryl iron and protein based radicals. Free Rad Res 1996; 25:117–123.

23. Esterbauer H, Gebicki J, Puhl H, Jurgens G. The role of lipid peroxidation and antioxidants in oxidative modification of LDL. Free Rad Biol Med 1992; 13:341–390.

24. Steinbrecher UP. Oxidation of human low density lipoprotein results in derivatization of lysine residues of apolipoprotein B by lipid peroxide decomposition products. J Biol Chem 1987; 262: 3603–3608.

25. Goldstein JL, Ho YK, Basu SK, Brown MS. Binding site on macrophages mediates uptake and degradation of acetylated LDL producing massive cholesterol deposition. Proc Natl Acad Sci 1979; 76:333–337.

26. Haberland ME, Fogelman AM, Edwards PA. Specificity of receptor mediated recognition of malondialdehyde modified low density lipoproteins. Proc Natl Acad Sci 1982; 79:1712–1716.

27. Keidar S, Rosenblat M, Fuhrman B, Dankner G, Aviram M. Involvement of the macrophage LDL receptor-binding domains in the uptake of oxidized LDL. Arterioscl Thromb 1992; 12:484–493.

28. Hoff HF, Whitaker TE, O'Neil J. Oxidation of low density lipoprotein leads to particle aggregation and altered macrophage recognition. J Biol Chem 1992; 267:602–609.

29. Fruebis J, Parthasarathy S, Steinberg D. Evidence for a concerted reaction between lipid hydroperoxides and polypeptides. Proc Natl Acad Sci 1992; 89:10,588–10,592.

30. Hodis HN, Kramsch DM, Avogaro P, Bittolo-Bon G, Cazzolato G, Hwang J, Peterson H, Sevanian A. Biochemical and cytotoxic characteristics of in-vivo circulating oxidized low density lipoprotein (LDL^-). J Lipid Res 1994; 35:669–677.

31. Hessler JR, Morel DW, Lewis LJ, Chisolm GM. Lipoprotein oxidation and lipoprotein-induced cytotoxicity. Arteriosclerosis 1983; 3:215–222.

32. Berliner JA, Heinecke JW. The role of oxidized lipoproteins in atherogenesis. Free Rad Biol Med 1996; 20:707–727.

33. Quinn MT, Parthasarathy S, Fong LG, Steinberg D. Oxidatively modified LDL: a potential role in recruitment and retention of monocyte/macrophages during atherogenesis. Proc Natl Acad Sci 1987; 84:2995–2998.

34. Berliner JA, Territo MC, Sevanian A, Ramin S, Kim JA, Esterson M, Fogelman AM. Minimally modified LDL stimulates monocyte endothelial interactions. J Clin Invest 1990; 85:1260–1266.

35. Parthasarathy S, Young SG, Witstum JL, Pittman RC, Steinberg D. Protocol inhibits oxidative modification of low-density lipoprotein. J Clin Invest 1986; 77:641–644.

36. Berliner JA, Heinecke JW. The role of oxidized lipoproteins in atherogenesis. Free Rad Biol Med 1996; 20:707–727.

37. Suzuki YJ, Forman HJ, Sevanian A. Reactive oxygen species as stimulators of signal transduction. Free Rad Biol Med 1996; 22:269–285.

38. Ricciarelli R, Tasinato A, Clement S, Ozer NK, Boscoboinik D, Azzi A. Alpha-tocopherol specifically inactivates cellular protein kinase C alpha by changing its phosphorylation state. Biochem J 1998; 334:243–249.

39. Ozer NK, Sirikci O, Taha S, San T, Moser U, Azzi A. Effect of vitamin E and probucol on dietary cholesterol-induced atherosclerosis in rabbits. Free Rad Biol Med 1998; 24:226–233.

40. Acheson RM, Williams DRR. Does consumption of fruit and vegetables protect against stroke? Lancet 1993; 1:1191–1193.

41. Armstrong BK, Mann JI, Adelstein Am, Eskin F. Commodity consumption and ischemic heart disease mortality, with special reference to dietary practices. J Chron Dis 1975; 28:455–469.

42. Verlangieri AJ, Kapeghian JC, el-Dean S, Bush M. Fruit and vegetable consumption and cardiovascular mortality. Med Hypoth 1985; 16:7–15.

43. Ginter E. Decline in coronary mortality in United States and vitamin C. Am J Clin Nutr 1979; 32:511–512.

44. Stampfer MJ, Hennekens CH, Manson JE, Colditz GA, Rosner B, Willett WC. Vitamin E consumption and the risk of coronary disease in women. N Engl J Med 1993; 328:1444–1449.

45. Rimm EB, Stampfer MJ, Ascherio A, Giovannucci E, Colditz, GA, Willett WC. Vitamin E consumption and the risk of coronary heart disease in man. N Engl J Med 1993; 328:1450–1456.

46. Kushi LH, Folsom AR, Prineas RJ, Mink PJ, Wu Y, Bostick RM. Dietary antioxidant vitamins and death from coronary heart disease in postmenopausal women. N Engl J Med 1996; 334:1156–1162.

47. Knekt P, Reunanen A, Jarvinen R, Seppanen R, Heliovaara M, Aromaa A. Antioxidant vitamin intake and coronary mortality in a longitudinal population study. Am J Epidemiol 1994; 139:1180–1189.

48. Losonczy KG, Harris TB, Havlik RJ. Vitamin E and vitamin C supplement use and risk of all-cause and coronary heart disease mortality in older persons: the Established Populations for Epidemiologic Studies of the Elderly. Am J Clin Nutr 1996; 64:190–196.

49. Manson JE, Stampfer MJ, Willett WC, Colditz GA, Rosner B, Speizer FE, Hennekens CH. A prospective study of vitamin C and incidence of coronary heart disease in women. Circulation 1992; 85:865.

50. Enstrom JE, Kanim LE, Breslow L. The relationship between vitamin C intake, general health practices, and mortality in Alameda County, California. Am J Public Health 1986; 76:1124–1130.

51. Pandey DK, Shekelle R, Selwyn BJ, Tangney C, Stamler J. Dietary vitamin C and β-carotene and risk of death in middle-aged men. Am J Epidemiol 1995; 142:1269–1278.

52. Lapidus L, Anderson H, Bengtsson C, Bosaeus I. Dietary habits in relation to incidence of cardiovascular disease and death in women: a 12-year follow-up of participants in the population study of women in Gothenburg, Sweden. Am J Clin Nutr 1986; 44:444–448.

53. Gale CR, Martyn CN, Winter PD, Cooper C. Vitamin C and risk of death from stroke and coronary heart disease in cohort of elderly people. Br Med J 1995; 310:1563–1566.

54. Enstrom JE, Kanim LE, Klein MA. Vitamin C intake and mortality among a sample of the United States population. Epidemiology 1992; 3:194–202.

55. Gaziano JM, Manson JE, Branch LG, Colditz GA, Willett WC, Buring JE. A prospective study of consumption of carotenoids in fruits and vegetables and decreased cardiovascular mortality in the elderly. Ann Epidemiol 1995; 5:255–260.

56. Manson JE, Stampfer MJ, Willett WC, Colditz GA, Rosner B, Speizer FE, Hennekens CH. A prospective study of antioxidant vitamins and incidence of coronary heart disease in women. Circulation 1991; 84:II-546.

57. Gey KF, Puska P, Jordan P, Moser U. Inverse correlation between plasma vitamin E and mortality from ischemic heart disease in cross-cultural epidemiology. Am J Clin Nutr 1991; 53:326S–334S.

58. Gey KF, Brubacher GB, Stahelin HB. Plasma levels of antioxidant vitamins in relation to ischemic heart disease and cancer. Am J Clin Nutr 1987; 45:1368–1377.

59. Riemersma RA, Oliver M, Elton RA, Alfthan G, Vartiainen E, Salo M, et al. Plasma antioxidants and coronary heart disease: vitamins C and E, and selenium. Eur J Clin Nutr 1990; 44:143–150.

60. Singh RB, Ghosh S, Niaz MA, Singh R, Beegum R, Chibo H, Shoumin Z, Postiglione A. Dietary intake, plasma levels of antioxidant vitamins, and oxidative stress in relation to coronary artery disease in elderly subjects. Am J Cardiol 1995; 76:1233–1238.

61. Simon JA, Hudes ES, Browner WS. Serum ascorbic acid and cardiovascular disease prevalence in U.S. adults. Epidemiology 1998; 9:316–321.

62. Kok FJ, de Bruijn AM, Vermeeren R, Hofman A, van Laar A, de Bruin M, Hermus RJJ, Valkenburg HA. Serum selenium, vitamin antioxidants, and cardiovascular mortality: a 9-year follow-up study in the Netherlands. Am J Clin Nutr 1987; 45:462–468.

63. Salonen JT, Salonen R, Penttilä I, Herranen J, Jauhiainen M, Kantola M, et al. Serum fatty acids, apolipoproteins, selenium and vitamin antioxidants and the risk of death from coronary heart disease. Am J Cardiol 1985; 56:226–231.

64. Street DA, Comstock GW, Salkeld RM, Schuep W, Klag MJ. Serum antioxidants and myocardial infarction: are low levels of carotenoids and α-tocopherol risk factors for myocardial infarction? Circulation 1994; 90:1154–1161.

65. Riemersma RA, Wood DA, Macintyre CCA, Elton RA, Gey KF, Oliver MF. Risk of angina pectoris and plasma concentrations of vitamins A, C, E, and carotene. Lancet 1991; 337:1–5.

66. Gey KF, Stahelin HB, Eichholzer M. Poor plasma status of carotene and vitamin C is associated with higher mortality from ischemic heart disease and stroke: Basel Prospective Study. Clin Invest 1993; 71:3–6.

67. Morris DL, Kritchevsky SB, Davis CE. Serum carotenoids and coronary heart disease: the Lipid Research Clinics Coronary Primary Prevention Trial and Follow-up Study. JAMA 1994; 272:1439–1441.

68. Nyyssonen K, Parviainen MT, Solonen R, Toumilehto J, Salonen JT. Vitamin C deficiency and risk of myocardial infarction: prospective population study of men from eastern Finland. Br Med J 1997; 314:634–638.

69. Ramirez J, Flowers NC. Leukocyte ascorbic acid and its relationship to coronary artery disease in man. Am J Clin Nutr 1980; 33:2079–2087.

70. Kok FJ, van Poppel G, Melse J, Verheul E, Schouten EG, Kruyssen DHCM, Hofman A. Do antioxidants and polyunsaturated fatty acids have a combined association with coronary atherosclerosis? Atherosclerosis 1991; 31:85–90.

71. Halevy D, Thiery J, Nagel D, Arnold S, Erdmann E, Hofling B, Cremer P, Seidel D. Increased oxidation of LDL in patients with coronary artery disease is independent from dietary vitamins E and C. Arterioscl Thromb Vas Biol 1997; 17:1432–1437.

72. Iribarren C, Folsom AR, Jacobs DR, Gross MD, Belcher JD, Eckfeldt JH. Association of serum vitamin levels, LDL susceptibility to oxidation, and autoantibodies against MDA-LDL with carotid atherosclerosis: a case control study. Arterioscl Thromb Vasc Biol 1997; 17:1171–1177.

73. Bonithon-Kopp C, Coudray C, Berr C, Touboul PJ, Feve JM, Favier A, Ducimetiere P. Combined effects of lipid peroxidation and antioxidant status on carotid atherosclerosis in a population aged 59–71 y: the EVA Study. Am J Clin Nutr 1997; 65:121–127.

74. Salonen JT, Myyssönen K, Parviainen M, Kantola M, Korpela H, Salonen R. Low plasma beta-carotene, vitamin E and selenium levels associate with accelerated carotid atherogenesis in hypercholesterolemic eastern Finnish men. Circulation 1993; 87:678.

75. Rapola JM, Virtamo J, Haukka JK, Heinonen OP, Albanes D, Taylor PR, Huttunen JK. Effect of vitamin E and beta carotene on the incidence of angina pectoris: a randomized, double-blind, controlled trial. JAMA 1996; 275:693–698.

76. Gillilan RE, Mondell B, Warbasse JR. Quantitative evaluation of vitamin E in the treatment of angina pectoris. Am Heart J 1977; 93:444–449.

77. Anderson TW, Reid DBW. A double-blind trial of vitamin E in angina pectoris. Am J Clin Nutr 1974; 27:1174–1178.

78. Blankenhorn DH, Nessim SA, Johnson RL, Sanmarco ME, Azen SP, Cashin-Hemphill L. Beneficial effects of combined colestipol-niacin therapy on coronary atherosclerosis and coronary venous bypass grafts. JAMA 1987; 257:3233–3240.

79. Cashin-Hemphill L, Mack WJ, Pogoda J, Sanmarco ME, Azen SP, Blankenhorn DH, and the CLAS Study Group. Beneficial effects of colestipol-niacin on coronary atherosclerosis: a 4-year follow-up. JAMA 1990; 264:3013–3017.

80. Blankenhorn DH, Selzer RH, Crawford DW, Barth JD, Liu CR, Liu CH, Mack WJ, Alaupovic P. Beneficial effects of colestipol-niacin therapy on the common carotid artery: two- and four-year reduction of intima-media thickness measured by ultrasound. Circulation 1993; 88:20–28.

81. Mack WJ, Selzer RH, Hodis HN, Erickson J, Crawford DW, Liu CR, Liu CH, Blankenhorn DH. One-year ultrasound detection of significant reduction in carotid intimal-medial thickness associated with colestipol/niacin therapy. Stroke 1993; 24:1779–1783.

82. Blankenhorn DH, Azen SP, Crawford DW, Nessim SA, Sanmarco ME, Selzer RH, Shircore AM, Wickham EC. Effects of colestipol-niacin therapy on human femoral atherosclerosis. Circulation 1991; 83:438–447.

83. Blankenhorn DH, Johnson RL, Nessim SA, Azen SP, Sanmarco ME, Selzer RH. The Cholesterol Lowering Atherosclerosis Study (CLAS): design, methods, and baseline results. Controlled Clin Trials 1987; 8:354–387.

84. Azen SP, Mack W, Cashin-Hemphill L, LaBree L, Shircore A, Selzer RH, Blankenhorn DH, Hodis HN. Progression of coronary artery disease predicts clinical coronary events: long-term follow-up from the Cholesterol Lowering Atherosclerosis Study. Circulation 1996; 93:34–41.

85. DeMaio SJ, King SB III, Lembo NJ, Roubin GS, Hearn JA, Bhagavan HN, Sgoutas DS. Vitamin E supplementation, plasma lipids and incidence of restenosis after percutaneous transluminal coronary angioplasty (PTCA). J Am Coll Nutr 1992; 11:68–73.

86. Tardif JC, Cote G, Lesperance J, Bourassa M, Lambert J, Doucet S, et al. Probucol and multivitamins in the prevention of restenosis after coronary angioplasty. N Engl J Med 1997; 337:365–372.

87. Yokoi H, Daida H, Kuwabara Y, Nishikawa H, Takatsu F, Tomihara H, et al. Effectiveness of an antioxidant in preventing restenosis after percutaneous transluminal coronary angioplasty: the Probucol Angioplasty Restenosis Trial. J Am Coll Cardiol 1997; 30:855–862.

88. Pignoli P, Tremoli E, Poli A, Oreste P, Paoletti R. Intimal plus medial thickness of the arterial wall: a direct measurement with ultrasound imaging. Circulation 1986; 74:1399–1406.

89. Mack WJ, Hodis HN, LaBree L, Liu CR, Liu CH, Selzer RH. Progression of carotid intima-media thickness correlates with angiographic progression of coronary disease. Circulation 1996; 94:I–122.

90. Hodis HN, Mack WJ, LaBree L, Selzer RH, Liu CL, Liu CH, Azen SP. The role of carotid arterial intima-media thickness in predicting clinical coronary events. Ann Intern Med 1998; 262–269.

91. Selzer RH, Hodis HN, Kwong-Fu Helenann, Mack WJ, Lee PL, Liu CR, Liu CH, Blankenhorn DH. Evaluation of computerized edge tracking for quantifying intima-media thickness of the common carotid artery from B-mode ultrasound images. Atherosclerosis 1994; 111:1–11.

92. Kritchevsky SB, Shimakawa T, Dennis B, Eckfeldt J, Carpenter M, Heiss G. Dietary antioxidants and carotid artery wall thickness: the ARIC Study. Circulation 1993; 87:679.

93. Blot WJ, Li JY, Taylor PR, Guo W, Dawsey S, Wang GQ, et al. Nutrition intervention trials in Linxian, China: supplementation with specific vitamin/mineral combinations, cancer incidence, and disease-specific mortality in the general population. J Natl Cancer Inst 1993; 85:1483–1492.

94. Wilson TS, Datta SB, Murrell JS, Andrews CT. Relation of vitamin C levels to mortality in a geriatric hospital: a study of the effect of vitamin C administration. Age Ageing 1973; 2:163–171.

95. Steering Committee of the Physicians' Health Study Research Group. Final report on the aspirin component of the ongoing Physicians' Health Study. N Engl J Med 1989; 321:129–135.

96. The HOPE Study Investigators. The HOPE (Heart Outcomes Prevention Evaluation) Study: the design of a large, simple randomized trial of an angiotensin-converting enzyme inhibitor (ramipril) and vitamin E in patients at high risk of cardiovascular events. Can J Cardiol 1996; 12:127–137.

97. Manson JE, Gaziano JM, Spelsberg A, Ridker PM, Cook NR, Buring JE, Willett WC, Hennekens CH. A secondary prevention trial of antioxidant vitamins and cardiovascular disease in women. Ann Epidemiol 1995; 5:261–269.

98. Women's Health Study Research Group. The Women's Health Study: summary of the study design. J Myocardial Ischemia 1992; 4:27–29.

99. Brown G, Zhao XQ, Chait A, Frohlich J, Cheung M, Heise N, et al. Lipid altering or antioxidant vitamins for patients with coronary disease and very low HDL cholesterol? The HDL Atherosclerosis Treatment Study Design. Can J Cardiol 1998; 14:6A–13A.

100. Brown G, Albers JJ, Fisher LD, Schaefer SM, Lin JT, Kaplan C, et al. Regression of coronary artery disease as a result of intensive lipid-lowering therapy in men with high levels of apolipoprotein B. N Engl J Med 1990; 323:1289–1298.

101. Hercberg S, Preziosi P, Briancon S, Galan P, Triol I, Malvy D, Roussel AM, Favier A. A primary prevention trial using nutritional doses of antioxidant vitamins and minerals in cardiovascular diseases and cancers in a general population: the SU.VI.MAX study-design, methods, and participant characteristics. Controlled Clin Trials 1998; 19:336–351.

102. Tribble DL. Antioxidant consumption and risk of coronary heart disease: emphasis on vitamin C, vitamin E, and β-carotene: a statement for healthcare professionals from the American Heart Association. Circulation 1929; 99:591–595.

7

Oxidative Stress and Antioxidants in Type 2 Diabetes

Srideri Devaraj and Ishwarlal Jialal

1. INTRODUCTION

Diabetes mellitus is a leading cause of morbidity and mortality mostly because of its vascular complications *(1,2)*. Diabetic complications can be broadly classified into microvascular (retinopathy, nephropathy) and macrovascular (coronary artery disease [CAD], cerebrovascular disease, peripheral vascular disease). This chapter focuses on the role of oxidative stress in the genesis of diabetic macrovascular disease.

The most common cause of death among people with diabetes today is atherosclerotic cardiovascular disease (CVD) *(3)*. Several studies have shown that mortality caused by CAD is 2–4× greater in individuals with diabetes than in those without. CVD can manifest as CAD, stroke, and peripheral vascular disease. Most studies have indicated that this excess risk for macrovascular complications cannot be explained by abnormal levels of conventional CV risk factors, such as dyslipidemia, hypertension (HT), and smoking. Therefore, the diabetic state, *per se*, confers an increased propensity to accelerated atherogenesis.

2. MECHANISMS OF DIABETIC MACROVASCULAR DISEASE

Numerous potential mechanisms that could mediate premature atherogenesis in diabetes are listed in Table 1. Briefly reviewed here are the other mechanisms, focusing mostly on oxidative stress in diabetes, i.e., glyco-oxidation and lipid peroxidation.

There is increased procoagulant activity in diabetes *(3–5)*, manifesting as increased factor VII activity, increase in factor X activity, and increased concentrations of plasminogen activator inhibitor-1. Levels of fibrinogen are also increased, and there is increased platelet aggregation in diabetes. Some of these abnormalities can be attributed to the hypertriglyceridemia (HTG).

The dyslipidemia of type 2 diabetes (the commonest type) includes HTG, low levels of high-density lipoprotein cholesterol (HDL-C), and alterations in the composition of low-density lipoprotein (LDL) *(6–8)*. HTG, reflecting increased plasma levels of very low-density lipoprotein (VLDL) and remnants, is common in both type 1 and type 2 diabetes. In nondiabetic individuals, most studies indicate an increased risk of CAD in univariate, but not in multivariate, analysis *(9)*. However, population studies of diabetic patients consistently suggest that HTG is a significant risk factor for CAD in type 1 and 2

From: *Primary and Secondary Preventive Nutrition*
Edited by: A. Bendich and R. J. Deckelbaum © Humana Press Inc., Totowa, NJ

Table 1
Mechanisms of Macrovascular Disease in Diabetes

Lipid and lipoprotein aberrations
    HTG; low HDL-C; small, dense LDL
Procoagulant state
    Increased platelet aggregation, increased factor VII and X activity, increased fibrinogen,
        increased PAI-1 synthesis and activity
Hyperinsulinism and IR syndrome
    IR; central obesity; increased apoB-100; decreased apoA1; small, dense LDL; abnormal glucose
        tolerance; HT
Microalbuminuria
Protein glycation
    AGE
Lipoprotein oxidation and antioxidant deficiencies
Cellular disturbances
    Decreased nitric oxide; increased superoxide cytokines; decreased superoxide dismutase

diabetics. HTG is chiefly related to the degree of diabetic control, and triglyceride levels tend to return to normal after therapy *(10,11)*. HTG in the diabetic patient is characterized by an increase in the concentration of chylomicron remnants and small, dense VLDL. Despite the lack of evidence for marked elevations of LDL cholesterol in diabetic patients, several studies *(10–12)* have shown that improved glycemic control can further reduce LDL-C levels. It is also known that, although levels of LDL may not be altered in diabetic subjects, the composition of the LDL particles is altered, resulting in a preponderance of small, dense LDL, which is more prone to oxidation *(13)*. Levels of HDL cholesterol (HDL-C) are uniformly low in untreated patients with type 2 diabetes. Most studies show an association between low levels of HDL-C and CAD in type 2 diabetic patients *(14)*. In the prospective data from the Framingham study, HDL-C levels were inversely related to CAD in the diabetic and nondiabetic population *(15)*.

The insulin resistance (IR) syndrome, as suggested by Reaven *(16)*, is also referred to as Syndrome X. The principal manifestations of this syndrome include hyperinsulinism and IR, increase in the waist-to-hip ratio (central or intra-abdominal obesity), HTG (increased apolipoprotein [apoB]-100), decreased HDL-C (decreased apoA1), small, dense LDL (pattern B), impaired glucose tolerance, and HT *(17)*. IR and hyperinsulinism mediate premature atherosclerosis (Athsc) via three potential mechanisms: hyperinsulinism caused by increased central obesity and decreased physical activity could lead to β-cell failure, and ultimately to diabetes; there is increase in certain risk factors for CAD, such as HT, HTG, and low levels of HDL-C; insulin could have a direct proatherogenic affect. Hyperinsulinism could also lead to HT via increased sodium resorption, increased sympathetic nerve activity, smooth muscle cell proliferation, and increased vascular sensitivity to vasoconstrictor amines (*see* Chapter 9).

Glycation (nonenzymatic glycosylation) involves the nonenzymatic binding of glucose to reactive amino groups located on lysine side chains and N-terminal amino acid residues of protein molecules *(18,19)*. The initial products of the reaction are Schiff's bases, which rearrange to form more stable Amadori products. These early glycation products are in reversible equilibrium with their precursors, and levels tend to rise and fall with ambient glucose concentrations. Amadori products are further degraded gradually into reactive carbonyls, such as 3-deoxyglucosone, methyl glyoxal, and so on, which can further react with free amino groups to form advanced glycation end products (AGEs), which are irreversible products of glycation and oxidation *(20–22)*. AGEs gradually accumulate on long-lived proteins during aging, and this process is accelerated in diabetes, even by modest elevations in blood glucose. AGEs are recognized by specific cell surface receptors, referred to as AGE receptors, which are present on circulating monocytes, lymphocytes, and endothelial and renal mesangial cells. AGE modification of proteins results in altered structure and function, and several studies have shown a strong relationship between AGE levels and the severity of diabetic microvascular complications. Uptake of AGE via the macrophage receptor leads to increased production of cytokines, such as interleukin 1 (IL-1), tumor necrosis factor (TNF), and insulin-like growth factor 1, resulting in proliferation of glomerular mesangial and arterial smooth muscle cells, and increased glomerular synthesis of type IV collagen. Uptake of AGE by endothelial cells results in the production of endothelin-1, tissue factor, resulting in thrombosis and vasoconstriction. AGEs have been shown to activate macrophages, resulting in increased chemotaxis and cholesterol ester accumulation, and to quench nitric oxide *(20–23)*. This implicates AGE in defective vascular relaxation and HT of diabetes and aging. Infusion of AGE albumin causes activation of the transcription factor, nuclear factor-КB, a pleiotropic regulator of many response-to-injury genes, including cytokines, tissue factor, and so on, the activation of which can be inhibited by pretreatment of animals with antibodies to the AGE receptor.

AGE also form on proteins in vivo. In erythrocytes, AGE hemoglobin in diabetic subjects is higher than in nondiabetics. Studies have established a close correlation between AGE formation and physicochemical changes on connective tissue taking place in diabetes and aging, such as collagen–collagen crosslinking and tissue rigidity. In addition, AGE moieties formed on matrix components, such as the vessel wall and kidney, crosslink and trap a variety of plasma proteins, most notably, lipoproteins and immunoglobulins. AGE has been demonstrated to modify LDL in both the lipid and apolipoprotein components and AGE-modified LDL, is more atherogenic than native LDL.

The formation of the Amadori product represents an important aspect of advanced glycosylation chemistry, because progression to protein crosslinks requires slow rearrangement reactions to create reactive intermediates that can react directly with additional amino groups. This understanding brought forward the possibility of pharmacological intervention. In 1986, a small nucleophilic compound, aminoguanidine, was shown to be a potent and specific inhibitor of glucose-mediated crosslinking and tissue damage in vivo *(24)*. The terminal amino group of aminoguanidine, because of a low pKa, reacts specifically with glucose-derived reactive intermediates and prevents formation of crosslinks. Diabetic rats treated with aminoguanidine exhibit significantly less collagen crosslinking, as assessed by fluorescence, and less crosslinking in the vascular wall; other studies have shown decrease in AGE accumulation in kidney, delay of retinal vascular lesions, and improved diabetic neuropathy.

3. LIPOPROTEIN OXIDATION

Several lines of evidence support a proatherogenic role for oxidized LDL (Ox-LDL) in Athsc *(25–27)*. Ox-LDL, but not native LDL, is taken up by the scavenger receptor pathway on macrophages, resulting in unregulated lipid accumulation and foam cell formation. Ox-LDL has several other biological consequences: It is chemotactic for circulating monocytes; inhibits resident macrophage motility; is cytotoxic to endothelial cells; may promote vasoconstriction; stimulates cytokines, such as IL-1β, and increases platelet aggregation and tissue factor production. Recently, it has been reported that Ox-LDL may also promote adhesion of monocytes to endothelial cells in vitro, an important early event in atherogenesis.

4. LDL OXIDATION AND DIABETES

Factors that may promote LDL oxidation in diabetes include antioxidant deficiencies, increased production of reactive oxygen species, glycation, and glycoxidation (28,29).

The most common antioxidant deficiency reported in diabetes is lower levels of ascorbate in diabetic plasma, as well as mononuclear cells (30). In addition to ascorbic acid concentrations being low in diabetes, the ratio of the oxidation product, dehydroascorbate, to ascorbate is increased in diabetic patients, compared to control. Also, low levels of reduced glutathione have been documented in diabetic neutrophils and monocytes. Superoxide dismutase activity in decreased in diabetic neutrophils and monocytes (31).

Increased reactive oxygen species, such as superoxide production, have been shown to be increased in diabetic monocytes and neutrophils. Also, superoxide production from mononuclear cells is enhanced in presence of attendant HTG.

Glycation and gluco-oxidation can also promote formation of reactive oxygen species, such as superoxide and hydrogen peroxide, which could, in turn, oxidize LDL (32,33). Increased gluco-oxidation products have been demonstrated in diabetic collagen, such as carboxymethyl lysine, carboxymethylhydroxylysine, and pentosidine. Glycated LDL, isolated from diabetic subjects, has also been found to stimulate release of thromboxane B_2 and platelet aggregation, providing another mechanism by which it may stimulate Athsc. Also, there is increased peroxidation of LDL by nonenzymatic glycated peptides, such as glycated polylysine–iron complexes (34,35). Several reports have shown that glycated LDL is more prone to oxidation. Bucala and Cerami (21) have shown increased AGE formation in diabetic LDL, with an increase in lipid peroxidation, as evidenced by MDA equivalents. Some studies have not found increased susceptibility of LDL to oxidation in diabetic subjects, but direct evidence for increased LDL oxidizability in diabetic subjects has been shown in at least five studies. Babiy et al. (36) have shown increased oxidizability of LDL exposed to irradiation in diabetic subjects, and another group has shown that both normo- and hypercholesterolemic diabetic subjects have increased LDL oxidizability. Beaudeaux et al. (37) have also reported enhanced oxidative susceptibility of LDL in 20 type 2 diabetic subjects, compared to matched controls. Cominacini et al. (38) have shown that, in both type 1 and type 2 diabetic patients, LDL is more susceptible to oxidation, as evidenced by a shortened lag phase of oxidation, measured by fluorescence. Furthermore, Yoshida et al. (39) have reported increased oxidative susceptibility of LDL in patients with diabetes, compared to normotriglyceridemic controls, and found that the vitamin E:lipid peroxide ratio of LDL is a major determinant of LDL lag time, and that diabetic subjects have a reduced ratio, compared to matched controls. Also, as mentioned before, diabetic subjects have small, dense LDL, which is more prone to oxidation than large, buoyant LDL.

Last, lipoprotein glycation and oxidation could result in lipoprotein immune complex formation. The detection of circulating autoantibodies to Ox-LDL is considered a biological signature of in vivo LDL oxidation. Increased concentrations of autoantibodies to both oxidized, glycated LDL and glycoxydated LDL have been documented in diabetes, suggesting that, in type 2 diabetic subjects, enhanced LDL oxidation occurs in vivo, and that LDL glycation may represent a predisposing event that facilitates subsequent oxidative modification (40). The presence of these circulating immune complexes has been associated with accelerated Athsc, presumably as a result of either macrophage foam cell formation in response to the uptake of these complexes or stimulation of atherogenic mechanisms in cells of the arterial wall (41). When stimulated with LDL immune complexes, monocyte macrophages have been shown to release more proathero-genic cytokines, such as IL-1 and TNF.

Numerous studies have shown increased plasma lipid peroxides in diabetes (42,43). However, a careful appraisal of the data reveals that, in most of these studies, increased lipid peroxides are prevalent only in patients who had angiopathy.

Direct evidence of increased oxidative stress and LDL oxidation in diabetes has also been reported. F2-isoprostanes are prostaglandin-like compounds formed in vivo from free-radical catalyzed peroxidation of arachidonic acid, and are emerging as novel and direct measures of oxidative stress. Urinary and plasma F2-isoprostane levels have been reported to be increased in type 2 diabetic subjects (44,45).

Thus, the diabetic state could promote atherogenesis via oxidation. Both glucose autoxidation and nonenzymatic glycation of LDL could promote lipid peroxidation (29,46–48). The HTG could promote increased release of superoxide anion, and could result in the production of small, dense LDL. The antioxidant deficiencies could also result in enhanced oxidation of LDL, thus contributing to accelerated Athsc in diabetic subjects.

5. TREATMENT OF DIABETIC MACROVASCULAR DISEASE

Regarding microvascular complications, there is overwhelming evidence, from the Diabetes Control and Complications Trial (49), that good glycemic control plays a major role in reducing microvascular complications of diabetes. Although this study was confined to type I patients, there is now good evidence, from the UK Prospective Diabetes Study (50), that good glycemic control in type II diabetic subjects will also reduce the development of microvascular complications. In general, it is best to take a stepped approach to the treatment of type II diabetes, starting with nonpharmacological approaches to improve diet, achieving weight reduction in obese patients, and increasing physical activity. If these measures are inadequate to obtain good metabolic control, oral antidiabetic medications should be added, such as sulfonylureas, metformin, α-glucosi-dase inhibitors, thiazolidinediones, and so on, alone or in combination. Finally, many type 2 diabetic subjects may also require insulin therapy, if the other measures fail to optimize diabetes control (HbA$_{1c}$ <7%). Another approach toward the management of diabetic macrovascular complications is to reduce all the traditional risk factors associated with CVD, such as cessation of cigarette smoking, use of antihypertensives that may improve the dyslipidemia of diabetes (such as α-adrenergic blocking agents) or reduce microalbuminuria (such as angiotensin-converting enzyme inhibitors), and aggressive treatment of dyslipidemia with lipid lowering agents.

6. ANTIOXIDANTS AND DIABETIC MACROVASCULAR DISEASE

The use of antioxidants in the prevention of Athsc is controversial, although some evidence from epidemiological, experimental, and clinical research suggests a beneficial effect. Nonetheless, it has been suggested, because of the antioxidant deficiencies in diabetes, that diabetic patients consume more than the recommended daily allowance of vitamin C, and supplement their diet with vitamin E.

Regarding improving glycemic control with α-tocopherol (AT) (vitamin E), the data is controversial. Ceriello et al. *(51,52)* and Jain et al. *(53)* showed that AT (600 mg/1200 mg/d and 100 mg/d, respectively) decreases protein glycation in type I diabetic subjects, without affecting plasma glucose disposition. However, Paolisso et al. *(54,55)* showed that supplementation with AT (900 mg/d) in type II diabetic subjects improved both glycemic control and insulin action. However, in two supplementation studies and one in vitro, the authors' group has failed to see any effect of AT on LDL glycation in type II diabetic subjects with and without macrovascular complications *(56–58)*. However, regarding advanced glycation end products, AT has been shown to inhibit the hyperglycemia-induced formation of AGE and reactive oxygen species *(19,59)*. Recently, Davi et al. *(45)* have shown, in diabetic subjects, that levels of urinary F2-isoprostanes, a marker of whole-body oxidation, could be significantly decreased, either by improving metabolic control or if the patients were treated with AT. Regarding the effect of AT on LDL oxidation in diabetics with macrovascular disease, the data is scanty. Reaven et al. *(60)* have shown that 1600 IU/d synthetic AT significantly reduced LDL oxidizability, as measured by lag phase of conjugated diene formation. Also, Fuller et al. *(58)* have shown that supplementation of type II diabetic subjects (1200 IU/d) with natural AT significantly decreased in vitro LDL oxidizability, without affecting protein glycation. Also, in a preliminary report, the authors showed that monocytes from type II diabetic patients with and without macrovascular disease exhibited greater proatherogenic activity, compared to matched controls (i.e., increased superoxide anion release, increased IL-1b, and increased adhesion to endothelium), and this was significantly decreased by AT therapy *(57)*. Furthermore, in these patients, AT supplementation significantly reduced levels of soluble adhesion molecules, s intercellular adhesion molecule, s vascular cell adhesion molecule, and sE-selectin.

One of the major causal risk factors for increased vascular disease in diabetic subjects is hyperglycemia, and it has been shown that one of the mechanisms by which hyperglycemia can cause adverse effects is via activation of diacylglycerol (DAG), a physiological activator of protein kinase C. AT, through activation of DAG kinase, can prevent increases in DAG levels following hyperglycemia, and thus reduce protein kinase activity in the retina, aorta, heart, and renal glomeruli or streptozotocin-induced diabetic rats *(61,62)*. Functionally, AT treatment in diabetic rats can prevent abnormalities in retinal blood flow and glomerular hyperfiltration in the kidney *(63)*. Also, more recently, AT supplementation has been shown to ameliorate diabetic microvascular complications, as evidenced by an improvement in retinal hemodynamic abnormalities and renal function *(64)*. Furthermore, AT supplementation decreases platelet aggregation in diabetes, and decreases levels of platelet thromboxane in type I diabetic subjects *(65,66)*. Thus, it is conceivable that AT supplementation in diabetic patients could also result in reduction in macrovascular disease. Further knowledge concerning the mechanisms of Athsc disease in the diabetic will no doubt lead to additional approaches to the management of diabetic macrovascular complications, and, perhaps, lead to a reduction in the alarming rate of accelerated Athsc in this population. A clinical trial examining the effect of high-dose AT on the progression of clinical Athsc is urgently needed.

7. RECOMMENDATIONS

There are currently no known placebo-controlled trials showing that antioxidants are beneficial in diabetic subjects, with respect to clinical end points. The only recommendation that appears to be reasonable, given the lower levels of ascorbate in plasma and cells of diabetic patients, is increasing the intake of vitamin C. Thus, the authors believe, that, in addition to consuming five servings of fruits and vegetables per day, diabetic subjects should ensure that their intake of vitamin C is around 250 mg/d. Vitamin E supplementation clearly has beneficial effects on surrogates of clinical Athsc, but recommendations with respect to supplementation must await results of clinical trials.

ACKNOWLEGMENTS

Work cited in this chapter was partially funded by NIH RO1-AT00005-01.

REFERENCES

1. Pyorala K, Laasko M, Uusitupa M. Diabetes and atherosclerosis: an epidemiologic view. Diabetes Metab Rev 1987; 3:463–524.
2. Everhart JE, Pettitt DJ, Knowler WC, et al. Medial arterial calcification and its association with mortality and complications of diabetes. Diabetologia 1988; 31:16–23.
3. Bierman E. Atherogenesis in diabetes. Arterioscl Thromb 1992; 12:647–656.
4. Banga JD, Sixma JJ. Diabetes mellitus, vascular disease and thrombosis. Clin Hematol 1986; 15:465–492.
5. Jones RL, Peterson CM. Hematologic alterations in diabetes mellitus. Am J Med 1981; 70:339–352.
6. Brunzell JD, Chait A, Bierman EL. Plasma lipoproteins in human diabetes mellitus. In: The Diabetes Annual, Vol 1. Albertini KG, eds. Amsterdam: Elsevier, 1985; 463–479.
7. Howard BV. Lipoprotein metabolism in diabetes mellitus. J Lipid Res 1987; 28:613–628.
8. Barakat HA, Carpenter JW, McLendon VD, et al. Influence of obesity, IGT and NIDDM on LDL structure and composition: possible link between hyperinsulinemia and atherosclerosis. Diabetes 1990; 39:1527–1533.
9. Hulley SB, Rosenman RH, Bawol RD, Brand RJ. Epidemiology as a guide to clinical decisions: association between TG and CHD. N Engl J Med 1980; 302:1383–1389.
10. Pietri AO, Dunn FL, Grundy SM, Raskin P. The effect of continuous subcutaneous insulin infusion on VLDL TG metabolism in Type 1 diabetes mellitus. Diabetes 1983; 32:75–81.
11. Taskinen MR, Kuusi T, Helve E, et al. Insulin therapy induces anti-atherogenic changes of serum lipoproteins in NIDDM. Arteriosclerosis 1988; 8:168–177.
12. Lyons TJ. Oxidized low density lipoproteins: a role in the pathogenesis of atherosclerosis in diabetes? Diabetic Med 1991; 8:411–419.
13. Chait A, Brazg R, Tribble D, Krauss R. Susceptibility of small, dense LDL to oxidative modification in subjects with pattern B. Am J Med 1993; 94:350–356.
14. Laasko M, Pyorala K, Sarlund H, Voutilainen E. Lipid and lipoprotein abnormalities associated with CAD in patients with IDDM. Arteriosclerosis 1986; 6:679–684.
15. Gordon T, Castelli WP, Hjortland MC, et al. Diabetes, blood lipids and role of obesity in CAD risk for women: The Framingham Study. Ann Intern Med 1977; 87:393–397.
16. Reaven G. Role of insulin resistance in human disease (syndrome X): an expanded definition. Annu Rev Med 1993; 44:121–131.
17. DeFronzo R, Ferrannini E. Insulin resistance. A Multifaceted syndrome responsible for NIDDM, obesity, hypertension, dyslipidemia, and atherosclerotic cardiovascular disease. Diabetes Care 1991; 14:173–194.
18. Lyons TJ, Jenkins AJ. Lipoprotein glycation and its metabolic consequences. Curr Opin Lipidol 1997; 8:174–180.
19. Brownlee M. Glycation products and the pathogenesis of diabetic complications. Diabetes Care 1992; 15:1835–1843.
20. Bucala R, Tracey K, Cerami A. Advanced glycosylation products quench nitric oxide and mediate defective endothelium-dependent vasodilatation in experimental diabetes. J Clin Invest 1991; 87:432–438.

21. Bucala R, Cerami, A. Advanced glycosylation: chemistry, biology, and implications for diabetes and aging. Adv Pharmacol 1992; 23:1–34.
22. Bucala R, Makita Z, Koschinski T, Cerami A, Vlassara H. Lipid advanced glycosylation: pathway for lipid oxidation in vivo. Proc Natl Acad Sci USA 1993; 90:6434–6438.
23. Lopes-Virella M, Klein R, Lyons T, Stevenson H, Witztum J. Glycosylation of low-density lipoprotein enhances cholesteryl ester synthesis in human monocyte-derived macrophages. Diabetes 1988; 37:550–557.
24. Brownlee M, Vlassara H, Kooney A, Ulrich P, Cerami A. Aminoguanidine prevents diabetes-induced arterial wall protein cross-linking. Science 1986; 232:1629–1632.
25. Witztum JL, Steinberg D. Role of Ox-LDL in atherogenesis. J Clin Invest 1991; 88:1785–1792.
26. Berliner JA, Heinecke JW. The role of oxidized lipoproteins in atherogenesis. Free Rad Biol Med 1992; 92:127–143.
27. Devaraj S, Jialal I. Oxidized LDL and atherosclerosis. Int J Clin Lab Res 1996, 26:178–184.
28. Strain J. Disturbances of micronutrient and antioxidant status in diabetes. Proc Nutr Soc 1991; 50: 591–604.
29. Baynes J. Perspectives in diabetes. Role of oxidative stress in development of complications in diabetes. Diabetes 1991; 40:405–412.
30. Sinclair A, Barnett A, Lunec J. Free radicals and antioxidant systems in health and disease. Br J Hosp Med 1990; 43:334–344.
31. Nath N, Chari S, Rath A. SOD in diabetic polymorphonuclear lymphocytes. Diabetes 1984; 33:586–589.
32. Kitahara M, Eyre H, Lynch R, Rallison M, Hill H. Metabolic activity of diabetic monocytes. Diabetes 1980; 29:251–256.
33. Hiramatsu K, Rosen H, Heinecke J, Wolfbauer G, Chait A. Superoxide initiates oxidation of low density lipoprotein by human monocytes. Arteriosclerosis 1987; 7:55–60.
34. Sakurai T, Tsuchiya S. Superoxide production from nonenzymatically glycated protein. Fed Eur Biochem Soc 1988; 236:406–410.
35. Sakurai T, Sugioka K, Nakano M. O_2 generation and lipid peroxidation during the oxidation of glycated polypeptide, glycated polylysine, in the presence of iron-ADP. Biochem Biophys Acta 1990; 1043:17–33.
36. Babiy A, Gebicki J, Sullivan DR, Willey K. Increased oxidizability of plasma lipoproteins in diabetic patients can be decreased by probucol therapy and is not due to glycation. Biochem Pharmacol 1992; 43:995–1000.
37. Beaudeaux J, Guillausseau P, Peynet J, Flourie F, et al. Enhanced susceptibility of LDL to in vitro oxidation in type 1 and 2 diabetic patients. Clin Chim Acta 1995; 239:131–141.
38. Cominacini L, Garbin U, pastorino AM, Pasini A, et al. Increased susceptibility of LDL to in vitro oxidation in patients with IDDM and NIDDM. Diabetes Res 1994; 26:173–184.
39. Yoshida H, Ishikawa T, Nakamura H. Vitamin E/Lipid peroxide ratio and susceptibility of LDL to oxidative modification in NIDDM. Arterioscl Thromb Vasc Biol 1997; 17:1438–1446.
40. Bellomo G, Maggi E, Poli M, Agosta FG, Bollati P, Finardi G. Autoantibodies against Ox-LDLD in NIDDM. Diabetes 1995; 44:60–66.
41. Witztum JL, Mahoney EM, Branks MJ, et al. Nonenzymatic glycation of LDL alters its biologic activity. Diabetes 1982; 31:283–291.
42. Nourooz-zadeh J, Sarmadi J, McCarthy S, Betteridge DJ, Wolff SP. Elevated levels of authentic plasma hydroperoxides in NIDDM. Diabetes 1995; 44:1054–1058.
43. Oranje WA, Wolffenbuttel BHR. Lipid peroxidation and atherosclerosis in Type 2 diabetes. J Lab Clin Med 1999; 134:19–32.
44. Gopaul NK, Anggard EE, Mallet AI, Betteridge DJ, Wolff SP, Nourooz-zadeh. Plasma 8-epi-PGF2alpha are elevated in individuals with NIDDM. FEBS Lett 1995; 368:225–229.
45. Davi G, Mezzett A, Vitacolonna E, Constantini F, et al. In vivo formation of 8-epi PGF2-alpha in diabetes mellitus: effect of tight control and vitamin E supplementation. Diabetes 1997; 46:13.
46. Bowie A, Owens D, Collins P, Johnson A, Tomkin G. Glycosylated low density lipoprotein is more sensitive to oxidation: implications for the diabetic patient? Atherosclerosis 1993; 102:63–67.
47. Mullarkey J, Edelstein D, Brownlee M. Free radical generation by early glycation products: a mechanism for accelerated atherogenesis in diabetes. Biochem Biophys Res Commun 1990; 173:932–939.
48. Hunt, JV, Smith, CCT, Wolf, SP. Autoxidative glycosylation and possible involvement of peroxides and free radicals in LDL modification by glucose. Diabetes 1990; 39:1420–1424.

49. The Diabetes Control and Complications Trial Research Group. The effect of intensive treatment of diabetes on the development and progression of long-term complications in insulin-dependent diabetes mellitus. New Engl J Med 1993; 329:977–986.
50. UK Prospective Diabetes Study Group. Intensive blood glucose control with sulphonylureas or insulin compared with conventional treatment and risk of complications in patients with type 2 diabetes (UKPDS 33). Lancet 1998; 352:837–853.
51. Ceriello A, Giugliano D, Quatraro A, Donzella C, Diaplo G, Lefevbre PJ. AT reduction of protein glycosylation in diabetics: new prospect for prevention of diabetic complications. Diabetes Care 1991; 14:68–72.
52. Ceriello A, Giugliano D, Quatraro A, Dello Russo P, Torella R. A preliminary note on inhibiting effect of alpha-tocopherol (vit. E) on protein glycation. Diab Metab 1988; 14:40–42.
53. Jain SK, McVie R, Jaramillo JJ, Palmer M, Smith T. Effect of modest vitamin E supplementation on blood glycated hemoglobin and triglyceride levels and red cell indices in type 1 diabetic patients. J Amer Coll Nutr 1996; 15:458–461.
54. Paolisso G, Giugliano D, D'Amore A, et al. Daily vitamin E supplementation improves control but not insulin secretion in elderly type 2 diabetic patients. Diabetes Care 1993; 16:433–437.
55. Paolisso G, D'Amore A, Galzerano D, Cacciapuoti F, Varricchio G, Varricchio M, D'Onfario F. Pharmacological doses of vitamin E and insulin action in elderly subjects. Am J Clin Nutr 1994; 59: 1291–1296.
56. Li DJ, Devaraj S, Fuller CJ, Bucala R, Jialal I. The effect of AT on LDL oxidation and glycation: in vitro and in vivo studies. J Lipid Res 1996; 37:1978–1986.
57. Devaraj S, Jialal I. The effect of AT supplementation on monocyte function in Type 2 diabetic subjects with and without macrovascular complications. Circulation 1998; 98:I601.
58. Fuller CJ, Chandalia M, Garg A, Grundy SM, Jialal I. RRR-AT acetate supplementation at pharmacological doses decreases LDL oxidation but nor protein glycation in patients with diabetes. Am J Clin Nutr 1996; 63:753–759.
59. Giardino I, Edelstein D, Brownlee M. BCL2 expression or antioxidants prevent hyperglycemia-induced formation of AGE in bovine EC. J Clin Invest 1996; 97:1422–1428.
60. Reaven PD, Herold DA, Barnett J, Edelman S. Effects of Vitamin E on susceptibility of LDL and LDL subfractions to oxidation and on protein glycation in NIDDM. Diabetes Care 1995; 18:807–816.
61. Kunisaki M, Bursell SE, Clermont AC, Ishii H, Ballas LM, Jirousek MR, et al. Vitamin E prevents diabetes-induced abnormal retinal blood flow via the DAG-PKC pathway. Am J Physiol 1995; 269:E239–246.
62. Koya D, Haneda M, Kikkawa R, King GL. D-alpha tocopherol prevents glomerular dysfunction in diabetic rats through inhibition of PKC-DAG pathway. Biofactors 1998; 7:69–76.
63. Kunisaki M, Bursell SE, Umeda F, Nawata H, King GL. Normalization of DAG-PKC activation by vitamin E in aorta of diabetic rats and cultured rat SMC exposed to elevated glucose levels. Diabetes 1994; 43:1372–1377.
64. Bursell S, Clermont AC, Aiello LP, Aiello L, Schlossman DK, Feener EP, Laffel L, King GL. High dose Vitamin E supplementation normalizes retinal blood flow and creatinine clearance in patients with Type I diabetes. Diabetes Case 1999; 22:1245–1251.
65. Jain SK, Krueger KS, McVie R, Jaramillo JJ, Palmer M, Smith T. Relationship of TxB2 with LPO and effect of vitamin E on these levels in type 1 diabetic patients. Diabetes Care 1998; 21:1511–1516.
66. Colette C, Herbute N, Monnier LH, Cartry E. Platelet function in type I diabetes: effects of supplementation with large doses of vitamin E. Am J Clin Nutr 1988; 47:256–261.

8

Hyperhomocysteinemia, Diabetes, and Cardiovascular Disease

Ellen K. Hoogeveen and Kenneth J. Rothman

1. INTRODUCTION

Cardiovascular disease (CVD), which accounts for more deaths globally than any other cause of death, is 2–4× higher in type 2 diabetic patients than in nondiabetic subjects *(1,2)*. The identification of risk factors that can explain the excess risk for CVD in diabetic patients may improve understanding of the pathophysiological mechanisms of atherosclerosis (Athsc), and allow the development of new preventive or therapeutic measures.

Only recently has the importance of hyperhomocysteinemia as a risk factor for CVD been recognized. It is a strong predictor of CV risk that is independent of other well-established risk factors, such as hypertension (HT), hypercholesterolemia, smoking, and, probably, diabetes *(3,4)*. Blood concentrations of homocysteine (Hcy) are governed by both genetic and environmental determinants, among which inherited enzymatic defects and nutritional deficiencies are most important. Lowering serum total homocysteine (tHcy) levels by increasing the intake of folate (FOL) (a B-vitamin), probably the most important dietary determinant of tHcy levels *(5,6)*, may be an effective means of decreasing CV risk.

Little is known about the impact of hyperhomocysteinemia on CVD among type 2 diabetic patients. This chapter provides a condensed overview of type 2 diabetes and its relation with CVD, especially in regard to the metabolism, regulation, and measurement of Hcy (*see* Chapter 13). It then reviews studies on the relation between hyperhomocysteinemia and CVD, the mechanisms through which hyperhomocysteinemia may cause atherothrombotic disease, and the interaction of hyperhomocysteinemia with other CV risk factors. Also a brief outline is given of the Hoorn Study, which offered the opportunity to evaluate the relation between hyperhomocysteinemia, diabetes, and both macro- and microangiopathy.

Hyperhomocysteinemia and diabetes are both common among the elderly. Understanding the possible interaction of these causes of vascular disease (VD) would provide greater biologic insight into the underlying pathophysiology. Interaction also opens the door to targeted prevention, if it allows the identification of populations that are especially susceptible to the effect of hyperhomocysteinemia. Finally, the chapter offers recommendations for Hcy-lowering therapy, and the authors evaluate the possible consequences for the treatment of type 2 (noninsulin-dependent) diabetes mellitus (DM).

From: *Primary and Secondary Preventive Nutrition*
Edited by: A. Bendich and R. J. Deckelbaum © Humana Press Inc., Totowa, NJ

2. TYPE 2 DIABETES AND CVD

CVD, with accelerated Athsc, is the most common complication of type 2 diabetes, and accounts for 75–80% of the mortality among diabetic subjects (7). CV morbidity and mortality (M&M) rates are 2–4× higher in diabetic patients than in nondiabetic subjects (2), but the underlying mechanisms for the accelerated Athsc in diabetes are still poorly understood (8). Despite their high prevalence in type 2 diabetes, established CV risk factors accounts for no more than half of the excess of CV M&M (8–10). Although accelerated Athsc appears to be the main explanation for excessive M&M among those with type 2 diabetes, microangiopathy may also play some role in the pathogenesis of their CVD (3). Clinically, diabetic microangiopathy leads to microalbuminuria (11). The prevalence of microalbuminuria varies from 5 to 20% among 25–75-yr-old people without diabetes, and from 20 to 40% among type 2 diabetic patients (12,13). The role of microangiopathy in the development of CVD is evidenced by greater CV M&M among those with microalbuminuria (14,15). Microalbuminuria may be a marker of endothelial or more generalized vascular dysfunction, and it is possible that microalbuminuria and atherothrombotic disease share pathogenic mechanisms (16,17). A common link in these mechanisms may be hyperhomocysteinemia. It is not clear whether hyperhomocysteinemia occurs more commonly among those with type 2 diabetes, but, even if it does not, if the effect of hyperhomocysteinemia interacts with the effects of diabetes, the resulting pathophysiology may explain, in part, the increased risk of CVD among type 2 diabetic patients.

3. HOMOCYSTEINE

3.1. Metabolism

Hcy is a sulfur-containing amino acid derived from dietary methionine (Met) by demethylation; its metabolism is at the intersection of two metabolic pathways: remethylation and transsulfuration (Fig. 1). In remethylation, Hcy acquires a methyl group from methyltetrahydrofolate (methyl-THF) or from betaine (trimethylglycine), to form Met. In most tissues, the remethylation of Hcy is catalyzed by methionine synthase (MS), which uses vitamin B_{12} as a co-factor and methyl-THF as a substrate. The reaction with betaine is confined mostly to the liver, and is independent of vitamin B_{12}. A considerable proportion of Met is then activated to form S-adenosylmethionine (SAM), which serves as a universal methyl donor to a variety of acceptors, including guanidinoacetate, neurotransmitters, nucleic acids, and hormones. In the transsulfuration pathway, Hcy condenses with serine to form cystathionine, in an irreversible reaction catalyzed by the vitamin B_6-dependent enzyme, cystathionine-β-synthase (CBS). When Met is in excess, Hcy is directed toward the transsulfuration pathway; under conditions of negative Met balance, Hcy is primarily remethylated, thus conserving Met. Selhub et al. (18) have suggested that the regulation of Hcy metabolism is coordinated by the level of SAM, which acts as an allosteric inhibitor of methylenetetrahydrofolate reductase (MTHFR) and an activator of CBS and methyl-THF (Fig. 1). According to Finkelstein (19), this switch function of SAM is an oversimplification, because there is evidence that Hcy metabolism is regulated by changes of the abundance of tissue-specific enzymes and their intrinsic kinetic properties.

Because Hcy is not a normal dietary constituent, the sole source of Hcy is Met. The Met content of animal proteins is generally 2–3× higher than that of plant proteins (20).

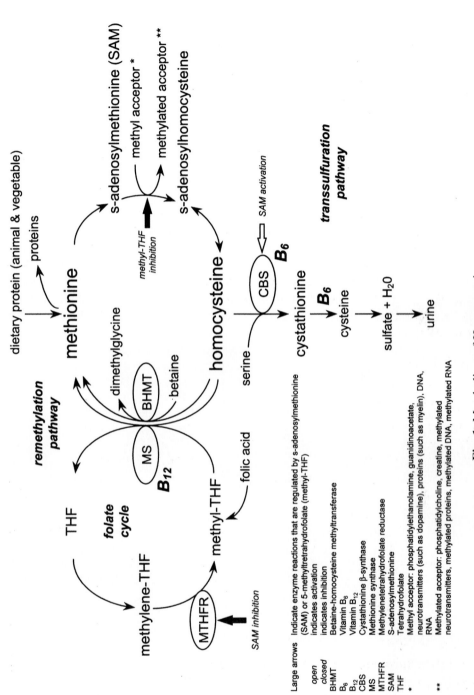

Fig. 1. Metabolism of Homocysteine.

dietary protein (animal & vegetable)

proteins

s-adenosylmethionine (SAM)

methyl acceptor *

methylated acceptor **

s-adenosylhomocysteine

methionine

methyl-THF
inhibition

*remethylation
pathway*

dimethylglycine

BHMT

betaine

homocysteine

serine

*transsulfuration
pathway*

SAM activation

CBS

B_6

cystathionine

B_6

cysteine

sulfate + H_2O

urine

MS

B_{12}

*folate
cycle*

THF

methylene-THF

MTHFR

methyl-THF

folic acid

SAM inhibition

Large arrows   Indicate enzyme reactions that are regulated by s-adenosylmethionine
                (SAM) or 5-methyltretrahydrofolate (methyl-THF)
  open   indicates activation
  closed   indicates inhibition
BHMT   Betaine-homocysteine methyltransferase
B_6 Vitamin B_6
B_{12} Vitamin B_{12}
CBS   Cystathionine β-synthase
MS   Methionine synthase
MTHFR   Methylenetetrahydrofolate reductase
SAM   S-adenosylmethionine
THF   Tetrahydrofolate
*   Methyl acceptor: phosphatidylethanolamine, guanidinoacetate,
                neurotransmitters (such as dopamine), proteins (such as myelin), DNA,
                RNA
**   Methylated acceptor: phosphatidylcholine, creatine, methylated
                neurotransmitters, methylated proteins, methylated DNA, methylated RNA

Red meat is an important source of Met. The recommended dietary allowance (RDA) of Met for U.S. adults is 0.9 g/d, and the estimated adult intake is about 2 g/d *(21)*.

The intracellular concentration of Hcy is kept within narrow bounds, and any increase in production results in increased export from cells *(21)*. The concentration of Hcy in blood is therefore an important reflection of its intracellular concentration, and of the integrity of the various pathways responsible for its metabolism. Values of serum tHcy in adult populations vary, but usually lie in the range of 5–15 μmol/L, in the fasting state. A level above 15 μmol/L is often referred to as hyperhomocysteinemia *(4)*. Hyperhomocysteinemia may be caused by inherited enzyme defects, acquired deficiencies of vitamin B_6, B_{12}, or FOL, by renal failure, and by certain drugs *(4)* (see below).

3.2. Measurement of Serum tHcy

Approximately 70% of Hcy in blood is bound to proteins, mostly albumin. The remaining unbound Hcy fraction combines by oxidation, either with itself, to form a dimer, or with cysteine, to form a mixed disulfide. Only a small proportion ($\approx 1\%$) circulates as free Hcy. The sum of all these Hcy forms is tHcy. It is not known which form(s) of Hcy are directly involved in pathological processes. In serum or plasma, free Hcy becomes protein-bound, even when samples are frozen immediately. Therefore, free Hcy varies much more than tHcy, which is comparatively constant. In 1985, Refsum et al. *(22)* developed an assay for the determination of tHcy. In the presence of blood cells, however, there is a time- and temperature-dependent increase of serum tHcy; at room temperature, tHcy increases by 5–15%/h *(23)*, because of the continuous production and release of Hcy from erythrocytes *(24)*. Therefore, when measuring tHcy, it is important to centrifuge the blood sample within 1 h of collection. The average concentration of tHcy in an individual remains relatively constant over a 12-mo period (within-person SD ≈ 1 μmol/L), showing little seasonal variation *(25)*.

3.3. Met Loading

Measuring tHcy after Met loading calls for the intake of a high dose of Met (0.1 g/kg), with tHcy level being measured immediately before Met loading, and again, typically, 4–6 h afterwards. A protein-rich meal (50 g protein) may increase serum tHcy levels for at least 8 h (mean increase 13.5 ± SD 7.5%), and may therefore represent a physiologic Met load *(26)*. The levels of tHcy after fasting and after a Met load are strongly correlated. The former may reflect vitamin B_{12}- and FOL-dependent remethylation, and the latter, vitamin B_6-dependent transsulfuration. Reliance on fasting tHcy level alone results in about 25% *(27)* fewer subjects classified as hyperhomocysteinemic, and thus fails to identify a substantial proportion of subjects who have normal fasting tHcy, but elevated tHcy after a Met load. Both the fasting and post-Met load serum tHcy levels are related to the risk of CVD *(27)*. The inconvenience of the Met loading test for the subject, however, makes it less suitable for epidemiologic studies.

4. DETERMINANTS OF TOTAL HCY LEVEL

4.1. Genetic Determinants

Homocystinuria and severe hyperhomocysteinemia (>100 μmol/L) are usually caused by rare inborn errors of Hcy metabolism, resulting in marked elevations of serum and urine Hcy concentrations. CBS deficiency is the most common genetic cause of severe hyperhomocysteinemia, with an estimated worldwide incidence of 1/300,000 live births (28). Heterozygotes (<1% of the general population [4]) have fasting tHcy concentrations in the range of 20–40 µmol/L. A homozygous deficiency of MTHFR (0–20% residual activity) may also lead to severe hyperhomocysteinemia (29).

In addition, Kang et al. (30) have reported a thermolabile variant of MTHFR that is caused by a point mutation (C677T) in the coding region for the methylene-THF-binding site, and is associated with decreased enzyme activity. This mutation was found in 5–15% of the general population of Canada, a frequency that is virtually identical to that observed in the Netherlands (31). This genetic variant predisposes to high tHcy concentrations under conditions of impaired FOL status. A recent meta-analysis, comprising about 6000 genotyped CVD patients and about 7000 control subjects, showed that subjects who are homozygous for this mutation (TT genotype) have 2.6 µmol/L (25%) higher tHcy levels than those with the CC genotype (32). The TT genotype, however, did not appear to have a strong association with CVD risk: the odds ratio (OR) comparing CVD risk among those with the TT genotype with those with the CC genotype was 1.12, and the 95% confidence interval (95% CI) was 0.92–1.37. Other abnormalities of the remethylation cycle that are associated with hyperhomocysteinemia include MS deficiency and disorders of vitamin B_{12} metabolism that impair MS activity.

4.2. Nutritional Determinants

Both plasma concentration and dietary intake of vitamins B_6, B_{12}, and FOL show a nonlinear inverse correlation with serum tHcy concentration (6). Individuals with low levels of each of these vitamins have high tHcy concentrations; those with moderate vitamin levels have substantially lower tHcy concentrations. The strongest association has been reported between FOL and tHcy. An inadequate plasma concentration of one or more B-vitamins was a contributing factor in approx two-thirds of all cases of hyperhomocysteinemia (>14 µmol/L) in an elderly population (6). Fasting hyperhomocysteinemia in vitamin B_6 deficiency may only occur if the deficiency is severe and sustained over a long time (33).

4.3. Other Determinants

Women have about 1 µmol/L lower tHcy concentrations than men, and tHcy increases with age (tHcy concentrations are about 1 µmol/L higher in older [70–74 yr] than in slightly younger [65–69 yr] individuals) (25). The difference between the sexes may be the result, in part, of vitamin intake (6), as well as the influence of sex hormones. Serum tHcy levels increase after menopause (34,35), and therefore result in a steeper age-related increase in women than in men. Further evidence for the influence of sex hormones on tHcy level comes from estrogen and androgen administration, which decreases and increases, respectively, tHcy levels (36,37). The sex difference may also be related to the formation of Hcy in connection with the creatine/creatinine synthesis, which is proportional to muscle mass, and therefore higher in men than in women (38).

There is a strong inverse correlation between creatinine clearance and tHcy (39). Impaired renal function causes a substantial increase in the half-life of tHcy, which is explained by a reduction in total body clearance, rather than reduced urinary excretion (40). The mechanism behind this relation is unclear (41), but the marked hyperhomocysteinemia and the 70% reduction of tHcy clearance in subjects with renal failure

(40) emphasize the importance of kidney function for Hcy homeostasis. The physiological decline in renal function may contribute to the increase of tHcy with aging.

The Hordaland Study, which comprised 12,000 healthy subjects aged 40–42 yr and 65–68 yr, showed that high serum cholesterol, high blood pressure, smoking, lack of exercise, and coffee and chronic high alcohol consumption are associated with high tHcy levels *(42–44)*. The association between chronic high alcohol consumption and tHcy is possibly mediated through its negative effect on B-vitamin status. Nonsmoking subjects with low coffee consumption and a high FOL intake had tHcy levels that were 3–4 μmol/L lower than in subjects who smoked, consumed coffee, and had a low FOL intake *(42)*. Methotrexate, phenytoin, theophyline, cyclosporine, and fenofibrate *(45)* are drugs that may induce hyperhomocysteinemia through interference in the Met metabolism.

5. HYPERHOMOCYSTEINEMIA AND ATHEROTHROMBOSIS

In 1969, McCully *(46)* noted that arterial and venous thromboembolic disease is a characteristic feature of homocystinuria, regardless of the site of the metabolic defect. This observation implies that Hcy may be a causal agent in Athsc disease. Approximately 50% of untreated patients with homocystinuria will have a thromboembolic event before the age of 30 yr *(47)*. On autopsy, the macroscopic findings included arterial and venous thrombosis, and Athsc lesions in arteries. These findings are the basis for McCully's theory that elevated tHcy concentrations cause Athsc, and therefore could be an important risk factor for CVD in the general population. In 1976, Wilcken and Wilcken *(48)* showed that moderate hyperhomocysteinemia is associated with premature coronary artery disease (CAD). In 1991, Clarke et al. *(49)* showed that moderate hyperhomocysteinemia is a risk factor for CVD, independent of HT, hypercholesterolemia, and smoking.

In 1995, Boushey et al. *(3)* published a meta-analysis based on 27 cross-sectional and prospective studies of tHcy and CVD. The analysis included about 3600 cases, and provided considerable evidence that elevated tHcy levels are associated with Athsc VD *(3)*. Boushey et al. assumed a linear relation between tHcy levels and risk of CVD. For each increment of 5 μmol/L (about 1 SD) serum tHcy, the risk increased by about 60% (OR = 1.6, 95% CI 1.4–1.7) in men and 80% in women (OR = 1.8, 95% CI 1.3–1.9) for CAD. For cerebrovascular disease, the risk increased by about 50% for men and women combined (OR = 1.5, 95% CI 1.3–1.9), and, for peripheral vascular disease, the OR was 6.8 (95% CI 2.9–15.8) for men and women combined. The proportion of deaths from CAD that were potentially preventable by lowering tHcy levels by 5 μmol/L was estimated to be 10% for U.S. men 45 yr and older, and 6% for women. Boushey et al. *(3)* concluded from their meta-analysis that a decrement of either 5 μmol/L tHcy or 0.5 mmol/L total cholesterol had equivalent effects in reducing CAD risk. Since the publication of this meta-analysis, the epidemiologic evidence supporting the Hcy theory has increased substantially. Another meta-analysis of five prospective nested-case–control studies, which comprised 1041 cases of CAD, provided an estimated OR of 1.3 (95%, CI 1.1–1.5)/5 μmol/L increment of tHcy *(50)*. In a prospective study among middle-aged British men, Perry et al. *(51)* found a monotonic positive relation between tHcy and the risk of stroke (ORs = 1.3, 1.9, 2.8 for the second, third, and fourth quartiles, relative to the first quartile). A tHcy concentration in the highest quartile, compared with the first quartile, was associated with a higher risk of stroke in hypertensive (OR = 3.7, 95% CI 1.0–13.1) than in normotensive subjects (OR = 1.8, 95% CI 0.6–5.5). A prospective study among patients with systemic lupus erythematosus, a condition known to be associated with premature atherothrombosis, showed convincingly that hyperhomocysteinemia (>14.1 µmol/L) was associated with stroke (OR = 2.44, 95% CI 1.04–5.75) (52). In addition, strong associations have been reported between hyperhomocysteinemia and both Alzheimer's disease and vascular dementia (53), possibly attributable to microvascular disease from high tHcy, or perhaps a direct neurotoxic effect.

The Physicians' Health Study comprised 22,071 U.S. male physicians, age 40–84 yr, who did not have a history of CVD, and were followed initially for 5 yr. After adjusting for major CV risk factors, the OR for ischemic stroke for subjects in the upper 20% of tHcy (>12.7 µmol/L), compared with those in the bottom 80% of tHcy levels, was 1.2 (95% CI 0.7–2.0). Among normotensive subjects, the effect was stronger than for HT subjects, with an OR of 2.0 (95% CI 1.0–4.0) among normotensives and 0.6 (0.3–1.5) among hypertensives (54). The OR for myocardial infarction (MI) for the highest 5% vs the bottom 90% of tHcy levels was 3.4 (95% CI 1.3–8.8) (55). After follow-up was extended to 7.5 yr, a much weaker relation was seen between hyperhomocysteinemia and MI (OR = 1.7, 95% CI 0.9–3.3) (56).

The Tromsø study (57) reported a nearly linear association between tHcy and risk for incident MI (123 cases, mean follow-up of 4 yr); per 5 µmol/L increment of tHcy, the OR was 1.41 (95% CI 1.06–1.87). A study (58) among middle-aged men provided a similar estimate: per 5 µmol/L increment of tHcy, the risk for MI rose 41% (OR = 1.41, 95% CI 1.20–1.65). Another study (59), with a mean follow-up of 3.3 yr reported a relation between hyperhomocysteinemia and CAD among middle-aged women (ORs = 0.76, 0.89, 1.71, and 2.53, in the second, third, fourth, and fifth quintiles, relative to the first quintile of the tHcy distribution). A Norwegian study that included 587 patients with CAD, after a median follow-up of 4.6 yr, found a strong relation with overall mortality (78% died from a CV cause), from a tHcy level below 5 µmol/L to above 20 µmol/L. The OR for overall mortality per 5 µmol/L increment tHcy was 1.6 between 10 and 15 µmol/L, and 2.5 between 15 and 20 µmol/L (60). This study shows that tHcy is also a risk factor among subjects with known Athsc disease. Two prospective studies found a clear relation between hyperhomocysteinemia and CVD among subjects with end-stage renal disease (61,62), thus providing evidence that the markedly elevated tHcy levels found in these patients may contribute to their excess risk for CVD, and may partially explain the accelerated Athsc that is a feature of end-stage renal disease.

There are three studies with a longer follow-up time. In a Finnish study of 7424 men and women, aged 40–64 yr at baseline, who were followed for 9 yr, during which there were 265 cases of MI and stroke, there was little association with serum tHcy level (63). In a Dutch study with a 10-yr follow-up among 878 elderly men, aged 64–84 yr at baseline, a tHcy concentration in the second and third tHcy tertile, compared with the first, showed a weak relation with CAD (relative risk = 1.23 and 1.58), but not with cerebrovascular disease (relative risk = 0.67 and 1.26) (64). The Multiple Risk Factor Intervention Trial, which involved a 17-yr follow-up, during which there were 240 cases of MI, found little association between tHcy and risk of MI in the second, third, and fourth quartile of the tHcy distribution, compared with the first (ORs = 1.03, 0.84, and 0.94) (65). A possible explanation for these results is the decreasing relevance of a single baseline tHcy level over a long period of follow-up.

The strongest evidence for a thrombotic effect of high Hcy levels come from prospective studies that estimated the risk for venous thrombosis (66,67). In a meta-analysis of 10 case–control studies, the pooled OR for venous thrombosis was 2.5 (95% CI 1.8–3.5) in subjects with fasting hyperhomocysteinemia, and 2.6 (95% CI 1.6–4.4) in subjects with elevated post-Met increase (both defined as tHcy concentration above 95th percentile of the control group) (68).

The European Concerted Action Project on Hcy and VD is a case–control study of 750 VD patients (coronary artery [CA], cerebrovascular, and peripheral arterial disease [PAD]) and 800 controls. Both males and females were included, and all subjects were younger than 60 yr of age (27). Hyperhomocysteinemia ($\geq$12.0 μmol/L) was associated with risk for VD (OR = 2.2, 95% CI 1.6–2.9). Subjects with diabetes were excluded. The interactions between tHcy and hypercholesterolemia, smoking, and HT were systematically investigated. An elevated tHcy level interacted strongly with HT and smoking, regarding risk of atherothrombotic disease.

6. PATHOPHYSIOLOGICAL MECHANISMS

There is no unifying hypothesis explaining the atherogenic and thrombogenic effects of circulating Hcy. Studies in humans and animals suggest that the atherogenic propensity associated with hyperhomocysteinemia results from endothelial dysfunction and injury, followed by smooth muscle cell proliferation, leukocyte and platelet activation, and thrombus formation. Impaired endothelium function is believed to be an early step in the pathogenesis of Athsc (69). Although the exact mechanism of endothelial dysfunction is unknown, there is growing evidence that Hcy exerts its effects by promoting oxidative damage (70). It may initiate lipid peroxidation and oxidation of low-density lipoprotein. Hcy also alters the normal antithrombotic phenotype of the endothelium by enhancing the activities of factor XII and factor V, and depressing the activation of protein C. Furthermore, Hcy inhibits the expression of thrombomodulin and heparan sulfate, and induces the expression of tissue factor by the endothelium (70). Finally, endothelial dysfunction, as assessed by reduced flow-mediated vasodilatation, caused by impaired nitric oxide release from the endothelium, has been demonstrated in children with homocysteinuria (71), in individuals aged 60–80 yr with moderate hyperhomocysteinemia ($\geq$16 μmol/L) (72), and during acute elevation of tHcy after an oral Met load (73,74). In addition, the association between hyperhomocysteinemia and von Willebrand factor (a marker of endothelial dysfunction) provides further in vivo evidence that hyperhomocysteinemia may induce endothelial dysfunction (75,76).

7. THE HOORN STUDY

The Hoorn Study is a prospective study of CV risk factors and complications in a 50–75-yr-old general Caucasian population. The baseline examination was conducted from October 1, 1989, until December 31, 1991, in the town of Hoorn, a town in the Netherlands with 59,000 inhabitants. From the registry office of Hoorn, a random sample of all inhabitants aged 50–75 yr was selected. Of the eligible subjects, 71% agreed to participate, resulting in a cohort of 2484 subjects. In all participants, an Oral Glucose Tolerance Test (OGTT: 75 g glucose load, according to the 1985 World Health Organization criteria [77]) was performed, except in type 2 diabetic patients treated with oral glucose-lowering agents or insulin, from whom only a fasting blood sample was taken.

An OGTT is a sensitive method to detect DM, and thus adds to the known diabetic population an additional group of about equal size that has undiagnosed diabetes. For a more reliable assessment of glucose tolerance, a second OGTT (participation rate 93%) was performed within 2–6 wk on all subjects with 2-h postload plasma glucose levels ≥7.5 mmol/L at the first test. An age- and sex-stratified random sample was taken, with five strata for both sexes (<55, 55–59, 60–64, 65–69, and >70 yr), from subjects with 2-h glucose levels <7.5 mmol/L. Finally, a second age-, sex-, and glucose tolerance-stratified random sample (n = 708) was drawn, to study the relation between hyper-homocysteinemia, diabetes, and both CVD and microalbuminuria.

7.1. Hyperhomocysteinemia, Type 2 Diabetes, and CVD

Because it is not known whether hyperhomocysteinemia is a risk factor for CVD among type 2 diabetic subjects, nor whether hyperhomocysteinemia and type 2 diabetes interact regarding CVD, one of us (E.H.) investigated these issues in the Hoorn Study, as previously reported (78). Although there was oversampling of diabetic subjects, the oversampling occurred before identification of CVD, and therefore introduced no bias. The authors also assessed whether the presence of type 2 diabetes itself is associated with higher tHcy levels. In addition, the three separate risk estimates of CA, cerebrovascular disease, and PAD were compared, because it was not known whether the strength of the relation of each of these outcomes with hyperhomocysteinemia is similar (3,79–81).

An extensive CV investigation was performed in the above-mentioned age-, sex-, and glucose tolerance-stratified random sample (n = 631; response rate 89.1%). CVD (n = 67) was defined as CA, cerebrovascular, and/or PAD. CAD (n = 40) was defined as a history of MI, CA bypass grafting, and/or Minnesota codes 1-1 or 1-2 on the electrocardiogram (82). Cerebrovascular disease (n = 19) was defined as a history of transient ischemic attack/stroke and/or a carotid artery stenosis of >80%. PAD (n = 17) was defined as a peripheral arterial reconstruction or limb amputation and/or an ankle brachial pressure index <0.50. Fasting blood samples were centrifuged within 1 h after collection. Serum was stored at –20°C for 4–6 yr. There is good evidence that frozen serum tHcy levels are stable for 10 yr or more (83,84). Serum tHcy level was measured by using tri-n-butylphosphine as the reducing agent and ammonium 7-fluorobenzo-2-oxa-1,3-diazole-4-sulphonate as the thiol-specific fluorochromophore, followed by high-performance liquid chromatography with fluorescence detection (85).

The authors conducted logistic regression analyses to study the association of serum tHcy with CA, cerebrovascular, and PAD, separately and combined (i.e., total CVD), and calculated OR and 95% CI per 5 µmol/L (about 1 SD) increment of serum tHcy (assuming a linear logistic relation between Hcy and risk of CVD). A multiple logistic equation was used to control for age, sex, HT, hypercholesterolemia, smoking, and DM. To evaluate a possible modifying role of glucose tolerance, the previous analysis was repeated in three strata.

The back-calculated prevalence (n = 2484) of fasting hyperhomocysteinemia (>14.0 µmol/L) was 25.8%. The medians and interquartile ranges for serum tHcy were 11.2 µmol/L (9.2–14.4) in subjects with normal glucose tolerance (NGT), 12.2 µmol/L (9.7–14.5) with impaired glucose tolerance (IGT), and 11.2 µmol/L (9.2–13.6) with type 2 diabetes. After adjustment for age and sex, there was little association between serum tHcy and fasting glucose, fasting insulin, HbA_{1c}, or duration of type 2 diabetes. Of all type 2 diabetic subjects, 96 (55.5%) were newly diagnosed. Ten (5.8%) were treated with diet

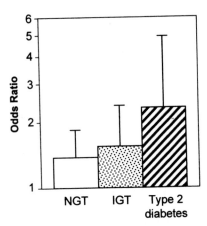

Fig. 2. Odds ratio for cardiovascular disease after stratification by glucose tolerance category. Odds ratios are calculated per 5 µmol/L increment of serum total homocysteine, adjusted for age, sex, hypertension, smoking, hypercholesterolemia, and serum creatine. The error bars represent the upper half of the 95% confidence intervals.

alone, and 67 (38.7%) with glucose-lowering agents: 15 (8.7%) with insulin, 51 (29.5%) with sulfonylureas, and 3 (1.7%) with metformin (2 of whom also used sulfonylureas). The median and interquartile range of duration of type 2 diabetes of those subjects treated with diet or glucose-lowering agents was 6.1 (2.5–11.2) yr. The prevalence of CVD was 7.3% in NGT, 11.2% in IGT, and 15.6% in type 2 diabetes. After adjustment for age, sex, HT, hypercholesterolemia, diabetes, and smoking, the ORs (95% CI) per 5 µmol/L tHcy increment were 1.44 (1.10–1.87) for peripheral arterial, 1.25 (1.03–1.51) for CA, 1.24 (0.97–1.58) for cerebrovascular, and 1.39 (1.15–1.68) for any CVD. After stratification by glucose tolerance category and adjustment for the classical risk factors and serum creatinine, the ORs per 5 µmol/L tHcy increment for any CVD were 1.38 (1.03–1.85) in NGT, 1.55 (1.01–2.38) in IGT, and 2.33 (1.11–4.90) in type 2 diabetes (Fig. 2).

Little is known about the impact of type 2 diabetes on serum tHcy levels. As in previous studies (86,87), the authors found no important difference in fasting serum tHcy level between diabetic and nondiabetic subjects. Although Araki et al. (88) and Munshi et al. (86) have demonstrated that diabetic subjects who also had macrovascular disease had a higher fasting and post-Met load tHcy level, respectively, than nondiabetic controls who were free of CVD, it is not clear from their studies that the higher tHcy levels were caused by the diabetic state *per se*. Although more than 55% of the diabetic subjects were newly diagnosed, the authors cannot rule out that changes of dietary habits of the 45% of diabetic patients who were aware of their disease may have improved their B-vitamin status, and thereby lowered the tHcy level. There is no indication that insulin or sulfonylureas alter tHcy metabolism (88). In contrast, metformin may induce vitamin B_{12} malabsorption, and thereby increase the serum tHcy level (89).

The magnitude of the association between hyperhomocysteinemia and CVD was similar for CA, cerebrovascular, and PAD in this 50–75-yr-old general population. A study among younger subjects (mean age, 45 yr) reached a similar conclusion (27). Furthermore, high serum tHcy may be a stronger (1.6-fold) risk factor for CVD in subjects with type 2 diabetes than in nondiabetic subjects. A 5-yr follow-up study of the entire cohort ($n = 2484$) showed that, after adjustment for major CV risk factors, hyperhomocysteinemia (defined as serum tHcy > 14.0 μmol/L) may be a stronger risk factor for overall mortality in type 2 diabetic patients (OR 2.51), compared with nondiabetic subjects (OR 1.34) *(90)*. Taken together, these results suggest that the strength of the relation between Hcy and CVD is stronger among those with diabetes than among those without diabetes.

7.2. Hyperhomocysteinemia, Protein Intake, and Microalbuminuria

A slightly elevated urinary albumin excretion rate, so-called microalbuminuria, is a strong predictor of CV M&M in both diabetic and nondiabetic individuals *(91,92)*. It is not known whether hyperhomocysteinemia is associated with, and thus a possible cause of, microalbuminuria. A high protein intake may increase the risk of developing microalbuminuria *(93,94)*, and may also increase serum tHcy levels *(26)*. It is thus a potential confounder of the relation between hyperhomocysteinemia and micro-albuminuria. Therefore, one of the authors (E.H.) specifically examined the relations among protein intake, serum tHcy, and presence of microalbuminuria, as described in the earlier paper in more detail *(95)*.

Fasting serum tHcy was measured in the previously described age-, sex-, and glucose tolerance-stratified random sample of a 50–75-yr-old general Caucasian population (*n* = 653; response rate 92.2%). The urinary albumin-to-creatinine ratio (ACR) was measured in an early morning, spot urine sample. An ACR ≤3.0 mg/mmol was defined as normo-albuminuria, and an ACR >3.0 mg/mmol as microalbuminuria. An ACR of 3–30 mg/mmol is approximately equivalent to an albumin excretion rate of 30–300 mg/24h *(96,97)*.

The authors conducted logistic regression analysis to study the association between serum tHcy and protein intake, on the one hand, and microalbuminuria on the other. A multiple logistic equation was used to control for possible confounders, and a possible dose-response relation was evaluated by calculating ORs for microalbuminuria for several ranges of Hcy concentrations, with values of serum tHcy equal to or less than 10 μmol/L as the reference category, and for several ranges of daily protein intake, with values of total protein intake equal to or less than 0.75 g/kg/d, as the reference category.

The prevalence of microalbuminuria was 4.3% (13/304) in subjects with NGT, 9.2% (17/185) in IGT, and 18.3% (30/164) in type 2 diabetes; it was 3.7% (15/402) in subjects without HT and 17.9% (45/251) in those with HT. After adjusting for age, sex, glucose tolerance category, HT, dyslipidemia, and smoking, the OR (95% CI) for micro-albuminuria per 5 μmol/L tHcy increment was 1.33 (1.08–1.63). Additional adjustment for protein intake and serum creatinine or creatinine clearance did not attenuate the association between microalbuminuria and tHcy (OR = 1.28, 95% CI 1.03–1.59). Risk of microalbuminuria increased with increasing serum tHcy levels (Fig. 3). A 0.1 g/kg/d increment of protein intake was also associated with an increased risk for microalbuminuria, after adjustment for age, sex, major CV risk factors, and serum tHcy (OR = 1.20, 95% CI 1.08–1.32). Risk of microalbuminuria increased with increasing daily total protein intake (Fig. 4).

This population-based study shows that serum tHcy is positively associated with the presence of microalbuminuria, independent of major determinants, i.e., DM, HT, protein intake, and renal function. For each 5 μmol/L increase in serum tHcy level, the risk of microalbuminuria being present increased by about 30%. This result is in line with a few cross-sectional studies *(39,98–100)* that reported a positive association between albu-minuria and tHcy level.

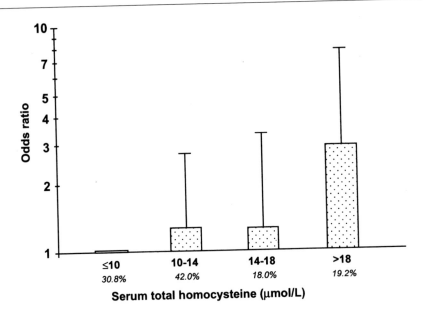

Fig. 3. Odds ratio for microalbuminuria according to serum total homocysteine leve adjusted for age, sex, impaired glucose tolerance/diabetes mellitus, hypertension and protein intake. The reference category was serum total homocysteine values equal or lower than 10 μmol/L. Percentages of the population under study for each serum total homocysteine range are presented. The error bars represent the upper half of the 95% confidence intervals.

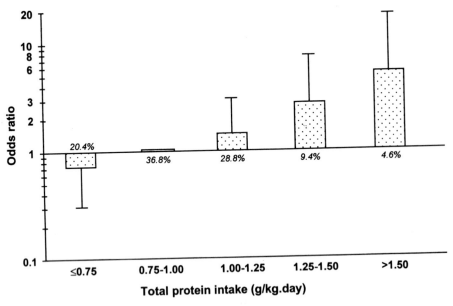

Fig. 4. Odds ratio for microalbuminuria according to total protein intake adjusted for age, sex, impaired gulcose tolerance/diabetes mellitus, hypertension and total homocysteine. The reference category was total protein intake 0.75–1.00 g/kg.day. Percentages of the population under study for each total protein intake range are presented. The error bars represent the lower or upper half of the 95% confidence intervals.

Microalbuminuria is thought to be caused by increased glomerular albumin filtration as a result of decreased glomerular charge selectivity, size selectivity, and/or increased intraglomerular pressure *(101,102)*, the regulation of which is affected by renal endothelial and mesangial cell function *(103,104)*. Mesangial cells have some properties in common with vascular smooth muscle cells *(104)*. Hyperhomocysteinemia may induce dysfunction of the vascular endothelium *(72)* and increase proliferation of vascular smooth muscle cells, possibly by increasing oxidative stress *(70)*. Therefore, it is conceivable that hyperhomocysteinemia is causally related to microalbuminuria through changes in renal endothelial and mesangial cell function, and may thus be one of the factors that link the presence of microalbuminuria to an increased risk of atherothrombotic disease.

An impaired renal function causes a substantial increase in the half-life of tHcy, explained by a reduction in total body clearance *(40)*, and is also a risk factor for microalbuminuria. Because the association between tHcy and microalbuminuria did not materially change after adjustment for serum creatinine or creatinine clearance, the authors consider it improbable that impaired renal function confounded the association between tHcy and the presence of microalbuminuria. The authors cannot exclude, however, that proximal tubular dysfunction in the presence of a normal glomerular filtration rate results in both decreased albumin reabsorption (and thus microalbuminuria) and impaired tHcy metabolism, but this appears unlikely.

There was an increased risk of microalbuminuria with increasing consumption of total protein, independent of serum tHcy levels. Dietary protein intake did not explain the relation between tHcy and microalbuminuria. A high protein intake may result in an increased glomerular filtration rate and renal workload, and therefore aggravate proteinuria *(105)*. In the present study, additional adjustment for total protein intake, if anything, strengthened the association between serum tHcy and risk of microalbuminuria. Taken together, it appears unlikely that hyperhomocysteinemia and high protein intake share a common causal pathway regarding risk of microalbuminuria: Therefore, both appear important determinants of microalbuminuria.

The authors conclude that both hyperhomocysteinemia and protein intake are related to microalbuminuria, independent of type 2 diabetes and HT. Hyperhomocysteinemia may partly explain the link between microalbumniuria and increased risk of CVD.

8. HCY-LOWERING THERAPY

Increased intake of FOL, vitamin B_{12}, and vitamin B_6 can probably reduce the tHcy level, in nearly all individuals, by 15–40%, dependent on their pretreatment tHcy level. FOL is the generic term for compounds that have vitamin activity similar to that of folic acid, the chemical that is added to supplements or fortified food. Folic acid is synthetic, heat-stable, and approximately twice as bioavailable as the FOL that occurs naturally in food *(106)*. A recent meta-analysis *(5)* showed that treatment with 0.5–5.0 mg/d folic acid can lower serum tHcy by 15–40% within approx 6 wk. Vitamin B_{12} (mean 0.5 mg/d) produced an additional 7% reduction of the tHcy level. Vitamin B_6 (mean 16.5 mg/d) did not have an important additional effect. The optimum dose of folic acid has not yet been defined, but a daily dose of as low as 400 µg may be sufficient for many individuals. The major sources of FOL in the diet are fortified breakfast cereals, fortified bread, and fruit and vegetables. The average FOL intake is approx 240 µg in U.S. adults *(107)*.

The addition of oral vitamin B_{12} to folic acid would be expected to avoid the theoretical risk of neuropathy, because of unopposed folic acid therapy in patients deficient in vitamin B_{12}, even if caused by intrinsic factor deficiency or malabsorption (108–110). The latter is relevant, because vitamin B_{12} deficiency is common among the elderly; prevalence estimates in the general population (65 yr and older) vary from 5 to 15% (111–113).

9. RECOMMENDATIONS

Lowering the markedly elevated Hcy levels (>150 µmol/L) found in patients with homocysteinuria reduces CV risk (114); whether lowering moderately elevated tHcy levels can have a similar effect on CV M&M risk has yet to be assessed. It has been estimated that lowering tHcy by 5 µmol/L (about 1 SD) may reduce risk of CV death by about 10% (3). This estimate may be even higher for diabetic subjects, because of the interaction between hyperhomocysteinemia and diabetes, regarding risk of CV morbidity and overall mortality (78,90). The presence of interaction may modify current approaches to VD prevention.

Type 2 diabetes frequently develops after the age of 40 yr, when development of Athsc has probably already taken place for decades. Type 2 diabetic patients are prone to accelerated development of Athsc. The B-vitamins are water-soluble, and poor diabetes control can result in excess excretion. Therefore, it may be argued that B-vitamin therapy, regardless of the initial Hcy level, should be an integral part of diabetes treatment. Slowing down of the progression of Athsc disease among type 2 diabetic patients, rather than prevention, may be a sensible goal.

Dietary supplementation with folic acid appears to be relatively safe, effective, and an inexpensive therapy for lowering blood Hcy levels, and hence affords great potential for the prevention of CVD, if the associations observed in epidemiological studies are causal. Only large-scale randomized trials of adequate dose and duration, in which subjects are allocated to either Hcy-lowering therapy or standard preventive approaches, can provide the necessary evidence that Hcy-lowering therapy is truly efficacious.

REFERENCES

1. Murray CJL, Lopez AD. Mortality by cause for eight regions of the world: Global Burden of Disease Study. Lancet 1997; 349:1269–1276.
2. Panzram G. Mortality and survival in type 2 (non-insulin-dependent) diabetes mellitus. Diabetologia 1987; 30:123–131.
3. Boushey CJ, Beresford SAA, Omenn GS, Motulsky AG. A quantitative assessment of plasma homocysteine as a risk factor for vascular disease. JAMA 1995; 274:1049–1057.
4. Refsum H, Ueland PM, Nygård O, Vollset SE. Homocysteine and cardiovascular disease. Annu Rev Med 1998; 49:31–62.
5. Homocysteine lowering trialists' collaboration. Lowering blood homocysteine with folic acid based supplements: meta-analysis of randomised trials. Br Med J 1998; 316:894–898.
6. Selhub J, Jacques PF, Wilson PWF, Rush D, Rosenberg IH. Vitamin status and intake as primary determinants of homocysteinemia in an elderly population. JAMA 1993; 270:2693–2698.
7. Pyörälä K, Laakso M, Uusitupa M. Diabetes and atherosclerosis: an epidemiologic view. Diabetes Metab Rev 1987; 3:463–524.
8. Nathan DM, Meigs J, Singer DE. The epidemiology of cardiovascular disease in type 2 diabetes mellitus: how sweet it is...or is it? Lancet 1997; 350(Suppl. I):4–9.
9. Wingard DL, Barrett-Connors E, Criqui MH, Suarez L. Clustering of heart disease risk factors in diabetic compared to nondiabetic adults. Am J Epidemiol 1983; 117:19–26.

10. Stamler J, Vaccaro O, Neaton JD, Wentworth D, for the Multiple Risk Factor Intervention Trial Research Group. Diabetes, other risk factors, and 12-yr cardiovascular mortality for men screened in the Multiple Risk Factor Intervention Trial. Diabetes Care 1993; 16:434–444.

11. Feener EP, King GL. Vascular dysfunction in diabetes mellitus. Lancet 1997; 350(Suppl. I):9–13.

12. Mogensen CE, Poulsen PL. Epidemiology of microalbuminuria in diabetes and in the background population. Curr Opin Nephrol Hypertens 1994; 3:248–256.

13. Gall M-A. Albuminuria in non-insulin-dependent diabetes mellitus. Dan Med Bull 1997; 44:465–485.

14. Dinneen SF, Gerstein HC. The association of microalbuminuria and mortality in noninsulin-dependent diabetes mellitus. Arch Intern Med 1997; 157:1413–1418.

15. Yudkin JS, Forrest RD, Jackson CA. Microalbuminuria as predictor of vascular disease in non-diabetic subjects. Islington Diabetes Survey. Lancet 1988; ii:530–533.

16. Deckert T, Kofoed-Enevoldsen A, Nørgaard K, Borch-Johnson K, Feldt-Rasmussen B, Jensen T. Microalbuminuria: implications for micro- and macrovascular disease. Diabetes Care 1992; 15: 1181–1191.

17. Stehouwer CDA, Nauta JJP, Zeldenrust GC, Hackeng WHL, Donker AJM, den Ottolander GJH. Urinary albumin excretion, cardiovascular disease, and endothelial dysfunction in non-insulin-dependent diabetes mellitus. Lancet 1992; 340:319–323.

18. Selhub J, Miller JW. The pathogenesis of homocysteinemia: interruption of the coordinate regulation by S-adenosylmethionine of the remethylation and transsulfuration of homocysteine. Am J Clin Nutr 1992; 55:131–138.

19. Finkelstein JD. The metabolism of homocysteine: pathways and regulation. Eur J Pediatr 1998; 157:S40–S44.

20. McCully KS. Homocysteine theory of arteriosclerosis: development and current status. Atheroscl Rev 1983; 11:157–252.

21. Mayer EL, Jacobsen DW, Robinson K. Homocysteine and coronary atherosclerosis. J Am Coll Cardiol 1996; 27:517–527.

22. Refsum H, Helland S, Ueland PM. Radioenzymic determination of homocysteine in plasma and urine. Clin Chem 1985; 31:624–628.

23. Ueland PM, Refsum H, Stabler SP, Malinow MR, Andersson A, Allen RH. Total homocysteine in plasma or serum: methods and clinical applications. Clin Chem 1993; 39:1764–1779.

24. Andersson A, Isaksson A, Hultberg B. Homocysteine export from erythrocytes and its implication for plasma sampling. Clin Chem 1992; 38:1311–1315.

25. Clarke R, Woodhouse P, Ulvik A, Frost C, Sherliker P, Refsum H, et al. Variability and determinants of total homocysteine concentrations in plasma in an elderly population. Clin Chem 1998; 44:102–107.

26. Guttormsen AB, Schneede J, Fiskerstrand T, Ueland PM, Refsum HM. Plasma concentrations of homocysteine and other aminothiol compounds are related to food intake in healthy human subjects. J Nutr 1994; 124:1934–1941.

27. Graham IM, Daly LE, Refsum HM, Robinson K, Brattström LE, Ueland PM, et al. Plasma homocysteine as a risk factor for vascular disease. JAMA 1997; 277:1775–1781.

28. Mudd SH, Levy HL, Skovby F. Disorders of transsulfuration. In: The Metabolic and Molecular Bases of Inherited Disease, 7th ed. Scriver CR, Beaudet AL, Sly WS, Valle D, eds. New York: McGraw-Hill, 1995; 1279–1327.

29. Carey MC, Donovan DE, FitzGerald O, McAuley FD. Homocystinuria. I. A clinical and pathological study of nine subjects in six families. Am J Med 1968; 45:7–25.

30. Kang SS, Zhou J, Wong PWK, Kowalisyn J, Strokosch G. Intermediate homocysteinemia: a thermolabile variant of methylenetetrahydrofolate reductase. Am J Hum Genet 1988; 43:14–21.

31. Kluijtmans LAJ, Kastelein JJP, Lindemans J, Boers GHJ, Heil SG, Bruschke AVG, et al. Thermolabile methylenetetrahydrofolate reductase in coronary artery disease. Circulation 1997; 96:2573–2577.

32. Brättström L, Wilcken DEL, Öhrvik J, Brudin L. Common methylenetetrahydrofolate reductase gene mutation leads to hyperhomocysteinemia but not to vascular disease: the result of a meta-analysis. Circulation 1998; 98:2520–2526.

33. Miller JW, Ribaya-Mercado JD, Russell RM, Shepard DC, Morrow FD, Cochary EF, et al. Effect of vitamin B6 deficiency on plasma homocysteine concentrations. Am J Clin Nutr 1992; 55: 1154–1160.

34. Andersson A, Brättström L, Israelsson B, Isaksson A, Hamfelt A, Hultberg B. Plasma homocysteine before and after methionine loading with regard to age, gender, and menopausal status. Eur J Clin Invest 1992; 22:79–87.

35. Wouters MGAJ, Moorrees MTEC, van der Mooren MJ, Blom HJ, Boers GHJ, Schellekens LA, et al. Plasma homocysteine and menopausal status. Eur J Clin Invest 1995; 25:801–805.

36. Giltay EJ, Hoogeveen EK, Elbers JMH, Gooren LJG, Asscheman H, Stehouwer CDA. Effects of sex steroids on plasma total homocysteine levels: a study in transsexual males and females. J Clin Endocrinol Metab 1998; 83:550–553.

37. Giri S, Thompson PD, Taxel P, Contois JH, Otvos J, Allen R, et al. Oral estrogen improves serum lipids, homocysteine and fibrinolysis in elderly men. Atherosclerosis 1998; 137:359–366.

38. Mudd SH, Poole JR. Labile methyl balances for normal humans on various dietary regimens. Metabolism 1975; 24:721–735.

39. Arnadottir M, Hultberg B, Nilsson-Ehle P, Thysell H. The effect of reduced glomerular filtration rate on plasma total homocysteine concentration. Scand J Clin Lab Invest 1996; 56:41–46.

40. Guttormsen AB, Ueland PM, Svarstad E, Refsum H. Kinetic basis of hyperhomocysteinemia in patients with chronic renal failure. Kidney Int 1997; 52:495–502.

41. van Guldener C, Donker AJM, Jakobs C, Teerlink T, de Meer K, Stehouwer CDA. No net renal extraction of homocysteine in fasting humans. Kidney Int 1998; 54:166–169.

42. Nygård O, Vollset SE, Refsum H, Stensvold I, Tverdal A, Nordrehaug JE, et al. Total plasma homocysteine and cardiovascular risk profile: the Hordaland Homocysteine Study. JAMA 1995; 274: 1526–1533.

43. Nygård O, Refsum H, Ueland PM, Stensvold I, Nordrehaug JE, Kvåle G, et al. Coffee consumption and plasma total homocysteine: the Hordaland Homocysteine Study. Am J Clin Nutr 1997; 65: 136–143.

44. Nygård O, Refsum H, Ueland PM, Vollset SE. Major lifestyle determinants of plasma total homocysteine distribution: the Hordaland Homocysteine Study. Am J Clin Nutr 1998; 67:263–270.

45. de Lorgeril M, Salen P, Paillard F, Lacan P, Richard G. Lipid-lowering drugs and homocysteine. Lancet 1999; 353: 209–210.

46. McCully KS. Vascular pathology of homocysteinemia: implications for the pathogenesis of arteriosclerosis. Am J Pathol 1969; 56:111–128.

47. Mudd SH, Skovby F, Levy HL, Pettigrew KD, Wilcken B, Pyeritz RE, et al. The natural history of homocystinuria due to cystathionine β-synthase deficiency. Am J Hum Genet 1985; 37:1–31.

48. Wilcken DEL, Wilcken B. The pathogenesis of coronary artery disease: a possible role for methionine metabolism. J Clin Invest 1976; 57:1079–1082.

49. Clarke R, Daly L, Robinson K, Naughten E, Cahalane S, Fowler B, et al. Hyperhomocysteinemia: an independent risk factors for vascular disease. N Engl J Med 1991; 324:1149–1155.

50. Danesh J, Lewington S. Plasma homocysteine and coronary heart disease: systematic review of published epidemiological studies. J Cardiovasc Risk 1998; 5:229–232.

51. Perry IJ, Refsum H, Morris RW, Ebrahim SB, Ueland PM, Shaper AG. Prospective study of serum total homocysteine concentration and risk of stroke in middle-aged British men. Lancet 1995; 346: 1395–1398.

52. Petri M, Roubenoff R, Dallal GE, Nadeau MR, Selhub J, Rosenberg IH. Plasma homocysteine as a risk factor for atherothrombotic events in systemic lupus erythematosus. Lancet 1996; 348:1120–1124.

53. Clarke R, Smith AD, Jobst KA, Refsum H, Sutton L, Ueland PM. Folate, vitamin B_{12}, and serum total homocysteine levels in confirmed Alzheimer Disease. Arch Neurol 1998; 55:1449–1455.

54. Verhoef P, Hennekens CH, Malinow MR, Kok FJ, Willett WC, Stampfer MJ. A prospective study of plasma homocyst(e)ine and risk of ischemic stroke. Stroke 1994; 25:1924–1930.

55. Stampfer MJ, Malinow MR, Willett WC, Newcomer LM, Upson B, Ullmann D, et al. A prospective study of plasma homocyst(e)ine and risk of myocardial infarction in US physicians. JAMA 1992; 268:877–881.

56. Chasan-Taber L, Selhub J, Rosenberg IH, Malinow MR, Terry P, Tishler PV, et al. A prospective study of folate and vitamin B_6 and risk of myocardial infarction in US Physicians. J Am Coll Nutr 1996; 15:136–143.

57. Arnesen E, Refsum H, Bønaa KH, Ueland PM, Førde OH, Nordrehaug JE. Serum total homocysteine and coronary heart disease. Int J Epidemiol 1995; 24:704–709.

58. Wald NJ, Watt HC, Law MR, Weir DG, McPartlin J, Scott JM. Homocysteine and ischemic heart disease: results of a prospective study with implications regarding prevention. Arch Intern Med 1998; 158:862–867.

59. Folsom AR, Nieto FJ, McGovern PG, Tsai MY, Malinow MR, Eckfeldt JH, et al. Prospective study of coronary heart disease incidence in relation to fasting total homocysteine, related genetic polymor-

phisms, and B vitamins. The Atherosclerosis Risk in Communities (ARIC) Study. Circulation 1998; 98:204–210.

60. Nygård O, Nordrehaug JE, Refsum H, Ueland PM, Farstad M, Vollset SE. Plasma homocysteine levels and mortality in patients with coronary artery disease. N Engl J Med 1997; 337:230–236.

61. Bostom AG, Shemin D, Verhoef P, Nadeau MR, Jacques PF, Selhub J, et al. Elevated fasting total plasma homocysteine levels and cardiovascular disease outcomes in maintenance dialysis patients: a prospective study. Arterioscl Thromb Vasc Biol 1997; 17:2554–2558.

62. Moustapha A, Naso A, Nahlawi M, Gupta A, Arheart KL, Jacobson DW, et al. Prospective study of hyperhomocysteinemia as an adverse cardiovascular risk factor in end-stage renal disease. Circulation 1998; 97:138–141.

63. Alfthan G, Pekkanen J, Jauhiainen M, Pitkäniemi J, Karvonen M, Tuomilehto J, et al. Relation of serum homocysteine and lipoprotein(a) concentrations to atherosclerotic disease in a prospective Finnish population based study. Atherosclerosis 1994; 106:9–19.

64. Stehouwer CDA, Weijenberg MP, van den Berg M, Jakobs C, Feskens EJM, Kromhout D. Serum homocysteine and risk of coronary heart disease and cerebrovascular disease in elderly men: a ten-year follow-up. Arterioscl Thromb Vasc Biol 1998; 18:1895–1901.

65. Evans RW, Shaten J, Hempel JD, Cutler JA, Kuller LH, for the MRFIT Research group. Homocyst(e)ine and risk of cardiovascular disease in the Multiple Risk Factor Intervention Trial. Arterioscl Thromb Vasc Biol 1997; 17:1947–1953.

66. den Heijer M, Koster T, Blom HJ, Bos GMJ, Briët E, Reitsma PH, et al. Hyperhomocysteinemia as a risk factor for deep-vein thrombosis. N Engl J Med 1996; 334:759–762.

67. Ridker PM, Hennekens CH, Selhub J, Miletich JP, Malinow MR, Stampfer MJ. Interrelation of hyperhomocyst(e)inemia, factor V Leiden, and risk of future venous thromboembolism. Circulation 1997; 95:1777–1782.

68. den Heijer M, Rosendaal FR, Blom HJ, Gerrits WBJ, Bos GMJ. Hyperhomocysteinemia and venous thrombosis: a meta-analysis. Thromb Haemost 1998; 80:874–877.

69. Ross R. Mechanisms of disease: atherosclerosis—an inflammatory disease. N Engl J Med 1999; 340:115–126.

70. Welch GN, Loscalzo J. Mechanisms of disease: homocysteine and atherothrombosis. N Engl J Med 1998; 338:1042–1050.

71. Celermajer DS, Sorensen K, Ryalls M, Robinson J, Thomas O, Leonard JV, et al. Impaired endothelial function occurs in the systemic arteries of children with homozygous homocysteinuria but not in their heterozygous parents. J Am Coll Cardiol 1993; 22:854–858.

72. Tawakol A, Omland T, Gerhard M, Wu JT, Creager MA. Hyperhomocyst(e)inemia is associated with impaired endothelium-dependent vasodilatation in humans. Circulation 1997; 95:1119–1121.

73. Chambers JC, McGregor A, Jean-Marie K, Kooner JS. Acute hyperhomocysteinaemia and endothelial dysfunction. Lancet 1998; 351:36–37.

74. Bellamy MF, McDowell IFW, Ramsey MW, Brownlee M, Bones C, Newcombe RG, et al. Hyperhomocysteinemia after an oral methionine load acutely impairs endothelial function in healthy adults. Circulation 1998; 98:1848–1852.

75. van den Berg M, Boers GHJ, Franken DG, Blom HJ, van Kamp GJ, Jakobs C, et al. Hyperhomocysteinaemia and endothelial dysfunction in young patients with peripheral arterial occlusive disease. Eur J Clin Invest 1995; 25:176–181.

76. de Jong SC, Stehouwer CDA, van den Berg M, Vischer UM, Rauwerda JA, Emeis JJ. Endothelial marker proteins in hyperhomocysteinaemia. Thromb Haemost 1997; 78:1332–1337.

77. World Health Organisation Study Group on Diabetes Mellitus. Technical Report Series No. 727. Geneva, WHO, 1985.

78. Hoogeveen EK, Kostense PJ, Beks PJ, Mackaay AJC, Jakobs C, Bouter LM, et al. Hyperhomocysteinemia is associated with an increased risk of cardiovascular disease especially in non-insulin-dependent diabetes mellitus: a population-based study. Arterioscl Thromb Vasc Biol 1998; 18:133–138.

79. Mölgaard J, Malinow MR, Lassvik C, Holm A-C, Upson B, Olsson AG. Hyperhomocyst(e)inaemia: an independent risk factor for intermittent claudication. J Intern Med 1992; 231:273–279.

80. Bergmark C, Mansoor MA, Swedenborg J, de Faire U, Svardal AM, Ueland PM. Hyperhomocysteinemia in patients operated for lower extremity ischaemia below the age of 50; effect of smoking and extent of disease. Eur J Vasc Surg 1993; 7:391–396.

81. Brattström L, Israelsson B, Norrving B, Bergqvist D, Thörne J, Hultberg B, et al. Impaired homocysteine metabolism in early-onset cerebral and peripheral occlusive arterial disease. Atherosclerosis 1990; 81:51–60.

82. Prineas RJ, Crow RS, Blackburn H. The Minnesota Code manual of electrocardiographic findings. In: Standards and procedures for measurement and classification. Boston, MA: John Wright, 1982.

83. Joosten E, van den Berg A, Riezler R, Naurath HJ, Lindenbaum J, Stabler SP, et al. Metabolic evidence that deficiencies of vitamin B-12 (cobalamin), folate, and vitamin B-6 occur commonly in elderly people. Am J Clin Nutr 1993; 58:468–476.

84. Savage DG, Lindenbaum J, Stabler SP, Allen RH. Sensitivity of serum methylmalonic acid and total homocysteine determinations for diagnosing cobalamin and folate deficiencies. Am J Med 1994; 96:239–246.

85. Ubbink JB, Vermaak WJH, Bissbort S. Rapid high-performance liquid chromatographic assay for total homocysteine levels in human serum. J Chromatogr 1991; 565:441–446.

86. Munshi MN, Stone A, Fink L, Fonseca V. Hyperhomocysteinemia following a methionine load in patients with non-insulin-dependent diabetes mellitus and macrovascular disease. Metabolism 1996; 45:133–135.

87. Genest JJ, McNamara JR, Salem DN, Wilson PWF, Schaeffer EJ, Malinow MR. Plasma homocyst(e)ine levels in men with premature coronary artery disease. J Am Coll Cardiol 1990; 16:1114–1119.

88. Araki A, Sako Y, Ito H. Plasma homocysteine concentrations in Japanese patients with non-insulin-dependent diabetes mellitus: effect of parenteral methylcobalamin treatment. Atherosclerosis 1993; 103:149–157.

89. Carlsen SM, Følling I, Grill V, Bjerve KS, Schneede J, Refsum H. Metformin increases total serum homocysteine levels in non-diabetic male patients with coronary heart disease. Scand J Clin Lab Invest 1997; 57:521–528.

90. Hoogeveen EK, Kostense PJ, Jakobs C, Dekker JM, Nijpels G, Heine RJ, et al. Hyperhomocysteinemia increases risk of death, especially in type 2 diabetes: 5-year follow-up of the Hoorn Study. Circulation 2000; 101:1506–1511.

91. Dinneen SF, Gerstein HC. The association of microalbuminuria and mortality in noninsulin-dependent diabetes mellitus. Arch Intern Med 1997; 157:1413–1418.

92. Yudkin JS, Forrest RD, Jackson CA. Microalbuminuria as predictor of vascular disease in non-diabetic subjects. Islington Diabetes Survey. Lancet 1988; ii:530–533.

93. Metcalf PA, Baker JR, Scragg RKR, Dryson E, Scott AJ, Wild CJ. Dietary nutrient intakes and slight albuminuria in people at least 40 years old. Clin Chem 1993; 39:2191–2198.

94. Pedrini MT, Levey AS, Lau J, Chalmers TC, Wang PH. The effect of dietary protein restriction on the progression of diabetic and nondiabetic renal diseases: a meta-analysis. Ann Intern Med 1996; 124: 627–632.

95. Hoogeveen EK, Kostense PJ, Jager A, Heine RJ, Jakobs C, Bouter LM, et al. Serum homocysteine level and protein intake are related to risk of microalbuminuria: the Hoorn Study. Kidney Int 1998; 54:203–209.

96. Rowe DJF, Dawnay A, Watts GF. Microalbuminuria in diabetes mellitus: review and recommendations for the measurement of albumin in urine. Ann Clin Biochem 1990; 27:297–312.

97. Bennett PH, Haffner S, Kasiske BL, Keane WF, Mogensen CE, Parving HH, et al. Screening and management of microalbuminuria in patients with diabetes mellitus: recommendations to the Scientific Advisory Board of the National Kidney Foundation from an Ad Hoc Committee of the Council on Diabetes Mellitus of the National Kidney Foundation. Am J Kidney Dis 1995; 25:107–112.

98. Hultberg B, Agardh E, Andersson A, Brattström, Isaksson A, Israelsson B. Increased levels of plasma homocysteine are associated with nephropathy, but not severe retinopathy in type I diabetes mellitus. Scand J Clin Lab Invest 1991; 51:277–282.

99. Chico A, Pérez A, Córdoba A, Arcelús R, Carreras G, de Leiva A, et al. Plasma homocysteine is related to albumin excretion rate in patients with diabetes mellitus: a new link between diabetic nephropathy and cardiovascular disease? Diabetologia 1998; 41:684–693.

100. Lanfredini M, Fiorina P, Grazia Peca M, Veronelli A, Mello A, Astorri E, et al. Fasting and post-methionine load homocyst(e)ine values are correlated with microalbuminuria and could contribute to worsening vascular damage in non-insulin-dependent diabetes mellitus patients. Metabolism 1998; 47:915–921.

101. Remuzzi G, Ruggenenti P, Benigni A. Understanding the nature of renal disease progression. Kidney Int 1997; 51:2–15.

102. Brenner BM, Hostetter TH, Humes HD. Molecular basis of proteinuria of glomerular origin. N Engl J Med 1978; 298:826–833.

103. Maddox DA, Brenner BM. Glomerular ultrafiltration. In: The Kidney, 4th ed. Philadelphia: WB Saunders, 1991; 205–244.

104. Deckert T, Kofoed-Enevoldsen A, Nørgaard K, Borch-Johnson K, Feldt-Rasmussen B, Jensen T. Microalbuminuria: implications for micro- and macrovascular disease. Diabetes Care 1992; 15: 1181–1191.
105. Schaap GH, Bilo HJG, Alferink THR, Oe PL, Donker AJM. The effect of a high protein intake on renal function of patients with chronic renal insufficiency. Nephron 1987; 47:1–6.
106. Oakley GP. Eat right and take a multivitamin. N Engl J Med 1998; 338:1060–1061.
107. Subar AF, Block G, James LD. Folate intake and food sources in the US population. Am J Clin Nutr 1989; 50:508–516.
108. Lindenbaum J, Healton EB, Savage DG, Brust JCM, Garrett TJ, Podell ER, et al. Neuropsychiatric disorders caused by cobalamin deficiency in the absence of anemia or macrocytosis. N Engl J Med 1988; 318:1720–1728.
109. Savage DG, Lindenbaum J. Folate-cobalamin interactions. In: Folate in Health and Disease. Bailey LB, ed. New York: Marcel Dekker, 1995; 237–285.
110. Campbell NRC. How safe are folic acid supplements? Arch Intern Med 1996; 156:1638–1644.
111. Joosten E, van den Berg A, Riezler R, Naurath HJ, Lindenbaum J, Stabler SP, et al. Metabolic evidence that deficiencies of vitamin B-12 (cobalamin), folate and vitamin B-6 occur commonly in elderly people. Am J Clin Nutr 1993; 58:468–476.
112. Pennypacker LC, Allen RH, Kelly JP, Matthews M, Grigsby J, Kaye K, et al. High prevalence of cobalamin deficiency in elderly outpatients. J Am Geriatr Soc 1992; 40:1197–1204.
113. Yao Y, Yao SL, Yao SS, Yao G, Lou W. Prevalence of vitamin B12 deficiency among geriatric outpatients. J Fam Pract 1992; 35:524–528.
114. Wilcken DEL, Wilcken B. The natural history of vascular disease and the effects of treatment. J Inherit Metab Dis 1997; 20:295–300.

9

Genetic and Environmental Influences on Obesity

David B. Allison, Patty E. Matz,
Angelo Pietrobelli, Raffaella Zannolli,
and Myles S. Faith

1. INTRODUCTION

This is an exciting time for research into genetic and environmental influences on obesity. Advances in molecular biology, pharmacology, and other fields are allowing rapid advances to be made in this arena. Knowledge that there is a genetic component to variations in body wt and composition is not new. Indeed, animal breeders and ranchers have known for centuries that animals could be selectively bred for traits related to body wt and composition (1). For example, the average pig used for pork production in the United States today has substantially more lean body mass and substantially less fat mass than its ancestors, thus demonstrating the influence of selective breeding (2). Many argue that the ability to induce species-wide changes in the average value of a trait by selective breeding provides the strongest evidence for a genetic effect on that trait (3), a phenomenon that has been demonstrated in livestock (4) and laboratory animals (5).

2. IS THERE GENETIC INFLUENCE IN HUMANS?

It had long been known that individuals grow up to resemble their parents, a phenomenon studied by Sir Francis Galton over 100 yr ago (6,7). As early as 1923, Davenport (8) demonstrated that, as adults, individuals tend to have relative body weights (RBWs) very similar to those of their parents. However, because family members typically share living environments, as well as genes, it has been difficult to tease apart the influences of these two factors. Therefore, scientists have looked to other types of information to assess the relative impact of genetic and environmental influences on RBW and obesity.

An amusing study by Mason (9) is illustrative of the type of data that has been brought to bear on the issue, and used to suggest that the familial resemblance for RBW is the result of shared common environmental influences. Mason examined the pet dogs of obese and nonobese owners, and classified the dogs as obese and nonobese. It was found that the dogs of obese owners were far more likely to be obese than were the dogs of nonobese owners. Because pet owners and their dogs are presumably genetically unrelated, one might interpret these data as demonstrating an environmental influence (at least on

From: *Primary and Secondary Preventive Nutrition*
Edited by: A. Bendich and R. J. Deckelbaum © Humana Press Inc., Totowa, NJ

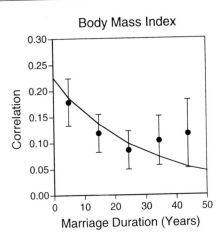

Fig. 1. Correlations of Interspousal BMI as a function of marriage duration. Adapted with permission from ref. *11*.

canine obesity). However, since people do not come to own particular dogs at random, this conclusion may not be valid. It is possible that owners tend to choose dogs with tendencies to gain weight that are comparable to their own.

More seriously, the same thinking has been applied to the observed similarity in RBW between husbands and wives. Allison et al. *(10)* provided an extensive tabulation of spousal correlations for body mass index (BMI: kg/m^2). Husband–wife correlation consistently averaged between approx .10 and .15, indicating a small but statistically significant resemblance among husbands and wives for BMI. Although some claim this as evidence for the household environment's influence on obesity, individuals do not marry each other at random. This leaves open the possibility of positive assortative mating, whereby individuals mate with/marry others who are similar with respect to a particular trait. To evaluate evidence for assortative mating, Allison et al. *(10)* examined the correlation in RBW among pairs of individuals prior to their mating/marriage and cohabitation. Among 296 couples, there was a statistically significant correlation ($r = .13$) for RBW, even before the couples were married and cohabitating, suggesting that people tend to pick mates who are similar in weight, rather than mates growing more similar over time. Similar conclusions were reached by Knuiman et al. *(11)*, who calculated the spousal correlation with respect to BMI as a function of marriage duration. As seen in Fig. 1, this correlation does not increase over time *(11)*. If anything, the correlation tends to decrease, further suggesting that the shared household environment may have little influence on adult BMI.

Stronger inferences about the nature of genetic and environmental influences on BMI can be drawn from the classical twin study *(12)* in which monozygotic (MZ) twins, who have virtually 100% of their genes in common, are compared to dizygotic (DZ) twins, who have, on average, 50% of the same genes. To the extent that MZ twins are more similar with respect to BMI than are DZ twins, this would suggest a genetic effect. Indeed, mathematical models can be fit to such data to estimate the proportion of variance caused by genetic and environmental effects, and to evaluate the extent to which those environmental effects result from shared common household influences or unique unshared

Table 1

Genetic and Familial Environmental Influences on Obesity in Parents vs Offspring
and in Siblings in Adulthood, as Estimated in Complete Adoption Studies

Study	Genetic influence	Familial environmental influence
Parent–adult offspring		
Danish	++++	0
Iowa	+++	+
Parent–offspring in childhood		
Danish	+++	+
Colorado	++++	0
Adult siblings		
Danish	++++	0
Siblings in childhood		
Danish	+++	+

Note: Expressed on a semiquantitative scale, from ++++ to 0, which add up to ++++ for the combined genetic and family environment effects.
Adapted with permission from ref. 15.
Reprinted with permission from Overview of the adoption studies. In: The Genetics of Obesity. Bouchard C, ed. Boca Raton, FL: CRC Press, 1994; 49–61.

influences among family members (12). One such study (13) of over 4000 adult twins found that genetic variations among individuals appeared to account for 60–75% of the variance in BMI, with the remaining variance attributable to unique environmental influences that are, on average, unshared among family members. The common household environment had no significant effect. This study is consistent with an enormous body of data. For example, Meyer (14) tabulated data from over 20 heritability estimates of BMI, and reported that all but four fell between .6 and .8, thus suggesting a strong genetic contribution to this phenotype.

Perhaps the strongest alternative to the twin design for testing genetic influences is the adoption study (3). Table 1, adapted from Sorenson and Stunkard (15), summarizes relevant adoption studies, and shows results that are mostly consistent with the twin literature, namely, that adoptees' BMIs tend to be correlated with their biological parents, but not their adoptive parents, suggesting again that most of the familial resemblance for BMI is the result of shared genetic influences.

3. WHAT IS THE HERITABILITY OF BMI?

Heritability can be defined as the proportion of within-population variance in a trait (e.g., BMI) that is attributable to within-population variations in genotype. That is, heritability is a ratio of the genetic variance to the total phenotypic variance. Twin studies have generally yielded heritability estimates of approx .70. In contrast, adoption and family studies have generally yielded lower estimates of heritability in the range of .25–.50. Why the discrepancy? Resolving this discrepancy is not a trivial matter, but is very important for obtaining a valid estimate of the magnitude of genetic influences on obesity. An extensive review of this question can be found in Maes et al. (16). Two major classes of reasons may explain the differences.

Table 2
Heritability of BMI Based on MZAs

Ref.	Sample	h^2
Stunkard et al. (22)	93 Swedish pairs	.66 (women)
		.70 (men)
Price and Gottesman (23)	34 English pairs	.61
Allison et al. (24)	17 Finnish pairs	.65
	10 Japanese pairs	.73
	26 U.S. and Danish pairs	.85

First, twin studies may yield upwardly biased estimates, because of a violation of the so-called "equal environments" assumption. This assumption states that the degree of similarity in treatment of MZ and DZ twins is equal. In contrast, if MZ twins were treated more similarly to one another than are DZ twins, with respect to environmental variables that affect their BMI, then this violation of the equal environments assumption would ultimately cause the heritability of BMI to be overestimated in twin studies. Concern about such violations (and therefore potentially inaccurate heritability estimates) has been raised repeatedly throughout the history of the use of twin studies (16). However, tests of the validity of this assumption suggest that the assumption is reasonable and tenable (16,17).

A second possible reason for the difference between twin and adoption studies concerns nonadditive genetic effects, which may occur in several ways. There can be dominance (18), age-by-gene interactions (19), gene-by-environment interactions (20), and gene-by-gene interactions (21). There is some evidence for each of these phenomena in the determination of interindividual variations in BMI. Of particular interest are gene-by-gene interactions, or epistasis (21), which occurs when the effect of the alleles at one genetic locus depends on the alleles present at another genetic locus. The simultaneous action of many genes in such a nonadditive epistatic fashion has been called emergenesis (21). Describing emergenesis, Lykken et al. (21) state, "Traits that depend on configurations of polymorphic genes that do segregate independently will be shared by MZ twins, who share all their genes and hence all gene configurations, but are much less likely to be shared by DZ twins, siblings, or parents and offspring. Such traits, although genetic, would not tend to run in families." Thus, emergenetic traits should have high heritabilities, but low correlations among all relatives, except MZ twins. This is precisely the pattern observed with respect to BMI. Such findings help to reconcile the high, but (in the authors' opinion) accurate, heritabilities from twin studies and low, but (again in the authors' opinion) incorrect, estimates from family and adoption studies.

Perhaps the most powerful and elegant alternative designs for estimating the heritability of RBW is the study of MZ twins reared apart (MZAs). MZAs share all of their genes in common, but, if separated at or shortly after birth, have no household environment in common. Therefore, if the household environment is truly of little influence, then the heritability estimates from studies of MZAs should be virtually identical to those from classical twin studies. There have now been at least three separate data sets reporting the correlation of BMI for MZAs (22–24). These studies are summarized in Table 2, and suggest two conclusions. First, like studies using the classical twin design, the heritability

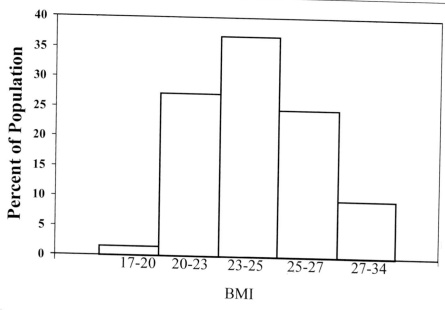

Fig. 2. BMI distribution of 720 runaway male Black slaves in 1860s. Adapted with permission from ref. 26.

of BMI from these studies appears to be on the order of approx .70. This means that approx 70% of the within-population variance in BMI results from within-population variations in genotype. Second, the correlation for these MZAs is virtually the same as the correlation for MZ twins reared in the same household, suggesting that the shared common environment of MZ twins reared together had a minimal enduring impact on BMI. Thus, studies of MZAs suggest that the high heritability observed in classical twin studies is accurate.

3.1. Interpreting the Heritability Coefficient

In the authors' experience, the statement that 70% of the variation in BMI is genetic is often misinterpreted in three ways: First, that 70% of obese people are genetically obese. Second, that 70% of the reason the average person is obese is genetic. Third, that 70% of an obese person's excess weight or fat is genetic weight or fat. None of these three interpretations is correct. However, regarding the first, it may be possible to find a distinction between obese people with respect to their degree of genetic predisposition, which, although arbitrary, is useful for everyday parlance. This approach was taken by Allison and Faith (25), who suggested that perhaps the person who is obese, even in an environment that allows less than or equal to 10% of the overall population to maintain an obese body wt, may be legitimately described as "genetically obese." The choice of this value of 10% is arbitrary, but it may actually have some validity. For example, Fig. 2 is a histogram of BMIs based on the measured heights and weights of 720 runaway, recaptured, male Black slaves in the southern United States in the 1860s (26). Clearly, these men were living under the harshest of environments, which were not obesegenic. Nevertheless, approx 10% of these individuals had BMIs greater than or equal to 27, a value that many expert bodies have considered overweight or obese (27). Thus, in this sample of 720 men, it appears that approx 10% had a sufficiently strong genetic predisposition toward having a high BMI that they were able to maintain a BMI in the overweight or obese range, despite this harshest of harsh environments.

Returning then to the question of what percent of obese Americans in the present day are genetically obese, using a total heritability estimate of .70, information on the overall BMI distribution, and an approximation based on statistical genetics, Allison and Faith *(25)* were able to estimate that about 21% of Americans with BMIs greater than 28 could be classified as genetically obese.

Yet another way of putting the heritability of BMI into perspective was provided by Hewitt *(28)*, who showed that, under the assumption of a heritability of .70, BMI could be written as a function of the genetic and environmental influences on BMI, as follows:

$$BMI = 5.8 \,(\sqrt{.7G} + \sqrt{1 - .7E}\,)$$

where 5.8 is approximately the standard deviation (SD) of adult BMI, G is an individual's score on a latent variable representing the composite of all the genetic influences on BMI, and E is an individual's score on a latent variable representing the composite of all those environmental influences on BMI. This equation implies that a one-SD decrease in the environmental factors that increase BMI would reduce BMI approx 3.2 units. For an average-height person (e.g., 5 ft 8 in.: 173 cm), this would correspond to a loss of about 21 lb (9.6 kg). This would clearly be a clinically significant weight loss, which could be achieved by either individuals or populations if changes were made to the environment equivalent to a one-SD reduction in the environmental risk for obesity.

3.2. Which Is Inherited, Thinness or Obesity?

Is the genetic influence on having an unusually high BMI as strong, stronger, or less strong than the genetic influence on having an unusually low BMI (i.e., being very thin)? One way to address this question is through the use of Risch's lambda (λ) statistic, a type of relative risk. Specifically, λ is the ratio of the probability of having a particular condition, such as obesity, given that one's relative has that condition, divided by the overall probability of having that condition in the population. For example, if the overall probability of being obese in a particular population were .2, and the probability of being obese, given that one's sibling is obese, were .6, then the λ for siblings would be 3 (i.e., .6 divided by .2). λ ratios can be calculated for different types of relatives, but are most commonly calculated for siblings *(29)*. Of course, sibling λ ratios are influenced by both genetic factors and shared common environmental factors. However, because shared common environmental influences on obesity are apparently trivial *(30)*, sibling λ ratios provide a reasonable index of the magnitude of genetic influence on BMI and obesity. In Fig. 3, sibling λ ratios are presented from a variety of populations on which data were obtained *(29,31–36)*. For each sample, the authors have calculated the sibling λ ratio for obesity, arbitrarily defined as having a BMI above the population-specific age- and sex-adjusted 90th percentile, and, for thinness, which the authors have defined as having a BMI below the population-specific age- and sex-adjusted 10th percentile. The figure illustrates that sibling λ ratios in most cases are just as high, if not higher, for thinness than for obesity, suggesting that extreme thinness is as much inherited as extreme obesity, and the potential of searching for genes for obesity resistance (if thinness = obesity resistance).

The concept that genes influence obesity resistance as much as obesity is consistent with knowledge from animal models. For example, Levin et al. *(37)* have shown that rats

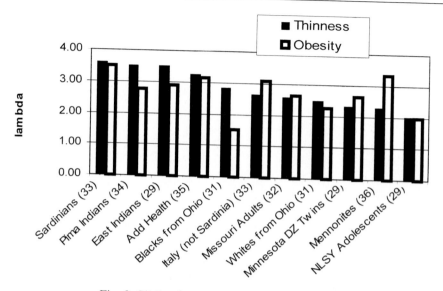

Fig. 3. Sibling λ values: thinness and obesity.

Table 3
Plausible Candidate Genes for Thinness or Leanness

	Ref.
RII β subunit of protein kinase A	(38)
Myostatin	(39)
Tumor necrosis factor-α	(40)
Pro12Ala substitution in peroxisome proliferator activated receptor γ2	(41)
Melanin-concentrating hormone	(42)
Protein tyrosine phosphatase-1B	(43)
Mahogany	(44)

can be bred for obesity resistance, as well as obesity susceptibility. Moreover, Table 3 lists seven specific genes that have been identified as producing nonhuman animals and humans that are resistant to obesity when these genes are knocked out or mutated, suggesting that loss of functional polymorphisms in these genetic loci could result in obesity resistance (38–44).

Consistent with a genetic hypothesis, one can also ask: "Is it true that individuals who are very thin at one point in time are very likely to be very thin at a subsequent point in time?" The answer appears to be yes. Figure 4 shows data from four different population-based samples measured longitudinally, with intervals ranging from 2 to 32 yr (45–48). As can be seen, the probability of being in the lower 10% of the BMI distribution at one point in time, given that one was in the lower 10% of the distribution at some prior point in time, is nearly as high as the probability of being in the upper 10% of the distribution, given that one was in the upper 10% of the distribution at some prior point in time. That is, extreme thinness is a rather stable trait, and is nearly as stable as is extreme fatness, further suggesting the potential value of studying the genetics of extreme thinness.

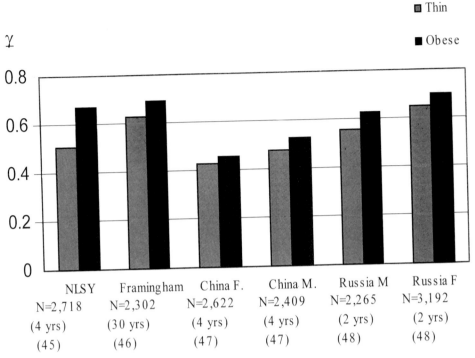

Fig. 4. Conditional probability of being in upper (obese) or lower (thin) decile at T2 given in same at T1.

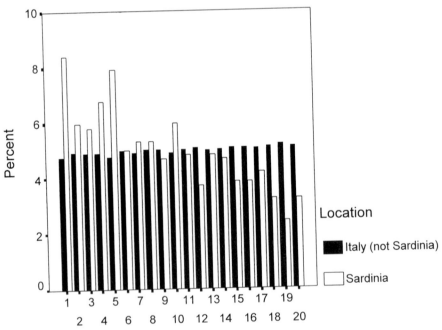

Fig. 5. Overrepresentation of extreme thinness among Sardinians. Taken from Allison DB, Zannolli R. Based on unpublished data from the Istituto Nazionale di Statistica. Indagine Multiscopo sulle Famiglie. Quinto Ciclo, 1987–1991.

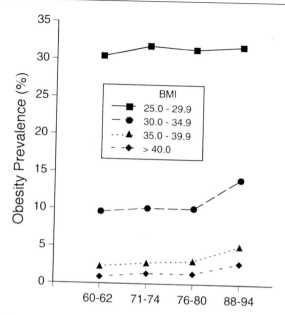

Fig. 6. Increase in obesity prevalence. Reprinted with permission from ref. *64.*

One place that may be especially interesting to conduct such studies is Sardinia, an island west of mainland Italy. Individuals living in Sardinia were traditionally geographically and socially isolated *(49–51)*. There is evidence to suggest increased inbreeding in Sardinia *(51,52)* and small and stable populations *(53)*. These factors are believed to produce greater genetic homogeneity and increased linkage disequilibrium, both of which are useful for gene-mapping studies *(54)*. All of these factors have been well documented previously *(55–60)*. However, what has not been previously reported is that, as illustrated in Fig. 5, there appears to be an overrepresentation of extreme thinness among Sardinians *(61)*. Thus, Sardinia may offer unique opportunities to study genetics of obesity resistance or thinness.

4. WHAT ABOUT ENVIRONMENT?

The recent and substantial rise in the prevalence of obesity clearly illustrates the importance of environmental influences on human obesity *(62,63)*. Particularly noteworthy is the fact that the increase in obesity appears to be focused on the upper end of the BMI distribution *(64;* Fig. 6), which suggests the possibility that genetically susceptible individuals are being pushed to ever greater degrees of obesity by an obesegenic environment, and less susceptible individuals remain relatively unaffected by the obesegenic environment. That broad-sweeping environmental changes may have a substantial impact on human biology is suggested by the increase in human stature over the past 2000 yr, and the decline in female age of menarche since 1800 *(65)*.

The potentially profound impact that the environment can have on individuals within the population can be seen by examining MZ twins that are discordant for obesity. For example, the authors' laboratory has studied one pair of 47-yr-old twins in which one twin had a BMI of 22 and the other twin had a BMI of 33. Assuming no somatic mutations, this difference is presumably environmental in origin (however, for alternative explanations, *see* ref. *66*). Another example showing the profound effect of the environment involves the Pima Indians of Arizona, one of the most obese populations in the world *(67)*. Recently, a tribe of related Pima Indians of similar descent were discovered in rural Mexico *(68)*. These Mexican Pima Indians lead an extremely rural lifestyle, and have few of the comforts of modern technology. In contrast to their counterparts in Arizona, the Pima Indians in Mexico have only modest rates of obesity and a mean BMI that is approximately equal to that seen among white Americans.

With respect to the specific environmental variables that may promote obesity in the population, decreased physical activity appears to play a role. Consider the amount of hours per day spent carrying water by women in third-world countries *(69)*. In Senegal, women spend an average of 2.5 h/d carrying water, clearly a vigorous physical activity. Even in Nepal, the average amount of time spent carrying water is approx 15 min/d, which is more vigorous physical activity than many Americans get. Moreover, carrying water is surely one of many vigorous physical activities conducted each day by individuals living in developing countries. The advent of modern technology has reduced the need to engage in physical activity, and, therefore, increased the ability to gain weight. One way to see the effects of modern Western lifestyle on the development of obesity is by examining differential obesity rates among immigrants to the United States and subsequent generations of their offspring. Individuals immigrating from parts of the world with lower rates of obesity than the United States (e.g., China, Japan) develop greater rates of obesity than members of the same national and ethnic groups who stay in the original country. In turn, the second generation offspring of such immigrants tend to have higher obesity rates than their parents born overseas. The third-generation offspring of these immigrants have even higher obesity rates *(70,71)*.

Finally, clarification of the nature and magnitude of environmental influences comes from behavioral genetic studies *(3)*. Such studies can tell about genetic effects, but they also tell us about the magnitude of environmental effects, whether they tend to be shared or unshared environmental influences, the extent to which these environmental influences have enduring or transitory impacts, and, in some cases, even what these specific environmental influences may be. For example, Fabsitz et al. *(19)* followed male twins from the age of approx 18 yr for the next 43 yr of adult life, during which time they obtained four BMI measurements on subjects. They examined the extent to which the genetic and environmental influences on BMI at one point in time had an enduring impact on BMI throughout adult life, or, in contrast, were more transient in their impact. This suggests that the majority of the tracking of BMI across the life-span results from the influence of a constant genotype across the life-span, and environmental influences seem to be more transient. Similar results were reported from the Colorado adoption project among young children *(72)*. Together, these data suggest that if one wishes to prevent obesity through environmental manipulations in current society, one must make changes to individuals' environments throughout life, and not only during childhood.

5. WHAT IS THE ROLE OF BEHAVIOR?

Individual variations in behavior, primarily food-intake and physical-activity behaviors, are believed to play a crucial role in promoting human obesity. Do data on the substantial heritability of obesity contradict this? The answer is no. Although earlier data suggested that obese people, on average, ate no more and, in fact, slightly fewer calories per day than did nonobese people (73), such conclusions were based on self-reported food-intake data. More recent studies, using doubly labeled water, a validated biochemical technique for determining energy expenditure (74), and thereby energy intake, have consistently shown that obese individuals clearly consume more calories per day, on average, than do nonobese individuals (74).

Thus, despite a strong genetic component to obesity, there is also a strong behavioral component. These two factors are not in conflict, and may in fact be quite overlapping. Consider the case of the ob/ob mouse, which becomes massively obese as the result of being homozygous for a recessive mutation in the leptin gene. Because of this mutation, the animal produces no leptin, behaves as though it were starving, eats voraciously, and gains weight to a level that is 2–3× that of its normal litter mates. However, if these same animals are pair-fed the same amount of food as their lean littermates, they will have relatively normal body wt that are only slightly elevated above that of the normal control animals (75). This illustrates how a genetically obese animal can achieve its ultimate weight mostly through ingestive behavior. However, it should also be noted that, despite being roughly normal in body wt, those ob/ob mice that are pair-fed to the levels of normal control mice still tend to have an abnormally large proportion of their body mass as adipose tissue (75), indicating that the effect of genotype depends on the manner in which the phenotype is operationalized.

6. SPECIFIC GENES

It is one thing to state that BMI has a strong genetic component, but another to say that there are specific genes that have an important independent effect on BMI. Is there indeed any evidence that such genes exist? Such evidence is available and comes from several sources. The first source is from murine models of obesity that are based on the effects of single major genes (76). Initially, five major obesity genes that were known to exist in mice were cloned in the early 1990s. The first such gene cloned was the agouti gene, which produces both yellow coat color and massive obesity in mice (77). Subsequently, in 1994, Friedman et al. (78) reported the cloning of the ob gene, now called the leptin gene or Lep, and its protein product, leptin (leptin derives from the Greek "leptos," meaning thin). Shortly thereafter, Tartaglia et al. (79) reported cloning the db gene, now referred to as ob receptor or lep-r. This is the gene producing the db syndrome in mice, which results from a homozygous mutation in the leptin receptor gene, rendering the leptin receptor nonfunctional. Because animals that are homozygous for this mutation cannot receive the signal of leptin, they function as though they have no leptin, despite high circulating levels. Therefore, animals (and humans) with leptin receptor mutations essentially recapitulate the phenotypic features of animals with leptin mutations. The gene in which a mutation produces the db (db for diabetes) syndrome in mice turned out to be the same gene in which mutations produce obesity in the Zucker fatty rat. That is, the same gene producing massive obesity in mice was shown, when mutated, to produce massive obesity in rats. The two other genes that were members of the original "big five" were the fat gene (now called carboxypeptidase E [CPE]), cloned in 1996 by Noben-Trauth et al. (80), and the Tubby (tub) gene cloned by Kleyn et al. (81). The tub and fat mutations are interesting because they produce, relative to mutations in the leptin and leptin receptor genes, relatively mild forms of obesity with slower onset, which more closely parallel much human obesity. The exact role that these genes play in human obesity is not clear. It now appears that at least one human Tubby-like homolog is in fact a gene for retinitis pigmentosa *(82)*. This may not be too surprising, because the Tubby mouse, in addition to becoming obese, also develops retinal and cochlear degeneration. These five syndromes (ob, db, agouti, fat, and Tubby) were the original "big five" mutations identified in mice, but numerous other genes have now been identified in mice, which, when disrupted, can lead to marked obesity or obesity resistance. These genes include the *melancortin-4 receptor (83), ICAM-1 (84), mahogany (44), PTP-1B (43)*, and others.

Genetic influences in animals are not limited to mice and rats. Consider the case of the myostatin gene, i.e., a gene for body composition and leanness. It is, so to speak, an antiobesity gene that was first realized to have this effect when it was being studied by a team at Johns Hopkins University *(39)*, who observed that the myostatin gene appeared to be expressed at various developmental phases of the life-span in which muscle growth and formation was under way. They suspected that knocking out this gene would produce an animal that had no muscle and was not viable. They conducted the crucial experiment of knocking out the myostatin gene, only to find that they had produced a mouse that was not only viable, but also massively muscled. Shortly thereafter, it was discovered that this gene may well be the long-sought-after double-muscling gene in cattle.

Certain strains of cattle, such as the Belgian Blue, had evidenced a spontaneous mutation that led to marked hypertrophy of lean tissue and minimal accretion of adipose tissue, i.e., cows that look like body builders. Upon examination, it became clear that the myostatin gene, which, when knocked out, produced massive muscling in mice, was the very same gene responsible for double-muscling in cattle *(85)*. This shows that genes for body composition can have important effects, not just, evolutionarily speaking, from mice to rats, but from mice through cows.

In addition, evidence for major genes influencing adiposity in other species, such as pigs *(86)* and sheep *(85)*, have also been reported. The report by Cockett et al. *(85)* on the callipyge sheep is especially interesting. Although this gene has yet to be cloned, it has been determined that mutations in this gene can produce a phenotype in sheep characterized by extreme leanness and muscle hypertrophy in the gluteus muscles and longismus dorsi. This hypertrophy gives the sheep very large, well-muscled, lean hind quarters, which, again, for ranchers, is a very desirable thing. An ordinary sheep is typically slaughtered at approx 120 lb, at which point it is already beginning to get somewhat fatty. In contrast, a callipyge sheep can often be fed to 150 pounds and slaughtered, at which point it is still fairly lean. Callipyge derives its name from the Greek words "calli" meaning beautiful and "pyge" meaning buttocks. The callipyge gene is interesting, because it is a gene for both body composition (i.e., leanness) and the anatomic distribution of body mass, which may have independent effects on health *(87)*. It is also especially interesting because of its pattern of inheritance. The callipyge phenotype is both imprinted and inherited in an overdominant fashion. By "imprinted" is meant that the effect of inheriting the mutant allele depends on the sex of the parent contributing that allele to the offspring. If a sheep inherits a callipyge allele from the ewe (mother), it will express a normal phenotype. In contrast, if a sheep inherits that same allele from the ram (father), then it will express the callipyge phenotype. By "overdominant" is meant that the callipyge phenotype is only expressed when the callipyge allele is inherited in heterozygous form. Animals receiving one, and only one, callipyge allele will express the callipyge phenotype. This points out the potential complexity that confronts study of the genetic influences on body composition.

6.1. Specific Genes in Humans

There is reason to believe that single genes can have considerable influence on obesity in humans. One source of evidence for this comes from rare syndromes that are caused by single genetic anomalies, such as Prader-Willi syndrome, a disorder resulting from an anomaly of chromosome (chr) 15. In approx 70% of cases, there is a deletion of chr material on the long (q11-q13) arm of chr 15; other cases derive from unipaternal disomy (i.e., two maternal copies of 15q and no paternal copies) *(88–90)*. Like the callipyge phenotype in sheep, the Prader-Willi phenotype is imprinted so that the phenotype is expressed only if the abnormal chr is inherited from the father. An individual inheriting what appears to be the same chr abnormality from the mother will not express Prader-Willi syndrome, but will instead express Angelman syndrome, a syndrome associated with profound mental retardation and normal body wt. A variety of other rare disorders, typically associated with mental retardation, have been reported to be inherited in Mendelian fashion *(91)*.

Further evidence for major genetic influences in humans comes through examination of the distribution of phenotypes such as BMI. If a phenotype were influenced by many genes and environmental influences of small effect, it would tend to have a normal distribution, following from the central limit theorem *(92)*. If a trait has a clearly nonnormal distribution, this implies the possibility that it is being influenced by specific genes with major effects. Therefore, it is noteworthy that the distribution of BMI is decidedly nonnormal (positively skewed), suggesting the possible mixture of several component normal distributions, each with an underlying distinct genotype. Numerous co-mingling analyses (e.g., ref. *93*) have shown that the observed distribution of BMI is consistent with such co-mingling.

Additional evidence for the possibility of major genes comes from linkage studies *(94)*, e.g., Comuzzie et al. *(95)*, Hager et al. *(96)*, Lee et al. *(97)*, and Norman et al. *(98)* have reported linkages with degrees of statistical significance that offer clear evidence for genes of major effect on obesity. The exact identity of these genes cannot yet be determined from these linkage studies.

Finally, perhaps the strongest evidence for obesity-promoting genes comes from the identification of individuals in whom obesity appears to result from a specific genetic anomaly. To date, just over 20 such individuals have been reported (*see* Table 4; *99–106*), and a number of other cases that one might more tentatively attribute to single gene effects can also be found (e.g., *107–109*). Virtually all of the genes listed in Table 4 were postulated *a priori* to play a role in obesity, based on research with rodent models.

9. CONCLUSION AND RECOMMENDATIONS

The past several decades of research have revealed strong genetic influences on body wt and composition in humans and other animals. Moreover, by finding rare cases of humans whose obesity results from specific mutations, a new era of treatment is beginning, based on knowledge of the underlying physiology. Consider the few cases of obesity caused by mutations of the leptin gene *(100,101)*. For these individuals, administration of exogenous leptin would seem to be the treatment of choice. In fact, such treatment has been applied to at least one of the individuals with these mutations, with excellent results *(110)*. Alternatively, although perhaps more disappointing for the clinician and patient, such knowledge also at times shows what not to do. Consider the case

Table 4

Ref	Gene	N Fam.	N Cases	Comments
Jackson et al. (99)	prohormone convertase 1 (PC1)	1	1	Apparently involved in same pathway as CPE (FAT)
Montague et al. (100)	OB (Lep)	1	2	Massively obese young children. Leptin is (theoretically) the tx of choice.
Strobel et al. (101)	OB (Lep)	1	3	Two were adults that never reached puberty.
Clement et al. (102)	OB-R (Lep-R)	1	3	No apparent onset of puberty. Leptin should (theoretically) have no effect.
Krude et al. (103)	POMC (pre-pro-opiomelanocortin)	2	2	Children (< age 8) with weight > 97th %ile and red hair
Ristow et al. (104)	PPARγ2	4	4	Morbid obesity w/ relatively low insulin. Mutation effective in heterozygous form.
Yeo et al. (105)	MC4R	1	2	Father & son w/ morbid obesity & marked hyperphagia. Mutation effective in heterozygous form.
Vaisse et al. (106)	MC4R	1	6	Mutation effective in heterozygous form.

of the three individuals with mutations in the leptin receptor gene *(102)*. It is unclear exactly what should be done for these individuals, but certainly leptin is not a reasonable treatment for them. They can then be spared any expense, discomfort, and possible side effects of leptin treatment, because it is known *a priori* that they do not have the ability to be responsive to it.

The past several decades of research have yielded enormous information on the genetic and environmental influences on obesity, thinness, and body wt regulation in humans. Although a great deal more is yet to be learned, progress has been outstanding, and we may be poised on the verge of true revolutions in clinical treatments based on increased molecular knowledge. At the same time, behavioral genetic studies clearly demonstrate the profound impact that the environment has on variations in adiposity, both within and across populations. If we are to be responsive to the obesity problem that the population has as a whole, the environment must be changed to become less obesegenic and more promoting of healthy diets and activity patterns.

REFERENCES

1. Comuzzie AG, Allison DB. The search for human obesity genes. Science 1998; 280:1374–1377.
2. Knott SA, Marklund L, Haley CS, Andersson K, Davies W, Ellegren H, et al. Multiple marker mapping of quantitative trait loci in a cross between outbred wild boar and large white pigs. Genetics 1998; 149:1069–1080.
3. Plomin R, DeFries JC, McClearn GE, Rutter M. Behavioral Genetics (3rd ed.) New York: Freeman, 1997.
4. Blott SC, Williams JL, Haley CS. Genetic variation within the Hereford breed of cattle. Animal Genet 1998; 29:202–211.
5. Levin BE, Keesey RE. Defense of differing body weight set points in diet-induced obese and resistant rats. Am J Physiol 1998; 274:R412–419.
6. Galton F. Natural Inheritance. London: Macmillan, 1889.
7. Johnson RC, McClearn GE, Yuen S, Nagoshi CT, Ahearn FM, Cole RE. Galton's data a century later. Am Psychol 1985; 40:875–892.
8. Davenport CB. Body Build and Its Inheritance. Washington DC: Carnegie Institution of Washington, 1923.

9. Mason E. Obesity in pet dogs. Vet Rec 1970; 86:612–616.

10. Allison DB, Neale MC, Kezis MI, Alfonso VC, Heshka S, Heymsfield SB. Assortative mating for relative weight: genetic implications. Behav Genet 1996; 26:103–111.

11. Knuiman MW, Divitini ML, Bartholomew HC, Wellborn TA. Spouse correlations in cardiovascular risk factors and the effect of marriage duration. Am J Epidemiol 1996; 143:48–53.

12. Neale MC, Cardon LR. Methodology for Genetic Studies of Twins and Families. Dordrecht, Netherlands: Kluwer Academic, 1992.

13. Allison DB, Heshka S, Neale MC, Lykken DT, Heymsfield SB. A genetic analysis of relative weight among 4,020 twin pairs, with an emphasis on sex effects. Health Psychol 1994; 13:362–365.

14. Meyer JM. Genetic studies of obesity across the life span. In: Behavior Genetic Approaches to Behavioral Medicine. Turner JR, Cardon LR, Hewitt JK, eds. New York: Plenum, 1995; 145–166.

15. Sorenson TIA, Stunkard AJ. Overview of the adoption studies. In: The Genetics of Obesity. Bouchard C, ed. Boca Raton: CRC, 1994; 49–61.

16. Maes HHM, Neale MC, Eaves LJ. Genetic and environmental factors in and human adiposity. Behav Genet 1997; 27:325–351.

17. Scarr S, Carter-Saltzman L. Twin method: defense of a critical assumption. Behav Genet 1979; 9: 527–542.

18. Price RA. The case for single gene effects in human obesity. In: The Genetics of Obesity. Bouchard C, ed. Boca Raton: CRC, 1994; 93–107.

19. Fabsitz RR, Carmelli D, Hewitt JK. Evidence for independent genetic influences on obesity in middle age. Int J Obes 1992; 16:657–666.

20. Heitmann BL. The influence of fatness, weight change, slimming history and other lifestyle variables on diet reporting in Danish men and women aged 35–65. Int J Obes 1999; 17:329–336.

21. Lykken DT, McGue M, Tellegen A, Bouchard TJ. Emergenesis. Genetic traits that may not run in families. Am Psychol 1992; 47:1565–1577.

22. Stunkard AJ, Harris JR, Pedersen NL, McLearn GE. The body-mass index of twins who have been reared apart. N Engl J Med 1990; 322:1483–1487.

23. Price RA, Gottesman II. Body fat in identical twins reared apart: roles for genes and environment. Behav Genet 1991; 21:1–7.

24. Allison DB, Kaprio J, Korkeila M, Koskenvuo M, Neale MC, Hayakawa K. The heritability of body mass index among an international sample of monozygotic twins reared apart. Int J Obes Related Metab Disord 1996; 20:501–506.

25. Allison DB, Faith MS. A proposed heuristic for communicating heritability estimates to the general public, with obesity as an example. Behav Genet 1997; 27:441–445.

26. Margo RA. Union Army Slave Appraisal Records from Mississippi, 1863–1865. Ann Arbor, MI: Inter-university Consortium for Political and Social Research, 1991.

27. Sichieri R, Everhart JE, Hubbard VS. Relative weight classifications in the assessment of underweight and overweight in the United States. Int J Obes Related Metab Dis 1992; 16:303–312.

28. Hewitt JK. The genetics of obesity: what have genetic studies told us about the environment. Behav Genet 1997; 27:353–358.

29. Allison DB, Faith MS, Nathan JS. Risch's lambda statistic for human obesity. Int J Obes 1996; 20: 990–999.

30. Grilo CM, Pogue-Geile MF. The nature of environmental influences on weight and obesity: a behavior genetic analysis. Psychol Bull 1991; 110:520–537.

31. Laskarzewski PM, Khoury P, Morrison JA, Kelly K, Mellies MJ, Glueck CJ. Familial obesity and leanness. Int J Obes 1983; 7:505–527.

32. Todorov AA, Siegmund KD, Genin E, Rao DC. Power of the affected sib-pair method in the presence of environmental factors. Genet Epidemiol 1997; 14:541.

33. Alison DB, Zannolli R. Analyses of the ISTAT (unpublished data). ISTAT, Istituto Nazionale di Statistica. Indagine Multiscopo sulle Famiglie. Quinto Ciclo, 1987–1991.

34. Ravussin E, Bogardus C. Personal communication, 1997.

35. Udry R, Popkin B. Analysis of The National Longitudinal Study of Adolescent Health (Add Health); 1997.

36. Chakravarti A, Puffenberger E, Allison DB. Calculated from raw data.

37. Levin BE, Dunn-Meynell AA, Balkan B, Keesey RE. Selective breeding for diet-induced obesity and resistance in Sprague-Dawley rats. Am J Physiol 1997; 273:R725–730.

38. Cummings DE, Brandon EP, Planas JV, Motamed K, Idzerda RL, McKnight GS. Genetically lean mice result from targeted disruption of the RII beta subunit of protein kinase A. Nature 1996; 382:622–626.

39. McPherron AC, Lee SJ. Double muscling in cattle due to mutations in the myostatin gene. Proc Natl Acad Sci 1997; 94:12,457–12,461.

40. Uysal KT, Wiesbrock SM, Marino MW, Hotamisligil GS. Protection from obesity-induced insulin resistance in mice lacking TNF-alpha function. Nature 1997; 389:610–614.

41. Deeb SS, Fajas L, Nemoto M, Pihlajamaki J, Mykkanen L, Kuusisto J, et al. A Pro12Ala substitution in PPARgamma2 associated with decreased receptor activity, lower body mass index and improved insulin sensitivity. Nat Genet 1998; 20:284–287.

42. Shimada M, Tritos NA, Lowell BB, Flier JS, Maratos-Flier E. Mice lacking melanin-concentrating hormone are hypophagic and lean. Nature 1998; 396:670–674.

43. Elchebly M, Payette P, Michaliszyn E, Cromlish W, Collins S, Loy AL, et al. Increased insulin sensitivity and obesity resistance in mice lacking the protein tyrosine phosphatase-1B gene. Science 1999; 283:1544–1548.

44. Nagle DL, McGrail SH, Vitale J, Woolf EA, Dussault BJ Jr, DiRocco L, et al. The mahogany protein is a receptor involved in suppression of obesity. Nature 1999; 398:148–152.

45. Baker PC, Keck Mott F, Quinlan SV. NLSY Child Handbook, revised ed. Columbus, OH: Center for Human Resource Research, the Ohio State University, 1993.

46. Dawber TR. The Framingham Study. Cambridge: Harvard University Press, 1980.

47. Popkin BM, Paeratakul S, Ge K, Zhai F. Body weight patterns among the Chinese: results from the 1989 and 1991 China Health and Nutrition Surveys. Am J Public Health 1995; 85:690–694.

48. Popkin BM, Zohoori N, Baturin A. The nutritional status of the elderly in Russia, 1992–1994. Am J Public Health 1996; 86:355–360.

49. Lopasic A. Family and economy among the Sardinian Shepherds (1986–1988). Acta Ethnographica Acad Sci Hung 1988; 34:217–227.

50. Vona G, Calo CM, Lucia G, Mameli GE, Succa V, Esteban E, Moral P. Genetics, geography, and culture: the population of S. Pietro Island (Sardinia, Italy). Am J Phys Anthropol 1996; 100:461–471.

51. Vona G, Francalacci P, Paoli G, Latini V, Salis M. Study of the matrimonial structure of the population of central Sardinia (Italy). Anthropol Anz 1996; 54:317–329.

52. McCullough JM, O'Rourke DH. Geographic distribution of consanguinity in Europe. Ann Hum Biol 1986; 13:359–367.

53. Workman PL, Lucarelli P, Agostino R, Scarabino R, Scacchi R, Carapella E, Palmarino R, Bottini E. Genetic differentiation among Sardinian villages. Am J Phys Anthropol 1975; 43:165–176.

54. Chapman NH, Wijsman EM. Genome screens using linkage disequilibrium tests: optimal marker characteristics and feasibility. Am J Hum Genet 1998; 63:1872–1875.

55. Caglia A, Novelletto A, Dobosz M, Malaspina P, Ciminelli BM, Pascali VL. Y-chromosome STR loci in Sardinia and continental Italy reveal islander-specific haplotypes. Eur J Hum Genet 1997; 5:288–292.

56. Piazza A, Mayr WR, Contu L, Amoroso A, Borelli I, Curtoni ES, et al. Genetic and population structure of four Sardinian villages. Ann Hum Genet 1985; 49:47–63.

57. Piazza A, Cappello N, Olivetti E, Rendine S. A genetic history of Italy. Ann Hum Genet 1988; 52:203–213.

58. Rendine S, Borelli I, Barbanti M, Sacchi N, Roggero S, Curtoni ES. HLA polymorphisms in Italian bone marrow donors: a regional analysis. Tissue Antigens 1998; 52:135–146.

59. Sartoris S, Varetto O, Migone N, Capello N, Piazza A, Ferrara GB, Ceppellini R. Mitochondrial DNA polymorphism in four Sardinian villages. Ann Hum Genet 1988; 52:327–340.

60. Vona G, Bitti PP, Succa V, Mameli GE, Salis M, Secchi G, Calo CM. HLA phenotype and haplotype frequencies in Sardinia (Italy). Coll Antropol 1997; 21:461–475.

61. Allison DB, Zannolli R. Based on unpublished data from the ISTAT. (ISTAT, Istituto Nazionale di Statistica. Indagine Multiscopo sulle Famiglie. Quinto Ciclo, 1987–1991).

62. Kuczmarski RJ, Flegal KM, Campbell SM, Johnson CL. Increasing prevalence of overweight among US adults. The National Health and Nutrition Examination Surveys, 1960 to 1991. JAMA 1994; 272:205–211.

63. Centers for Disease Control and Prevention. Update: Prevalence of Overweight Among Children, Adolescents, and Adults—United States, 1988–1994. MMWR 1997; 46(9).

64. Taubes G. As obesity rates rise, experts struggle to explain why. Science 1998; 280:1367–1368.

65. Heymsfield SB, Pietrobelli A. Morbid obesity: the price of progress. Endocr Pract 1997; 3:320–323.

66. Hall JG. Twinning: mechanisms and genetic implications. Curr Opin Genet Dev 1996; 6:343–347.

67. Sakul H, Pratley R, Cardon L, Ravussin E, Mott D, Bogardus C. Familiarity of physical and metabolic characteristics that predict the development of non-insulin-dependent diabetes mellitus in Pima Indians. Am J Hum Genet 1997; 60:651–656.

68. Ravussin E, Valencia ME, Esparza J, Bennett PH, Schulz LO. Effects of a traditional lifestyle on obesity in Pima Indians. Diabetes Care 1994; 17:1067–1074.
69. Ferro-Luzzi A, Martino L. Obesity and physical activity. In: The Origins and Consequences of Obesity. Chadwick DJ, Cardew G, eds. England: John Wiley, 1996; 207–227.
70. Curb DJ, Marcus EB. Body fat and obesity in Japanese Americans. Am J Clin Nutr 1991; 53:1552S–1555S.
71. Popkin BM, Udry JR. Adolescent obesity increases significantly in second and third generation U.S. immigrants: the National Longitudinal Study of Adolescent Health. J Nutr 1998; 128: 701–706.
72. Cardon LR. Genetic influences on body mass index in early childhood. In: Behavior Genetic Approaches in Behavioral Medicine. Turner JR, Cardon LR, Hewitt JK, eds. New York: Plenum, 1995; 133–143.
73. Wooley SC, Wooley OW, Dyrenforth SR. Theoretical, practical, and social issues in behavioral treatments of obesity. J Appl Behav Anal 1979; 12:3–25.
74. Schoeller DA. How accurate is self-reported dietary energy intake? Nutr Rev 1990; 48:373–387.
75. Bray GA. Mechanisms for development of genetic, hypothalamic, and dietary obesity. In: Pennington Center Nutrition Series: Molecular and Genetic Aspects of Obesity, Vol. 5. Bray GA, Ryan DA, eds. Baton Rouge, LA: Louisiana State University Press, 1996; 3–66.
76. Chua SC Jr. Monogenic models of obesity. Behav Genet 1997; 27:277–284.
77. Miltenberger RJ, Mynatt RL, Wilkinson JE, Woychik RP. The role of the agouti gene in the yellow obese syndrome. J Nutr 1997; 127:1902S–1907S.
78. Zhang Y, Proenca R, Maffei M, Barone M, Leopold L, Friedman JM. Positional cloning of the mouse obese gene and its human homologue. Nature 1994; 372:425–432.
79. Tartaglia L, Dembski M, Weng X, Deng N, Culpepper J, Devos R, et al. Identification and cloning of a leptin receptor, OB-r. Cell 1995; 83:1263–1271.
80. Noben-Trauth K, Naggert JK, North MA, Nishina PM. A candidate gene for the mouse mutation tubby. Nature 1996; 380:534–538.
81. Kleyn PW, Fan W, Kovats SG, Lee JJ, Pulido JC, Wu Y, et al. Identification and characterization of the mouse obesity gene tubby: a member of a novel gene family. Cell 1996; 85:281–290.
82. Banerjee P, Kleyn PW, Knowles JA, Lewis CA, Ross BM, Parano E, et al. TULP1 mutation in two extended Dominican kindreds with autosomal recessive retinitis pigmentosa. Nat Genet 1998; 18: 177–179.
83. Yeo GS, Farooqi IS, Aminian S, Halsall DJ, Stanhope RG, O'Rahilly S. A frameshift mutation in MC4R associated with dominantly inherited human obesity. Nat Genet 1998; 20:111–112.
84. Dong ZM, Gutierrez-Ramos JC, Coxon A, Mayadas TN, Wagner DD. A new class of obesity genes encodes leukocyte adhesion receptors. Proc Natl Acad Sci USA 1997; 94:7526–7530.
85. Cockett NE, Jackson SP, Shay TL, Farnir F, Berghmans S, Snowder GD, Nielsen DM, Georges M. Polar overdominance at the ovine callipyge locus. Science 1996; 273:236–238.
86. Andersson L, Haley CS, Ellegren H, Knott SA, Johansson M, Andersson K, et al. Genetic mapping of quantitative trait loci for growth and fatness in pigs. Science 1994; 263:1771–1774.
87. Vague J. La Différentiation, sexuelle, facteur déterminant des formes de l'obésité. Presse Médicale 1947; 55:339–340.
88. Butler MG. Prader Willi Syndrome: current understanding of cause and diagnosis. Am J Med Genet 1990; 35:319–332.
89. Butler MG, Palmer CG. Parental origin of chromosome 15 deletion in Prader Willi syndrome. Lancet 1983; 1285–1286.
90. Nicholls RD, Glenn CC, Jong MTC, Saitoh S, Mascari MJ, Driscoll DJ. Molecular pathogenesis of Prader-Willi syndrome. In: Molecular and Genetic Aspects of Obesity. Bray GA, Ryan DH, eds. Baton Rouge, LA: Louisiana State University Press, 1996; 560–577.
91. Allison DB, Packer-Munter W, Pietrobelli A, Alfonso VC, Faith MS. Obesity and developmental disabilities: pathogenesis and treatment. J Dev Phys Dis 1998; 10:215–255.
92. Schork NJ, Allison DB, Thiel B. Mixture distributions in human genetics research. Stat Methods Med Res 1996; 5:155–178.
93. Allison DB, Heshka S, Gorman BS, Heymsfield SB. Evidence of commingling in human eating behavior. Obes Res 1993; 1:339–344.
94. Allison DB, Heo M. Meta-analysis of linkage data under worst-case conditions: a demonstration using the human *OB* region. Genetics 1998; 148:859–865.

95. Comuzzie A, Hixson J, Almasy L, Mitchell BD, Mahaney MC, Dyer TD, et al. A major quantitative trait locus determining serum leptin levels and fat mass is located on human chromosome 2. Nat Genet 1997; 15:273–276.

96. Hager J, Dina C, Francke S, Dubois S, Houari M, Vatin V, et al. A genome-wide scan for human obesity genes reveals a major susceptibility locus on chromosome 10. Nat Genet 1998; 20:304–308.

97. Lee JH, Reed DR, Li WD, Xu W, Joo EJ, Kilker RL, et al. Genome scan for human obesity and linkage markers in 20q13. Am J Hum Genet 1999; 64:196–209.

98. Norman RA, Tataranni PA, Pratley R, Thompson DB, Hanson RL, Prochazka M, et al. Autosomal genomic scan for loci linked to obesity and energy metabolism in Pima Indians. Am J Hum Genet 1988; 62:659–668.

99. Jackson RS, Creemers JW, Ohagi S, Raffin-Sanson ML, Sanders L, Montague CT, Hutton JC, O'Rahilly S. Obesity and impaired prohormone processing associated with mutations in the human prohormone convertase 1 gene. Nat Genet 1997; 16:303–306.

100. Montague CT, Faroqi IS, Whitehead JP, Soos MA, Rau H, Wareham NJ, et al. Congenital leptin deficiency is associated with severe early-onset obesity in humans. Nature 1997; 387:903–908.

101. Strobel A, Issad T, Camoin L, Ozata M, Stosberg AD. A leptin missense mutation associated with hypogonadism and morbid obesity. Nat Genet 1998; 18:213–215.

102. Clement K, Vaisse C, Lahlou N, Cabrol S, Pelloux V, Cassuto D, et al. A mutation in the human leptin receptor gene causes obesity and pituitary dysfunction. Nature 1998; 392:398–401.

103. Krude H, Biebermann H, Luck W, Horn R, Brabant G, Gruters A. Severe early-onset obesity, adrenal insufficiency and red hair pigmentation caused by POMC mutations in humans. Nat Genet 1998; 19:155–157.

104. Ristow M, Muller-Wieland D, Pfeiffer A, Krone W, Kahn CR. Obesity associated with a mutation in a genetic regulator of adipocyte differentiation. N Engl J Med 1998; 339:953–959.

105. Yeo GS, Farooqi IS, Aminian S, Halsall DJ, Stanhope RG, O'Rahilly S. A frameshift mutation in MC4R associated with dominantly inherited human obesity. Nat Genet 1998; 20:111–112.

106. Vaisse C, Clement K, Guy-Grand B, Froguel P. A frameshift mutation in human MC4R is associated with a dominant form of human obesity. Nat Genet 1998; 20:113–114.

107. Gu W, Tu Z, Kleyn PW, Kissebah A, Duprat L, Lee J, et al. Identification and functional analysis of novel human melanocortin-4 receptor variants. Diabetes 1999; 48:635–639.

108. Nothen MM, Cichon S, Hemmer S, Hebebrand J, Remschmidt H, Lehmkuhl G, et al. Human dopamine D4 receptor gene: frequent occurrence of a null allele and observation of homozygosity. Hum Mol Genet 1994; 3:2207–2212.

109. Pérusse L, Chagnon YC, Weisnagel J, Bouchard C. The human obesity gene map: the 1998 update. Obes Res 1999; 7:111–129.

110. Faroqi IS, Jebb S, Cook G, Cheetham CH, Lawrence E, Prentice A, et al. Treatment of congenital leptin deficiency in man. Presentation at the Eighth International Congress of Obesity, Paris, 1998; (Abstract).

10   Obesity and Insulin Resistance in Childhood and Adolescence

Erik Bergström and Olle Hernell

1. OBESITY

The objective of this review is to examine certain aspects of obesity in children and adolescents. This chapter focuses particularly on the etiology and pathology of insulin resistance (IR), but also discusses possible preventive measures.

1.1. Epidemiology

Obesity is an increasing health problem in both industrialized and developing countries. In developing countries, obesity co-exists with undernutrition, with prevalence rates higher in urban than in rural populations. Women generally have higher rates of obesity than men in both developed and developing countries. In adults, obesity is associated with increased mortality and morbidity (M&M) in a number of diseases, the most common being cardiovascular diseases (CVD) and noninsulin dependent diabetes mellitus (NIDDM) *(1)*.

1.2. Etiology

Obesity is the consequence of an energy imbalance in which energy intake has exceeded energy expenditure over considerable time. The amount of stored energy equals the difference between energy intake and energy expenditure, i.e., resting metabolic rate and physical activity. Although it is evident that obese individuals eat more than they need, there is increasing evidence to support the idea that there are genetically determined metabolic differences between individuals who gain extensive weight and those who do not *(2–4)*.

1.2.1. REGULATION OF BODY WT

Body wt is regulated by complex interactions of endocrine and neural signals from adipose tissue and the endocrine, neural, and gastrointestinal systems (Fig. 1). Afferent neural (vagal and cholinergic) and hormonal stimuli (insulin, cholecystokinin, leptin, glucocorticoids [GCs]) related to metabolic status are received in the hypothalamus, where they modulate the release of peptides known to affect food-intake and efferent signals to the hypothalamic–pituitary axis, resulting in energy expenditure and insulin release *(4)*. In the normal state, body wt is regulated so that energy expenditure equals energy intake. If energy intake exceeds expenditure for a long time period, the surplus of energy is stored as fat mass, and, if the energy imbalance continues, the result is obesity.

From: *Primary and Secondary Preventive Nutrition*
Edited by: A. Bendich and R. J. Deckelbaum © Humana Press Inc., Totowa, NJ

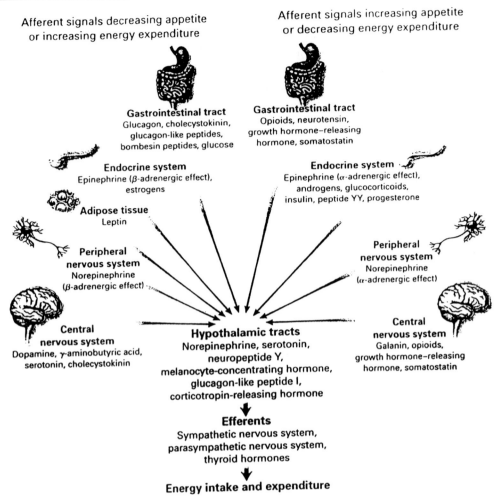

Fig. 1. Molecules that affect energy intake and expenditure. (Adapted with permission from ref. *4.*)

Once the obese state is established, the new weight appears to be defended, resulting in an involuntary, physiologically driven increase in energy intake and difficulties in loosing weight *(5)*.

1.2.2. GENETICS

During the past decade, it has become apparent that regulation of body wt is under strong genetic influence. Obesity, diabetes, and CVD aggregate in some families, but family members do not only share the same genes, but also, to various extent, the same environment and habits. However, studies on twins, adoptees, and families show a strong correlation between body wt of relatives, also, when they have not shared the same environment. The results indicate that as much as 80% of the variance in body mass index (BMI) may be attributable to genetic factors. The heritage of obesity is mediated through factors such as resting metabolic rate, changes in energy expenditure in response to overeating, lipoprotein lipase activity, maximal insulin-stimulated glyceride synthesis, basal rates of lipolysis, adipose tissue distribution, certain aspects of eating behavior, food preferences, and level of physical activity *(4,6)*. Although there are examples of cases of obesity in rodents, resulting from single-gene mutations in metabolic pathways, obesity in humans is rarely attributable to a single gene. Because disturbance of energy balance is the central pathology of obesity, the search for candidate genes has focused on those that have a role in energy metabolism, i.e., genes that program the β_3-adrenergic receptor, the glucocorticoid receptor, and Na^+/K^+-adenosine triphosphatase (ATPase), obesity syndromes in human, as well as obesity genes in rodents, e.g., genes coding for leptin and the leptin receptor, and genes involved in regulation of response to an obesity-promoting environment *(4,6,7)* (*see* Chapter 8).

1.2.3. THRIFTY GENOTYPE AND THRIFTY PHENOTYPE

Even if there seems to be a stronger genetic influence in the etiology of obesity than previously thought, epidemiological data showing large differences in obesity prevalence, and trends between countries demonstrate the additional contribution of environmental factors. This is further supported by variation in rates by ethnicity and socioeconomic status, and the shift in rates seen in migrant populations *(1)*. One hypothesis to explain the epidemics of lifestyle-related diseases, e.g., CVD and NIDDM, is the thrifty genotype. As stated by Neel, "Genes and combinations of genes which were at some time an asset may in the face of environmental change become a liability" *(8)*. An energy-saving genotype, and preference for energy-dense food, i.e., rich in fat and sugar, is a survival and reproductive advantage, given an environment with shortage of food, but not when confronted with the surplus of Western lifestyle and society. This hypothesis is given support by the absence of CVD and obesity in native populations still unaffected by Western lifestyle, and also by the fact that the highest obesity and NIDDM prevalences are found in populations that have undergone rapid alterations in lifestyle, e.g., Australian Aborigines, Native Americans, Pacific Islanders, and some migrant populations, such as Asian Indians *(1,9–11)*.

No doubt, the chief cause of NIDDM and CVD, besides genetics, is excess intake of food in adult life. Another hypothesis is that poor prenatal and infant nutrition, resulting in growth retardation, may predispose to development of atherosclerosis and other metabolic disturbances, such as IR and NIDDM later in life. This hypothesis has been named the "thrifty phenotype hypothesis" *(12)*. In the 1970s, reporting from Norway, Forsdahl *(13)* was the first to propose that fetal and infant exposures could influence the risk of subsequent adult chronic diseases, showing regional associations between infant mortality and CVD mortality in adults a generation later in the same regions. Later retrospective and ecological studies *(14–17)* have confirmed the associations between reduced physical growth in early life and CVD mortality in adulthood, extending this also to associations between poor fetal and infant growth and elevated serum lipids, higher blood pressure (BP), impaired glucose tolerance, higher fibrinogen levels, higher incidence of NIDDM, and also the metabolic syndrome. Other reports have shown that low birth wt (LBW), in conjunction with rapid childhood gain in weight, especially as subcutaneous fat, is associated with reduced glucose tolerance in childhood, and consequent increased susceptibility, making them susceptible to development of NIDDM later in life *(18–20)*. Further, stunted children seem to have a higher risk of developing obesity *(21)*. Contrasting with this are reports that adolescents with high serum insulin levels were heavier and taller at birth, during infancy, and childhood, compared to those with lower serum insulin values (Fig. 2; *22*). Possible explanations for this finding may be that high insulin values

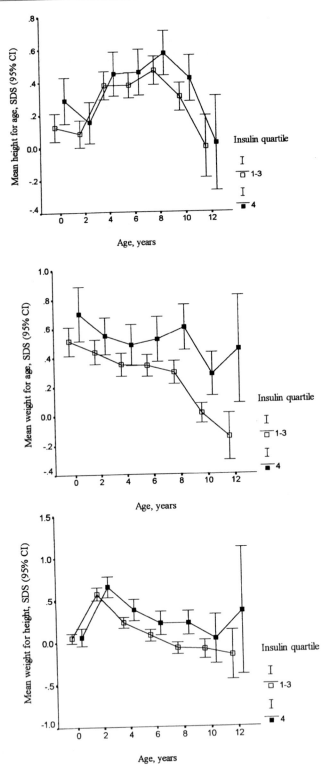

Fig. 2. Relationship between s-insulin levels in adolescence and previous attained heights and weights during infancy and childhood. (Adapted with permission from ref. 22.)

stimulate growth. Alternatively, tall and heavy children may have higher insulin values. A corresponding finding, also illustrating the positive association between physical growth and glucose metabolism, showed higher linear growth prior to the onset of insulin-dependent diabetes in children (23).

Referring to animal experiments, Barker (15) has proposed a biological explanation for the association between LBW and infant growth and later metabolic diseases, i.e., that fetal malnutrition may result in a permanent underdevelopment of certain organs, e.g., liver and pancreas, or alternatively, an early metabolic or nutritional programming. Both alternatives could result in difficulties in coping with a nutritional overload later in life. If fetal malnutrition results in increased risk of CVD, the low occurrence of adult CVD in developing countries, with concurrent malnutrition and high rates of intrauterine and infant growth retardation, may look paradoxical. This could, however, partly be explained by a shorter life-span in developing countries (too short for chronic diseases to appear) and by adult populations in these countries not yet having been exposed to nutritional overload. According to Barker (15), transition from nutritional insufficiency to nutritional overload may be particularly harmful. This mechanism could be an alternative, or additional, explanation to genetic susceptibility, for the rapid increase in obesity and CVD in native populations (15).

The molecular mechanisms underlying the suggested links between fetal and infant malnutrition and later metabolic disorders are unknown, but it has been demonstrated that supraphysiological doses of GCs retard fetal growth, and that human intrauterine growth retardation is associated with elevated cortisol levels. Exposing rats to excessive GCs *in utero* reduces birth wt and causes permanent hypertension in the adult offspring. Hence, GCs could be one link between LBW and later disease (24).

The programming hypothesis has been disputed; the main criticism being the lack of proper control for confounding by later dietary and other socially determined environmental factors (25). Even if the programming hypothesis suggests that experiences *in utero* or in early life may permanently affect the risk of developing CVD in adulthood, this hypothesis does not exclude that the risk may be affected also by environmental factors or lifestyle later in life.

1.3. Obesity in Childhood and Adolescence

Compared to adult obesity, it seems that obesity during childhood or adolescence, in its mild and moderate form, is less related to significant somatic health problems. The psychological and social consequences, i.e., poor self-esteem and peer problems, may, however, be severe (26). Obesity in childhood and adolescence tracks into adulthood, and is related to M&M in CVD in adult life (27). The association between childhood and adult obesity is rather weak, but increases with the age of the child, the degree of obesity, and the presence of a family history of obesity. Most infants and young children who are overweight become nonobese adults without treatment (28,29).

1.4. Assessment of Obesity

Several suggestions have been made on how to assess obesity in children, e.g., standard deviation (SD) scores of weight, weight:height ratios or indices, and skinfold measurements and ratios. All these anthropometric measurements depend on sex, age, and physical development of the individual. Because weight is closely related to height, it is necessary, when evaluating obesity, always to consider height and weight at the same time. The easiest way to judge if an individual is overweight or obese is simply by inspection.

The growth chart is the most commonly used instrument in the evaluation of obesity in children and adolescents (30). The weight of a child is considered normal if it falls between ±2 SD (SDs of the mean for the corresponding age and sex). If the weight exceeds height with +2–4 SD, the child is regarded as overweight, and as obese if the weight exceeds height with >4 SD. In adults, the BMI (kg/m²) has become the standard index for assessing obesity, and this index has become increasingly used also in children and adolescents. BMI values in children and adolescents need to be assessed using age-related reference curves. Such curves have been produced by a number of countries (31–33). When using BMI in developing countries, it is also important to consider the effect of stunting, because the lower height of the child results in a relatively higher BMI without presence of obesity.

The current lack of consistency and agreement between different studies on classification of obesity in children and adolescents makes it difficult to estimate global prevalence and trends of obesity for younger age groups. The only integrated data currently available are those compiled by the World Health Organization Program of Nutrition (9). Whatever classification system is used, studies investigating obesity during childhood and adolescence have reported increasing prevalence of obesity, illustrating that children and adolescents are part of the worldwide epidemic of obesity. Childhood obesity is not confined to industrialized countries (29,34,35).

1.5. Social Environment

Obesity is related to low socioeconomic status. The chief explanations are dietary and physical activity habits. To varying degrees, obesity is a social handicap (36). One explanation of the association between low socioeconomic status and obesity could be a downward social mobility of obese individuals, resulting in a higher prevalence of obesity in low socioeconomic groups. Social class differences, with higher CVD mortality in underprivileged groups of the population, have been demonstrated from most industrialized countries. The decline in CVD mortality seen in recent decades has not occurred in the lower social classes, which has resulted in widening social inequality (37). The difference in trends in smoking in different social classes is regarded as a major explanation of social differences in CVD mortality. Other social factors, e.g., lack of social network and social support, have an additional independent effect. Abdominal fat deposition is one result of what has been termed the "civilization syndrome." Stress, increased activity of the hypothalamic–pituitary–adrenal axis, increased cortisol levels, and a variety of current social situations have been linked to the increased prevalence of obesity and its metabolic consequences (38).

The mortality and health of young children seem to follow the pattern of their parents, with increasing mortality and health problems with decreasing socioeconomic status, but this pattern is less obvious in adolescence. In both boys and girls, low socioeconomic status and educational level of the parents are related to a greater prevalence of smoking, higher BMI, higher dietary fat intake, and, in girls, to lower physical fitness. The quality of the diet in the family relates to the educational level of the mother, with higher fat intake in families in which the mother has a low educational level (39).

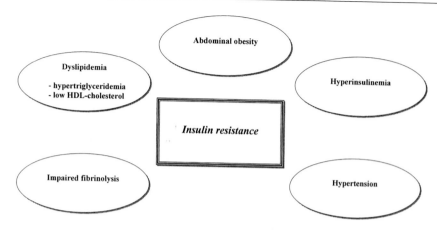

Fig. 3. Insulin resistance syndrome.

2. IR SYNDROME

The clinical entity of obesity, dyslipidemia, and hyperinsulinemia combined with hypertension, is sometimes called the "insulin resistance syndrome" or the "metabolic syndrome" (Fig. 3). The syndrome was first described in 1966 by Camus *(40)*, and popularized by Reaven in 1988 *(41)*. Although the pathogenesis of this syndrome is multifactorial, genetic factors, in combination with a sedentary lifestyle, including a high-energy diet, rich in saturated fat, and low physical activity leading to obesity, are regarded as major determinants *(40,41)*.

Obesity is related to increased cellular resistance to insulin, which in turn affects glucose and lipid metabolism, resulting in a secondary hyperglycemia, a compensatory hyperinsulinemia and dyslipidemia, i.e., hypertriglyceridemia and hypo-high-density lipoproteinemia (high-density lipoprotein [HDL] cholesterol). Insulin-stimulated glucose uptake and utilization in liver, skeletal muscle, and adipose tissue is impaired and coupled to impaired suppression of hepatic glucose output *(42–44)*. IR also affects the regulation of BP and the fibrinolysis system. The exact molecular mechanisms behind IR remain unclear, but there seems to be a genetic component. Changes in free fatty acids (FFAs) may be an important link between obesity and IR *(45–48)*. The metabolic disturbances caused by IR are related to increased risk of CVD and NIDDM. One important mechanism could be that IR leads to inadequate intracellular glucose concentration, which in turn leads to insufficient amounts of ATP, needed for ion transfer and energy-requiring reactions *(49)*. Degree of overweight, the change in weight, and the duration of overweight are all separate predictors of NIDDM. The metabolic syndrome seems to be more related to obesity than to heredity of IR, but it should also be noted that IR is related to CVD, regardless of obesity *(45,50,51)*.

2.1. Visceral Fat

The metabolic disturbances seen in the metabolic syndrome are especially related to abdominal obesity, or, more precisely, increased visceral fat, even in normal-weight individuals. Genes and/or familial nongenetic factors seem to influence both visceral fat mass and plasma insulin levels *(52–54)*.

2.2. Leptin

Leptin is the adipocyte-specific product of the *ob* gene (*Lep* gene). The leptin gene was first identified in the leptin-deficient, obese *ob/ob* mouse, by positional cloning technique *(55)*. The leptin receptor has at least five splice variants; the long form of the receptor is primarily expressed in the hypothalamus, and is thought to be the predominant signaling isoform. Leptin is synthesized in and secreted from adipose tissue, and is an afferent signal of fat stores to the brain, resulting in subsequent efferent signals to regulate food intake and whole-body energy expenditure via central and peripheral mechanisms. Leptin receptors are expressed in most tissues, and in vitro evidence suggests that leptin may have direct effects on some tissues, such as adipose tissue, the adrenal cortex, and the pancreatic β cells.

Mutations in the leptin, or leptin receptor genes, results in morbid obesity, infertility, and IR in rodents and humans, but most obese humans do not have any abnormalities in the gene coding sequences for leptin or the leptin receptor. Plasma leptin concentrations are increased in obese humans in direct proportion to body fat mass, and leptin is thought to influence whole-body glucose homeostasis and insulin action, and may be involved in the pathogenesis of the metabolic syndrome *(56–58)*.

Although leptin has been regarded as a critical link between somatic energy stores, on the one hand, and growth and fertility, on the other, the role of leptin in the pathogenesis and treatment of human obesity is still unclear. Current knowledge of leptin suggests that its primary role may be to indicate whether somatic fat stores are sufficient for growth and reproduction. If the fat stores are inadequate, as reflected by a decline in plasma leptin concentrations to a level below a threshold that may be genetically and developmentally set, the result is hyperphagia, low energy expenditure, and infertility. In contrast to this, increased levels of leptin have little or no physiologic effects, i.e., they do not result in hypophagia or hypermetabolism *(4)*.

2.3. Body Iron

Iron (Fe) deficiency is still a major health problem in many developing countries, but, in industrialized countries, an increasing concern regarding the potential hazards of body Fe excess has emerged. In high concentrations, Fe is toxic, with potentially negative health consequences, partly by being a pro-oxidant promoting formation of free radicals, which in turn increase pathological processes, such as oxidization of low-density lipoprotein cholesterol (LDL-C) *(59)*. There are no data to support the proposition that high Fe stores are beneficial. On the contrary, it has been claimed by Sullivan *(60)* that Fe stores constitute a sign of Fe excess, and therefore should be kept low. High levels of stored Fe, estimated as serum ferritin, have been reported to be associated with an increased risk of myocardial infarction in men, and also of cancer, but the evidence is controversial and inconclusive *(61–63)*. Differences in Fe stores between adult men and women have been suggested to contribute to the sex differences in CVD M&M *(64)*. If so, one explanation could be that large body Fe stores relate to high BMI, and thus to elevated blood glucose and insulin levels, suggesting that there may be a relationship between high Fe stores and obesity and IR *(65,66)*. Obesity in individuals with the iron-loading gene (genetic hemochromatosis) may therefore be particularly hazardous, and they are especially vulnerable to Fe overload *(67)*.

2.4. IR in Children and Adolescents

Information on the early stages of obesity-related IR in children and adolescents is scarce, but there is increasing evidence to support the view that the metabolic aberrations seen in the adult metabolic syndrome can be identified early in childhood and tracked into young adulthood (22,68,69). Heredity, as well as ethnicity, seem to have an impact, with a stronger effect of obesity on IR in black, compared to white, American adolescents (70). However, it is not yet known at what levels serum insulin or serum lipids, BP, or overweight increase the risk of later adult disease. Indices of obesity (BMI, skinfold, waist circumference), independent of age, correlate positively to serum insulin and an atherogenic serum lipid profile, i.e., high total cholesterol, high LDL-C, high triglycerides, and high apolipoprotein B and low HDL-C. Waist:hip or subscapular:triceps ratios seem to have no advantage to BMI or waist circumference measurement alone, as indicators of unfavorable metabolic or physiologic values. BMI and waist circumference are also easy to obtain, making these measurements particularly suitable for epidemiological studies (22,71; Table 1).

There are no available reference values for serum insulin in healthy children and adolescents. Serum insulin levels increase during puberty, probably resulting from a combination of higher secretion, reflecting a higher demand of insulin during the pubertal growth spurt, and increased cellular resistance to insulin (72). The physiological explanation for increased cellular resistance to insulin in puberty is, however, not known. Still, insulin is known to have a growth-hormone-like effect, and increased levels may result from increased secretion of insulin related to the pubertal growth spurt. At any given age, girls have higher values, compared to boys, probably reflecting differences in maturation (22). There is also an intraindividual diurnal variation in serum insulin, partly caused by variation in daily dietary intake. These variations make comparisons between different studies difficult. Insulin growth factor binding protein-1 level is strongly associated with insulin sensitivity, and may be a useful predictor for early identification of development of IR in prepubertal obese children (73).

3. TREATMENT AND PREVENTION

Despite various pharmacological and surgical therapies used over several decades, obesity continues to increase in both adults and children. Treatment of obesity is disappointing, with very few programs showing lasting weight reduction. Weight loss can, at least in the short term, act to decrease the risk of developing diabetes, by reducing IR, and thus relieving β-cell stress (50). The best concept is that treatment and prevention of obesity must focus on increasing physical activity and changing the diet (74–76). Also, in children, it is generally accepted that, besides genetics, characteristics of family life, e.g., diet, physical activity, and social support, are closely linked to the development and maintenance of obesity (77,78).

3.1. Diet

The increase in obesity in various populations is associated with a change to Western diet. Compared to traditional diets of native populations, such diet contains increased amounts of total fat, particularly animal fat, animal protein, and sugar, and decreased

Table 1
Associations Between Different Anthropometric Measurements and S-Insulin, S-Lipids, and Systolic Blood Pressure

	Insulin	TG	TC	HDL-C	LDL-C	Apo A-I	Apo B	Lp(a)	SBP
Boys									
Weight	.28[a]	.25[a]	.09	−.15[a]	.11[c]	−.11[c]	.16[a]	−.01	.18[a]
BMI	.36[a]	.28[a]	.15[a]	−.13[b]	.17[a]	−.06	.23[a]	.02	.16[a]
Waist circumference	.36[a]	.33[a]	.17[a]	−.16[a]	.17[a]	−.06	.24[a]	.00	.16[a]
Waist:hip ratio	.27[a]	.26[a]	.15[a]	−.12[b]	.18[a]	.02	.24[a]	−.01	.10[c]
Subscap skinfold	.38[a]	.33[a]	.17[a]	−.13[b]	.20[a]	−.02	.27[a]	.02	.09[c]
Subscap:triceps ratio	−.02	.09	.06	−.06	.04	−.08	.05	.00	.09[c]
Girls									
Weight	.24[a]	.14[b]	.11[c]	−.17[b]	.15[b]	−.05	.12[c]	.09	.05
BMI	.25[a]	.21[a]	.19[a]	−.21[a]	.24[a]	−.05	.23[a]	.11	.03
Waist circumference	.25[a]	.23[a]	.18[a]	−.17[a]	.20[a]	−.03	.20[a]	.09	.01
Waist:hip ratio	.06	.15[b]	.11[c]	−.04	.10	.01	.13[c]	.01	−.01
Subscap skinfold	.23[a]	.21[a]	.19[a]	−.17[a]	.22[a]	−.05	.23[a]	.07	.04
Subscap:triceps ratio	.06	.14[b]	.05	−.13[c]	.07	−.10[c]	.11[c]	.03	.02

[a] $p \leq 0.001$, [b] $p \leq 0.01$, [c] $p \leq 0.05$.

amounts of vegetable fat, vegetable protein, and complex carbohydrates. This implies a change both in composition and energy density of the diet (9).

3.1.1. ENERGY INTAKE

It is indisputable that a high-energy diet, exceeding energy demands, especially in combination with low level of physical activity, results in obesity. However, most dietary studies show no, or an inverse, correlation between reported energy intake and body wt (3). The common explanation for this has been a higher degree of underreporting of dietary intake in obese individuals. Studies in children indicate that obese children do report a relatively lower energy intake than lean children. Obese adolescents underreported their dietary intake more than adolescents of normal weight, when their 7-d self-reported records were compared with estimated energy expenditure, using the double-labeled water method (79,80). Comparing three dietary surveys in Sweden in the past 20 yr, mean energy and fat intakes seemed to decrease, which is a trend also reported from other countries (81,82). Thus, another possible explanation for increased obesity prevalence could be a gradual reduction in physical activity over the past few decades. However, even if the relatively low energy intakes found in obese individuals is an effect of underreporting, it may also be a reflection of metabolic differences between lean and obese individuals.

3.1.2. METABOLIC EFFECTS OF COMPOSITION OF DIET

There are some characteristics of macronutrients that may explain part of the difficulties of regulating food intake when food is available in excess. Humans seem to have a poor defense against excess intake of fat. Compared to carbohydrates, fat has a lower ability to suppress hunger and bring eating to an end, and there are limited metabolic pathways transferring excess intake of fat to other compartments, including a low ability to stimulate increased oxidation on intake. At the same time, fat is energy-dense, and is easily stored at low energy cost (1). Further, there is some evidence to support the contention that high intake of protein in the Western diet could, through a specific effect on hormonal status, contribute to the metabolic disturbances behind obesity. Together with a genetic susceptibility for weight gain, this specific effect of high protein intake could partly explain why obese individuals tend to have energy intakes lower than would be expected from their degree of obesity, even when the underreporting of energy intake is accounted for. In rats, there is a more persistent increased secretion of glucagon after protein intake, compared with the transient increase of insulin and increased glycogenolysis (83,84). However, although the composition of the food may have some specific effects on development of obesity, the most significant contributing factor appears to be the high energy density of the diet.

There are also reports showing that IR and hyperinsulinemia may occur prior to other manifestations of the metabolic syndrome, indicating that high fat and refined-sugar diets may have a more direct effect. Monosaccharides, disaccharides, and starch are defined as digestible carbohydrates, because they are digested and absorbed in the human small intestine. A second category of carbohydrates, defined as "nondigestible" (i.e., dietary fibers), cannot be digested by intestinal enzymes. This latter category of carbohydrates, including a fraction of starch called "resistant starch," may still have an important nutritional role, because of its inhibitory role on food intake and possible role in weight management. Among the various dietary constituents, the one with the strongest influence on blood glucose levels in the postprandial period is the amount of digestible carbohydrate in the diet. The glycemic index is defined as the incremental blood glucose area after a test product has been ingested, expressed as a percentage of the corresponding area after a carbohydrate-equivalent amount of white bread.

Dietary factors are able to delay the process of digestion and/or absorption of carbohydrates in the intestine, thus reducing the glycemic response to carbohydrate-rich foods, i.e., flattening the glycemic index. Such dietary fibers may prevent, or may be used to treat, obesity, through the lower energy density of the high-fiber foods, their satiety effects, and by slowing the rate of food ingestion, gastric emptying, digestion, lower insulin levels, and more favorable plasma lipid profiles (85). Although well documented in adults, there are few useful studies of these effects of fibers in children. Switching to a diet rich in complex carbohydrates and dietary fiber increases peripheral insulin sensitivity (86–88); lowering fat in the diet to 25% of total energy reduces platelet aggregation and increases fibrinolytic activity significantly (89). Elevations of plasma FFA levels produce peripheral, and probably also hepatic, IR in obese healthy and diabetic subjects. It also increases glucose-stimulated insulin secretion, and this effect seems to be dependent also on chain length and degree of saturation. The longer and more saturated the FA, the more pronounced insulin response (48,90).

Even if there is substantial agreement that diet, predominantly the amount and type of fat intake, affects s-lipoproteins, and ultimately the occurrence of CVD, it has been difficult to demonstrate a direct association between dietary fat intake and serum lipid levels. In infants and younger children, the association seems to be stronger than in older children (91,92). However, ecological studies comparing different countries have shown clear correlation between fat intake in the population and the level of total cholesterol and LDL-C in adolescents. A reduction of fat intake, or a modification of fat composition with respect to atherogenic FAs, have, in experimental studies, been shown to lower serum lipids in children (93,94).

There are several possible explanations for the difficulties in showing an association between individual fat intakes and serum lipid levels, e.g., poor dietary data, genetically determined differences in responsiveness to fat intake, or a threshold effect, i.e., that the effect of fat intake on s-lipids is more pronounced in the low range of fat intake, and therefore difficult to show when the population level of fat intake is comparatively high and homogenous (95,96). It should also be considered that atherosclerosis develops over decades, and the variation in food consumed would, of course, be greater, if the exposure time, and hence the cumulative exposure, of different diets was considered. Alternatively, there may be other dietary factors, e.g., antioxidants, that may prove more important than fat intake, or at least equally important, for protection against CVD (97).

3.2. Physical Activity

The major part of daily energy expenditure is explained by basic metabolic energy expenditure, or basic metabolic rate, constituting 50–70% of daily energy expenditure. Voluntary physical activity accounts for less that 25%. The increase in obesity in society parallels the increase in sedentary lifestyles. There are large differences between individuals with respect to spontaneous physical activity (fidgeting) (3).

3.2.1. EFFECTS OF PHYSICAL ACTIVITY ON INSULIN, LIPID, AND FE METABOLISM

Physical exercise, even of short duration, especially when combined with a low-fat, high-complex-carbohydrate diet, increases insulin sensitivity, decreases serum insulin and triglyceride levels, and increases HDL-C (Fig. 4). Increased participation in

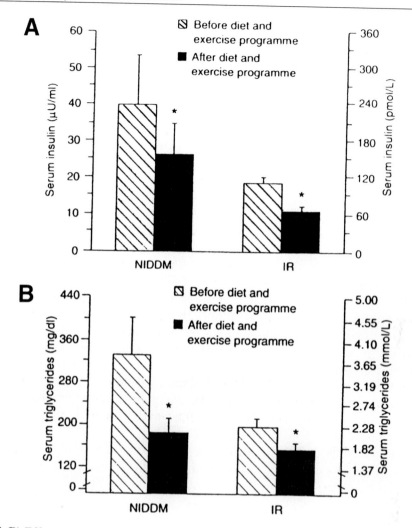

Fig. 4. (A,B) Effects of high-complex-carbohydrate diet and daily aerobic exercise on s-insulin and s-triglyceride level. (Adapted with permission from ref. *76*.)

nonvigorous, as well as overall and vigorous, physical activity significantly reduces the risk of developing NIDDM *(76,98)*. Physical activity is thought to influence the FA composition of phospholipids in skeletal muscle, affecting skeletal muscle membrane fluidity and peripheral insulin sensitivity. Skeletal muscle glucose uptake and metabolism are major determinants of whole-body glucose metabolism in response to exercise and insulin stimulation *(99–102)*.

High levels of physical activity and physical fitness, most often not discussed as separate entities, have, in epidemiological studies in adults, been associated with lower prevalence of CVD risk factors and a lower incidence of coronary heart disease *(103)*. The positive effect of physical activity on the CVD process is not fully understood, but increase in HDL-C, decrease in very-low-density lipoprotein cholesterol and triglycerides, and a lowering of BP, are thought to contribute. Information on the effect of physical activity and physical fitness on CVD risk indicators in children and adolescents indicate that a high level of physical activity and physical fitness have a favorable effect on serum lipids and serum insulin concentrations, especially in obese children (65,104).

Hypothetically, one benefit from physical exercise on CVD could be a reduction in body Fe (105). Physical activity reduces concentrations of hemoglobin and serum ferritin. This has been regarded mostly as a consequence of increased Fe losses, leading to Fe deficiency, the so-called "sports anemia." However, alternatively, the lower hemoglobin concentration and Fe stores found in physically fit individuals could indicate a physiological adaptation, including a redistribution or utilization of body Fe. That sports anemia is not caused by Fe deficiency is supported by the findings that, in most studies, Fe supplements given to athletes with supposed Fe deficiency have not been effective unless the subjects were also anemic (106). Therefore, it is possible that the lower Fe stores found in slimmer individuals are in fact beneficial, and, also, that high Fe stores are a sign of a metabolic disturbance caused by a sedentary lifestyle and obesity (65,66).

3.3. Treatment and Prevention of Obesity in Children and Adolescents

There is evidence that treatment of obesity with modification of energy intake and expenditure, i.e., decreased energy intake and exercise programs, can be successfully managed from childhood through adolescence to adulthood (107). A prerequisite for successful treatment of obesity in children is a strongly motivated child. Therefore, when treating children and adolescents, it is advisable to concentrate on those with severe adiposity or, when the obesity is less severe, those who seek help voluntarily. A family history of obesity is an important argument to intervene and involvement of the family is also an important component in most programs. Because of favorable prognosis of moderate forms of childhood obesity, it is advisable that dieting programs should be avoided until after puberty (28,107). It is also important to consider that treatment of obesity in children and adolescents may have serious side effects on growth (82,91,108). Some adolescents, mostly girls, are concerned with their body wt, and are often responsive to advice about healthy lifestyles. As part of anorectic behavior, some of these girls already have low intake of energy and fat, and further reduction could have a negative influence on their growth and health (109) (see Chapter 10).

4. SUMMARY AND RECOMMENDATIONS

Obesity has been classified as a modern epidemic, evolving during recent decades in both industrialized and developing countries. The epidemic also includes children and adolescents. Obesity is related to increased M&M in a number of diseases, the most important being NIDDM and CVD. The clinical entity of obesity, hyperglycemia, dyslipidemia, and hypertension, also seen in children and adolescents, is referred to as the "metabolic syndrome." Increased resistance to insulin in liver, muscle, and adipose tissue is regarded as an important explanation behind the disturbances in glucose and lipid metabolism. IR is closely related to obesity, and visceral fat accumulation seems to have a particularly harmful effect. Even if genetic and early nutritional factors influence the susceptibility to gain weight, the major underlying cause of the obesity epidemic is the spread of a sedentary Western lifestyle, i.e., a combination of low physical activity and consumption of high-fat, high-sugar, high-animal protein diets, with energy intake exceeding energy expenditure. Attempts to achieve lasting weight reductions in obese adults have been disappointing, implying that preventive efforts promoting physical activity and healthy diets in children and adolescents is the "drug of choice."

Even if it seems easier to treat obesity in children than in adults, it is obvious that the best strategy would be primary prevention, targeting all children. However, as obesity can be regarded as an epidemic caused by modern lifestyle, effective preventive measures should not focus only on individual behavior, but also on the social and physical environment for children, supporting more daily physical activities (not only sports) and healthy diets. This will not be an easy task, because there are a number of factors operating in the opposite direction: motorization; restricting physical activities, both for convenience and safety reasons; pursuit of sedentary recreations during leisure time, such as computers, video games, and TV; and easy access to high-fat/high-sugar fast foods.

REFERENCES

1. World Health Organization. Obesity. Preventing and managing the global epidemic, Report of a WHO Consultation on Obesity. Geneva: WHO, 1997.
2. Bouchard C, Tremblay A, Després JP, Nadeau A, Lupien PJ, Thériault G, et al. The response to long-term overfeeding in identical twins. N Engl J Med 1990; 322:1477–1482.
3. Ravussin E, Swinburn BA. Pathophysiology of obesity. Lancet 1992; 340:404–408.
4. Rosenbaum M, Leibel RL, Hirsch J. Obesity. N Engl J Med 1997; 337:396–407.
5. Leibel RL, Rosenbaum M, Hirsch J. Changes in energy expenditure resulting from altered body weight. N Engl J Med 1995; 332:1201–1205.
6. Bouchard C. The Genetics of Obesity. Boca Raton: CRC, 1994.
7. Montague CT, Farooqi IS, Whitehead JP, et al. Congenital leptin deficiency is associated with severe early-onset obesity in humans. Nature 1997; 387:903–908.
8. Neel JV. Diabetes mellitus: a "thrifty genotype rendered detrimental by progress"? Am J Hum Genet 1962; 14: 353–362.
9. World Health Organization. Diet, nutrition, and the prevention of chronic diseases. Geneva: WHO Tech Rep Ser 1990; 797.
10. Drenowski A. Human preference for sugar and fat. In: Appetite and Body Weight Regulation: Sugar, Fat and Macronutrient Substitutes. Fernström JD, Miller GD, eds. Boca Raton: CRC, 1994; 137–147.
11. Lindeberg S, Nilsson-Ehle P, Terént A, Vessby B, Schersten B. Cardio-vascular risk factors in a Melanesian population apparently free from stroke and ischemic heart disease: the Kitava study. J Intern Med 1994; 236:331–340.
12. Hales CN, Barker DJP. Type 2 (non-insulin-dependent) diabetes mellitus: the thrifty phenotype hypothesis. Diabetologia 1992; 35:595–601.
13. Forsdahl A. Are poor living conditions during childhood and adolescence an important risk factor for arteriosclerotic heart disease? Br J Prev Med 1977; 31:91–95.
14. Barker DJP, Hales CHD, Osmond C, Phipps K, Clark PMS. Type 2 (non-insulin dependent) diabetes mellitus, hypertension and hyperlipidemia (syndrome X): relation to reduced fetal growth. Diabetologia 1993; 36:62–67.
15. Barker DJP. Fetal origins of coronary heart disease. Br Med J 1995; 311:171–174.
16. Lithell HO, McKeigue PM, Berglund L, Mohsen R, Lithell UB, Leon DA. Relation of size at birth to non-insulin dependent diabetes and insulin concentrations in men aged 50–60 years. Br Med J 1996; 312:406–410.
17. Phillips DI. Birth weight and the future development of diabetes. Diabetes Care 1998; 21(Suppl. 2): B150–155.
18. Law CM, Gordon GS, Shiell AW, Barker DJP, Hales CN. Thinness at birth and glucose tolerance in seven-year-old children. Diabet Med 1994; 1224–1229.
19. Yajnik CS, Fall CHD, Vaidya U, Pandit AN, Bavdekar A, Bhat DS, et al. Fetal growth and glucose and insulin metabolism in four-year-old Indian children. Diab Med 1995; 12:330–336.
20. Crowther NJ, Cameron N, Trusler J, Gray IP. Association between poor glucose tolerance and rapid post natal weight gain in seven-year-old children. Diabetologia 1998; 41:1163–1167.
21. Popkin BM, Richards MK, Montiero CA. Stunting is associated with overweight in children of four nations that are undergoing the nutritional transition. J Nutr 1996; 126:3009–3016.
22. Bergström E, Hernell O, Persson LÅ, Vessby B. Insulin resistance syndrome in adolescents. Metabolism 1996; 45:908–914.

23. Blom L, Persson LÅ, Dahlquist G. A high linear growth is associated with an increased risk of childhood diabetes mellitus. Diabetologia 1992; 35:528–533.

24. Nyirenda MJ, Seckl JR. Intrauterine events and the programming of adulthood disease: the role of fetal glucocorticoid exposure. Int J Mol Med 1998; 2:607–614.

25. Paneth N. Early origin of coronary heart disease (the "Barker hypothesis"). Br Med J 1995; 310:411–412.

26. Hill AJ, Silver EK. Fat, friendless and unhealthy: 9-year old children's perception of body shape stereotypes. Int J Obes 1995; 19:423–430.

27. Must A, Jacques PF, Dallal GE, Bajema CJ, Dietz WH. Long-term morbidity and mortality of overweight adolescents. New Engl J Med 1992; 327:1350–1355.

28. Whitaker RC, Wright JA, Pepe MS, Seidel KD, Dietz WH. Predicting obesity in young adulthood from childhood and parental obesity. N Engl J Med 1997; 337:869–873.

29. Kotani K, et al. Two decades of annual medical examinations in Japanese obese children: do obese children grow into obese adults? Int J Obes Related Met Dis 1997; 21:912–921.

30. Vital and health statistics. NCHS growth curves for children, birth-18 years. Hyattsville, MD: Department of Health, Education and Welfare; United States series 11-No 165; DHEW Publication No (PHS) 78-1650, 1977.

31. Rolland-Cachera MF, et al. Body mass index variations: centiles from birth to 87 years. Eur J Clin Nutr 1991; 45:13–21.

32. Hammer LD, et al. Standardized percentile curves of body mass index for children and adolescents. Am J Dis Child 1991; 145:259–263.

33. Lindgren G, et al. Swedish population reference standards for height, weight and body mass index attained at 6 to 16 years (girls) or 19 years (boys). Acta Paediatr 1995; 84:1019–1028.

34. Mo-suvan L, Junjana C, Puetpaiboon A. Increasing obesity in school children in a transitional society and the effect the weight control program. Southeast Asian J Trop Med Publ Health 1993; 24:590–594.

35. Freedman DS, et al. Secular increases in relative weight and adiposity among children over two decades: the Bogalusa Heart Study. Pediatrics 1997; 99:420–426.

36. Gortmater SL, Must A, Perrin JM, Sobol AM, Dietz WH. Social and economic consequences of overweight in adolescence and young adults. N Engl J Med 1993; 329:1008–1012.

37. Marmot M. Socioeconomic determinants of CHD mortality. Int J Epidemiol 1989; 18(Suppl. 1):196–202.

38. Björntorp P. Visceral fat accumulation: the missing link between psychosocial factors and cardiovascular disease? J Int Med 1991; 230:195–201.

39. Bergström E, Hernell O, Persson LÅ. Cardiovascular risk indicator cluster in girls from families of low socioeconomic status. Acta Paediatr 1996; 85:1083–1090.

40. Camus JP. (Gout, diabetes, hyperlipidemia: a metabolic trisyndrome). Rev Rhum Mal Osteoartic 1966; 33:10–14 (in French).

41. Reaven GM. Banting Lecture 1988. Role of insulin resistance in human disease. Diabetes 1988; 37:1595–1607.

42. Hunter SJ, Garvey WT. Insulin action and insulin resistance: diseases involving defects in insulin receptors, signal transduction, and the glucose transport effector system. Am J Med 1998; 105:331–345.

43. Bloomgarden ZT. Insulin resistance: current concepts. Clin Ther 1998; 20:216–231.

44. Reaven GM. Hypothesis: muscle insulin resistance is the ("not so") thrifty genotype. Diabetologia 1998; 41:482–484.

45. Shaw JT, Levy JC, Turner RC. The relationship between the insulin resistance syndrome and insulin sensitivity in the first-degree relatives of subjects with noninsulin dependent diabetes mellitus. Diabetes Res Clin Pract 1998; 42:91–99.

46. Turner NC, Clapham JC. Insulin resistance, impaired glucose tolerance and noninsulin-dependent diabetes, pathological mechanisms and treatment: current status and therapeutic possibilities. Prog Drug Res 1998; 51:33–94.

47. Fendri S, Roussel B, Lormeau B, Tribout B, Lalau JD. Insulin sensitivity, insulin action, and fibrinolysis activity in nondiabetic and diabetic obese subjects. Metabolism 1998; 47:1372–1375.

48. Boden G. Free fatty acids (FFA), a link between obesity and insulin resistance. Front Biosci 1998; 3:D169–175.

49. Fournier AM. Intracellular starvation in the insulin resistance syndrome and type II diabetes mellitus. Med Hypotheses 1998; 51:95–99.

50. Ferrannini E, Camastra S. Relationship between impaired glucose tolerance, noninsulin-dependent diabetes mellitus and obesity. Eur J Clin Invest 1998; 28(Suppl. 2):3–6.

51. Yip J, Facchini FS, Reaven GM. Resistance to insulin-mediated glucose disposal as a predictor of cardiovascular disease. J Clin Endocrinol Metab 1998; 83:2773–2776.
52. Carey DG. Abdominal obesity. Curr Opin Lipidol 1998; 9:35–40.
53. Ruderman N, Chisholm D, Pi-Sunyer X, Schneider S. The metabolically obese, normal-weight individual revisited. Diabetes 1998; 47:699–713.
54. Hong Y, Rice T, Gagnon J, Despres JP, Nadeau A, Perusse L, et al. Familial clustering of insulin and abdominal visceral fat: the HERITAGE Family Study. J Clin Endocrinol Metab 1998; 83: 4239–4245.
55. Zhang Y, Proenca R, Maffei M, Barone M, Leopold L, Friedman JM. Positional cloning of the mouse obese gene and its human homologue. Nature 1994; 372:425–432 (Erratum, Nature 1995; 374:479).
56. Considine RV, Considine EL, Williams CJ, et al. Evidence against either a premature stop codon or the absence of obese gene mRNA in human obesity. J Clin Invest 1995; 95:2986–2988.
57. Rosenbaum M, Nicolson M, Hirsch J, et al. Effects of gender, body composition, and menopause on plasma concentrations of leptin. J Clin Endocrinol Metab 1996; 81:3424–3427.
58. Houseknecht KL, Portocarrero CP. Leptin and its receptors: regulators of whole-body energy homeostasis. Domest Anim Endocrinol 1998; 15:457–475.
59. Fuhrman B, Oiknine J, Aviram M. Iron induces lipid peroxidation in cultured macrophages, increases their ability to oxidatively modify LDL, and affects their secretory properties. Atherosclerosis 1994; 111:65–78.
60. Sullivan Conference on cardiovascular disease epidemiology and prevention. American Heart Health Association. Santa Fe. Food Chem News 1993; 19.
61. Salonen JT. The role of iron as a cardiovascular risk factor. Curr Opin Lipidol 1993; 4:277–282.
62. Stevens RG, Graubard BI, Micozzi MS, Neriishi K, Blumberg BS. Moderate elevation of body iron level and increased risk of cancer occurrence and death. Int J Cancer 1994; 56:364–369.
63. Ascherio A, Willet WC. Are body iron related to the risk of coronary heart disease? N Engl J Med 1994; 330:1152–1153.
64. Sullivan JL. Iron and the sex difference in heart risk. Lancet 1981; 1:1293–1294.
65. Bergström E, Hernell O, Persson LÅ. Endurance running performance in relation to cardiovascular risk indicators in adolescents. Int J Sports Med 1997; 18:300–307.
66. Fernandez-Real JM, Ricart-Engel W, Arroyo E, Balanca R, Casamitjana-Abella R, Cabero D, Fernandez-Castaner M, Soler J. Serum ferritin as a component of the insulin resistance syndrome. Diabetes Care 1998; 21:62–68.
67. Edwards CQ, Kushner JP. Screening for hemochromatosis. N Engl J Med 1993; 328:1616–1620.
68. Bao W, Srinivasan SR, Wattigney WA, Berensson GS. Persistence of multiple cardiovascular risk clustering related to syndrome X from childhood to young adulthood. Arch Intern Med 1993; 154: 1842–1847.
69. Vanhala M, Vanhala P, Kumpusalo E, Halonen P, Takala J. Relation between obesity from childhood to adulthood and the metabolic syndrome: population based study. Br Med J 1998; 317:319.
70. Srinivasan SR, Elkasabani A, Dalferes ER Jr, Bao W, Berenson GS. Characteristics of young offspring of type 2 diabetic parents in a biracial (black-white) community-based sample: the Bogalusa Heart Study. Metabolism 1998; 47:998–1004.
71. Becque MD, Hattori K, Katch VL, et al. Relationship of fat patterning to coronary artery disease risk in obese adolescents. Am J Phys Anthropol 1986; 71:423–429.
72. Amiel SA, Sherwin RS, Simonsson DC, Lauritano AA, Tamborlane WT. Impaired insulin action in puberty. Contributing factor to poor glycemic control in adolescents with diabetes. N Engl J Med 1986; 315:215–219.
73. Travers SH, Labarta JI, Gargosky SE, Rosenfeld RG, Jeffers BW, Eckel RH. Insulin-like growth factor binding protein-I levels are strongly associated with insulin sensitivity and obesity in early pubertal children. J Clin Endocrinol Metab 1998; 83:1935–1939.
74. NIH Technology Assessment Conference Panel: Consensus Development Conference, 30 March to 1 April, 1992. Methods for voluntary weight loss and control. Ann Intern Med 1993; 119:764–770.
75. Wadden TA. Treatment of obesity by moderate and severe caloric restriction: results of clinical research trials. Ann Intern Med 1993; 229:688–693.
76. Barnard RJ, Wen SJ. Exercise and diet in the prevention and control of the metabolic syndrome. Sports Med 1994; 18:218–228.
77. Dietz WH. Prevention of childhood obesity. Pediatr Clin North Am 1986; 33:823–833.

78. Lissau I, Sørensen TIA. Parental neglect during childhood and increased risk of obesity in young adulthood. Lancet 1994; 343:324–327.

79. James WPT, Sahakian BJ. Energetic significance in relation to obesity. In: Nutrition and Child Health. Perspectives for the 1980s. Tsang RC, Nichols BL, eds. New York: Alan R Liss, 1981; 25–33.

80. Schoeller DA, Bandini LG, Dietz WH. Inaccuracies in self-reported intake identified by comparison with the double labelled water method. Can J Physiol Pharmacol 1990; 68:941–949.

81. Whitehead RG, Paul AA, Cole TJ. Trends in food energy intakes throughout childhood from one to 18 years. Hum Nutr Appl Nutr 1982; 36:57–62.

82. Bergström E, Hernell O, Persson LÅ. Dietary changes in Swedish adolescents. Acta Paediatr 1993; 82:472–480.

83. Gannon MC, Nuttall FQ. Physiological doses of oral casein affect hepatic glycogen metabolism in normal food-deprived rats. J Nutr 1995; 125:1159–1166.

84. Rolland-Cachera MF, Deheeger M. Nutrient balance and android body fat distribution: why not a role for protein? Am J Clin Nutr 1997:64:663–664.

85. Saris WHM, Asp NGL, Björck I, Blaak E, Bornet F, Brouns F, et al. Functional food science and substrate metabolism. Br J Nutr 1998; 80(Suppl. 1):S47–S75.

86. Grey N, Kipnis DM. Effect of diet composition on the hyperinsulinemia of obesity. N Engl J Med 1971; 285:827–831.

87. Fukagawa NK, Anderson JW, Hogeman G, et al. High-carbohydrate, high-fiber diets increase peripheral insulin sensitivity in healthy young and old adults. Am J Clin Nutr 1990; 52:524–528.

88. Barnard RJ, Roberts CK, Varon SM, Berger JJ. Diet-induced insulin resistance precedes other aspects of the metabolic syndrome. J Appl Physiol 1998; 84:1311–1315.

89. Marckman P, Sandström B, Jespersen J, Favorable long-term effect of a low-fat/high-fiber diet on human blood coagulation and fibrinolysis. Arterioscl Thromb 1993; 3:306–318.

90. Stein DT, Stevenson BE, Chester MW, Basit Majid, Daniels MB, Turley SD, McGarry, JD. The insulinotropic potency of fatty acids is influenced profoundly by their chain length and degree of saturation. J Clin Invest 199; 100:398–403.

91. ESPGAN Committee on Nutrition: Aggett PJ, Haschke F, Heine W, Hernell O, Koletzko B, Lafeber H, et al. Committee report: Childhood diet and prevention of coronary heart disease. J Pediatr Gastroenterol Nutr 1994; 19:261–269.

92. Hornstra G, Barth CA, Galli C, Mensink RP, Mutanen M, Riemersma RA, et al. Functional food science and the cardiovascular system. Br J Nutr 1998; 80(Suppl. 1):S113–146.

93. Knuiman JT, et al. Determinants of total and high lipoprotein cholesterol in boys from Finland, The Netherlands, Italy, The Philippines and Ghana with special reference to diet. Hum Nutr Clin Nutr 1983; 37C:237–254.

94. Lapinleimu H, Viikari J, Jokinen E, Salo P, Routi T, Leino A, et al. Prospective randomised trial in 1062 infants of diets low in saturated fat and cholesterol. Lancet 1994; 345:471–476.

95. Pesonen E, Viikari J, Räsänen L, Moilanen T, Turtinen J, Åkerblom HK. Nutritional and genetic contributions to serum cholesterol concentration in a children follow-up study. Acta Paediatr 1994; 83:378–382.

96. Lehtimäki T, Moilanen T, Porkka K, Åkerblom HK, Rönnemaa T, Räsänen L, et al. Associations between serum lipids and apolipoprotein E phenotype is influenced by diet in a population-based sample of free-living children and young adults: the Cardiovascular Risk in Young Finns Study. J Lipid Res 1995; 36:653–661.

97. Lorgeril M, Renaud S, Mamelle N, Salen P, Martin JL, Monjaud I, et al. Mediterranean alpha-linolenic acid-rich diet in secondary prevention of coronary heart disease. Lancet 1994; 343:1454–1459.

98. Helmrich SP, Ragland DR, Leung RW, Paffenbarger RS Jr. Physical activity and reduced occurrence of non-insulin diabetes mellitus. N Engl J Med 1991; 325:147–152.

99. Mayer-Davies EJ, D'Agostino R Jr, Karter AJ, Haffner SM, Rewers MJ, Saad M, Bergman RN. Intensity and amount of physical activity in relation to insulin sensitivity; the Insulin Resistance Atherosclerosis Study. JAMA 1998:279:669–674.

100. Andersson A, Sjodin A, Olsson R, Vessby B. Effects of physical exercise on phospholipid fatty acid composition in skeletal muscle. Am J Physiol 1998; 274:E432–438.

101. Goodyear LJ, Kahn BB. Exercise, glucose transport, and insulin sensitivity. Annu Rev Med 1998; 49:235–261.

102. Hargraves M. 1997 Sir William Refshauge Lecture. Skeletal muscle glucose metabolism during exercise: Implications for health and performance. J Sci Med Sport 1998; 1:195–202.

103. Bouchard C, Despres JP. Physical activity and health: atherosclerosis, metabolic and hypertensive diseases. Res Q Exerc Sport 1995; 66:268–275.

104. Sallis JF, Patterson TL, Buono MJ, Nader PR. Relation of cardiovascular fitness and physical activity to cardiovascular disease risk factors in children and adults. Am J Epidemiol 1988; 127:933–941.

105. Lauffer RB. Exercise as prevention: Do the health benefits derive in part from lower iron levels? Med Hypothesis 1991; 35:103–107.

106. Cook JD. The effect of endurance training on iron metabolism. Semin Hematol 1994; 31:146–154.

107. Epstein LH, Valoski A, Wing RR, McCurley J. Ten-year follow-up of behavioral, family-based treatment for obese children. JAMA 1990; 264:2519–2523.

108. Olson RE. The dietary recommendations of the American Academy of Pediatrics. Am J Clin Nutr 1995; 61:271–273.

109. Wardle J, Beales S. Restraint, body image and food attitudes in children 12 to 18 years. Appetite 1986; 7:209–217.

11   Can Childhood Obesity Be Prevented?

Christine L. Williams

1. INTRODUCTION AND RATIONALE

Obesity has reached epidemic proportions in the United States in the past several decades. Prevalence rates have increased sharply among adults, reflecting an average weight gain of 8 lb over a single decade. Recent national survey data (National Health and Nutrition Examination Survey III [NHANES III]) indicates that more than 1/3 of American adults are obese (1). The health implications of this mounting problem are significant, because obesity is now considered to be a chronic disease that is associated with other chronic conditions, such as coronary heart disease, type II diabetes mellitus, hypertension, dyslipidemia, gallbladder disease, respiratory disease, and some types of cancer, gout, and arthritis (2). As such, direct health care costs related to obesity annually exceed $68 billion, or about 6% of total health care expenditures in the United States (3).

Obesity has also increased dramatically among children and youth in the United States. Surveys indicate that the number of overweight children 6–17 yr of age has doubled within three decades (4–6). In the decade between the late 1970s (NHANES II:1976–1980) and the early 1990s (NHANES III:1988–1994), the prevalence of overweight increased from 7.6 to 13.7% for 6–11-yr-old children, and from 5.7 to 11.5% for adolescents 12–19 yr old (4–6).

National surveys also indicate that the prevalence of childhood obesity has increased even among preschool children less than 5 yr of age. The problem is especially acute among minority preschoolers, with highest prevalence rates among Mexican-American children, intermediate rates among non-Hispanic black children, and lowest rates in non-Hispanic White children. Obesity has also increased among low-income preschool children.

Increasing prevalence of childhood obesity has serious implications for child health, because it is associated with co-morbidity, even during early childhood. This includes elevated blood pressure (BP), abnormal blood lipid concentrations, insulin resistance, type II diabetes mellitus, orthopedic disorders, skin problems, and psychological problems (7–13).

Treatment of human obesity at any age is very difficult, rarely successful, and is characterized by repeated recidivism over time (14). Prevention of obesity must therefore be the cornerstone of a widespread public health campaign to control overweight, and to reverse the growing epidemic. Such prevention efforts can be targeted simultaneously on several levels, with appropriately different goals: primordial prevention, to prevent children from becoming at-risk of overweight; primary prevention, to prevent at-risk children from becoming overweight; and secondary prevention, to prevent increasing severity of obesity and reduce co-morbidity among overweight children (Fig. 1). Within this frame

From: *Primary and Secondary Preventive Nutrition*
Edited by: A. Bendich and R. J. Deckelbaum © Humana Press Inc., Totowa, NJ

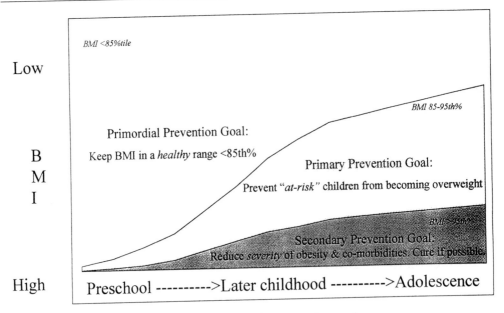

Fig. 1. Childhood obesity prevention goals.

of reference, it is possible to identify key priorities for action, as well as potentially successful prevention strategies. Because primordial and primary obesity prevention strategies are most likely to be effective if initiated before school age, and sustained during childhood and adolescence, the primary focus of this chapter is on obesity prevention efforts aimed at young children in the first decade of life (*see* Chapters 8 and 9).

2. PREVALENCE OF OBESITY IN YOUNG CHILDREN

The increase in childhood obesity has been observed in U.S. children as young as 4 yr of age, and, in some gender- and ethnic-specific subgroups, as young as 2 yr of age (*14,15*). This increase has been demonstrated in national health examination surveys, such as the NHANES studies, which have been conducted since the early 1970s (*4*).

Currently, almost 8% of 4- and 5-yr-old children in the United States are overweight, i.e., above the 95th percentile of the weight for height growth reference. This represents a significant increase in the past 20 yr, especially among girls. The percent of 4- and 5-yr-old girls who were overweight increased from 5.8% in the early 1970s to over 10% recently (NHANES III, 1988–1994). Overweight among 4–5-yr-old boys also increased, but not as much as for girls (*14*; Fig. 2). This gender difference is true for older children and adults, as well.

There are also significant differences by ethnicity. For both boys and girls, overweight is highest among Mexican-American children, intermediate among non-Hispanic black children, and lowest in non-Hispanic white children (Figs. 3 and 4). For specific gender/ethnicity groups, non-Hispanic white boys have the lowest prevalence of overweight, at 4.3%, and Mexican-American girls have the highest rates, at 13.2% (*14*).

For even younger, 2–3-yr-old children, prevalence estimates of overweight for most gender and race/ethnicity groups (based on NHANES I–III surveys) were less than the expected 5% (Fig. 5). One notable exception was for 2–3-yr-old Mexican-American girls, 10.5% of whom were overweight, more than twice the expected number (*14*).

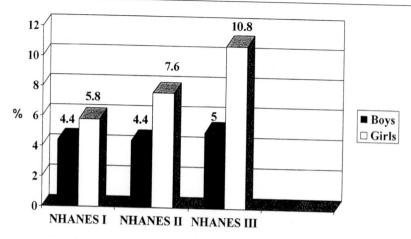

Fig. 2. Percentage of 4 and 5-yr-old boys and girls above the 95th percentile of the weight-for-length growth reference: First, Second, and Third National Health and Nutrition Examination Survey (1971–1994).

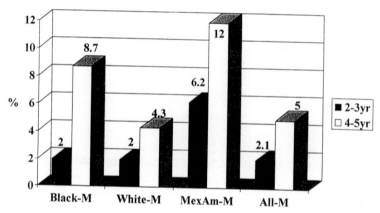

Fig. 3. Percentage of 2–3 and 4–5-yr-old boys above the 95th percentile of the weight-for-length growth reference: Third National Health and Nutrition Examination Survey (1971–1994).

The prevalence of overweight depends on the selection of the reference population and the overweight criteria. The Centers for Disease Control (CDC) defines the prevalence of overweight as the percent of children whose weight-for-height is above the 95th percentile cutoff in the original 1979 National Center for Health Statistics (NCHS) reference growth curves. For 3–6-yr-old preschool children, the weight-for-height charts were based on data from NHANES I (1971–1974). The NCHS and modified NCHS/CDC growth curves represent smoothed versions of the data; thus, prevalence estimates of overweight for 3–6-yr-olds for NHANES I are not exactly the expected 5% (at the 95th percentile cutoff point). Although there is some concern about using the original NCHS charts, choice of this reference will not affect trend estimates over time *(4,5,14)*.

The increase in obesity is also significant among low-income preschool children in the United States, as reported in data from CDC's Pediatric Nutrition Surveillance System *(15)*. The proportion of low-income children, under 5 yr of age, who are above the 85th and 95th percentile cutoff of the height-for-weight growth reference, has increased

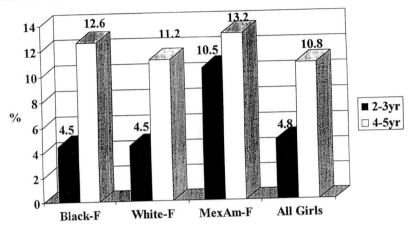

Fig. 4. Percentge of 2–3 and 4–5-yr-old girls above the 95th percentile of the weight-for-length growth reference: Third National Health and Nutrition Examination Surveys (1988–1994).

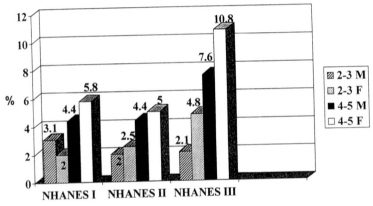

Fig. 5. Percentage of 2–3 and 4–5-yr-old boys and girls above the 95th percentile of the weight-for-length growth reference: First, Second, and Third National Health and Nutrition Examination Surveys (1971–1994).

significantly between 1983 and 1995. At present, 21.6% are above the 85th percentile cutoff (compared with 18.6% in 1983), and 10.2% are above the 95th percentile cutoff (compared with 8.5% in 1983) (Fig. 6). The increase was observed in all races/ethnicities; however, low-income 2–4-yr-old Hispanic children had the highest prevalence, both in 1983 and 1995; black children were intermediate, and white children had the lowest rates. The greatest increase in overweight has been among the low-income 4-yr-olds (48–59 mo of age), a finding similar to that reported in the NHANES-III survey, which included children of all income levels (15; Fig. 7).

In a recent survey by Williams et al. (16) of 1239 2–5-yr-old children in nine upstate New York Head Start Centers in 1995–1996 (part of a 3-yr National Heart, Lung, and Blood Institute funded cardiovascular risk reduction project named "Healthy Start"), 12.1% of the children (age 3.5 yr) had body mass index (BMI) levels above the 95th percentile for age, sex, and ethnicity, based on NHANES-III data. Hispanic preschoolers had the greatest prevalence of overweight, black children were intermediate, and white children

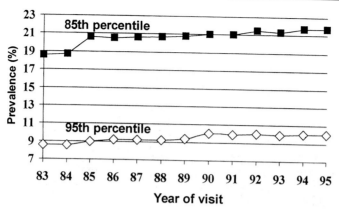

Fig. 6. Prevalence of overweight among U.S. low-income children under 5 yr of age, adjusted by race or ethnicity, sex ratio, and age in months. The CDC Pediatric Nutrition Surveillance, 1983–1995.

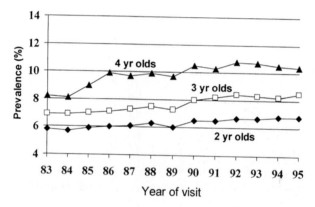

Fig. 7. Prevalence of overweight among U.S. low-income children 2–4 yr of age, adjusted by race or ethnicity, sex ratio, and age in months; the CDC Pediatric Nutrition Surveillance, 1983–1995.

the lowest (16.5% Hispanic; 10.7% black; and 8.8% white): similar to the CDC data for low-income children. Measures of triceps skinfold gave lower prevalence estimates of obesity, with 4.9% above the NHANES III 95th percentile level: about what would be expected. There were no significant differences by age, race, or gender. Thus, the prevalence of overweight is increasing among preschool children in the United States, indicating that prevention strategies are needed before 3 yr of age.

3. PHYSICAL AND MENTAL CO-MORBIDITIES

The increase in preschool obesity is of public health concern, because childhood obesity is linked to a number of other adverse health conditions, both physical and mental. Many of these may have serious implications for future child health.

In the Healthy Start preschool project, both diet and cardiovascular risk factors were monitored in preschool children attending nine Head Start Centers in New York over a period of 3 yr. Thirty-eight percent of the children had elevated total cholesterol levels, and 21% had borderline low or low levels of good cholesterol (high-density lipoprotein

[HDLs]) *(16)*. Overweight children had significantly lower levels of good cholesterol than leaner children, especially comparing those greater than the 95th percentile BMI cutoff with those below the 85th percentile. Almost half (44%) of those who were above the 95th percent cutoff level for BMI had low HDL-C levels (<35 mg%), compared with 31% of those who were below the 85th percent for BMI. In addition, BMI was positively and significantly correlated with both systolic and diastolic BP in this population of predominantly low-income minority preschoolers ($n = 1226$). The higher the BMI, the higher the BP. The relative risk of borderline high or high systolic and/or diastolic BP more than doubled for preschoolers with BMI above the 95th percentile, compared to those below the 85th percentile. Thus, obesity affects cardiovascular disease risk status, even in preschool children.

Childhood obesity also takes a toll on mental health, with reported negative effects on self esteem and peer relationships. Several studies have shown that children are negatively sensitized to obesity at a young age, and develop cultural preferences for leanness. In one study of 10–11-yr-olds, children preferred handicapped children as friends, more so than obese children, and ranked obese children lowest among those with whom they would like to be friends *(17)*. Others reported that children as young as 6–10 yr of age already associated laziness and sloppiness with obesity *(18)*.

Self-esteem is negatively affected by obesity more so in older children and teens, compared with young children, probably reflecting the increasing role of peers, rather than parents, as sources of self-esteem during adolescence *(19–21)*. As obese children grow older, they are less likely than their lean peers to be chosen as best friend, invited to birthday parties, selected for team sports, or become members of child-initiated clubs. Repeated rejection leads to feelings of unworthiness, withdrawal, passivity, and, sometimes, depression. Obesity in young women has been shown to be an important determinant of lower socioeconomic status (SES) rather than a consequence. Obese women earn, on average, $6710 less annually, are 10% more likely to have income below poverty level, and 20% less likely to be married *(22)*.

There is substantial evidence that increasing early childhood obesity has serious implications for future child health. It is associated with adverse changes in physiological measures, such as BP and cholesterol, which may increase risk of future chronic diseases, and also tends to decrease self-esteem and jeopardize mental health.

4. OBESITY PREVENTION STRATEGIES

Effective primordial, primary, and secondary prevention of obesity in childhood will require a combination of effective public health, population-based community approaches, and individualized or high-risk approaches to the problem. Both will need to consider what may be the most critical or vulnerable periods for developing obesity in childhood and adolescence (Fig. 8).

Primordial prevention aims to prevent children with desirable BMI levels (<85th percentile) from advancing into the "at-risk of obesity" BMI range (85–95th percentile). Because obesity eventually affects one-fourth of children, primordial prevention initiatives require a broad-based population approach that includes as many infants and toddlers as possible. Prevention goals would aim to help young children (and their parents and teachers) adopt a healthy, fat-controlled, balanced, and nutritionally adequate diet, and engage in an adequate amount of physical activity each day.

- <u>Prenatal period</u>: Early undernutrition may impair the regulation of food intake, and predispose to later obesity. Third trimester and later undernutrition may influence adipose tissue cellularity and protect against or promote later.

- <u>Period of Adiposity Rebound</u>: BMI increases during infancy then decreases. Early timing of the second increase in BMI (adiposity rebound) has been associated with increased fatness in adolescence.

- <u>Adolescence</u>: Individuals who become obese during adolescence, particularly girls, are at significant risk of adult obesity. Adult morbidity is increased among persons who were overweight as adolescents, even if subsequent normal weight is achieved.

Fig. 8. Critical periods in childhood for the development of childhood obesity.

Primary prevention aims to prevent children who are at risk of obesity (85–95th percentile BMI) from progressing to frank obesity (>95th percentile BMI). Achievement of this goal may require a high-risk or individual approach, in addition to a background of population-based programs that encourage healthy eating and activity patterns. Primary prevention strategies would be especially applicable for at-risk children of obese parent(s), and for other children who experience accelerated weight gain after 3 yr of age. High-risk approaches aimed at primary prevention will also be facilitated by population-based programs, in preschools and elementary schools, that facilitate increased physical activity, and encourage/serve heart healthy meals and snacks in appropriate child-size portions.

Secondary prevention aims to prevent children who are already obese (BMI >95th percentile) from becoming more severely affected, and ameliorating co-morbidities associated with obesity. As such, secondary prevention initiatives include traditional obesity treatment approaches and require weight-control strategies that target weight loss, weight maintenance (with continued height increase), or decreasing the rate of weight-for-height increase (fewer pounds gained for inches grown).

5. PREVENTION GOALS AND STRATEGIES

5.1. Primordial Prevention

The most desirable prevention goal would be the primordial prevention of obesity, i.e., preventing children with desirable BMI (less than 85th percentile) from becoming at-risk of overweight (BMI between the 85 and 95th percentile). Success in achieving this goal is most likely to occur if prevention strategies and interventions are initiated in the first few years of life, perhaps even beginning during the prenatal period and infancy.

There are several reasons for emphasizing primordial prevention, the most significant of which are related to adipocyte physiology, adiposity rebound, and the limited potential for reversing metabolic changes associated with obesity.

During fetal life, babies begin to develop fat cells (adipocytes) at around 15 wk gestation *(23)*. Rapid increase in fat cell number and size, especially during the third trimester of pregnancy, results in an increase in percent body fat, from about 5 to 15% *(24)*. Thus, by term, birth about one-sixth of the infant's weight is fat (a 6-lb baby would have about 1 lb fat). This translates into about 5 billion adipocytes, or 16% of the 30 billion found in adults.

During infancy, fat cells increase primarily in size, rather than number. Between 2 and 14 yr of age, there is little change in fat cell size in lean children, and only a small increase in fat cell number from age 2 and 10 yr (25–27). Among obese children, however, fat cells continue to increase in size (28). Eventually, this triggers an increase in fat cell number, when adipocyte lipid content exceeds about 1 µg lipid per cell (29,39). During therapeutic weight loss, the rate at which new fat cells are formed (from pericapillary fibroblasts) slows down in obese children, but still continues at a rate that is greater than lean children (31). Thus, once obesity has developed in childhood, it may be restrained, but perhaps not reversed, giving added impetus for primordial prevention.

5.1.1. INFANT WEIGHT GAIN, ADIPOSITY, AND OBESITY

A number of studies have demonstrated an association between caloric intake and adiposity in infancy. Dewey and Lonnerdal (32) found that caloric intake was related to weight for length at 2 mo of age, but not at 4 or 6 mo. Average energy intake over the first 6 mo of life correlated significantly with weight gain and weight-for-length at 6 mo. Others reported (33) that British infants consumed significantly more calories and demonstrated twice the prevalence of overweight than comparable Swedish infants. For 6–9-mo-old infants, no correlation was found between adiposity and caloric intake, using 3-d food intake records (34).

Rate of weight gain during the first year of life, however, is a powerful predictor of adiposity at 7 yr of age, in both boys and girls. Weight gain above the 90th percentile during infancy was associated with a relative risk of obesity at age 7 yr of 3.3 for boys and 1.7 for girls (35).

Some studies suggest that mode of infant feeding (i.e., breast vs bottle, early vs later introduction of solids) is an important determinant of childhood obesity. Evidence is mixed, however, since studies are confounded by problems, including the fact that many infants get mixed feedings of both bottle and breast; bottle-fed babies often get solids added earlier, and lack of control for SES, maternal age, and race. Many studies suggest that the bottle-fed infant tends to take in more calories and gains weight more rapidly than the breast-fed infant (36). Kramer et al. (37), in a study that controlled for SES, maternal age, and race, found that breast feeding conferred a significant long-term protective effect against obesity in childhood. Breast feeding, combined with delayed introduction of solid foods, exerted a protective effect against obesity to age 2 (38). Although others have not found any differences between bottle-fed and breast-fed infants in development of adiposity (39), advocating breast feeding has other benefits, and can be recommended for these reasons in addition to the possible benefit in preventing accelerated weight gain.

5.1.2. FEEDING AND ACTIVITY PATTERNS OF OBESE AND LEAN INFANTS AND TODDLERS

A number of investigators have explored differences in feeding and activity patterns of lean and obese infants, in an effort to determine the earliest times at which clear-cut differences can be identified, and also to determine which factors may be etiologically more important in the initiation of childhood obesity.

Roberts et al. (40) measured both energy intake and expenditure at 6, 9, and 12 mo of age, among infants of normal-weight and overweight mothers. Infants of overweight mothers consumed 42% more calories than infants of normal weight mothers at 6 mo of age. At 9 and 12 mo of age, there was no difference. With respect to energy expenditure, infants of obese mothers, at 3 mo of age, who were becoming overweight, already had total energy expenditure that was 20.7% lower, on average, than all normal infants combined. Griffith et al. *(41,42)* studied energy intake and expenditure in preschool children, and similarly found that the children of obese parents had a significantly lower total energy expenditure (22% lower), compared with children of normal-weight parents. In this study, however, self-reported energy intake was also lower. Collectively, these data suggest that perhaps both early overfeeding and reduced energy expenditure contribute to infant obesity, or that infants and children who are susceptible to obesity have a variety of mechanisms for providing the surplus energy for excessive weight gain, including excess intake of energy, as well as low energy expenditure in physical activity.

Other investigators have reported evidence that the feeding behaviors of heavier infants differ from that of leaner infants soon after birth *(43)*. Heavier infants suck faster and consume more formula, if sweetened, compared with lighter infants. Babies with medium or increased adiposity showed increased sucking rate and pressures (greater avidity of feeding) for sweet-tasting fluids, compared with thinner babies, who demonstrated a relative aversion for sweet taste. This behavior predicted relative weight at 3 yr of age. Overall, sucking studies found that infants who suck more frequently at higher pressures, with shorter intervals between bursts of sucking, consume more calories and tend to be fatter. These characteristics explained about 25% of the variance in adiposity (triceps skinfold thickness) at age 2 yr, in a multiple regression analysis. The strongest positive correlation was between sucking pressure and triceps skinfold thickness at 2 yr of age. Number of feeds per day was negatively correlated with adiposity, with fewer feeds associated with greater triceps skinfold thickness *(43)*.

Tracking studies indicate that the obese infant has an increased risk of becoming an obese older child, although, overall, only one-fourth to one-third tend to show persistence of the problem, and the most significant predictor is parental obesity *(35,44–46)*. In general, the longer the obesity persists, and the more severe the problem, the greater the likelihood it will persist into adulthood. Parental obesity increases the likelihood of all of these factors occurring.

5.1.3. ADIPOSITY REBOUND

The importance of primordial prevention is also supported by studies of adiposity rebound (AR) in childhood. Normally BMI increases from birth to age 1 yr, then falls, and reaches a low point at around 6 yr of age, before rebounding again. In several studies to date, the timing of adiposity rebound in childhood is related to risk of adolescent and adult obesity. Rolland-Cachera et al. *(47)* studied the pattern of BMI changes during childhood for 151 children, age 1 mo to 16 yr of age. She reported that early AR before age 5.5 yr of age (vs later AR) was associated with significantly greater adiposity at age 16 yr *(47)*. She noted that infants who eventually became obese by age 14 yr were slightly heavier at birth, reached a higher peak BMI slightly later in infancy (14 mo of age vs 12 mo), showed less of a decline in BMI at about 2 yr of age, and began AR at a mean age of 4 yr (50 mo) vs 6 yr (70 mo) for lean children/teens. Figure 9 illustrates changes in BMI for an overweight 6-yr-old in whom AR occurred at 3 yr of age.

Whitaker et al. *(44)* conducted a retrospective cohort study using lifelong height and weight measures recorded in outpatient medical records. He found that a younger age at AR was associated with an increased risk of adult obesity, and that the risk was independent of BMI at AR, and of parent obesity *(46)*. Thus, the earlier the age at which AR

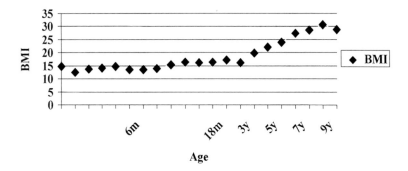

Fig. 9. Adiposity rebound before 3 yr of age.

occurs, the more likely a child will become an obese adult. Thus, one of the most compelling arguments for initiating obesity prevention in the first few years of life is the desire to delay AR.

Although AR was first described 15 yr ago, little is known about what triggers early AR. It is likely to be influenced by a complex interaction of both genetic and environmental factors. One may also expect that the mean age of AR may be decreasing in the United States, in view of the increasing prevalence of the condition among children and adolescents. To date, however, no data have reported temporal trends for AR in the United States or other developed countries. Additional studies are also needed to determine if dietary factors (e.g., high fat) promote early AR, or if inactivity also plays a role.

There are some clues that accelerated weight gain in preschool children may be associated with an increasing proportion of calories from fat in the diet. This may be expected, because fat is very energy-dense relative to protein and carbohydrate; thus, foods high in fat are typically higher in total energy and smaller in volume (an important satiety cue). High-fat foods are also very palatable (which encourages overeating), but not highly satiating, so that children may be less likely to adjust subsequent dietary intake to compensate for having consumed a high-fat (high-calorie) meal. Dietary fat is stored more efficiently than dietary protein or carbohydrate; and oxidation of dietary fat does not increase as dietary fat intake increases, in a manner similar to carbohydrate and protein.

Klesges et al. *(48)* evaluated determinants of accelerated weight gain over 3 yr in a cohort of 146 preschool children. Higher baseline levels of % energy from fat were associated with greater increases in adiposity and BMI, as were recent increases in % energy from fat. Total caloric intake did relate to weight gain; however, when fat kcal were entered into the regression equation, it explained more of the variance in weight gain than total energy intake. This suggests that, for preschool children, the % calories from total fat is an important contributor to accelerated weight gain. Baseline aerobic activity and increased leisure activity were also significant predictors of change in BMI. These modifiable diet/activity variables together accounted for 33% more of the variance in body mass change than the combined set of nonmodifiable variables (such as parental obesity). Eck et al. *(49)*, in the same study, found that percent of calories from fat, but not total calories, were higher on a high-risk group of 3–4-yr-old children who gained more weight over a 1 yr period of time.

Robertson et al. *(50)* also found that total energy intake was higher among preschool children who had accelerated weight gain over a 2-yr period of time, compared with children whose weight gain for height was normal. Children with accelerated weight gain also consumed a greater proportion of their calories from fat *(50)*. Daheeger et al. *(51)* reported that number of calories from dietary fat was a significant predictor of fat mass for 4–7-yr-old boys (even after controlling for total caloric intake), but not for girls.

Obese preschool children are also prompted by their parents to eat more at mealtimes. Klesges et al. *(52)* sent trained meal observers into homes to observe families at mealtimes, and found that obese children were prompted to eat more, offered more food, presented with more food, and encouraged to eat more food, twice as often or more, compared with lean children.

A major rationale for very early primordial and primary prevention is that obesity in children 3 yr of age and older is an important predictor of adult obesity. Whitaker et al. *(32)* found that this was true, regardless of whether the parents were obese. In addition, parental obesity more than doubled the risk of adult obesity among both obese and nonobese children less than 10 yr of age. In contrast, obese children younger than 3 yr of age, whose parents were not obese, were not at increased risk of adult obesity. The fact that parental obesity is a powerful predictor of child obesity has been known for several decades. With the currently increasing rates of adult obesity, however, the prevalence of parental obesity increases, as does the risk that children of these obese parents will also become obese.

5.2. Secondary Prevention

Secondary prevention is also important, because both duration and severity of childhood obesity are critical predictors of eventual adult obesity and related health problems. In other words, the longer obesity persists during childhood and adolescence, and the more severe it becomes, the greater the likelihood that the problem will persist into adult life. Thus, there is good rationale for believing that obesity prevention efforts should be initiated in the preschool period for maximum effectiveness.

6. OBESITY PREVENTION STRATEGIES IN PRESCHOOL AND DAY CARE SETTINGS

An underutilized, potentially effective, but low-cost public health approach to primordial and primary obesity prevention in the preschool period would involve dissemination and implementation of comprehensive preschool health education programs in nursery schools, daycare, and Head Start centers in the United States. In 1995, almost two-thirds of mothers with children <6 yr old were working outside the home (nearly double the rate 20 yr ago), and an increasing proportion of their children (about 3 million at present) are cared for in preschool or day care centers. The idea of providing universal preschool for all children is gaining momentum.

Health education and interventions aimed at preschoolers are important from a developmental point of view, since health habits are acquired and practiced during the preschool period, health knowledge is gained, and early attitudes about health begin to be established at this time, as well. So comprehensive health education should be part of every preschool program, as the basic minimal obesity prevention program for all children and parents.

Preschool children actually acquire a large number of health behaviors: safety behaviors (seatbelts, helmets, hats and sunscreen, avoiding danger); dietary behaviors (food preferences and choices); physical activity behaviors (preference for active or inactive play); hygiene behaviors (washing hands, brushing teeth, and so on).

It is important for disease prevention that health education programs are comprehensive in nature, because such programs include health education curriculum for the children, teacher training, parent education, cook training, and adequate physical activity. This is in addition to legal and specific program requirements for medical and dental checkups, immunizations, safety policies, smoking policies, medication and emergency policies, and health professional staff support.

An example of a comprehensive preschool health education program is the Healthy Start program *(53)*. The Healthy Start children's curriculum was developed with a basis in social learning theory *(54)*, and was designed to be developmentally appropriate for 3- and 4-yr-old children. The curriculum has 12 units, covering a wide variety of health topics, including nutrition, physical activity, self-esteem, and drug abuse prevention, designed to be taught in nursery school for 20 min 3× a week throughout the school year. The emphasis is on exploratory hands-on activities, games, and acquisition of new skills, knowledge, and healthy attitudes *(55)*. In addition, there is teacher training, take-home education materials for parents, a food service modification manual, and a computer-assisted knowledge quiz for evaluation *(55–60)*.

The effectiveness of preschool health education programs in preventing childhood obesity is likely to be significantly enhanced, if they are part of a larger national public health campaign focused on reduction of obesity for the population as a whole. For children, a more global public health campaign would also include identification and early treatment of at-risk and already obese children and adolescents, carried out by pediatricians and other health professionals in a variety of settings.

Obesity results from a positive net energy balance (more calories are consumed than expended), and the major modifiable factors in the equation are caloric intake (diet) and caloric expenditure (physical activity). Thus, the primary goals of a preschool prevention strategy must be to help children, parents, and teachers achieve a fat-controlled heart healthy diet, as well as daily physical activity goals (at least 30 min/d for children over 2 yr of age) *(61)*. Dietary goals include reducing the total and saturated fat in preschool meals and snacks, and increasing dietary fiber with more grains, vegetables, fruits, and legumes, and helping parents and teachers do the same at home. Physical activity goals include helping preschool centers develop adequate and developmentally appropriate physical activity programs for the children, as well as helping parents and teachers initiate more personal and family physical activities for themselves and their families.

The dietary fat goals are consistent with the 1998 American Academy of Pediatrics Guidelines, which recommend that children 2 yr of age and older consume no more than 30% (and no less than 20%) of their daily energy intake (kcal/d) as fat, and less than 10% of energy intake as saturated fat *(62)*. Most preschool children are still not meeting these goals, however. Data from NHANES-III (ph1) indicate that 77–85% of 2–19-yr-olds exceed recommended intake of total fat; and 91–93% exceed recommended intake of saturated fat *(63)*. In the 1995 Continuing Survey of Food Intakes by Individuals *(64)*, two-thirds of children still exceed recommended goals (63–69% exceeded the total fat goal of <30%E; and 62–77% exceeded the saturated fat goal of <10%E.

Dietary fiber is also important in childhood, since dietary fiber often replaces some of the fat. According to the age + 5 dietary fiber rule *(65,66)*, 3–5-yr-old children should be consuming 8–10 g of fiber as a minimum (Fig. 10). Only 54% of children this age meet

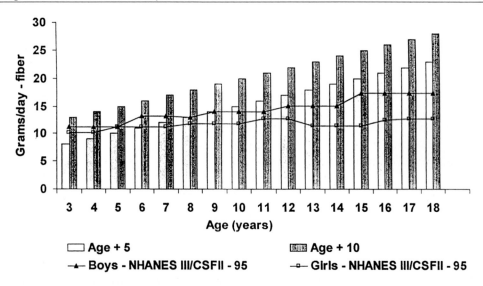

Fig. 10. Current vs recommended fiber intake children 3–18 yr of age "age + 5" minimal to "age + 10" maximal.

this goal. The Bogalusa Heart Study also found that 10-yr-olds in the top quartile for dietary fiber intake also had the lowest intake of fat *(67)*.

In the Healthy Start project *(68)*, saturated fat in preschool meals and snacks was reduced from about 10 to 9% of energy in intervention sites (compared with an increase from 10 to 12% in control sites), resulting in lower blood cholesterol levels among preschool children. Growth rates were not affected, because calorie intake remained normal. Other studies, such as the STRIP study in Finland, have proved that growth is dependent on total energy intake, and not on fat intake, and that preschool children grow normally, as long as a balanced diet with adequate energy and essential nutrients is provided *(69,70)*.

Young children also need more and better physical activity programs. If obesity is increasing among preschool children, greater effort is needed to improve the duration and intensity of daily physical activity. In preschool centers, there is a tendency to try to make the children sit down and be quiet! Even at recess in the playground, children are generally left to their own devices to run around and play. Experts suggest that preschool children should be actively taught new motor skills, and then helped to practice and perfect them *(71)*. This includes motor skills such as running, jumping, hopping, throwing, kicking, standing on one foot, doing a somersault, and riding a tricycle. Children who acquire these skills develop a sense of accomplishment, and enjoy being physically active *(72)*. We also need to encourage communities to help their children be more physically active, and to provide neighborhoods that are safe for our children.

7. OBESITY PREVENTION STRATEGIES
FOR FAMILIES WITH YOUNG CHILDREN

The Food Guide Pyramid for young children, from the U.S. Department of Agriculture, more clearly defines the number of servings of foods from each area of the pyramid that should be consumed by young children *(74)*. More importantly, it clarifies portion size for this age group, since, in the past, there has been confusion as to what constitutes a portion size for a young child. For most 2–6-yr-olds, energy requirements, as well as macronutrient and micronutrient needs, will be met if, over an average of 3 d they consume six servings of the grain groups, three servings of vegetables, two servings of the fruit group, two servings of the milk group, and two servings of the meat group. In general, 2–3-yr-olds will consume fewer calories and smaller portions (about two-thirds a regular portion size) than older children. By 4 yr of age, regular portion sizes apply. The key features of healthy food-pyramid eating for preschool children could be summarized as follows:

- A good estimate of a serving for a 2–3-yr-old child is about one-third of what counts as a regular Food Guide Pyramid serving.
- Children 2–3 yr of age need the same variety of foods as older children, but usually need fewer calories.
- Younger children eat smaller portions than older children. They should be offered smaller servings and allowed to ask for more. This will satisfy their hunger, and not waste food.
- By the time children are 4 yr old, they can eat amounts that count as regular Food Guide Pyramid servings eaten by older family members, i.e., one-half cup fruit or vegetable, one-fourth cup juice, one slice of bread, 2–3 oz of cooked lean meat, poultry, or fish.
- New foods should be offered in small "try me" portions (1–2 tbsp). Children may not begin to like a new food until they have tasted it many times and become familiar with it.
- Eating a variety of foods every day is important for the whole family. Offer children a variety of foods from the five major food groups, and let them decide how much to eat.
- 2–6-yr-old children need two servings from the milk group each day. After 2 yr of age, drinking low-fat (1% or skim) milk will help preschoolers achieve a heart-healthy diet, and avoid excessive intake of saturated fat.
- Young children's appetites can vary widely from day to day, depending on growth rates, environmental factors, and energy expenditure in play.
- As long as children have plenty of energy, are healthy, are growing well, and are eating a variety of foods, they are probably getting enough of the nutrients they need from the foods they eat.

The USDA food guide pyramid does not specify a recommended fat content for milk and cheese, or recommend lean vs fattier meats or grain products. Guidelines from the American Heart Association recommend a fat-modified diet after age 2 yr of age. The Academy of Pediatrics (62) recommends that preschool children gradually adopt a fat-modified diet after age 2, which provides no more than 10% of energy from saturated fat by 5 yr of age. One of the easiest ways to achieve this goal is for healthy children over 2 yr of age to consume low-fat dairy products, such as 1% low-fat milk (73). This strategy, coupled with adequate consumption of vegetables, fruits, and fiber-containing grain products, and limiting intake of added sugars and fats (the tip of the pyramid) will result in an energy-adequate, calorically balanced, and fat-controlled diet (74). In addition to a low-saturated fat, healthy pyramid eating plan for preschoolers, daily physical activity is essential (30 minutes a day of active play). These three key heart healthy themes for preschool diet and physical activity form the basis for educational messages for parents and teachers of young children, as well (Fig. 11).

Parents can be helped to establish diet and physical activity patterns that become healthy habits in the home, which promote health, rather than increase risk of future chronic diseases, such as obesity, cardiovascular disease, diabetes, and cancer.

RECOMMENDATION	THEME	RATIONALE
Drink Low-fat milk.	"If your age is over 2, Low-Fat milk's the one for you ! "	As a single strategy for reducing dietary fat, use of non-fat milk alone may be sufficient to meet dietary goals for preschool children.
Eat vegetables, fruits and grains every day.	"Vegetables, fruits and grains are best. (Can you pass the fiber test?)" (*Age+5 g/day dietary fiber for kids over 2)	Achieving "5-a-day" and fiber goals for kids will help them replace excess fat & sugar calories with more nutritious foods; achieve RDA's for more nutrients; and help them meet dietary fat goals as well.
Play hard	"Play hard to keep your body strong. Run and jump and skip along."	Kids >2 yrs old need 30 minutes active play each day. Energy expenditure increases; helps prevent obesity.

Fig. 11. 3 Key "heart healthy" themes for preschool diet and physical activity.

8. PRINCIPLES OF PREVENTION/RECOMMENDATIONS

The programs and activities described in this chapter include potential strategies that could be incorporated into an effective childhood obesity prevention campaign. Such strategies should benefit the vast majority of children, as a population approach to the problem, including those at increased risk of obesity, as well as those at low risk. Based on scientific and behavioral considerations, childhood obesity prevention initiatives should:

- Begin early, at least by 2 yr of age, if not earlier.
- Have no deleterious effects.
- Be relatively inexpensive.
- Benefit all children, even those at low risk of obesity.
- Have a strong child health education component (behavioral orientation).
- Include a Child Healthy Diet (and Heart Healthy) at home and at preschool (Fig. 12).
- Include adequate daily physical activity ("Active play—half hour a day").
- Limit inactivity (television viewing time, and so on).
- Involve the whole family: healthy home environments.
- Educate and involve parents, teachers, and older children as role models.
- Involve preschool centers in heart-healthy nutrition and physical activity initiatives.

1
Keep up caloric intake for normal growth

2
Keep total fat to 30% or less of calories (20-30%);
keep saturated fat below 10% of calories;
keep cholesterol intake below 300 mg/day

3
Eat at least 5 vegetables and fruits each day
(3 vegetables; 2 fruits)

4
Keep-up adequate calcium intake for bone health.

5
Increase carbohydrates to 50-55% of calories; eat a mix of starches, high
fiber carbohydrates, and whole grains

6
Eat at least "AGE + 5" grams of dietary fiber each day

7
Increase protein from vegetable sources (soy, grains, etc);
Decrease protein from animal sources

8
Eat fish at least once a week.

9
Limit added sugar and salt

10
Serve appropriate portion sizes for age and activity of child;
Smaller portions for preschool children;
Larger portions for very active children and teens

Fig. 12. The child-healthy diet.

Prevention of childhood obesity should begin as early in life as possible, but at least by 2–3 yr of age. Preschool programs that include health education, daily physical activity, and a child-healthy diet could be an effective public health intervention strategy.

REFERENCES

1. Kuczmarski RJ, Flegal KM, Campbell SM, Johnson CL. Increasing prevalence of overweight among US adults: the National Health and Nutrition Examination Surveys, 1960–1991. JAMA 1994; 272:205–211.
2. Wolf AM. What is the economic case for treating obesity? Obesity Res 1998; 6:2S–7S.
3. Pi-Sunyer FX. Medical hazards of obesity. Ann Intern Med 1993; 119:655–660.
4. Troiano RP, Flegal KM, Kuczmarski RJ, Campbell SM, Johnson CL. Overweight prevalence and trends for children and adolescents. Arch Pediatr Adolesc Med 1995; 149:1085–1091.
5. Troiano RP, Flegal KM. Overweight children and adolescents: Description, epidemiology, and demographics. Pediatrics 1998; 101(Suppl.):497–504.

6. National Institutes of Diabetes and Digestive and Kidney Diseases. Statistics Related to Overweight and Obesity. NIH Publication 96–4158. Rockville, MD: National Institutes of Health; July 1, 1996.

7. Dietz WH. Health consequences of obesity in youth: clinical predictors of adult disease. Pediatrics 1998; 101(Suppl.):518–525.

8. Williams DP, Going SB, Lohman TG, Harsha DW, Srinivasan SR, Webber LS, Berenson GS. Body fatness and risk for elevated blood pressure, total cholesterol, and serum lipoprotein ratios in children and adolescents. Am J Public Health 1992; 82:358–363.

9. Baranowski T, Stone R, Klesges RC, Basch C, Ellison RC, Iannottii R, et al. Studies of child activity and nutrition (SCAN): longitudinal research on CVD risk factors and CVH in young children. Cardiovasc Risk Factors 1993; 2:4–16.

10. Salbe AD, Fontvielle AM, Harper IT, Ravussin E. Low levels of physical activity in 5 year old children. J Pediatr 1997; 131:423–429.

11. NHLBI Research Group. Obesity and cardiovascular disease risk factors in Black and White girls: the NHLBI Growth and Health Study. Am J Public Health 1992; 82:1613–1620.

12. Must A, Jacques PF, Dallal GE, Bajema CJ, Dietz WH. Long term morbidity and mortality of overweight adolescents: a follow-up of the Harvard Growth Study of 1922 to 1935. N Engl J Med 1992; 327:1350–1355.

13. Stunkard A, Burt V. Obesity and the body image. II. Age at onset of disturbances of the body image. Am J Psychiatry 1967; 123:1443–1447.

14. Ogden C, Troiano RP, Briefel R, Kuczmarski RJ, Flegal KM, Johnson CL. Prevalence of overweight among preschool children in the United States, 1971 through 1994. Pediatrics 1997; 99:e1–e13.

15. Mei Z, Scanlon KS, Grummer-Strawn LM, Freedman DS, Yip R, Trowbridge FL. Increasing prevalence of overweight among US Low-income preschool children: The Centers for Disease Control and Prevention Pediatric Nutrition Surveillance, 1983–1995. Pediatrics 1998; 101:e12–e23.

16. Williams CL, Squillace M, Strobino BA, Brotanek J, Campanaro L. Cardiovascular Risk Factors in Low Income Preschool Children: Project Healthy Start. Presented at the 4th International Congress on Preventive Cardiology, Montreal, Canada, June 29–July 3, 1997.

17. Richardson SA, Goodman N, Hastorf AH, Dornbusch SM. Cultural uniformity in reaction to physical disabilities. Am Soc Rev 1961; 26:241–247.

18. Staffieri JR. A study of the social stereotypes of body image in children. J Perspect Soc Psychol 1967; 7:101–104.

19. Stunkard A, Burt V. Obesity and the body image. II. Age at onset of disturbances in the body image. Am J Psychiatry 1967; 123:1443–1447.

20. Sallade J. A comparison of the psychological adjustment of obese vs non-obese children. J Psychosom Res 1973; 17:89–96.

21. Kaplan KM, Wadden TA. Childhood obesity and self esteem. J Pediatr 1986; 109:367–370.

22. Gortmaker SL, Must A, et al. Social and economic consequences of overweight in adolescence and young adulthood. N Engl J Med 1993; 329:1008–1012.

23. Knittle J. Adipose tissue development in man. In: Human Growth, Vol 2. Postnatal Growth. Faulkner F, Tanner JM, eds. New York: Plenum, 1978; pp. 1–38.

24. Rosso P. Prenatal nutrition and fetal growth and development. Ped Ann 1981; 10:21–30.

25. Johnston F. Sex differences in fat patterning in children and\ youth. In: Fat Distribution During Growth and Later Health Outcomes. Bouchard C, Johnston F, eds. New York: Liss, 1988; 85–102.

26. Forbes C. Body composition in adolescence. In: Human Growth: A Comprehensive Treatise. Vol 2. Faulkner F, Tanner JM, eds. New York: Plenum, 1986.

27. Liebel R, Berry E, Hirsch J. Biochemistry and development of adipose tissue in man. In: Health and Obesity. Conn HL Jr, DeFelice EA, Kuo P, eds. New York: Raven, 1983; pp. 134–139.

28. Knittle J, Timmrs K, Ginsberg-Fellner F. The growth of adipose tissue in children and adolescents. J Clin Invest 1979; 63:239–246.

29. Doglio A, Amri E, Dani C, et al. Effects of growth hormone in the differentiation process of preadipose cells. In: Growth Hormone: Basic and Clinical Aspects. Isaksson O, Binder C, Hall K, eds. Amsterdam, The Netherlands: Elsevier, 1987.

30. Faust I, Miller WJ. Hyperplastic Growth of Adipose Tissue in Obesity. New York: Raven, 1983; 41–51.

31. Hagar A, Sjostrom I, Arvidsson V. Adipose tissue cellularity in obese school girls before and after dietary treatment. Am J Clin Nutr 1978; 31:68–75.

32. Dewey KG, Lonnerdal B. Milk and nutrient intake of breast-fed infants from 1–6 months; relation to growth and fatness. J Pediatr Gastroenterol Nutr 1983; 3:497–506.

33. Sveger T, Lindberg T, Weibull B, Olsson UL. Nutrition, overnutrition and obesity in the first year of life in Malmo, Sweden. Acta Pediatr Scand 1975; 64:635–640.

34. Shapiro LR, Crawford PB, Clark MJ, Pearson DL, Raz J, Huenemann RL. Obesity prognosis: a longitudinal study of children from age 6 months to 9 years. Am J Public Health 1984; 74:968–972.

35. Melbin T, Vuille JC. The relative importance of rapid weight gain in infancy as a precursor of childhood obesity. In: The Adipose Child. Laron Z, Dickman Z, eds. Basel, Karger, 1976 W1PE 163H v.1 1975.

36. Fomon S, Thomas L, Filer L, et al. Food consumption and growth of normal infants fed milk-based formulas. Acta Pediatr Scand 1971; 223:1–36.

37. Kramer MS. Do breast-feeding and delayed introduction of solid foods protect against subsequent obesity? J Pediatr 1981; 98:883–887.

38. Kramer MS, Barr RG, Leduc DG, Boisjoly C, Pless IB. Infant determinants of childhood weight and adiposity. J Pediatr 1985; 107:104–107.

39. Dine MS, Gartside PS, Glueck CJ, et al. Where do the heaviest children come from? A prospective study of white children from birth to 5 years of age. Pediatrics 1979; 63:1–7.

40. Roberts, SB, Savage J, Coward WA, Chew B, Lucas A. Energy expenditure and energy intake in infants born to lean and overweight mothers. N Engl J Med 1988; 318:461–466.

41. Griffiths M, Payne PR. Energy expenditure in small children of obese and non-obese parents. Nature 1976; 260:698–700.

42. Griffiths M, Payne PR, Stunkard AJ, Rivers JPW, Cox M. Metabolic rate and physical development in children at risk of obesity. Lancet 1990; 336:76–78.

43. Agras WS, Kraemer HC, Berkowitz RI, Hammer LD. Influence of early feeding style on adiposity at 6 years of age. J Pediatr 1990; 116:805–809.

44. Mack RW, Johnston FE. The relationship between growth in infancy and growth in adolescence: report of a longitudinal study among urban black adolescents. Hum Biol 1976; 48:493–711.

45. Garn S, Levelle M. Two decade follow-up of fatness in early childhood. Am J Dis Child 1985; 139:181–185.

46. Whitaker RC, Wright JA, Pepe MS, Seidel KD, Dietz WH. Predicting obesity in young adulthood from childhood and parental obesity. N Engl J Med 1997; 337:869–872.

47. Rolland-Cachera MF, Deheeger M, Bellisle F, Sempe M, Guilloud-Bataille M, Patois E. Adiposity rebound in children: a simple indicator for predicting obesity. Am J Clin Nutr 1984; 39:129–135.

48. Klesges RC, Klesges LM, Eck LH, Shelton ML. A longitudinal analysis of accelerated weight gain in preschool children. Pediatrics 1995; 95:126–130.

49. Eck LH, Klesges RC, Hanson CL, Slawson D. Children at familial risk for obesity: an examination of dietary intake, physical activity and weight status. Int J Obes 1992; 16:71–78.

50. Robertson AM, Cullen KW, Baronowski J, Baranowski T, Hu S, deMoor C. Factors related to adiposity among three to seven year old children. (Personal communication, 1999).

51. Deheeger M, Rolland-Cachera M, Fontvieille A. Physical activity and body composition in 10 year old French children: linkages with nutritional intake? Int J Obes 1997; 21:372–379.

52. Klesges R. Parental influences in children's eating behavior and relative weight. J Appl Behav Anal 1983; 16:3731–3718.

53. Williams CL, Spark A, Strobino BA, Bollella M, D'Agostino C, Brotanek J, et al. Cardiovascular risk reduction in a preschool population: the Healthy Start Project. Prev Cardiol 1998; 2:45–55.

54. Bandura A. Social learning theory. Englewood Cliffs, NJ: Prentice-Hall, 1977.

55. D'Agostino C, D'Andrea T, Lieberman L, Sprance L, Williams CL. Healthy Start: a new comprehensive preschool health education program. J Health Educ 1999; 30:9–12.

56. D'Agostino C, D'Andrea T, Nix S, Williams CL. Nutrition knowledge in preschool children: the Healthy Start Project Year 1. J Health Educ 30:217–221.

57. D'Agostino C, Nix S, Williams CL. Development and reliability of the healthy start knowledge computer quiz for preschool children. J School Health 1999; 69:9–11.

58. Spark A, Pfau J, Nicklas T, Williams CL. Reducing fat in preschool meals: description of the food service intervention component of healthy start. J Nutr Educ 1998; 30:170–177.

59. Bollella M, Boccia L, Nicklas T, Lefkowitz K, Pittman B, Zang E, Williams CL. Dietary assessment of children in preschool: Healthy Start. Nutr Res 1999; 19:37–48.

60. Bollella M, Boccia L, Nicklas T, Lefkowitz K, Pittman B, Zang E, Williams CL. Sources of nutrient intake in diets of Head Start children: home vs school. J Am College Nutr 1999; 18:108–114.

61. Centers for Disease Control and Prevention. Guidelines for school and community programs to promote lifelong physical activity among young people. MMWR 1997; 46(No. RR-6):1–36.

62. American Academy of Pediatrics, Committee on Nutrition. Statement on cholesterol. Pediatrics 1998; 101:141–147.
63. Kennedy E, Goldberg J. What are American children eating? Implications for public policy. Nutr Rev 1995; 53:111–126.
64. CFSII, 1989–91: U.S. Department of Agriculture. Food and nutrient Intakes by Individuals in the United States, 1 Day, 1989–1991. NFS Report No. 91-2. Washington DC: US GPO, 1995.
65. Williams CL, Bollella M, Wynder E. A new recommendation for dietary fiber in childhood. Pediatrics 1995; 96S:985–988.
66. Williams CL. Importance of dietary fiber in childhood. J Am Diet Assoc 1995; 95:1140–1146.
67. Nicklas T, Myers L, Berenson GS. Impact of ready to eat cereal on the total dietary intake of children. JADA 1994; 94:316–318.
68. Williams CL, Bollella MC, Spark A, Strobino BA. Promoting a heart healthy diet among preschool children: Outcome of the "Healthy Start" nutrition education and food service intervention. Abstract presented at the 40th Annual Conference on Disease Epidemiology and Prevention, March 1–4, 2000, San Diego, CA.
69. Lapinleimu T, Vikari J, Jokinen E, et al. Prospective randomized trial in 1062 infants of a diet low in saturated fat and cholesterol. Lancet 1995; 345:471–476.
70. Lagstrom H, Seppanen R, Jokinen E, Niinikoski H, Ronnemaa T, Viikari J, Simell O. Influence of dietary fat on the nutrient intake and growth of children from 1 to 5 years of age: the Special Turku Coronary Risk Factor Intervention Project. Am J Clin Nutr 1999; 69:516–523.
71. Gutteridge MA. A study of the motor achievement of young children. Arch Psychol 1939; 244:1–178.
72. Bredenkamp S, ed. Developmentally Appropriate Practice in Early Childhood Programs Serving Children from Birth Through Age 8. Washington DC. National Association for the Education of Young Children.
73. Sigman-Grant M, Zimmerman S, Kris-Etherton PM. Dietary approaches for reducing fat intake in preschool children. Pediatrics 1993; 91:955–960.
74. United States Department of Agriculture. Center for Nutrition Policy and promotion. Tips for Using the Food Guide Pyramid for Young Children 2 to 6 years old. USDA Program Aid 1647. Washington DC, 1999.

12 Obesity and Chronic Disease
Impact of Weight Reduction

Henry I. Frier and Harry L. Greene

1. INTRODUCTION

"Opinion is a flitting thing but truth outlasts the sun"
—Emily Dickinson

Diet and poor eating habits continue to play a significant role in the health of individuals. Improvements in public health, low-cost food production, transportation, and food processing have eliminated most nutrient deficiencies in this country and replaced them with diseases of excess calories. The *Surgeon General's Report on Nutrition and Health* (1988) ranked the 10 leading causes of death in the United States *(1)*. Several were strongly related to dietary excess, including coronary heart disease (CHD), cancer, stroke, diabetes mellitus, and atherosclerosis. Despite the recommendations in the *Surgeon General's Report (1)* to maintain a desirable weight and a caloric intake pattern in keeping with energy expenditure, Americans have experienced a substantial increase in body wt and obesity related morbidity and mortality. In fact, the prevalence of overweight and obesity is currently estimated at 54% of the adult population *(2)*. The greatest increase is in those classified as obese and morbidly obese. These are represented by the heaviest individuals (now estimated at 22%) with a body mass index (BMI) of >30 and >40 kg/m^2, respectively *(3;* Fig. 1). Of greatest concern is the increased incidence of obesity in children. Evidence suggests that they will be the next generation of obese adults, with the accompanying disease risks. This incidence is currently estimated at 14%, using the 95th percentile of weight *(4;* Fig. 2).

Wolf and Colditz *(5)* estimated the annual direct cost of obesity and its related co-morbidities, in 1995 U.S. dollars, to be 52 billion. This accounted for 5.7% of the U.S. national health expenditure. These authors again echoed the recommendations of the *Surgeon General's Report* to improve the diet and avoid overweight and obesity as the most important step in containing the rising costs of health care.

This chapter reviews the association between excess body wt and its major co-morbid conditions, as well as to review the impact of weight reduction on the improvement in obesity-related diseases. Five major co-morbidities are discussed: type 2 diabetes, hypertension (HT), cardiovascular disease (CVD), dyslipidemia, and certain types of cancer.

Obesity results from an imbalance in energy consumed and energy expended; however, the causes for this imbalance is more speculative. It is believed that there is a permissive component that is genetic, but is promoted by the societal and environmental

From: *Primary and Secondary Preventive Nutrition*
Edited by: A. Bendich and R. J. Deckelbaum © Humana Press Inc., Totowa, NJ

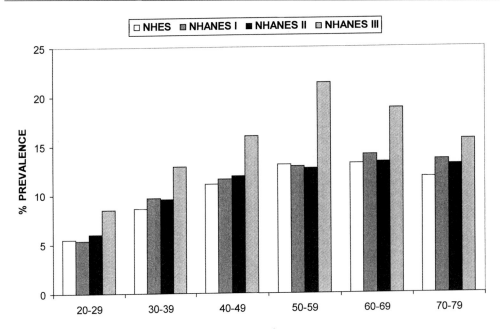

Fig. 1. Trends in Class I obesity (BMI 30–34.9 kg/m^2) at different age ranges (yr). Adapted with permission from ref. *3*.

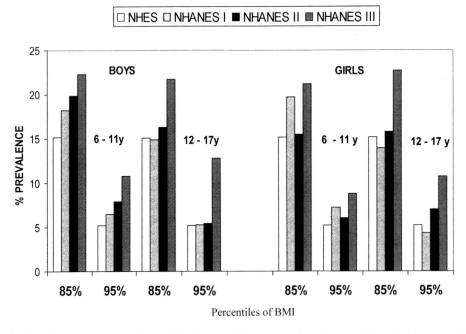

Fig. 2. Trends in obesity in 6–11 and 12–17-yr-old boys and girls. Adapted from Troiano et al. *(4)*.

changes in dietary patterns and reductions in physical activity. There is little doubt that a 5–10% decrease in body wt can significantly improve several risk factors associated with chronic disease *(2)*. What is not as clear is whether there is an improvement in mortality associated with the reduction in risk factors. Intuitively, one would expect that reductions in the risk factors, i.e., blood lipids, blood pressure (BP), and glycemic control, would improve the health of the population, hence, improving mortality rates. Additionally, because the positive relationship of weight gain and mortality has been established (6), logic would suggest that reversing this gain would decrease mortality.

Several recent reviews (7–9) critically evaluated the epidemiological studies on the association of weight loss and increased longevity. Williamson and Pamuk (7) concluded that the prospective studies reporting a positive benefit of weight loss on mortality were not justified by the data. Drawing on a series of published reports from diverse populations in the United States and Europe, Andres et al. (8) concluded that moderate weight gain was associated with the lowest rates of all-cause mortality.

The majority of the studies evaluated by Williamson and Pamuk (7) may have been misleading, in that no consideration was given to whether the observed weight loss was intentional or caused by an underlying illness associated with the weight loss (7,9). Second, habitual smoking may have contributed to the weight loss and increased mortality. Andres et al. (8) made several adjustments to account for weight and smoking. Additionally, the effect of weight reduction on mortality was analyzed in several ways, with the same conclusion, i.e., Cox regression coefficients with adjustments for multiple variables and quadratic analysis. Pamuk et al. (9) analyzed data from a cohort of men and women in the National Health and Nutrition Examination Survey (NHANES I), reporting weight loss, and correcting for smoking and premature death. As the percent of weight loss increased, there was a greater relative risk (RR) of death for both sexes at each BMI category evaluated between 26 and 29 kg/m^2, but this decreased for those individuals with a BMI > 29 kg/m^2.

Contrasting with the above reports on mortality are several studies supporting the role of weight loss in improving mortality risk. Lean et al. (10) retrospectively analyzed mortality data in diabetics, and found that weight loss *per se*, and its relationship with initial BMI, actually improved survival. They estimated a 3–4 mo increased survival with each 1 kg body wt lost. Goldstein (11) reviewed the available clinical studies reporting weight losses ≤ 10% in obese individuals with type 2 diabetes, HT, or hyperlipidemia, and also concluded that modest weight loss decreased risk factors, and should therefore increase longevity. Goldstein theorized that a decrease in BMI from 40 to 38 kg/m^2 would improve mortality risk by 12%, and that decreasing the BMI from 30 to 28.5 kg/m^2 would improve mortality by 7.5% (Fig. 3, shaded areas; 11). These data suggest that even the morbidly obese can reduce the mortality risk with as little as a 5% weight reduction.

To understand the association between intentional weight loss and longevity, Williamson et al. (12) analyzed prospective data from overweight and obese women in the Cancer Prevention Study I. Exclusions were a BMI ≤ 27, smokers, and ages >64 and <40 yr. Women who had an obesity-related health condition, and who intentionally lost weight, had a 20% lower all-cause mortality. Diabetes-associated mortality was also reduced by 44% and CVD mortality by 9%. Weight loss of >9 kg in women without a preexisting disease was associated with a 25% decrease in cancer and CVD mortality (12).

The benefit of weight loss on mortality remains controversial. Several critical evaluations of the published observational data challenge the conventional wisdom that weight loss improves mortality. On the other hand, the weight of clinical trials, e.g., cholesterol reduction (*see* Subheading 2.3. and 4.) and more recent observational studies (12) would suggest otherwise.

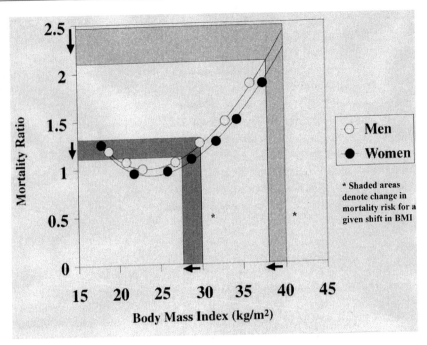

Fig. 3. Relationship between all cause mortality and BMI. Theoretical changes in mortality risk with decreases in BMI are denoted by arrows. Reproduced from Goldstein *(18)*.

2. OBESITY-RELATED HEALTH RISKS AND THE BENEFITS OF WEIGHT LOSS

2.1. Impaired Glucose Tolerance and Type 2 Diabetes Mellitus

The medical consequences of obesity can be classified as metabolic, e.g., diabetes mellitus and dyslipidemia, or mechanical, e.g., joint pain and osteoarthritis. The role of obesity in the development of the diabetic state is well established. Type 2 diabetes, via impaired glucose tolerance and insulin resistance, is also related to the development of several additional risk factors (e.g., HT and dyslipidemia). This relationship plays a key role in the progression to increased risk of macro- and microvascular diseases, such as kidney failure and blindness *(13)*. As an example, Ohlson et al. *(14)* observed that obese middle-aged Swedish men with impaired glucose tolerance were more likely to have increases in systolic BP and an elevation in plasma triacylglycerols.

The prediabetic state is marked by an increased level of fasting circulating insulin and a diminished response of peripheral insulin-sensitive tissues to oxidize and store glucose (insulin resistance) *(15)*. Increased circulating insulin in the obese individual is insufficient to maintain normal blood glucose, because of increased hepatic glucose production coupled with a reduced glucose uptake by muscle and adipose tissue. How adiposity is related to this pathological state is speculative. One early theory *(16)*, "the glucose fatty acid cycle," suggests that, in obesity, an excess of circulating free fatty acids (FFAs) inhibit glucose uptake by muscle, inducing glucose intolerance. It is thought that an imbalance exists between rates of FA esterification in adipose tissue and an accelerated glyceride breakdown in muscle, caused by the insulin insensitivity of this tissue (*see* Chapter 9).

2.1.1. BMI and Diabetes Risk

Campbell and Gerich *(17)* measured both insulin sensitivity, by half-maximal glucose disposal rates (EC_{50}), and insulin responsiveness in subjects with varying BMI and normal glucose tolerance. Those investigators found that BMI must exceed a critical threshold before insulin action is impaired. Using a broken-line regression model, they estimated a breakpoint in BMI of 26.8 kg/m², which corresponds to 120% of ideal body wt. In a follow-up study, Campbell and Carlson *(18)*, using similar techniques, compared normal lean subjects to obese type 2 diabetics (52 ± 2 yr, BMI of 28.1 ± 0.8 kg/m²). The results strengthen the earlier findings of a relationship between increased BMI and decreased insulin sensitivities in type 2 diabetics. Additionally, hepatic glucose production was correlated with BMI only in the type 2 diabetics. These findings are consistent with the epidemiological data and the long-held clinical association between obesity and type 2 diabetes.

2.1.2. Visceral Adiposity and Diabetes Risk

Several lines of evidence suggest that increased visceral adiposity is more likely to be associated with abnormal glycemic control and subsequent development of diabetes than simply with an increased body wt. Several prospective studies have shown an increased relative risk of diabetes, in both men and women, with increased central (visceral) obesity. The Gothenburg studies *(19,20)* focused on the importance of central adiposity and the increased incidence of diabetes; both men and women had significant correlations with waist:hip ratio (WHR) and total body fat. Cassano et al. *(21)*, utilizing a cohort from the Normative Aging Study, found a 2.4-fold increase in diabetic risk with increasing WHR, when adjustments were made for age, BMI, and smoking. Those authors also found a positive association between blood glucose and abdominal fat that was independent of total body fat.

2.1.3. Metabolic Alterations and Insulin Resistance

Other metabolic alterations are commonly associated with obesity and insulin resistance. Dyslipidemia manifested as hypertriglyceridemia, decreased high-density lipoprotein-cholesterol (HDL-C), increased very low density (VLDL) triglyceride and reduction in low-density lipoprotein (LDL) particle size (increased atherogenic potential) increases the risk for age-related CHD *(22)*. Although type 2 diabetics with good glycemic control have normal concentrations of LDL-C, the concentrations of fasting and postprandial triglyceride-rich particles (VLDL) are often elevated and HDL-C levels are decreased *(23)*.

2.1.4. Weight Loss and Glycemic Control

Weight loss has been shown repeatedly to improve glycemic control in both obese diabetic and nondiabetic patients *(2,15)*. These improvements have been observed early during therapy, suggesting that the caloric reduction is the primary promoter for the observed changes. Wing et al. *(24)* attempted to separate the effects of caloric restriction and weight loss, in obese type 2 diabetic patients. Those investigators used two levels of caloric restriction (400 vs 1000 kcal/d). At the point of an 11% weight loss, assessment of subjects showed that individuals consuming fewer calories per day had greater reductions in fasting blood glucose and greater insulin sensitivities. Hence, the degree of calorie restriction, independent of the magnitude of weight loss, appeared to play a dominant role in improvements in glycemic control. Additional support for the primary

Table 1
Metabolic Improvements in Patients with Type II Diabetes Following Weight Loss Over 1 Yr

	Before	13.6 kg	6.9–13.6 kg	2.4–6.8 kg	0–2.3 kg	Wt gain
RBW%	159	121[a]	143[a]	152[a]	157[b]	164[a]
HbA$_1$ (%)	9.7	7.1[b]	8.7[a]	9.8	10.4	10.6[c]
Glucose (mg/dL)	190	109[a]	162[b]	185	197	217[c]
Insulin (mU/mL)	20	2.9[a]	10.5[c]	11.8[c]	14.6	14.9
TG (mg/dL)	195	87[a]	155[b]	165[c]	175	204
HDL-C (mg/dL)	28.2	48.8[a]	41.3	40.3	38.4	39.7

p values: [a]0.001; [b]0.01; [c]0.05.
Reproduced with permission from ref. 28.

role of calorie reduction is provided by a report in type 2 diabetic patients undergoing gastric bypass surgery for weight loss (25). These patients showed an early correction of hyperglycemia before the appearance of weight loss. The authors relate these changes to the immediate reduction of food intake following surgery. They were also able to rule out the interaction of more traditional treatment approaches, i.e., exercise, sulfonylureas, and insulin, which were not part of the surgical recovery regimen.

2.1.5. DIABETES AND CHD

Controversy exists as to the association between CHD mortality and type 2 diabetes. Observational and prospective studies have not demonstrated a clear relationship between the hyperglycemia in type 2 diabetics and CHD (23). However, several studies showed an association between glucose-intolerant populations and increased risk of CHD. Singer et al. (26) also found a significant relationship between hemoglobin A$_1$C (HbA$_{1c}$) and CVD in female survivors of the original cohort of the Framingham Heart Study. In addition, HbA$_{1c}$ was strongly related to HT and the ratio of LDL-C to HDL-C. An analysis of the Framingham Offspring Study (27) found several associated metabolic abnormalities. For example, obesity was associated with HT and an elevation in fasting insulin, low HDL-C, and elevated triacylglycerol (TG) concentrations and a wide range of impaired glucose tolerances.

2.1.6. WEIGHT LOSS AND IMPROVEMENT IN RISK FACTORS

Clinically, improvements in glycemic control accompanying body wt loss are also mirrored by improvements in plasma insulin concentrations and lipid profiles (28). Long-term weight loss in type 2 diabetics, ranging from 2.3 to 13.6 kg, was associated with significant graded improvements in fasting blood glucose, HbA$_{1c}$, insulin, TGs, and HDL-C (Table 1). Weinsier et al. (29) found that 10 d of energy restriction (800 kcal/d) produced significant decreases in plasma total cholesterol (TC), TG, LDL-C, and insulin (all at $p < 0.05$). Strong correlations existed between insulin concentrations and triglycerides. Several reports have evaluated the efficacy of very low calorie diets in type 2 diabetic patients (40% or more above their ideal weight) for periods of 4–20 wk (30–32). Serum cholesterol and triglycerides were significantly reduced, and were associated with improvements in the fasting blood glucose and glycosylated hemoglobin. In one of these studies (31), the improvements in the lipid profiles during active treatment were negated, because of a partial weight regain. However, the regain in weight was not of sufficient magnitude to dampen the improvements observed in glycemic control and HDL-C.

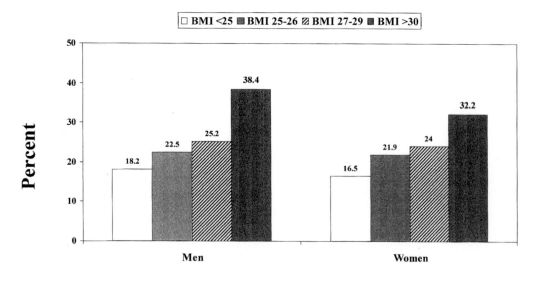

BMI Levels

Fig. 4. Age-adjusted prevalence of hypertension with increasing BMI in men and women. Reproduced from NHLBI Report *(3)*.

2.2. Hypertension

HT (>140 mmHg systolic/>90 mmHg diastolic) *(33)* afflicts over 60 million Americans, and as such is the most common CVD in the United States. The regulation of BP is complex, and involves the interaction of a number of mechanical and hormonal control mechanisms *(34)*. HT from obesity is associated with both increased cardiac output and peripheral arteriolar resistance. It is also strongly associated with the male obesity pattern of upper body adiposity *(35)*.

2.2.1. Increased Risk of HT from Obesity

Population comparisons indicate that HT is strongly associated with societies that also exhibit excess body wt. The Hypertension Detection and Follow-up Study *(36)* found that 60% of HT participants were at least 120% of normal body wt, with BMIs approximating 27 kg/m^2. On further analysis, this study *(37)* found that, in the 30–39 yr age group, a threefold greater incidence of HT occurred at body wts ≥20% of normal. A 6-yr follow-up analysis of the Multiple Risk Factor Intervention Trial *(38)* reported a strong independent relation between increasing BMI and systolic and diastolic BP. The most recent NHANES survey estimated that age-adjusted BP increases progressively with increasing BMI in both sexes *(2;* Fig. 4).

2.2.2. Effects of Weight Loss on BP

The benefits of weight loss on BP in obese HT and non-HT patients has been well established *(2,15,39)*. A 10-kg body wt loss in obese HT subjects was accompanied by a significant fall in both systolic and diastolic pressures, and was associated with decreases in several cardiac parameters, e.g., heart rate, cardiac output, and cardiopulmonary volume *(40)*. A meta-analysis *(41)* found an average fall of 6 and 3 mmHg in systolic and diastolic BPs with a 9-kg weight loss. Large patient multicenter trials, the Trial of Nonpharmacologic Intervention in the Elderly *(42)* and the Trials of Hypertension Prevention (TOPH) *(43)*, demonstrated significant and independent effects of weight loss on BP. Elderly individuals maintaining a weight loss of approx 4 kg over 30 mo had significantly lower clinical end points (HT, resumption of medication) than controls *(42)*. Subjects in TOPH who lost weight exhibited half the incidence of HT of the control group *(43)*.

The public health impact of a small downward shift in the population distribution of BP was shown to reduce the community burden related–CVD risk *(44)*. In 35–64-yr-olds, a decrease of 2 mmHg in diastolic BP was estimated to decrease the prevalence of HT by 17%, and to decrease the annual incidence of clinically relevant coronary artery disease and stroke by 6 and 14%, respectively *(44)*.

2.3. Cardiovascular Disease

2.3.1. DYSLIPIDEMIA

Analysis of the NHANES surveys found that serum TC levels, over the past 30 yr, have been declining in the U.S. adult population *(45)*. This finding suggests that the public health programs designed to lower serum cholesterol have been effective *(46)*. Still, there is some debate regarding the relationship of serum TC and all-cause and CV mortality in women *(47,48)*.

2.3.1.1. Obesity and CV Risk. The relationship between obesity, CVD risk factors, and increased risk of CHD and stroke has been demonstrated in several observational and prospective studies in both men and women *(49–55)*. Analysis of NHANES III data demonstrates the increasing prevalence of high serum TC (Fig. 5) and low HDL-C (Fig. 6) with increasing BMI *(5)*. Denke et al. *(52,53)*, utilizing data from NHANES II, found that excess body wt resulted in deleterious changes in the lipoprotein profile of both men and women. A linear trend analysis showed that increased BMI was significantly related to elevations in serum TG, TC, and LDL concentrations in both sexes.

Several recent prospective analyses of the Nurses' Health Study *(49–51,54)* estimated the risk of CHD and stroke, with increased body wt, in over 121,000 women. Similar relative risks of nonfatal myocardial infarction (MI) and fatal CHD in 8- *(54)* and 14- *(51)* yr follow-ups, were 3.3 and 3.6 for a BMI of ≥ 29 kg/m^2. Of greater interest were the changes in RR with body wt gain. Women who gained 8–10.9 kg from 18 yr of age doubled their risk of CHD and nonfatal MI, compared to stable-weight controls *(51)*. Higher WHR and waist circumference were independently associated with greater CHD risk in a cohort of women 40–65 yr of age in the Nurses' Health Study *(49)*.

2.3.1.2. Obesity and Risk of Stroke. Examination of the risk of stroke with increasing BMI and weight change *(50)*, in a cohort of registered nurses, found that women with a BMI ≥ 27 kg/m^2 had a significantly increased risk of ischemic stroke. Weight gain from age 18 yr was positively associated with ischemic stroke and was 1.7× greater in women who gained from 11 to 19 kg, compared to stable-weight controls.

Additional evidence for association of increases in body wt, blood lipids, BP, and mortality is provided in the Framingham Heart Study *(55,56)*. Elevation in serum cholesterol, systolic and diastolic BP, and blood glucose was positively associated with increasing weight gain in both men and women. Although total mortality did not increase until the highest quintile of BMI, CHD mortality increased linearly with increasing BMI. Two cross-sectional studies in Swedish women and men *(57,58)* provide additional

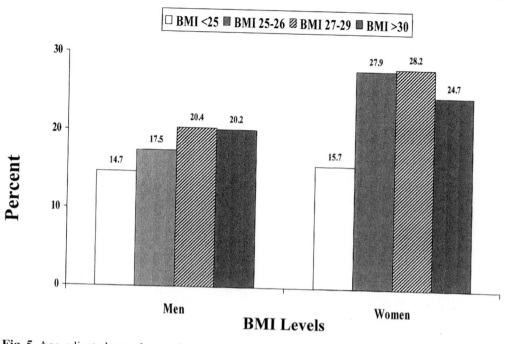

Fig. 5. Age-adjusted prevalence of high serum cholesterol (≥340 mg/dL) with increasing BMI in men and women. Reproduced from NHLBI Report *(3)*.

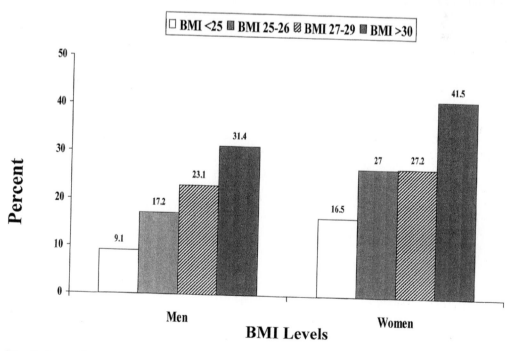

Fig. 6. Age-adjusted prevalence of low HDL-C (<35 mg/dL) with increasing BMI in men and women. Reproduced from NHLBI Report *(3)*.

Table 2
Associated Risk Factors and Definite CHD
with Increasing Tertiles of Subscapular Skinfold Thickness

	Tertile of subscapular skinfold		
Covariate	Lowest	Middle	Highest
BMI (kg/m^2)	21.2 (2.2)	24.1 (2.1)	26.3 (2.6)
Total cholesterol (mg/dL)	210.1 (37.7)	220.4 (37.2)	223.6 (38.1)
Glucose (mg/dL)	151.7 (52.6)	159.4 (57.2)	169.3 (62.9)
Triglycerides (mg/dL)	185.1 (168.8)	250.6 (211.2)	278.8 (218.3)
Incidence of CHD (no. events)	97	161	190

Adapted with permission from ref. 59.

support for this association. In women (57), WHR was significantly and positively associated with the 12-yr incidence of MI, stroke, and death. Similar associations were present for Swedish middle-aged men (58). Central obesity, as measured by subscapular skinfold thickness in the Honolulu Heart Program, was linearly related to the 12-yr incidence of CHD (59). A twofold increase in risk was estimated in those men with the highest skinfold thickness, compared to the lowest. Other CVD risk factors also increased with increasing tertiles of subscapular skinfold thickness (Table 2).

Modest reductions in body wt are paralleled by significant improvements in plasma lipids. Several reviews of the literature (2,11,15,60) have found consistent improvements in plasma TG and TC and LDL-C. Changes in HDL-C varied from study to study. Goldstein (11) reviewed six studies using various methods of weight reduction, and found HDL-C improved in half of those studies. The changes in HDL-C seem to be dependent on the magnitude of weight loss and gender. A 5% body wt loss was insufficient to raise HDL-C, unless coupled with an extensive exercise program (60). Weinser et al. (29) in a carefully controlled study to evaluate lipid and insulin changes in postmenopausal women found significant improvements in TC and LDL-C and TGs. No improvement in either HDL-C or LDL:HDL, with weight loss of 17% of initial body wt, was observed.

2.3.2. Thrombogenesis

The Northwick Park Heart Study (61) established a separate role for several hemostatic factors in ischemic heart disease. Increasing levels of clotting factor VII is an independent risk factor for CVD, and is associated with obesity and elevated plasma triglycerides (60). Landin et al. (62) measured components of the fibrinolytic system involved in the pathogenesis of CHD and atherosclerosis, in matched obese women with gluteofemoral or abdominal obesity. They found increased fibrinogen and plasminogen activator inhibitor-1 (PAI-1) in those obese women with a WHR of ≥ 0.8. PAI-1 was strongly correlated with fasting glucose and insulin levels, and negatively correlated with insulin sensitivity (euglycemic clamp). A reduction in PAI-1 has been demonstrated with energy restriction and weight reduction in obese patients (61).

2.4. Cancer

The rate of breast cancer (BC) has been steadily increasing in the United States, and is the second leading cause of cancer death in women (63). There is substantial evidence linking BC to obesity, the attendant hormonal changes, and the causes of obesity itself, i.e., excess dietary fat and caloric intakes and decreased physical activity. There is, however, considerable debate over cause and effect.

2.4.1. OBESITY AND RISK OF BC

The available case–control studies and large prospective studies are at variance over the association of BMI and BC (64). Twelve/13 case–control studies found a RR >1 in postmenopausal women, when the highest BMI (>32 kg/m^2) was compared to the lowest (≤19 kg/m^2). However, large prospective studies do not support this relationship. The authors (64) cited a large Norwegian study in which the observed RR of 1.2 for a 10 kg/m^2 increase in Quetelet's index was considered insignificant, given the large BMI change.

Reviewing the associations between site-specific cancers and several anthropometry measures, Ballard-Barbash (65) concluded that the observed associations for weight gain after 18 yr of age and central body fat exhibit stronger associations than weight or BMI. Because developed societies have a more sedentary lifestyle and a higher caloric intake, weight gain and increased fat mass, especially visceral, are better predictors of BC. Most, but not all, studies have shown a doubling of BC risk with expanding stores of visceral fat in postmenopausal, but not premenopausal, women (65).

As stated, obesity can be caused by diet (excess energy intake) and/or decreased physical activity. The evidence for the role of diet is beyond the scope of this chapter, but the controversy that exists is worthy of mention. Hunter and Willett (64) critically evaluated the strength of the studies implicating the amount of dietary fat as a major factor in BC incidence. The strongest evidence comes from studies based on national food disappearance estimates and those based on dietary recall. In contrast, several large prospective studies, which are not subject to recall bias, found no relation to BC (RR ≤1), when the highest deciles of total fat intake were compared to the lowest. A recent analysis of the Nurses' Health Study (66) found no difference in RR for BC in subjects consuming 20% dietary fat, compared to those consuming 30–35%. RR did not differ for type of fat consumed.

A central debate also concerns the relative carcinogenic effect of individual FAs vs the energy content of fat intake. Excess fat calories could promote primary BC by expanding centrally located adipose tissue, which in turn could increase the levels of circulating estrogens (higher conversion of adrenal androgens to estrone in female adipose tissue). The increased levels of estrogens have been implicated in the etiology of some breast and reproductive cancers, i.e. endometrial cancer (67,68). Recent studies have also implicated insulin and insulin-like growth factors, which are elevated in obesity, as direct promoters of tumor growth, or indirectly, by their actions on estrogen and estrogen receptors (65).

The evidence for a relationship between specific FAs or classes of TGs and BC is equivocal. In a pooled analysis of case–control studies, the overall association of BC with total fat was related to saturated fat intake. However, a pooled analysis of several large prospective studies found no relation of an increased risk (69). Case–control and prospective cohort studies failed to find a relationship with BC (69) for specific FAs, i.e., long-chain n-3 FAs and 18:2n-6 (linoleic acid).

2.4.2. BC SURVIVAL AND OBESITY

Once BC is diagnosed, women with higher BMIs exhibited poorer survival rates and increased reoccurrence of disease. In large population cohorts, obese women with stage I

or stage II disease have an increased risk of dying from BC: 70 and 40%, respectively
(65). Obesity is also associated with more advanced cancers at the time of diagnosis.
In Dutch women, a greater incidence of metastatic disease in axillary nodes was associated with significantly heavier body wt in the 50–69-yr age group *(63)*.

The data suggest that adult weight gain, whatever the cause, is associated with greater
risks of BC, and that the extent of the disease is more highly pronounced in patients with
the highest quintile of BMI.

2.4.3. WEIGHT LOSS AND CANCER

No prospective human trials have been conducted for the purpose of demonstrating a
reduction in risk of cancer from weight loss maintenance. It is hoped that such studies can
be performed when methods for sustained weight loss are more predictive.

3. INTERVENTION THERAPIES: MANAGEMENT OF OBESE PATIENTS

A review of clinical studies concerning diet and diet plus increased physical activity
has demonstrated successful 1–2-yr weight loss, ranging from 5 to 13% *(2)*. In these
studies, reductions in plasma lipids ranged from 0 to –18% for TC, –2 to –44% for TG,
–2 to –22% for LDL-C, and –7 to +27 for HDL-C.

Significant reductions in diameter stenosis of coronary arteries occurred in patients
making intensive lifestyle changes (diet, physical activity, stress management, and smoking cessation), compared to controls not making changes, –5.3 vs +2.7% *(70)*. Associated
risk factors, BMI, serum TC, and LDL-C were significantly reduced. A 5-yr follow-up
of these patients *(71)* showed continued improvement in regression of stenosis in the
intervention group, and worsening of the stenosis in the control group, –7.9 vs +27.7%.

A 10-wk multicenter trial *(72)* compared a prepackaged meal program, based on the
National Academy of Science–National Research Council (NAS-NRC) dietary recommendations, to a self-selection diet based on the American Heart Association (AHA) Step
I/II diets, in 560 patients suffering from dyslipidemia, HT, or diabetes. Weight loss was
significant for both groups (–4.7 kg in the NAS-NRC diet, and –3.2 kg in the AHA diet),
and was accompanied by significant reductions in major CVD risk factors, i.e., BP, TC,
glycemic control, and blood lipids. Similar findings in key risk factors occurred in a group
of patients identified with acute MI or unstable angina *(73)*. After 1 yr, those patients
randomized to a low-fat, high-fruit, grain, and vegetable diet lost 6.3 kg body wt, and had
significantly decreased cardiac events and mortality, compared to a control group, who
were simply advised to follow a low-fat diet *(see* Chapter 12).

Improvement in health risk associated with long-term weight loss was studied by
Ditschuneit et al. in a randomized controlled trial *(74)*. Those authors reported on a
2-yr follow-up of 100 obese patients (average BMI of 33 kg/m^2). Average weight loss
of patients, randomized to a traditional low-calorie diet group, was 1.3 kg, with no
improvements in markers of disease risk over the first 3 mo. By contrast, the group
receiving the same prescribed calorie intake, but with two meals replaced with a Slim·Fast
liquid meal replacement lost an average of 7.1 kg. These patients showed significant
improvements in BP, plasma insulin, glucose, and TG concentrations. A 24-mo follow-up of patients replacing an average of one meal per day with a Slim·Fast shake demonstrated continued improvement in these biomarkers, with associated weight losses of

5–11.5% of their initial body wt. The authors followed these patients for another 2 yr *(75)*, and found sustained weight loss and maintenance of the improvements in biomarkers.

The use of gastric bypass surgery *(25)* as a primary method for weight loss (10 yr) in morbidly obese is also instructive. In addition to the improvements in glycemic control, the sustained weight loss also corrected or alleviated a number of other co-morbid conditions associated with obesity, i.e., HT, sleep apnea, arthritis, cardiopulmonary failure, and infertility.

4. SUMMARY, CONCLUSIONS, AND RECOMMENDATIONS

The short-term and intermediate benefits of weight loss in the obese have been well-established *(2)*. Improvements in glycemic control in patients with type 2 diabetes occurs early in the weight loss regimen, and mostly results from the reduction in calories ingested *(24,25)*.

Weight losses of 5–15% of initial body wt is beneficial for the reduction of CVD risk factors *(60)*. Cardiac patients making major lifestyle changes have shown significant regression in aortic stenosis and cardiac events *(70–73)*. A program of reduced dietary fat intake, smoking cessation, stress management, and increased physical activity were essential to the improvements observed. It is difficult to isolate the individual impact that each one of these changes had; however, the decrease in BMI in these patients is consistent with improvements in several of the risk factors.

Although it is obvious that weight loss will reduce risk factors for disease, the relationship to mortality remains tentative. The published conclusions discussed earlier in this chapter are troublesome, since they suggest that the greater majority of individuals who attempt weight loss may be at an increased risk for all-cause mortality. It further implies that the assumption of weight loss on improvements in mortality may not be as clear-cut as simply reducing risk factors *(76)*.

However, insight can be gained from clinical trials demonstrating improvements in CHD mortality with reductions in blood lipids. In a review of 22 clinical trials on cholesterol reduction *(77)*, there was a 23% risk reduction in CHD events (nonfatal MI and cardiac death). A meta-analysis of six primary prevention trials found mortality from CHD tended to be lower in men receiving interventions to reduce cholesterol. When analyzed separately, a significant decrease in mortality was found in each study *(78)*. The Scandinavian Simvastin Survival Study *(79)* showed significant improvement in lipid profiles in patients taking the drug. During 6 yr follow-up, there were significantly more coronary deaths in the placebo group, compared to the simvastin group (189 vs 111; relative risk of 0.58). Hence, the reduction of blood lipids that occur with weight loss should provide similar changes in CHD risk.

Williamson et al.'s *(12)* 12-yr prospective study on weight loss and mortality adds significantly to the expectation that weight loss, via improvements in risk factors, will improve mortality. Women with obesity-related co-morbidities showed significant reductions in all-cause and diabetes-related mortality with weight loss. Preliminary evidence from Williamson would suggest the same for men *(2)*. Although there is limited data supporting improved mortality rates with weight loss *(80)*, the positive changes in biomarkers for disease risk justifies the public health objective to reduce the weight of the nation.

Recently, the National Institutes of Health *(2)* created a panel to assess the scientific literature regarding the severity of the medical problem and the benefits to weight loss.

Based on the evidence, they concluded that obesity is a major public health problem that can and should be addressed. The panel further established the evidence-based guidelines to help physicians and associated health professionals manage the overweight and obese patient *(2)*.

REFERENCES

1. The Surgeon General's Report on Nutrition and Health. DHHS (PHS) Publ No. 88–50210 Washington DC, 1988.
2. National Heart, Lung, and Blood Institute. NIH. Clinical guidelines on the identification, evaluation, and treatment of overweight and obesity in adults. Obes Res 1998; 6:51S–180S.
3. Flegal KM, Carroll MD, Kuczmarski RJ, Johnson CL. Overweight and obesity in the United States: prevalence and trends, 1960–1994. Int J Obes 1998; 22:39–47.
4. Troiano RP, Flegal KM, Kuczmarski RJ, Campbell SM, Johnson CL. Overweight prevalence and trends for children and adolescents. Arch Pediatr Adolesc Med 1995; 149:1085–1091.
5. Wolf AM, Colditz GA. Current estimates of the economic cost of obesity in the United States. Obes Res 1998; 6:97–106.
6. Bender R, Jöckel K-H, Trautner C, Spraul M, Berger M. Effect of age on excess mortality in obesity. JAMA 1999; 281:1498–1504.
7. Williamson DF, Pamuk ER. The association between weight loss and increased longevity. Ann Intern Med 1993; 119:732–736.
8. Andres R, Muller DC, Sorkin JD. Long-term effects of change in body weight on all-cause mortality. Ann Intern Med 1993; 119:737–743.
9. Williamson DF. "Weight cycling" and mortality: how do the epidemiologists explain the role of intentional weight loss. J Am Coll Nutr 1996; 15:6–13.
10. Lean MEJ, Powrie JK, Anderson AS, Garthwaite PH. Obesity, weight loss and prognosis in type 2 diabetes. Diabetic Med 1990; 7:228–233.
11. Goldstein DJ. Beneficial health effects of modest weight loss. Int J Obes 1992; 16:397–415.
12. Williamson DF, Pamuk E, Thun M, Flanders D, Byers T, Heath C. Prospective study of intentional weight loss and mortality in never-smoking overweight US white women aged 40–64 years. Am J Epidemiol 1995; 141:1128–1141.
13. Blake GH. Control of type II diabetes: reaping the rewards of exercise and weight loss. PostGrad Med 1992; 92:129–137.
14. Ohlson L, Larrson B, Eriksson H, Svärdsudd K, Welin L, Tibblin G. Diabetes mellitus in Swedish middle-aged men: the study of men born in 1913 and 1923. Diabetologia 1987; 30:386–393.
15. Pi-Sunyer FX. Short-term medical benefits and adverse effects of weight loss. Am Coll Phys 1993; 119:722–726.
16. Randle PJ, Garland PB, Hales CN, Newsholme EA. The glucose fatty-acid cycle. Its role in insulin sensitivity and the metabolic disturbances of diabetes mellitus. Lancet 1963; 21:785–789.
17. Campbell PJ, Gerich JE. Impact of obesity on insulin action in volunteers with normal glucose tolerance: demonstration of a threshold for the adverse effect of obesity. J Clin Endocrinol Metab 1990; 70:1114–1118.
18. Campbell PJ, Carlson MG. Impact of obesity on insulin action in NIDDM. Diabetes 1993; 42:405–410.
19. Lundgren H, Bengtsson C, Blohme G, Lapidus L, Sjöström L. Adiposity and adipose tissue distribution in relation to incidence of diabetes in women: results from a prospective population study in Gothenberg, Sweden. Int J Obes 1987; 13:413–423.
20. Ohlson L-O, Larsson B, Svardsudd K, Welin L, Eriksson H, Wilhelmsen L, Björntorp P, Tibblin G. The influence of body fat distribution on the incidence of diabetes mellitus. Diabetes 1985; 34:1055–1058.
21. Cassano PA, Rosner B, Vokonas PS, Weiss ST. Obesity and body fat distribution in relation to the incidence of non-insulin-dependent diabetes mellitus. Am J Epidemiol 1992; 136:1474–1486.
22. Syvänne M, Taskinen M-R. Lipids and lipoproteins as coronary risk factors in non-insulin-dependent diabetes mellitus. Lancet 1997; 350:20–23.
23. Nathan DM, Meigs J, Singer DE. The epidemiology of cardiovascular disease in type 2 diabetes mellitus: how sweet it is…or is it? Lancet 1997; 350:4–9.
24. Wing RR, Blair EH, Bononi P, Marcus MD, Watanabe R, Bergman RN. Caloric restriction per se is a significant factor in improvements in glycemic control and insulin sensitivity during weight loss in obese NIDDM patients. Diabetes Care 1994; 17:30–36.

25. Pories WJ, Swanson MS, MacDonald MD, Long SB, Morris PG, Brown BM, et al. Who would have thought it? An operation proves to be the most effective therapy for adult-onset diabetes mellitus. Ann Surg 1995; 222:339–352.

26. Singer DE, Nathan DM, Anderson KM, Wilson PW, Evans JC. Association of HbA$_{1c}$ with prevalent cardiovascular disease in the original cohort of the Framingham Heart Study. Diabetes 1992; 41: 202–208.

27. Meigs JB, Singer DE, Nathan DM, Cupples LA, Wilson PWF. Metabolic abnormalities associated with glucose intolerance extend across the spectrum of prevalent glucose tolerance in 3297 Framingham offspring study subjects. Diabetes 1995; 44:5A.

28. Bosello O, Armellini F, Zamboni M, Fitchet M. The benefits of modest weight loss in type II diabetes. Int J Obes 1997; 21:S10–S13.

29. Weinsier RL, James D, Darnell BE, Wooldrigde NH, Birch R, Hunter GR, Bartolucci AA. Lipid and insulin concentrations in obese postmenopausal women: separate effects of energy restriction and weight loss. Am J Clin Nutr 1992; 56:44–49.

30. Inoue S, Okamura A, Okamoto M, Tanaka K, Sugimasa T, Takamura Y. Effects of very low calorie diet (VLCD) on body weight, blood glucose and serum lipid metabolism in severe obesity with glucose intolerance. Int J Obes 1989; 13:183–184.

31. Wing RR, Marcus MD, Salata R, Epstein LH, Miaskiewicz S, Blair EH. Effects of a very-low-calorie diet on long-term glycemic control in obese type 2 diabetic subjects. Arch Intern Med 1991; 151: 1334–1340.

32. Uusitupa M, Laakso M, Sarlund H, Majander H, Takala J, Penttilä I. Effects of a very-low-calorie diet on metabolic control and cardiovascular risk factors in the treatment of obese non-insulin-dependent diabetics. Am J Clin Nutr 1990; 51:768–773.

33. 1984 Joint National Committee. The 1984 report of the Joint National Committee on the detection, evaluation, and treatment of high blood pressure. Arch Int Med 1984; 144:1045–1057.

34. Frolich ED. Mechanisms contributing to high blood pressure. Ann Int Med 1983; 98:709–714.

35. Bray GA. Obesity. In: Present Knowledge in Nutrition. Ziegler EE, Filer LJ, eds. Washington DC: ILSI Press, 1996; 19–32.

36. Hypertension Detection and Follow-Up Program Cooperative Group. Race education and prevalence of hypertension. Am J Epidemiol 1977; 106:351–361.

37. Havlik RJ, Hubert HB, Fabsitz RR, Feinleib M. Weight and hypertension. Ann Intern Med 1983; 98:855–859.

38. Stamler J, Caggiula AW, Grandits GA. Relation of body mass and alcohol, nutrient, fiber and caffeine intakes to blood pressure in the special intervention and usual care groups in the multiple risk factor intervention trial. Am J Clin Nutr 1997; 65:338S–365S.

39. Björntorp P. Obesity. Lancet 1997; 350:423–426.

40. Reisin E, Frohlich ED, Messerli FH, Dreslinski GR, Dunn FG, Jones MM, Batson HM. Cardiovascular changes after weight reduction in obesity hypertension. Ann Intern Med 1983; 98:315–319.

41. MacMahon S, Cutler J, Brittain E, Higgins M. Obesity and hypertension: epidemiological and clinical issues. Eur Heart J 1987; 8:57–70.

42. Whelton PK, Appel LJ, Espeland MA, Applegate WB, Ettinger WH, Kostis JB, et al. Sodium reduction and weight loss in the treatment of hypertension in older persons: a randomized controlled trial of nonpharmacologic interventions in the elderly. JAMA 1998; 279:839–846.

43. Whelton PK, Kumanyika SK, Cook NR, Cutler JA, Borhani NO, Hennekens CH, et al. Efficacy of nonpharmacologic interventions in adults with high-normal blood pressure: results from phase 1 of the Trials of Hypertension Prevention. Am J Clin Nutr 1997; 65:652S–660S.

44. Cook NR, Jerome C, Hebert PR, Taylor JO, Hennekens CH. Implications of small reductions in diastolic blood pressure for primary prevention. Arch Intern Med 1995; 155:701–709.

45. Johnson CL, Rifkind BM, Sempos CT, Carroll MD, Bachorik PS, Briefel RR, et al. Declining serum total cholesterol levels among US adults. JAMA 1993; 269:3002–3008.

46. Expert Panel on Detection, Evaluation, and Treatment of High Blood Pressure in Adults. Summary of the second report of the National Cholesterol Education Program (NCEP) Expert Panel on detection, evaluation, and treatment of high blood cholesterol in adults (adult treatment panel II) JAMA 1993; 269:3015–3023.

47. Jacobs D, Blackburn H, Higgins M, Reed D, Iso H, McMillan G, et al. Report of the conference on low blood cholesterol: mortality associations. Circulation 1992; 86:1046–1060.

48. Hulley SB, Walsh JMB, Newman TB. Health policy on blood cholesterol: time to change directions. Circulation 1992; 86:1026–1029.

49. Rexrode KM, Carey VJ, Hennekens CH, Walters EE, Colditz GA, Stampfer MJ, Willett WC, Manson JE. Abdominal adiposity and coronary heart disease in women. JAMA 1998; 280:1843–1848.

50. Rexrode KM, Hennekens CH, Willett WC, Colditz GA, Stampfer MJ, Rich-Edwards JW, Speizer FE, Manson JE. A prospective study of body mass index, weight change, and risk of stroke in women. JAMA 1997; 277:1539–1545.

51. Willett WC, Manson JE, Stampfer MJ, Colditz GA, Rosner B, Speizer FE, Hennekens CH. Weight, weight change, and coronary heart disease in women. JAMA 1995; 273:461–464.

52. Denke MA, Sempos CT, Grundy SM. Excess body weight: an under-recognized contributor to dyslipidemia in white American women. Arch Intern Med 1994; 154:401–410.

53. Denke MA, Sempos CT, Grundy SM. Excess body weight: an under-recognized contributor to high blood cholesterol levels in white American men. Arch Intern Med 1993; 153:1093–1103.

54. Manson JE, Colditz GA, Stampfer MJ, Willett WC, Rosner B, Monson RR, Speizer FE, Henneken CH. A prospective study of obesity and risk of coronary heart disease in women. N Engl J Med 1990; 322:882–889.

55. Higgins M, Kannel W, Garrison R, Pinsky J, Stokes J III. Hazards of obesity: the Framingham experience. Acta Med Scand 1988; 723:23–36.

56. Hubert HB, Feinleib M, McNamara PM, Castelli WP. Obesity as an independent risk factor for cardiovascular disease: a 26-year follow-up of participants in the Framingham Heart Study. Circulation 1983; 67:968–976.

57. Lapidus L, Bengtsson C, Larsson B, Pennert K, Rybo E, Sjostrom L. Distribution of adipose tissue and risk of cardiovascular disease and death: a 12 year follow up of participants in the population study of women in Gothenburg, Sweden. Br Med J 1984; 289:1257–1261.

58. Larsson B, Svärdsudd K, Welin L, Wilhlemsen L, Björntorp P, Tibblin G. Abdominal adipose tissue distribution, obesity, and risk of cardiovascular disease and death: 13 year follow up of participants in the study of men born in 1913. Br Med J 1984; 288:1401–1404.

59. Donahue RP, Bloom E, Yano K, Abbott RD, Reed DM. Central obesity and coronary heart disease in men. Lancet 1987; 2:821–824.

60. Van Gaal LF, Wauters MA, De Leeuw IH. The beneficial effects of modest weight loss on cardiovascular risk factors. Int J Obes 1997; 21:S5–S9.

61. Meade TW, Brozovic M, Chakrabarti RR, Haines AP, Imeson JD, Mellows S, et al. Haemostatic function and ischaemic heart disease: principal results of the Northwick Park heart study. Lancet 1986; 2:533–537.

62. Landin K, Stigendal L, Eridsson E, Krotkiewski M, Risberg B, Tengborn L, Smith U. Abdominal obesity is associated with an impaired fibrinolytic activity and elevated plasminogen activator inhibitor-1. Metabolism 1990; 39:1044–1048.

63. Nixon DW, Rodgers K. Breast cancer. In: Nutritional Oncology. Heber D, Blackburn GL, Go VLW, eds. New York: Academic, 1999; 447–451.

64. Hunter DJ, Willett WC. Diet, body build, and breast cancer. Ann Rev Nutr 1994; 14:393–418.

65. Ballard-Barbash R. Energy balance, anthropometry, and cancer. In: Nutritional Oncology. Heber D, Blackburn GL, Go VLW, eds. New York: Academic, 1999; 137–151.

66. Holmes MD, Hunter DJ, Colditz GA, Stampfer MJ, Hankinson SE, Speizer FE, Rosner B, Willett WC. Association of dietary intake of fat and fatty acids with risk of breast cancer. JAMA 1999; 281:914–920.

67. Bjöntorp P. The associations between obesity, adipose tissue distribution and disease. Acta Med Scand 1988; 723:121–134.

68. Heber D, Blackburn G, Go VLW. Introduction: the principles of nutritional oncology. In: Nutritional Oncology. Heber D, Blackburn GL, Go VLW, eds. New York: Academic, 1999; 1–4.

69. Willett WC. Specific fatty acids and risks of breast and prostate cancer: dietary intake. Am J Clin Nutr 1997; 66:1557S–1563S.

70. Ornish D, Brown SE, Scherwitz LW, Billings JH, Armstrong WT, Ports TA, et al. Can lifestyle changes reverse coronary heart disease? Lancet 1990; 336:129–133.

71. Ornish D, Scherwitz LW, Billings JH, Gould KL, Merritt TA, Sparler S, et al. Intensive lifestyle changes for reversal of coronary heart disease. JAMA 1998; 280:2001–2007.

72. McCarron DA, Oparil S, Chait A, Haynes B, Kris-Etherton P, Stern JS, et al. Nutritional management of cardiovascular risk factors. Arch Intern Med 1997; 157:169–177.

73. Singh RB, Rastogi SS, Verma R, Laxmi B, Singh R, Ghosh S, Niaz MA. Randomised controlled trial of cardioprotective diet in patients with recent acute myocardial infarction: results of one year follow up. Br Med J 1992; 304:1015–1019.

74. Ditschuneit HH, Flechtner-Mors M, Johnson TD, Adler G. Metabolic and weight-loss effects of a long-term dietary intervention in obese patients. Am J Clin Nutr 1999; 69:198–204.

75. Ditschuneit HH, Flechtner-Mors M, Johnson TD, et al. Metabolic and weight loss effects of long-term dietary intervention in obese patients. Obes Res 2000; 8(5):399–402.

76. Kassirer JP, Angell M. Losing weight-an ill fated New Year's resolution. N Engl J Med 1998; 338:52–54.

77. Yusuf S, Wittes J, Friedman L. Overview of the results of randomized clinical trials in heart disease. II. Unstable angina, heart failure, primary prevention with aspirin, and risk factor modification. JAMA 1988; 260:2259–2263.

78. Muldoon MF, Manuck SB, Matthews KA. Lowering cholesterol concentrations and mortality: a quantitative review of primary prevention trials. Br Med J 1990; 301:309–314.

79. Scandinavian Simvastin Survival Group. Randomized trial of cholesterol lowering in 4444 patients with coronary heart disease: The Scandinavian Simvastin Survival Study (4S). Lancet 1994; 344:1383–1389.

80. Willett WC, Dietz WH, Coditz GA. Guidelines for healthy weight. N Engl J Med 1999; 341:427–434.

13

Meal Replacement Products and Fat Substitutes in Weight Control and Maintenance

Allan Geliebter, Amy Funkhouser, and Steven B. Heymsfield

1. OVERVIEW

With a surplus of nutritious and palatable foods and a reduced need for occupational physical labor, most Americans are finding weight control a major problem. The national mean body mass index (BMI) rises with each new survey, and obesity-related co-morbidities, such as type II diabetes mellitus, are reaching epidemic proportions *(1)*.

This weight-gain-promoting environment is leading many to seek means of controlling their food intake, while still maintaining a nutritious and flavorful diet that potentially promotes longevity and minimizes the risks of chronic conditions, such as osteoporosis. This chapter reviews two such available dietary measures, meal replacements and fat substitutes. Additional related topics, such as artificial sweeteners, are reviewed in other reports *(2)*.

2. MEAL REPLACEMENT PRODUCTS

Meal replacement products became a popular weight loss and maintenance option in the early 1990s. However, the safety, effectiveness, and patient compliance of meal replacement products have rarely been studied or critically evaluated by the scientific community. For example, the major report, "Clinical Guidelines on the Identification, Evaluation and Treatment of Overweight and Obesity in Adults: the Evidence Report" *(3)*, did not mention the use of meal replacement products (*see* Chapter 11).

Meal replacement products are designed primarily for overweight individuals seeking dietary measures for weight loss. Other individuals use meal replacement products as a means of maintaining their body weight within the normal range. The strategy behind the use of meal replacement products is threefold: to reduce the choices or options for a particular meal; to provide a portion controlled, nutritious alternative; and to help patients adhere to a hypocaloric diet with minimal effort.

A characteristic feature of meal replacement products as a group is their nutrient composition. Meal replacements are usually moderately high in protein and low in fat, with varying amounts of carbohydrates. Products are often fortified with vitamins and

From: *Primary and Secondary Preventive Nutrition*
Edited by: A. Bendich and R. J. Deckelbaum © Humana Press Inc., Totowa, NJ

minerals. Ice cream shakes or peanut butter cookies therefore cannot be included in the meal replacement category.

Early meal replacement products were often beverages designed for replacing a self-selected regular-food meal. Today the term "meal replacement" encompasses a range of products, such as beverages, prepackaged entrées, and meal/snack bars. These products can be used as the sole energy source for a meal, or in combination with fresh foods, as well. Products are available at medically supervised weight-loss clinics, commercial weight loss centers, and over the counter. Most over-the-counter meal replacement products include a package insert or label with instructions on how to incorporate the product into a weight control regime.

2.1. Beverages

Meal replacement beverages replace one or two regular food meals a day. These products provide a lower caloric alternative to self-selected meals, while being well-balanced and satisfying. Meal replacement beverages are typically fortified with vitamins and minerals to allow a daily energy intake of 1200–1500 kcal, while still meeting the recommended dietary allowance (RDA) for vitamins and minerals.

Under some circumstances, meal replacement beverages can be used in a clinical setting, such as a medical or nutritional office, to facilitate weight loss or maintenance. The low purchase cost and availability of these products makes this approach attractive. The cost of a beverage meal may be comparable or less expensive than a regular meal purchased at commercial establishments. The beverages may be in dehydrated powder form or already reconstituted in a ready-to-drink container. There are few contra-indications to the use of such beverages, and at present there are no BMI (wt [kg]/ht^2 [m^2]) criteria established for their purchase or use. This is distinct from pharmacotherapy or very low calorie diets (VLCDs), for which patient selection and monitoring procedures are well established and stringent. Meal replacement beverages may therefore be particularly useful in overweight patients (i.e., those with BMI = 25–29.9 kg/m^2), who do not qualify for pharmacologic or VLCD treatments (i.e., BMI $\geq$ 30 kg/m^2 or BMI $\geq$ 27 kg/m^2 with co-morbidities).

Research is limited regarding the efficacy of and adherence to meal replacement beverages. The chief studies are with the use of the Ultra-SlimFast product (Slim-Fast Foods, West Palm Beach, FL). Phase one of a study by Ditschuneit et al. (4) compared an energy-restricted diet incorporating two Ultra-SlimFast meal replacements and snack replacements with an isoenergetic diet composed of self-selected conventional foods over a 3-month weight-loss period. Phase two of the study was a 24-month, case-controlled, weight-maintenance period, with an energy-restricted diet in which one meal and one snack were replaced daily for all subjects.

In phase one, subjects using the food replacements lost significantly more in percentage of weight (mean $\pm$ SD; 11.3 $\pm$ 6.8%) than did the group using the conventional restricted diet (5.9 $\pm$ 5.0%). In phase two, initial weight loss was maintained, with additional losses (0.07% of initial body weight/month) observed. This study provides support for the use of beverage meal replacement products for both weight loss and maintenance.

Heber et al. (5) evaluated a simplified weight loss program that provided subjects with Ultra-SlimFast and package insert information. Nonphysicians carried out weekly follow-up visits over 12 wk. A subgroup was then followed biweekly. At 116 wk, 44% of subjects remained in the study, and had lost an average of 5–6 kg. The study did not include a control group, however.

2.1.1. FORMULA DIETS

Specially designed meal replacement products have been developed as complete beverage-only regimens, usually referred to as formula diets. The formula diets restrict energy intake and eliminate food choices. There are two types of formula diets, VLCDs and low calorie diets (LCDs). VLCDs are extensively reviewed elsewhere (6,7). The transition from VLCD to LCD is not a formal one, but typically VLCDs provide 300–800 kcal/d, LCDs ~800–1200 kcal/d; nonmedically supervised beverage meal replacement products/programs ~1200–1500 kcal/d.

VLCDs and LCDs are usually provided in powdered form, with 100% of the RDA for essential nutrients, and can be mixed with water or low-fat milk. The formulation is designed to be high in protein (>70 g/d), to help limit the loss of lean tissue. Fiber is often supplemented to maintain adequate bowel movements. The patient is generally instructed to drink 3–6 formula beverages per day, and to abstain from other caloric foods and beverages. At least 2–3 liters of noncaloric fluids should be consumed daily, including formula. The LCD energy intake prescribed can be held constant or can depend on the subject's initial BMI, and then be adjusted upward or downward, based on the observed rate of weight change and the patient's tolerance and compliance. LCDs usually avoid the VLCD-associated metabolic adjustments, such as ketosis, and do not require the intensive medical follow-up of a VLCD. However, monthly or bimonthly blood chemistry evaluations are often recommended. Formula diets can be safely administered under medical supervision for up to 3 months to patients with co-morbid conditions (e.g., diabetes).

During the entire formula program, the patient should receive nutritional and behavioral counseling, either individually or in a group, to promote healthy eating and exercise habits to help achieve and maintain the weight loss. The behavioral program should continue with an experienced nutritionist and psychologist, ideally for several months after food is reintroduced. As the frequency of visits diminish to biweekly and monthly, the patient should be encouraged to return for up to a year or longer. The estimated total cost for such a year long program can exceed $3000.

Currently, VLCDs are no longer recommended for weight loss, because of safety concerns (8,9) and lack of long-term efficacy in the majority of treated patients. Weight loss with LCDs is usually not as large as with VLCDs (10). In controlled clinical trials, 90% of patients treated with VLCDs lost 10 kg or more; only 60% of patients treated with LCDs lost 10 kg or more (11). However, in a randomized comparison of three formula regimens of 420, 660, and 800 kcal, over 6 mo, there was no significant difference in weight loss or body composition change (12). With respect to weight maintenance, Wadden et al. (13) compared weight-loss maintenance after a VLCD and a hypocaloric regular-food LCD over 26 wk. During the maintenance phase, VLCD-treated subjects regained significantly more weight than did those who lost weight on the regular-food LCD. In four randomized controlled trials comparing VLCDs with LCDs, although weight loss during the active treatment phase was greater with a VLCD, because of poorer weight maintenance on the VLCD, long-term weight loss (>1 yr) did not differ between the diets (9).

2.2. Prepackaged Entrées

Single meals composed of frozen or shelf-stable food items represent another meal replacement group. These products differ from traditional frozen food entrées in that they are designed to provide low energy intake. These food entrées can be purchased at local grocery stores, or can be provided as part of a structured weight-loss program, such as Jenny Craig. Prepackaged entrées can now be ordered over the internet for home delivery.

These packaged entrées are low in fat, and some are low in sodium; but, they are not usually nutritionally balanced. Less than one serving of vegetables is provided in some dishes. Addition of fresh vegetables and fruit is often necessary to meet nutritional requirements. By referring to the nutrient label, the dieter can plan to adhere to a nutrient exchange pattern as developed by the American Diabetes Association. Meal replacement frozen entrées often use a familiar and traditionally high-fat meal (e.g., lasagna with ricotta and chopped meat), then prepare it with less fat and in a small portion. However, use of these entrées alone is not sufficient to allow the dieter to learn adequate nutrition or behavior modification, such as how to prepare lasagna with vegetables (e.g., spinach and zucchini), instead of meat, how to use low-fat cheeses, or how to eat fewer energy-dense foods.

Often, nonmedical professionals and successful weight-loss participants staff the clinics that provide these meal replacement entrées. The client can come to the center or order meals via the telephone or internet. The meals usually provide a 1-day food allotment that can range from 1000 to 2300 kcal. A vitamin supplement is also encouraged. The cost of a single meal replacement entrée may be comparable to or slightly higher than a traditional frozen meal entrée. The ease in use of prepackaged entrées makes this an appealing weight-loss approach. The products are safe, although their efficacy for weight loss remains understudied. Meal replacement use, administered as prepackaged meals over 10 wk, in the study by McCarron et al. *(14)*, led to weight loss and improved cardiovascular risk factors, including blood pressure, serum lipids, and insulin. Subjects consuming meal replacement entrées lost significantly more weight and were more compliant than subjects consuming a self-selected American Heart Association diet (men, –4.5 vs 3.5 kg; and women, –4.8 vs 2.8 kg).

For a highly motivated individual, these products may be a useful means for achieving weight loss and maintenance, especially within the framework of a program for behavior modification.

2.3. Sports and Meal Bars

Sports bars were originally used to provide extra energy before or after a bout of exercise. Currently, sports bars are often used as meal replacements that are convenient, palatable, and quick to ingest. Meal bars are similar to sports bars, but they were not intended to provide extra energy for exercise. Meal bars provide energy typical of a small meal, 150–300 kcal, and usually have more vitamins and minerals. Several bars use the popular "Zone" formulation of 40% energy from carbohydrate, 30% from protein, and 30% from fat. Other bars offer a more traditional energy distribution with 60% from carbohydrate, 10% from fat, and 30% from protein. There are numerous flavors and varieties, such as vegan bars made with soy or whey protein, or bars fortified with herbs and antioxidants such as ginseng or chromium picolinate. Sports/meal bars are widely available in health food stores as a meal replacement alternative. Meal bars typically cost more than the traditional candy bar, but their nutritional value is usually superior. Efficacy and adherence to meal bars are difficult to assess, because the outpatient clinics providing meal replacements often do not publish data regarding treatment outcomes.

2.4. Clinical Application

Nutrition education and reduced energy intake are cornerstones of obesity treatment. At one end, patients can be prescribed a self-selected, energy-restricted diet consisting of regular foods combined with various beverage, prepackaged entrée, and sports bar, meal replacement products. At the other end, patients can be recommended LCD and VLCD formula. The first alternative is relatively inexpensive, safe, convenient, and provides a nutritionally complete energy-restricted program. This approach, used widely in the weight-loss field, is appropriate for subjects who are not in need of rapid weight loss and comfortable managing their food selections. The LCD and VLCD formulas are usually reserved for patients who require rapid and medically significant weight loss over relatively short time periods. Some patients also request a "food holiday" when they have previously failed to lose weight with self-selected regular foods. Varying degrees of medical supervision and laboratory tests increase the cost of formula diet programs. The practitioner must weigh these considerations when recommending one or another of these approaches to patients.

With all meal replacement products, whether beverage or prepackaged entrée, long-term use may lead to monotony and boredom. If this is the only weight loss strategy implemented, the individual may not be learning the necessary behavior modification techniques nor developing plans for managing the inevitable situations involving conventional foods. The use of these products alone should therefore not be regarded as a panacea for patients who need to achieve significant long-term weight loss.

3. FAT SUBSTITUTES

A relatively new method for reducing dietary fat intake is by incorporating a noncaloric fat substitute into food, analogous to reducing sugar intake with sugar substitutes such as saccharin or aspartame. By using a fat substitute, a person can obtain the benefits of the taste and texture of fat without the extra calories. Although there have been a number of low-calorie fat substitutes, only one noncaloric substitute has reached the marketplace: sucrose polyester. Given the 25 yr it required to obtain U.S. Food and Drug Administration (FDA) approval, it is unlikely that another new class of such noncalorie substitutes will become available in the near future.

Mattson and Volpenheim serendipitously discovered sucrose polyester, or olestra, in 1968 at Procter & Gamble (P&G) while trying, paradoxically, to develop a more digestible fat for infants (15). The compound they synthesized, with fatty acids esterified to a sucrose molecule, cannot be digested by lipases, and pass virtually unabsorbed through the gastrointestinal (GI) tract (16–18). Because each olestra molecule consists predominantly of 6–8 long-chain fatty acids, olestra's sensory and physical characteristics are similar to edible oil, and can be used for frying and cooking. Early problems with anal leakage (19,20) were remedied by increasing the length and saturation of the fatty acids, to raise the viscosity of olestra. P&G obtained a patent in 1971, and originally filed a petition in 1975 for olestra as a drug to lower serum cholesterol, but the effect was not sufficient to warrant this use. In 1987, P&G filed a petition for olestra to be used to replace up to 35% of cooking oil and shortening for home use, and up to 70% for commercial use. This petition was amended and resubmitted in 1990 to replace 100% of fat in savory or salty snacks. This last petition finally received FDA approval in 1996, for limited use of olestra in such snacks as potato chips, tortilla chips, and crackers (20,21).

The FDA requires that the product packaging display a label that olestra may cause abdominal cramping and loose stools. Controlled clinical studies of daily ingestion of olestra for 8 and 16 wk have revealed increased reports of loose stools or diarrhea and flatulence, with larger doses of olestra, 20 and 32 g *(17,22)*. However, a double-blind study of a single eating period of potato chips (mean = 60 g) with olestra (mean = 17.5 g), during a movie, found no difference in GI reports between those eating chips with olestra or regular chips *(23*. Similarly, in a rechallenge test of consumers who reported having GI symptoms after consumption of olestra products, there was no difference in symptoms after either chips with olestra (<16.5 g) or regular chips *(24)*. This implies that some of the reports of GI symptoms may result from suggestibility from label warnings. Thus, GI symptoms following olestra consumption are more likely with chronic use and a dose exceeding 20 g/d. Consistent with this, a recent large field trial *(25)*, with 3181 subjects who were given regular and olestra chips, all labeled as olestra chips, significantly more GI symptoms, such as frequent bowel movements and looser stools, were reported only by those consuming more than 2.34 oz of chips with 19.3 g olestra.

The FDA has also required addition of the fat-soluble vitamins A, D, E, and K to olestra products, given the potential loss of these vitamins, which can combine with olestra, a highly lypophilic compound, as it moves through the digestive tract. P&G has been required to continue to monitor the safety and side effects postmarketing. Consumers can call an 800 number listed on packages with their comments. Comments about side effects are forwarded to P&G, which compiles the information, and submits quarterly summaries to the FDA. P&G has also initiated cross-sectional studies in samples of free-living individuals in various communities, before and after olestra products were marketed. Some of these individuals are also being followed in a cohort study. The chief purpose of these studies is to assess blood levels, in relation to product use, of fat-soluble vitamins and carotenoids, to ensure that adequate vitamin replacements have been made *(26)*. In July, 1998, 2.5 yr postapproval, the FDA Advisory Committee reviewed the results gathered from postmarketing surveillance. The Committee reconfirmed the safety of olestra for use in savory snacks, but denied the request by P&G to remove the warning label *(27)* on foods with olestra (brand name, Olean). Additional reviews are available on olestra's safety and interaction with other nutrients *(16,22)*, GI effects *(17,22)*, and effects on cholesterol *(28)*.

Although the FDA could require more rigorous postmarketing studies, it regards olestra as a food additive, and not a drug *(29)*. As a food additive, olestra does not require a demonstration of its benefits, only its safety. There are, therefore, relatively few studies on whether use of olestra leads to reduction of fat and energy intake, and, subsequently, body wt in overweight individuals.

3.1. Caloric Compensation

Most of the studies on caloric compensation with olestra-substituted foods are with normal-weight subjects. It is likely that overweight subjects would compensate less well, as suggested by early studies of covert caloric dilution of a liquid formula diet obtained freely from a feeding machine *(30)*. In those studies, obese inpatients failed to compensate over several weeks; normal-weight subjects did so within a few days. For obese individuals with extra energy reserves as body fat, survival is not imminently threatened by food restriction, and hunger signals may be muted *(31)*. In contrast, lean individuals with less body fat are more prone to lose lean tissue during food restriction, and may experience greater hunger, and therefore compensate better calorically than obese individuals (31).

3.1.1. SHORT-TERM STUDIES

Compared to adults, children appear to regulate energy intake more accurately (32), consistent with their higher metabolic requirements and smaller body fat depots. In one study, 29 normal-weight children, ages 2–5 yr, had 14 g olestra substituted throughout all meals of the first day (33). Although energy intake was somewhat reduced that day, nearly complete compensation for the missing calories occurred by the end of the second day. In a study of normal-weight young men, when olestra was substituted into 1 d's meals, leading to a reduction in fat intake from 32 to 10% of daily energy intake, most (74%) of the energy was compensated for by the end of the next day (34).

When olestra is substituted into specific meals, energy compensation appears best after it is substituted into breakfast. Following substitution of 0, 20, or 32 g olestra in the breakfast of lean young men, appropriate energy compensation occurred at dinner (35,36). However, when 24 g of sucrose polyester similar to olestra (SPE) was substituted into lunch meal croissants, the mean caloric compensation later in the day averaged only 22% in normal-weight young men and women (37). In another study, compensation also did not occur when olestra was introduced into either lunch or dinner (38). Compensation after breakfast may be more accurate, because there is more opportunity within the same day to increase intake, or because the body is more sensitive to calories following food deprivation overnight (39). Even when appropriate caloric compensation occurred, fat replacement did not lead to a specific increase in fat intake, and daily fat consumption was therefore lowered. These studies suggest that fat replacement in later meals may be desirable if the goal is to reduce both energy and fat intake.

3.1.2. INTERMEDIATE-TERM STUDIES

In 12-d crossover studies in normal-weight young men and women, with 52 g SPE replacing most of the fat in dinner meals, energy compensation averaged only 21%, with no apparent improvement over days (40). The mean daily reduction in energy intake, 1.5 mJ (360 kcal), during the SPE period, led to a small weight loss of about 0.15 kg. Similarly, in a study of 10 obese inpatients (41), who consumed 60 g/d olestra in foods during one of two 20-d periods, energy compensation was only 23%. However, subjects did not lose significantly more weight during the olestra period. Hill et al. (42) recently studied both lean and obese subjects who ingested a daily total of 26 g olestra in breakfast and dinner over a 2-wk period, in the laboratory. The mean compensation, 20% for energy intake and 15% for fat intake, was similar for both weight groups, and did not improve over days. Despite a mean daily reduction of 987 kJ/d (236 kcal), there was no impact on body wt.

In these intermediate-term studies, there was poor compensation for the displaced energy and dietary fat. The authors recognize, however, that even periods of 12–20 d are too short to assess whether subjects will eventually compensate for energy. To infer what might happen in longer periods, one must rely on related studies using low-fat diets, rather than olestra.

3.1.3. LONG-TERM STUDIES

Kendall et al. (43) studied 13 slightly overweight women, mean age 34 yr, during 11-wk crossover periods of either reduced, 20–25% fat, or conventional 35–40% fat.

The 15% difference in fat intake would be similar to substituting 35–40 g/d olestra. By the end of 11 wk, energy compensation on the low-fat diet reached 35%. Weight loss on the low-fat diet was significantly greater, by 1.28 kg, than the conventional diet. The authors note that the slopes for the regression lines of energy compensation over time for the two periods did not vary significantly. Nevertheless, the low-fat group significantly improved in energy regulation over weeks, as indicated from their regression equation, $y = -0.52x + 16.3$, where y represents the error (in %) from perfect compensation, and x represents the week. From this equation, one can calculate that, at 31 wk, compensation would be perfect (when $y = 0$). Studies with even longer periods than 11 wk would be needed to address this issue empirically.

In the Women's Health Trial Feasibility study, slightly overweight women (BMI = 25.5) were divided into two groups: 171 to receive an intervention, and 105 as controls *(44)*. The intervention group received behavioral and nutritional counseling to promote low fat intake, with the goal of reducing fat intake from 39 to 20%. The subjects met in small groups, at first weekly, then biweekly, and finally monthly for 2 yr. After 6 mo, the intervention group lost 2.8 kg more than the control group. After 1 yr, the weight difference diminished to 2.6 kg, and after 2 yr to 1.8 kg. If the increase in protein and carbohydrate intake over time is considered to be the result of energy compensation, then, after 6 mo, compensation was 14%; after 1 yr, 18%; and, after 2 yr, 19%. If the additional fat intake that occurs at 2 yr, compared to 6 mo, is regarded as further energy compensation, the compensation at 2 yr would be 25%. Thus, energy compensation slowly increased over 2 yr even in overweight individuals who ended up with only a small weight loss.

3.2. Covert Substitution

In most studies with olestra or SPE, fat substitution was done covertly. However, in everyday experience, individuals would usually be aware of the fat substitution. In the few studies that compared covert and overt labeling of olestra snacks, there was a tendency to overeat with overt labeling, especially among restrained or dieting individuals *(40,45)*. Other groups that might be susceptible to overconsumption are children and adolescents, who were unfortunately not included in the clinical studies. Some young individuals may feel a license to eat snacks with olestra, even after having previously avoided such snack foods. They may then consume olestra snacks at the expense of more nutritious foods, such as fruits and vegetables. The clinical studies also excluded individuals with eating disorders, such as bulimia nervosa and binge eating disorder, for whom olestra products could hold appeal as potential binge foods, given their reduced energy content *(46)*.

Criticism also comes from some researchers *(47)* whose main concern is the induced loss of carotenoids, such as lycopene, which may have protective effects for certain cancers and coronary heart disease *(48)*. There is less concern about the carotenoid, β-carotene, a precursor for Vitamin A, because Vitamin A is added with D, E, and K, as required by the FDA. The FDA has accepted the argument by P&G that snack foods are generally not eaten together with fruits and vegetables, the main source of carotenoids.

Hypothetically, if it is assumed that consumers obtained all their savory snacks with olestra substituted for fat, it is estimated that, for 18–44-yr-old adults, mean daily intake of olestra would be only 3.7 g *(23,49)*. At these doses, it is unlikely that overweight individuals would have benefits for either weight or cholesterol reduction. If we assume, furthermore, that overweight individuals are consuming snacks at the 90th percentile for all young adults, or 8.1 g olestra, it is unlikely to yield a weight or cholesterol benefit, because the studies that show such benefits used still larger amounts of olestra. To substantially reduce fat intake, e.g., from 40 to 30%, would require a 25-g fat reduction, possible only with much more extensive use of olestra.

To extend the use of olestra into other foods, P&G would need to petition the FDA again (20). Should olestra eventually be permitted into other foods, such as sweet snacks, nonsnack foods, oils and spreads, cheeses, and baked goods, there would be increased potential for both benefits and risks. The benefits could include some weight loss and cholesterol reduction, but the risks may include greater loss of carotenoids, because of more potential interaction in the gut (23). Given that side effects appear related to dose of olestra, it would be desirable to list the amount of olestra in a food product, as is done for protein, fat, and carbohydrate. For example, each ounce of olestra potato chips, considered one serving, contains 8.25 g olestra (24).

3.3. Olestra: Conclusion and Recommendation

During the past 25 yr, increased use of sugar substitutes has unfortunately not led to a reduction in obesity. In fact, the prevalence of obesity has increased over the same period (1,50,51). During just the past decade, while fat intake has decreased in several countries, obesity prevalence has increased, implicating other factors, such as a decline in physical activity (52,53). One can therefore predict with assurance that the limited availability of a fat substitute alone will not reverse the current trend toward more obesity. However, for a well-motivated group of individuals who are either trying to lose or maintain weight, and are already in the habit of eating salty snacks, olestra products may make it easier to limit energy and fat intake as part of an overall weight management plan.

REFERENCES

1. Kuczmarski RJ, Flegal KM, Campbell SM, Johnson CL. Increasing prevalence of overweight among US adults. The National Health and Nutrition Examination Surveys, 1960 to 1991. JAMA 1994; 272: 205–211.
2. Krenkel J, Read M. Dietetic products and supplements. In: Obesity Assessment: Tools, Methods, Interpretations. St. Jeor ST, ed. New York: Chapman & Hall, 1997; 268–280.
3. Clinical guidelines on the identification, evaluation and treatment of overweight and obesity in adults: the evidence report. Obesity Res 1998; 6(Suppl. 2):51S–209S.
4. Ditschuneit H, Fletchner-Mors M, Johnson T, Adler G. Metabolic and weight loss effects of a long term dietary intervention in obese patients. Am J Clin Nutr 1999; 69:198–204.
5. Heber D, Ashley J, Wang H, Elashoff R. Clinical evaluation of a minimal intervention meal replacement regimen for weight reduction. J Amer Coll Nutr 1994; 13:608–614.
6. Position of the American Dietetic Association: weight management. J Am Diet Assoc 1997; 97: 71–74.
7. Bray GA. Contemporary Diagnosis and Management of Obesity. Handbooks in Health Care. PA: Newtown, 1998; 192–224.
8. Van Itallie TB, Yang MU. Cardiac dysfunction in obese dieters: a potentially lethal complication of rapid massive weight loss. Am J Clin Nutr 1984; 39:695–702.
9. National Task Force on the Prevention and Treatment of Obesity, National Institutes of Health. Very low-calorie diets. JAMA 1993; 270:967–974.
10. Wadden TA, Stunkard AJ, Brownell KD. Very low calorie diets: their efficacy, safety, and future. Ann Intern Med 1983; 99:675–684.
11. Wadden TA, Sternberg JA, Letizia KA, Stundard AJ, Foster GD. Treatment of obesity by very low calorie diet, behavior therapy, and their combination: a five year perspective. Int J Obes 1989; 13(Suppl. 2): 39–46.

12. Foster GD, Wadden TA, Peterson FJ, Letizia KA, Bartlett SJ, Conill AM. A controlled comparison of three very-low-calorie diets: effects on weight, body composition, and symptoms. Am J Clin Nutr 1992; 55:811–817.
13. Wadden TA, Foster GD, Letizia KA. One-year behavioral treatment of obesity: comparison of moderate and severe caloric restriction and the effects of weight maintenance therapy. J Consul Clin Psych 1994; 62:165–171.
14. McCarron D, et al. Nutritional management of cardiovascular risk factors. Arch Internal Med 1997; 157:169–177.
15. Mattson FH, Volpenheim RA. Hydrolysis of fully esterified alcohols containing from one to eight hydroxyl groups by the lipolytic enzymes of rat pancreatic juice. J Lipid Res 1972; 13:325–328.
16. Lawson KD, Middleton SJ, Hassall CD. Olestra, a nonabsorbed, noncaloric replacement for dietary fat: a review. Drug Metab Rev 1997; 29:651–703.
17. Freston JW, Ahnen DJ, Czinn SJ, Earnest DL, Farthing MJ, Gorbach SL, et al. Review and analysis of the effects of olestra, a dietary fat substitute, on gastrointestinal function and symptoms. Reg Toxicol Pharmacol 1997; 26:210–218.
18. Bergholz CM. Safety evaluation of olestra, an on-absorbed, fatlike fat replacement. Crit Rev Food Sci Nutr 1992; 32:141–146.
19. Bernhardt CA. Olestra- a non-caloric fat replacement. Food Tech Intl Europe 1988; 176–178.
20. Institute of Food Science and Technology. Current Hot Topics: Olestra. Position Statement, 1996.
21. Prince DM, Welschenbach MA. Olestra: a new food additive. J Am Diet Assoc 1998; 98:565–569.
22. Peters JC, Lawson KD, Middleton SJ, Triebwasser KC. Assessment of the nutritional effects of olestra, a nonabsorbed fat replacement: summary. J Nutr 1997; 127:1719S–1728S.
23. Cheskin LJ, Miday R, Zorich N, Filloon T. Gastrointestinal symptoms following consumption of olestra or regular triglyceride potato chips: a controlled comparison. JAMA 1998; 14:150–152.
24. Zorich NL, Biedermann D, Riccardi KA, Bishop LJ, Filloon TG. Randomized, double-blind, placebo-controlled, consumer rechallenge test of Olean salted snacks. Regul Toxicol Pharmacol 1997; 26: 200–209.
25. Sandler RS, Zorich NL, Filloon TG, Wiseman HB, Lietz DJ, Brock MH, Royer MG, Miday RK. Gastrointestinal symptoms in 3181 volunteers ingesting snack foods containing olestra or triglycerides. A 6-week randomized, placebo-controlled trial. Ann Intern Med 1999; 130:253–261.
26. Rock CL, Thornquist MD, Kristal AR, Patterson RE, Cooper DA, Neuhouser ML, Neumark-Sztainer D, Cheskin LJ. Demographic, dietary and lifestyle factors differentially explain variability in serum carotenoids and fat-soluble vitamins: baseline results from the sentinel site of the Olestra Post-Marketing Surveillance Study. J Nutr 1999; 129:855–864.
27. Josefson D. Fat substitute declared safe. Br Med J 1998; 316:1926.
28. Glueck CJ. Sucrose polyester, cholesterol, and lipoprotein metabolism. In: Carbohydrate Polyesters as Fat Substitutes. Akoh CC, Swanson BG, eds. New York: Marcel Dekker, 1994;169–182.
29. Blackburn H. Olestra and the FDA. N Engl J Med 1996; 334:984–986.
30. Campbell RG, Hashim SA, Van Itallie TB. Studies of food-intake regulation in man. Responses to variations in nutritive density in lean and obese subjects. N Engl J Med 1971; 16:1402–1407.
31. Yang MU, Van Itallie TB. Effect of energy restriction on body composition and nitrogen balance in obese individuals. In: Treatment of the Seriously Obese Patient. Wadden TA, Van Itallie TB, eds. New York: Guilford, 1992; 83–106.
32. Birch LL, Deysher M. Caloric compensation and sensory specific satiety: evidence for self regulation of food intake by young children. Appetite 1986; 7:323–331.
33. Birch LL, Johnson SL, Jones MB, Peters JC. Effects of a non-energy fat substitute on children's energy and macronutrient intake. Am J Clin Nutr 1993; 58:326–333.
34. Cotton JR, Weststrate JA, Blundell JE. Replacement of dietary fat with sucrose polyester: effects on energy intake and appetite control in nonobese males. Am J Clin Nutr 1996; 63:891–896.
35. Rolls BJ, Pirraglia PA, Jones MB, Peters JC. Effects of olestra, a noncaloric fat substitute, on daily energy and fat intakes in lean men. Am J Clin Nutr 1992; 56:84–92.
36. Burley VJ, Blundell JE. Evaluation of the action of a nonabsorbable fat on appetite and energy intake in lean healthy males. In: Obesity in Europe 91. Ailhaud G, et al., eds. London: John Libbey, 1992; 63–65.
37. Hulshof T, de Graaf C, Weststrate JA. Short-term satiating effect of the fat replacer sucrose polyester (SPE) in man. Br J Nutr 1995; 74:569–585.
38. Cotton JR, Burley VJ, Weststrate JA, Blundell JE. Fat substitution and food intake: effect of replacing fat with sucrose polyester at lunch or evening meals. Br J Nutr 1996; 75:545–556.

39. Geliebter A. Effects of equicaloric loads of protein, fat and carbohydrate on food intake in the rat and man. Physiol Behav 1979; 22:267–273.

40. De Graaf C, Hulshof T, Weststrate JA, Hautvast JG. Nonabsorbable fat (sucrose polyester) and the regulation of energy intake and body weight. Am J Physiol 1996; 270:R1386–1393.

41. Glueck CJ, Jandacek R, Hogg E, Allen C, Baehler L, Tewksbury M. Sucrose polyester: substitution for dietary fats in hypocaloric diets in the treatment of familial hypercholesterolemia. Am J Clin Nutr 1983; 37:347–354.

42. Hill JO, Seagle HM, Johnson SL, Smith S, Reed GW, Tran ZV, et al. Effects of 14 d of covert substitution of olestra for conventional fat on spontaneous food intake. Am J Clin Nutr 1998; 67:1178–1185.

43. Kendall A, Levitsky DA, Strupp BJ, Lissner L. Weight loss on a low-fat diet consequence of the imprecision of the control of food intake in humans. Am J Clin Nutr 1991; 53:1124–1129.

44. Sheppard L, Kristal AR, Kushi LH. Weight loss in women participating in a randomized trial of low-fat diets. Am J Clin Nutr 1991; 54:821–828.

45. Miller DL, Castellanos VH, Shide DJ, Peters JC, Rolls BJ. Effect of fat-free potato chips with and without nutrition labels on fat and energy intakes. Am J Clin Nutr 1998; 68:282–290.

46. Hampl JS, Sheeley AE, Schnepf MI. Sounding the alarm for misuse of olestra-containing foods in binge-eating disorders J Am Diet Assoc 1998; 98:971.

47. Stampfer MJ, Willett WC. Olestra and the FDA. N Engl J Med 1996; 335:669–670.

48. Weststrate JA, van het Hof KH. Sucrose polyester and plasma carotenoid concentrations in healthy subjects. Am J Clin Nutr 1995; 62:591–597.

49. Middleton SJ, Dwyer J, Peters JC. An indirect means of assessing potential nutritional effects of dietary olestra in healthy subgroups of the general population. J Nutr 1997; 127:1710–1718S.

50. Flegal KM, Carroll MD, Kuczmarski RJ, Johnson CL. Overweight and obesity in the United States: prevalence and trends, 1960–1994. Int J Obes Related Metab Disord 1998; 22:39–47.

51. Kuczmarski RJ, Carroll MD, Flegal KM, Troiano RP. Varying body mass index cutoff points to describe overweight prevalence among U.S. adults: NHANES III (1988 to 1994). Obes Res 1997; 5:542–548.

52. Astrup A, Toubro S, Raben A, Skov AR. The role of low-fat diets and fat substitutes in body weight management: what have we learned from clinical studies? J Am Diet Assoc 1997; 97:S82–87.

53. Prentice AM, Jobb SA. Obesity in Britain. Gluttony or sloth. Br Med J 1995; 311:437–439.

IV GROWTH, IMMUNITY, AND INFECTION

14

Role of Long-Chain Polyunsaturated Fatty Acids in Infant Growth and Development

Berthold Koletzko and Tamás Decsi

1. INTRODUCTION

Long-chain polyunsaturated fatty acids (LCPUFAs) have potential roles and functional effects during early human growth and development, under the perspective of preventive nutrition. LCPUFA sources and the metabolism of essential fatty acids (EFA) and their metabolites, and differences between breast-fed and formula-fed infants, are addressed. Available information is reviewed on the influence of LCPUFAs on infant growth and the development of visual and other neural functions in healthy, full-term infants. Although LCPUFAs play delicate and important roles in the nutrition of preterm infants, data obtained in preterm infants is discussed only when parallel data obtained in full-term infants are not available.

2. BIOCHEMICAL ASPECTS OF EFA METABOLISM IN INFANCY

Linoleic acid (C18:2ω-6, LA) and α-linolenic acid (C18:3ω-3, ALA) (Fig. 1) are EFAs because humans, like other higher mammals, cannot insert double bonds in the ω-6 and ω-3 position of a FA, i.e., at 6 or 3 carbon atoms from the methyl end of the molecule. The precursor EFAs, LA and ALA, are the precursors of ω-6 and ω-3 LCPUFA, i.e., PUFAs with 20 and 22 C atoms (Fig. 2). The biologically most important LCPUFAs are dihomo-γ-linolenic acid (C20:3ω-6, DGLA) and arachidonic acid (C20:4ω-6, AA) of the ω-6 and eicosapentaenoic acid (C20:5ω-3, EPA) and docosahexaenoic acid (C22:6ω-3, DHA) of the ω-3 series. Enzymatic conversion of LA to AA is a relatively short metabolic pathway consisting of one chain elongation and two desaturation steps (Fig. 2, left panel). In contrast, DHA is synthesized from ALA via several consecutive desaturation and elongation steps (Fig. 2, right panel), involving also indirect steps via FAs with 24 C atoms (1).

AA and DHA are indispensable components of plasma membranes, and are incorporated in large amounts in membrane-rich tissues, such as the brain and retina, during early human growth (2). The analysis of tissue composition from deceased neonates and fetuses of different gestational ages has demonstrated a very rapid incorporation of AA and DHA into structural lipids of the brain, retina, and other tissues during the latter part of pregnancy

From: *Primary and Secondary Preventive Nutrition*
Edited by: A. Bendich and R. J. Deckelbaum © Humana Press Inc., Totowa, NJ

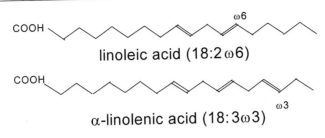

Fig. 1. Tertiary structure of LA (18:2ω-6) and ALA (18:3ω-3).

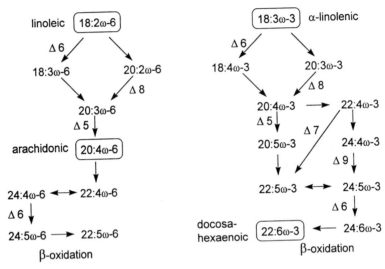

Fig. 2. Current concept of the biochemical conversion of the EFAs, LA (18:2ω-6) and ALA (18:3ω-3), to their long-chain polyunsaturated metabolites.

(3,4). Phospholipids (PLs) of membranes with high fluidity, such as synaptosomal membranes and retinal photoreceptors, have particularly high LCPUFA concentrations. Moreover, DGLA, AA, and EPA serve as precursors for the formation of prostaglandins, prostacyclins, thromboxanes, leukotrienes, and other lipid mediators that are powerful regulators of various cell and tissue processes, such as thrombocyte aggregation, leukocyte function, and inflammation *(5)*.

3. SOURCES OF EFAS AND LCPUFAS IN PERINATAL PERIOD

3.1. EFA and LCPUFA Supply **In Utero**

Fetal supply of EFA and LCPUFA depends entirely on the placental transfer. By studying the FA composition of the major plasma lipid classes in pairs of mothers and their healthy full-term infants, using high-resolution capillary gas-liquid chromatography (GLC), the median percentages of LA and ALA were found to be markedly lower in cord, than in maternal, plasma lipids *(6)*. In contrast, percentage values for both AA and DHA were significantly higher in infants than in their mothers. These results corroborate previous findings *(7)*, and point to a preferential and selective materno-fetal LCPUFA transfer *in utero*. Consequences of premature disruption of this LCPUFA transfer should be taken into consideration when designing postnatal LCPUFA supply to preterm infants (8–10).

3.2. EFA and LCPUFA Supply with Breast-Feeding

Human milk, as the single food source of exclusively breast-fed infants, is expected to generally meet the substrate requirements of healthy, growing infants. Human milk contains both the precursor EFA, LA, and ALA, as well as a variety of preformed LCPUFA metabolites. The medians and ranges for EFA and LCPUFA contents in human milk were calculated from the results of 14 European and 10 African studies on the FA composition of mature human milk (11). Median LA values were 11% w/w in Europe and 12% in Africa, ALA 0.9 and 0.8%, AA 0.5 and 0.6%, and DHA 0.3 and 0.3%, respectively. Thus, values were similar in European and in African human milk samples. However, the overall ranges of reported values were wide (LA, 5.7 to 17.2%; ALA, 0.1 to 1.44%; AA, 0.2 to 1.2%; DHA, 0.1 to 0.9%), which appear to reflect not only biological variation, but also methodological differences, because different analytical approaches were used, with the majority of the 24 studies using packed column chromatography with limited sensitivity and precision.

To exclude some of the methodological bias, the authors calculated data from eight relatively recently published studies that determined the FA composition of mature human milk, with modern methods based on capillary GLC (12–19). In these investigations, AA values were within a very narrow range, and the variability of LA values was also relatively small (Table 1). In contrast, there were more than fourfold differences between the lowest and highest ALA and DHA values, respectively. Thus, the relative variability of ω-3 FA contents in human milk seems to be larger than that of ω-6 FAs.

The pronounced biological variability in the contribution of DHA to the FA composition of mature human milk has been corroborated by a study investigating, in the same laboratory, milk samples from five groups of lactating women living in five geographically different regions of China (20). Mean LA values were within narrow ranges (18.43–20.57%), and mean AA and ALA values showed only moderate variability (AA, 0.80–1.22%; ALA, 2.08–3.03%). In contrast, mean DHA values ranged from 0.44 to 2.78%, thus exhibiting a more than sixfold variance. Again, the relative variability of ω-3 FA exceeded that of ω-6 FAs.

The observed variability of human milk FA composition highlights the need for caution in using such data as the basis to define infant substrate requirements. However, the considerable uncertainties in defining the LCPUFA content characteristic to mature human milk should not mask the fact that all lactating women provide some amount of preformed dietary LCPUFA to their infants.

3.3. Sources of EFA and LCPUFA in Human Milk

The cited data indicate that milk LCPUFA content may be influenced by maternal dietary intakes. However, compositional studies have also provided indications for some degree of metabolic control of human milk LCPUFA content. In previous studies carried out in Germany, as well as in Nigeria, the authors did not find any correlation between LA and ALA and their respective LCPUFA metabolites in mature human milk (21,22). Moreover, women with very low dietary intakes of preformed AA still maintained high AA milk contents (22). These observations suggest that the LCPUFA content in human milk is not linearly related to the maternal dietary intake of EFA and LCPUFA.

Table 1

Contribution of Linoleic Acid (C18:2ω-6), Arachidonic Acid (C20:4ω-6),
α-Linolenic Acid (C18:3ω-3), and Docosahexaenoic Acid (C22:6ω-3) to FA Composition of Mature Human Milk

Country and reference	Australia (12)	Canada (13)	Congo (14)	France (15)	Germany (16)	Italy (17)	Norway (18)	Spain (19)
Linoleic acid	14.06	11.8	13.65	13.23	11.33	9.79	11.60	12.02
Arachidonic acid	0.41	0.4	0.44	0.50	0.45	0.47	0.40	0.50
α-Linolenic acid	0.97	1.5	1.19	0.57	0.90	0.36	0.93	0.78
Docosahexaenoic acid	0.21	0.3	0.55	0.38	0.23	0.12	0.46	0.34

Data are % w/w, medians or means from recently published studies using high-resolution capillary GLC.

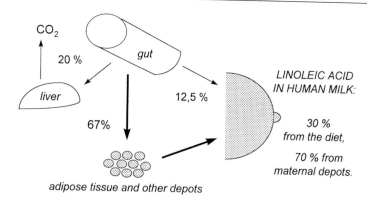

Fig. 3. Schematic depiction of LA (C18:2ω-6) flux in healthy breast-feeding women. Data are based on results of a stable-isotope study with oral application of 1 mg/kg body wt of U-^{13}C-labeled LA, and measurements of its oxidation from breath-gas analyses and its transfer into milk by analysis of milk samples collected over 5 d. Data are taken with permission from ref. 24; graphics are adapted with permission from ref. 68.

Understanding of the sources of EFA and LCPUFA in human milk has been enhanced by metabolic investigations using stable-isotope techniques, which are safe and without adverse effects (23). In a recent study on EFA metabolism during lactation, the authors gave an oral dose of 1 mg/kg body wt of uniformly ^{13}C-labeled LA to six apparently healthy lactating women, and estimated LA oxidation from analysis of breath gas enrichment and LA transfer into milk by analysis of milk samples collected over 5 d (24). From the data obtained in this study, the authors estimate that, over a period of 5 d, only about 30% of milk LA was directly transferred from the dietary LA intake; during the same time period, about 11% of milk DGLA and 1.2% of milk AA originated from direct endogenous conversion of dietary LA. In contrast, the major portion of EFA and LCPUFA in human milk lipids was derived from maternal body stores, and not directly from the maternal diet (Fig. 3). Thereby, the influence of maternal dietary intake on milk composition was moderated by the quantitatively larger contribution of FAs from body compartments with slow turnover, thus resulting in a relatively constant milk LCPUFA supply to the recipient infant.

3.4. LCPUFA Sources in Formula-Fed Infants:
Diet, Body Stores and Endogenous Synthesis

Conventional infant formulae based on vegetable oils contain both LA and ALA in amounts that are often similar to those typically found in mature human milk, but such conventional infant formulae do not contain appreciable amounts of AA and DHA (2,25,26). Infants fed such formulae without LCPUFA depend on utilization of body stores accreted during intrauterine growth, endogenous synthesis from the precursor EFA, or a combination thereof, to obtain the LCPUFA deposited in structural lipids of newly formed cell membrane systems.

It has previously been questioned whether infants would be capable of synthesizing LCPUFA themselves. Recent refinements of isotope techniques rendered it possible to investigate FA turnover in vivo, even in infants (27). The availability of uniformly ^{13}C-labeled, highly enriched tracer FAs, and the high sensitivity and precision of gas chromatography isotope ratio mass spectrometry, have made it possible to perform accurate measurements on ^{13}C-enrichment in precursor and product FAs from very small

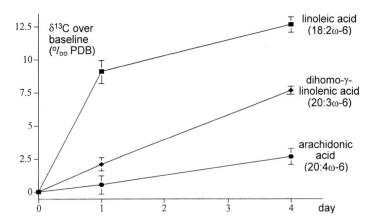

Fig. 4. Change of ^{13}C-enrichment (δ^{13}C over baseline) in plasma FAs of healthy, full-term infants aged 18 ± 4 d (mean ± SD), fed a diet with increased ^{13}C-enrichment of LA (C18:2ω-6). The increase of ^{13}C-contents in the LA metabolites, DGLA (C20:3ω-6) and AA (C20:4ω-6), indicates endogenous synthesis of these LCPUFA. Adapted with permission from ref. 28.

volumes of blood. With these techniques, the authors estimated LA conversion in healthy, full-term infants given a diet providing LA with an increased content of the stable isotope [13]C *(28)*. In the plasma lipids, the authors determined the ^{13}C-contents in different ω-6 FAs, and found a clear increase of ^{13}C-content, not only in the precursor LA, but also in ω-6 LCPUFA after the diet change (Fig. 4). These data showed that there was an active endogenous LA conversion in full-term infants, but the rate of conversion appears to be low. Using a simplified isotope-balance equation, the authors estimate that the contribution of AA synthesis to the total plasma AA pool is only on the order of about 6%/d in early infancy. More recent results indicate that endogenous AA synthesis occurred as early as the first week of life, but, again, the contribution of LA conversion to the total plasma pool was very small *(28a)*. Thus, endogenous synthesis may not be preferred to meet the needs of LCPUFA for incorporation into critical membranes during phases of rapid growth.

4. FA STATUS IN INFANTS FED HUMAN MILK OR FORMULA WITHOUT AND WITH LCPUFAS

EFA and LCPUFA status can be evaluated on the basis of the FA composition of plasma, red blood cell (RBC) membrane lipids, and the lipid composition of other tissues. FA composition of plasma and erythrocyte membrane lipid classes, in full-term infants fed human milk or formula without LCPUFA, was reported, at times as a minor part of a more complex data set, in several studies *(29–46)*. AA and DHA values in plasma or RBC membrane lipids were found to be significantly higher in breast-fed infants than in those receiving formula at ages of 2 mo *(33,38)*, 3 mo *(35,36,41)*, 4 mo *(34,37,39, 42,45)*, 6 mo *(40)*, 8 mo *(37,40)*, 9 mo *(49)*, and 12 mo *(42,45)*. These results indicate that, in infants fed formula without LCPUFA, endogenous synthesis of LCPUFA from the parent EFA and mobilization of tissue LCPUFA stores are insufficient to maintain similar plasma and RBC LCPUFA contents, as typically found in breast-fed infants. Moreover, not only plasma and RBC, but also tissue LCPUFA contents appear to be affected.

Cerebral and retinal DHA contents were found to be higher in infants who died from sudden infant death syndrome, if they had been breast-fed, compared to those fed formula without preformed LCPUFA *(47,48)*.

The reported differences in LCPUFA status between breast-fed and formula-fed full-term infants prompted investigations on the effect of the supplementation of infant formulae with LCPUFA. Studies evaluating the supplementation with DHA alone *(37,39,43–45)*, or in combination with AA *(34,35,42,45,49,50)*, indicated the potential to normalize LCPUFA status in the recipient infants, compared to reference groups fed human milk.

5. LCPUFAS AND PERINATAL GROWTH

Since early reports on EFA deficiency demonstrated growth failure as one of the chief clinical consequences of an EFA depletion *(9)*, the relationship of different EFAs and LCPUFAs to parameters of growth has been investigated. Birth weights are known to be greatly influenced by a large variety of variables, but overall show only a relatively small variation in healthy, full-term infants; therefore, the possible relationship of LCPUFAs to perinatal growth was first raised in studies on preterm infants, who tend to show a wider relative variation of growth parameters *(51,52)*. Koletzko and Braun *(51)* first reported a statistically significant and positive correlation of plasma triglyceride AA values on d 4 of life to birth weight; no correlations were seen either between birth weights and LA values or between AA values and gestational ages. Similar relationships were reported by Leaf et al. *(52)* for birth weights of preterm infants and FAs in umbilical vein plasma choline phosphoglycerides. These data suggest that, during early life, AA may have a growth-promoting effect that could be related either to its role as an eicosanoid precursor or to its structural function in membrane lipids *(53)*.

These earlier observations have been corroborated by findings of a recent prospective feeding trial *(54)*. On d 10 of life, RBC AA contents were significantly and positively related to standard deviation scores of weight, length, and head circumference, in a sizeable group of preterm infants fed five different infant formulae, including three without and two with dietary LCPUFA. RBC AA values at the age of 10 d were also significantly and positively related to birth weights, and there was no correlation between anthropometric data and RBC AA values at the age of 42 d. The authors concluded that early neonatal AA status is related to intrauterine rather than to postnatal growth *(54)*.

However, the putative relationship between AA status and postnatal growth has been seen in some studies. Prolonged depletion of AA levels throughout the first year of life was associated with poor growth in preterm infants fed a preterm infant formula supplemented with oils comprising high amounts of EPA (C20:5ω-3), compared to DHA, and containing no preformed AA or other ω-6 LCPUFA *(55)*. On the other hand, a preliminary report indicates that enhanced weight gain during the hospital stay, and higher body wt at 2 and 4 mo corrected age, was seen when premature infants received a preterm infant formula with both DHA and AA, compared to infants fed formulae containing no LCPUFA, or only DHA *(56)*. These results suggest that formulae containing both ω-6 and ω-3 LCPUFA may be best for the promotion of growth in preterm infants.

The much smaller rate of postnatal growth in full-term, compared to preterm infants, renders it methodologically more difficult to address the question of LCPUFA supply and somatic growth in full-term infants. Comparison of growth between breast-fed and formula-fed infants is obviously biased by the considerably higher protein intake with formula feeding than with feeding human milk. The published prospective feeding trials on full-term infants fed the same formula, without and with LCPUFA (*vide infra*), usually did not include sufficient numbers of subjects to allow evaluation of the presumably subtle differences in somatic development *(57)*.

6. EFFECT OF DHA STATUS ON VISUAL FUNCTION IN HEALTHY, FULL-TERM INFANTS

After indications for a causal relationship between DHA status and visual functions had been reported in animal studies, as well as in human premature infants *(58)*, nonrandomized comparative studies investigated the relationship between dietary LCPUFA supply and the development of visual functions in healthy full-term infants. Makrides et al. *(59)* studied groups of infants fed human milk or formula without added DHA, at the age of 5 mo. The formula-fed group had significantly lower DHA content in the membrane lipids of RBCs; these infants also had significantly poorer responses in standardized visually evoked potential tests, indicating a poorer visual acuity of term infants with a low DHA status. The visually evoked potential method measures the electroencephalographic responses over the visual cortex when the infant is exposed to a changing checkerboard pattern presented on a monitor under standardized conditions. Depending on the methodological details applied, this approach allows for a precise physiological assessment of visual acuity and other parameters of the visual process.

Another measure was used by Birch et al. *(60)*, who followed a group of children from a middle-class population in Texas, and tested visual acuity at the age of 3 yr, following then earlier participates in an infant feeding study designed for a different purpose. This earlier study data had determined the RBC FA composition at the age of 3 mo. When followed-up at the age of 3 yr, previously breast-fed children had a significant advantage in both random dot stereo acuity and letter-matching ability, over children who had been fed formula containing neither AA nor DHA. The stereo-acuity performance at 3 yr was significantly correlated with an index of ω-3 FA sufficiency calculated from RBC lipid composition at 3 mo of age *(60)*. These two studies suggested a positive effect of breast-feeding (which provided preformed DHA), compared to formula-feeding (without DHA) on visual and possibly other neural functions, which persisted beyond the duration of breast-feeding.

Other studies, however, have not detected such effects. Innis et al. *(36)* assessed visual acuity in healthy full-term infants who had been fed either human milk or formula. They used a behavioral test, called the Teller visual acuity card procedure. In this test, the investigator monitors the forced choice preferential looking of the tested infants, who tend to look preferentially at areas with grated black and white stripes with different widths, relative to a gray background on the cards. When the limit of resolution is reached, the black and white stripes are perceived as a gray area by the infants. With this test, Innis et al. found no group difference in visual acuity at the age of 3 mo between full-term infants fed human milk or formula, despite substantially higher DHA contents in RBC membranes and plasma lipids in the breast-fed group *(36)*.

The apparent discrepancy of results between the cited studies may be related to differences in study design and methodology applied, as well as to differences between populations studied and their ω-3 FA supply. Innis et al. studied infants from the area of Vancouver, BC, located on the Pacific coast, where mothers may have had a higher habitual fish intake, and hence higher DHA. These mothers could have provided a higher supply of DHA to their infants, both through the placenta and via breast milk, than in some other areas of the world. However, even if differences are detected between breast- and formula-fed populations, this does not provide conclusive evidence for a causal effect of the dietary DHA supply on visual function, because breast- and formula-fed infants differ in many aspects, and it is obviously impossible to randomize infants to breast or formula feeding.

These limitations in study design were overcome in double-blind, randomized clinical trials in which all full-term infants have been given formulae containing, or without, preformed DHA (37,42,44,45,50). These studies differed, however, in the amount and composition of LCPUFA supplied, in the duration of feeding the respective diets, and in the methodologies used for measuring visual functions. Most of these studies also enrolled a nonrandomized reference group of breast-fed babies. These studies designs validated the comparison between the test and the control formulae, but they obviously do not exclude bias caused by confounding factors in the nonrandomized breast-fed group.

Makrides et al. (37) investigated full-term infants in Australia, randomly assigned to receive either an experimental formula with 0.36% DHA (% w/w) or a control formula without DHA. Both at the ages of 16 and 30 wk, infants fed the formula with DHA exhibited significantly better visually evoked potential acuity than infants fed the control formula; there was no difference of visual acuity between infants fed formula with DHA and breast-fed infants. The differences in visual acuity corresponded to the DHA content in RBC membrane lipids. As age increased from 16 to 30 wk, the differences in visual acuity between infants fed the DHA, compared to the control formulae, became even more marked.

Carlson et al. (50) performed another controlled, randomized clinical trial, and determined visual acuity with the Teller Acuity Card procedure, repeated at the ages of 2, 4, 6, 9, and 12 mo in a cohort of full-term infants (from Memphis, Tennessee), randomized to formula either without or with a relatively low DHA content of only 0.1% (% w/w of all formula FAs) and 0.43% AA. Those authors also included a nonrandomized reference group of breast-fed infants. At the age of 2 mo, infants fed the DHA-supplemented formula had a significantly better grating visual acuity than controls, and matched the results of the breast-fed reference group, but, at the later time-points, there were no group differences in visual acuity, despite a persistent significant difference in DHA levels in plasma and RBC lipids. In agreement with these findings, a recently published trial from Denmark evaluated full-term infants fed formula supplemented with DHA alone (0.32% w/w), or in combination with GLA (C18:3ω-6), and did not detect any influence on steady-state visually evoked potential values at 4 mo of age (44).

In a large, multicenter trial involving more than 100 infants, Auestad et al. (42) investigated infants receiving formula supplemented with DHA alone (0.23% w/w) or with DHA and AA (0.12 and 0.43%, respectively), as well as infants fed formula without LCPUFA, and also included a nonrandomized, breast-fed reference infant group. Using a different methodology at each of the four study sites, visual acuity was assessed with either an acuity card procedure or a visually evoked potential methodology from the ages of 2 to 12 mo. The authors reported no group differences in visual functions. Because the study formula used was the same as the one used by Carlson et al. (50), who did find an effect on visual function, it appears possible that the differences in results of the two studies are related to the methodology applied.

In contrast to Auestad et al. *(42)*, Birch et al. *(45)* found a lasting effect of a DHA-enriched formula on visual acuity, in a study that also involved more than 100 infants. These investigators used an infant formula with a higher DHA content, either alone (0.35% DHA, w/w) or in combination with AA (0.36% DHA and 0.72% AA). Compared to infants receiving a control formula without DHA, those who received one of the two DHA-containing formulae had significantly better sweep visually evoked potential acuity at the ages of 6, 17, and 52 wk, i.e., the provision of DHA improved visual function up to 1 yr of age.

Although some studies could not detect effects of DHA-containing formula on visual function in healthy infants, which may result from relatively low contents of DHA in some of the studies, and/or specific aspects of the methodologies applied, recent trials have clearly documented that the addition of preformed DHA to infant formula may improve visual acuity up to the age of 1 yr. Whether or not this effect persists beyond the age of 1 yr, and varies in extent in specific subpopulations, may be determined by future research. However, these results clearly document that the provision of DHA during early human development enhances information transfer in neural tissue.

7. EFFECT OF DHA AVAILABILITY ON PERFORMANCE IN DEVELOPMENTAL TESTS IN HEALTHY, FULL-TERM INFANTS

Several authors have proposed that breast-fed infants have a better performance on some developmental tests and a lower rate of neurological handicaps than formula-fed infants, even after mathematical correction for potential confounding factors, such as socioeconomic status of the family *(58)*. However, one cannot assign infants at random to breast and formula feeding; therefore, a selection bias cannot be excluded, and these studies do not provide indisputable evidence of an advantage of breast-feeding for infant development. Nonetheless, these observations have sparked interest in investigating whether DHA, which is provided by breast milk, may enhance specific neurodevelopmental functions.

Innis et al. *(61)* used a behavioral preferential-looking test, in an open, nonrandomized study, to assess the behavior of breast-fed and formula-fed infants at the age of 9 mo. This test presents familiar and novel pictures to the tested infants, and monitors their looking preference, which reflects recognition-memory and information-processing abilities. The authors reported no difference between breast-fed and formula-fed infants, but, again, nonrandomized observational studies of breast- and formula-feeding may be biased by recognized and unrecognized genetic, socioeconomic, and other confounding factors.

In the previously cited randomized multicenter trial of Auestad et al. *(42)*, using a formula with low DHA content, the authors also found no beneficial effect on development. Rather, the authors reported a poorer performance of the DHA-supplemented infants on vocabulary repertoire *(42)*. Whether or not this is a causal effect or a spurious finding has been debated, but results of two presently unpublished studies have not detected any effect of DHA supplementation on infant verbal development (unpublished information).

Global psychomotor development, in relation to LCPUFA status in full-term infants, was tested by Agostoni et al. *(62)*, who performed the Brunet-Lézine test of neurodevelopment in a sizeable group ($n = 90$) of healthy infants, who were randomly assigned to formula supplemented with DHA and AA from egg PLs (0.30% DHA and 0.44% AA), or to a control formula without LCPUFA, or were part of a nonrandomized reference group who were fed human milk. At the age of 4 mo, developmental quotients were significantly lower in infants fed formula without LCPUFA than in those receiving the LCPUFA-supplemented formula or human milk (Fig. 5). Psychomotor development was correlated with the percentage contribution of DHA to RBC phospholipids. When data obtained in all infants participating in the study were evaluated as a combined group, developmental quotient values were significantly and positively related to the DHA content of RBC PLs (63). The majority of the infants (81/90) could be followed-up at the age of 24 mo. At that time, no group differences in the Brunet-Lézine psychomotor test results were detected. However, the developmental quotients at age 2 yr were still significantly and positively correlated with both AA and DHA content of RBC phosphatidyl-choline lipids at the age of 4 mo (64).

The ability to solve a complex task also has been related to early LCPUFA supply, in a recently published study by Willats et al. (65). Infant cognitive behavior was assessed by a battery of problem-solving tests at the age of 10 mo, in infants who had been randomly assigned in a double-blind study to feeding during the first postnatal months with formula without or with both DHA and AA from egg PLs, providing 0.15–0.25% DHA and 0.30–0.40% AA, respectively (65). The test evaluated the intentional execution of a sequence of steps, in order to find a hidden toy. The test is considered to be specially applicable for studying early development of complex cognitive functions, since tests results at the age of 9 mo were reported to correlate closely with intelligence quotients and vocabulary scores at the age of 3 yr (66). At the age of 10 mo, the tested infants who had received preformed dietary LCPUFA during early infancy had significantly more intentional solutions and better intention scores than infants whose formula was devoid of LCPUFA (Fig. 6).

Considering that positive effects of early DHA provision on global development at the corrected age of 1 yr were also reported in preterm infants (67), the authors conclude that feeding of conventional infant formulae, providing only LA and ALA, but no preformed LCPUFA, can impair the functional development of the infant nervous system.

8. CONCLUSIONS AND RECOMMENDATIONS

Preformed LCPUFA are provided to the fetus *in utero* through the placenta, and to the breast-fed infant after birth, as an integral component of human milk lipids. In contrast, conventional vegetable oil-based infant formulae provide only the precursor EFAs, LAs, and ALAs, and no appreciable levels of LCPUFA. Human infants can convert precursor EFAs into LCPUFA, but the capacity of this endogenous LCPUFA synthesis is low, and does not prevent LCPUFA depletion of plasma and tissue lipids in infants fed conventional formulae. Breast-feeding provides preformed LCPUFA, and, for this and a larger number of further reasons, is highly recommended as the first choice for feeding healthy babies.

If breast-feeding is not possible, the use of formulae that provide a balanced supply of LCPUFA appears advantageous over conventional formulae without LCPUFA. However, each of the various possible approaches of LCPUFA supplementation needs to be closely evaluated in terms of safety and efficacy. Moreover, further research is required to better define the appropriate composition and amounts of LCPUFA in infant diets, the appropriate duration of supplementation, and the longer-term effects of early LCPUFA

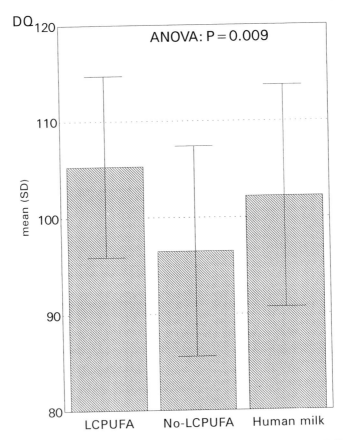

Fig. 5. Brunet-Lézine test developmental quotient (DQ) values in 4-mo-old, full-term infants fed formula supplemented with LCPUFAs, unsupplemented formula (No-LCPUFA), and human milk. Drawn with permission from ref. *62*.

supply, which may extend beyond infancy. Today, a number of different formulas, providing a spectrum of different types and amounts of preformed LCPUFA, are available in approx 60 countries of the world. An adequate LCPUFA enrichment can normalize the recipient infant's biochemical LCPUFA status, as measured by the analysis of lipids in plasma, RBCs, and mucosa cells. Some, but not all, randomized, double-blind, placebo-controlled clinical trials, in healthy full-term infants, have demonstrated that formula, supplemented with DHA alone or in combination with AA, may be beneficial for physical growth, the increased development of visual acuity up to the age of 1 yr, and the enhancement of complex neural and cognitive functions. Taken together, these data furnish evidence for considering LCPUFA conditionally essential substrates for human infants who should be provided with the postnatal diet to allow for optimal growth and development.

REFERENCES

1. Sauerwald TU, Hachey DL, Jensen CL, Chen H, Anderson RE, Heird WC. Intermediates in endogenous synthesis of C22:6ω3 and C20:4ω6 by term and preterm infants. Pediatr Res 1997; 41:183–187.
2. Koletzko B. Lipid supply for infants with special needs. Eur J Med Res 1997; 2:69–73.

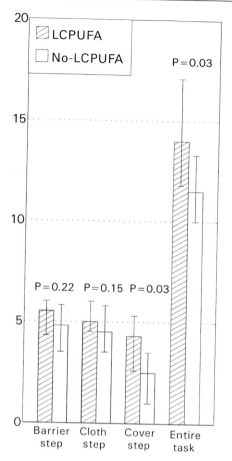

Fig. 6. Problem-solving scores in 10-mo-old, full-term infants fed formula supplemented with LCPUFA or unsupplemented formula (No-LCPUFA). The infant was able to reach a small toy (the goal object) by removing a barrier block (barrier step), pulling a cloth to retrieve the toy from the far end of the table (cloth step), and removing the cover from the toy (cover step). Drawn with permission from ref. 65.

3. Clandinin MT, Chappell JE, Leong S, Heim T, Swyer PR, Chance GW. Intrauterine fatty acid accretion in human brain: implications for fatty acid requirements. Early Hum Dev 1980; 4:121–129.
4. Martinez M. Tissue levels of polyunsaturated fatty acids during early human development. J Pediatr 1992; 120:S129–S138.
5. Keicher U, Koletzko B, Reinhardt D. Omega-3 fatty acids suppress the enhanced production of 5-lypoxygenase products from polymorph neutrophil granulocytes in cystic fibrosis. Eur J Clin Invest 1995; 25:915–919.
6. Berghaus T, Demmelmair H, Koletzko B. Fatty acid composition of lipid classes in maternal and cord plasma at birth. Eur J Pediatr 1998; 157:763–768.
7. Koletzko B, Müller L. Cis- and trans-isomeric fatty acids in plasma lipids of newborn infants and their mothers. Biol Neonate 1990; 57:172–178.
8. Koletzko B, Decsi T, Dürr U, Edenhofer S. Milk formulae for preterm infants: special lipid requirements. In: Common Food Intolerances 2: Milk in Human Nutrition and Adult-Type Hypolactasia. Auricchio S, Semenza G, eds. Basel: S. Karger AG, 1993; 5–19.
9. Decsi T, Koletzko B. Polyunsaturated fatty acids in infant nutrition. Acta Paediatr 1994; 395(Suppl.): 31–37.

10. Koletzko B, Diener U, Fink M, Berghaus T, Demmelmair H, von Schönaich P, Bernsau U. Supply and biological effects of long-chain polyunsaturated fatty acids (LCPUFA) in premature infants. In: Nutrition of the Extremely Low Birthweight Infant. Ziegler E, Lucas A, Moro G, eds. Philadelphia: Lippincott-Raven, 1999.

11. Koletzko B, Thiel I, Abiodun PO. The fatty acid composition of human milk in Europe and Africa. J Pediatr 1992; 120:S62–S70.

12. Makrides M, Neumann MA, Gibson RA. Effect of maternal docosahexaenoic acid (DHA) supplementation on breast milk composition. Eur J Clin Nutr 1996; 50:352–357.

13. Cherian G, Sim JS. Changes in breast milk fatty acids and plasma lipids of nursing mothers following consumption of n-3 polyunsaturated fatty acid enriched eggs. Nutrition 1996; 12:8–12.

14. Rocquelin G, Tapsoba S, Dop MC, Mbemba F, Traissac P, Martin-Prével Y. Lipid content and essential fatty acid (EFA) composition of Congolese breast milk are influenced by mothers' nutritional status: impact on infants' EFA supply. Eur J Clin Nutr 1998; 52:164–171.

15. Guesnet P, Antoine J-M, Rochette de Lempdes J-B, Galent A, Durand G. Polyunsaturated fatty acid composition of human milk in France: changes during the course of lactation and regional differences. Eur J Clin Nutr 1993; 47:700–710.

16. Genzel-Boroviczény O, Wahle J, Koletzko B. Fatty acid composition of human milk during the 1st month after term and preterm delivery. Eur J Pediatr 1997; 156:142–147.

17. Serra G, Marletta A, Bonacci W, Campone F, Bertini I, Lentieri BP, Risso D, Ciangherotti S. Fatty acid composition of human milk in Italy. Biol Neonate 1997; 72:1–8.

18. Helland IB, Saarem K, Saugstad OD, Drevon CA. Fatty acid composition in maternal milk and plasma during supplementation with cod liver oil. Eur J Clin Nutr 1998; 52:839–845.

19. Presa-Owens S, López-Sabater MC, Rivero-Urgell M. Fatty acid composition of human milk in Spain. J Pediatr Gastroenterol Nutr 1996; 22:180–185.

20. Chulei R, Xiaofang L, Hongsheng M, Xiulan M, Guizheng L, Gianhong D, DeFrancesco CA, Connor WE. Milk composition in women from five different regions of China: the great diversity of milk fatty acids. J Nutr 1995; 125:2993–2998.

21. Koletzko B, Mrotzek M, Bremer HJ. Fatty acid composition of mature human milk in Germany. Am J Clin Nutr 1988; 47:954–959.

22. Koletzko B, Thiel I, Abiodun PO. Fatty acid composition of mature human milk in Nigeria. Z Ernährungswiss 1991; 30:289–297.

23. Koletzko B, Sauerwald T, Demmelmair H. Safety of stable isotope use. Eur J Pediatr 1997; 156(Suppl. 1): S12–S17.

24. Demmelmair H, Baumheuer M, Koletzko B, Dokupil K, Kratl G. Metabolism of U[13]C-labelled linoleic acid in lactating women. J Lipid Res 1998; 39:1389–1396.

25. Koletzko B, Bremer HJ. Fat content and fatty acid composition of infant formulae. Acta Paediatr Scand 1989; 78:513–521.

26. Decsi T, Behrendt E, Koletzko B. Fatty acid composition of Hungarian infant formulae revisited. Acta Paediatr Hung 1994; 34:107–116.

27. Demmelmair H, Sauerwald T, Koletzko B, Richter T. New insights into lipid and fatty acid metabolism via stable isotopes. Eur J Pediatr 1997; 156(Suppl. 1):S70–S74.

28. Demmelmair H, Schenck U, Behrendt E, Sauerwald T, Koletzko B. Estimation of arachidonic acid synthesis in full term neonates using natural variation of ^{13}C content. J Pediatr Gastroenterol Nutr 1995; 21:31–36.

28a. Szitanyi P, Koletzko B, Mydlilova A, Demmelmair H. Metabolism of ^{13}C-labeled linoleic acid in newborn infants during the first week of life. Ped Res 1999; 45:669–673.

29. Olegard R, Svennerholm L. Effects of diet on fatty acid composition of plasma and red cell phosphoglycerides in three-month-old infants. Acta Paediatr Scand 1971; 60:505–511.

30. Putnam JC, Carlson SE, DeVoe P, Barness LA. The effect of variations in dietary fatty acids on the fatty acid composition of erythrocyte phosphatidylcholine and phosphatidylethanolamine in human infants. Am J Clin Nutr 1982; 36:106–114.

31. DeLucchi C, Pita ML, Faus MJ, Molina JA, Uauy R, Gil A. Effects of dietary nucleotides on the fatty acid composition of erythrocyte membrane lipids in term infants. J Pediatr Gastroenterol Nutr 1987; 6:568–574.

32. Gil A, Lozano E, De-Lucchi C, Maldonado J, Molina JA, Pita M. Changes in the fatty acid profiles of plasma lipid fractions induced by dietary nucleotides in infants born at term. Eur J Clin Nutr 1988; 42:473–481.

33. Ponder DL, Innis SM, Benson JD, Siegman JS. Docosahexaenoic acid status of term infants fed breast milk or infant formula containing soy oil or corn oil. Pediatr Res 1992; 32:683–688.

34. Agostoni C, Riva E, Bellu R, Trojan S, Luotti D, Giovannini M. Effects of diet on the lipid and fatty acid status of full-term infants at 4 months. J Am Coll Nutr 1994; 13:658–664.

35. Kohn G, Sawatzki G, Van Biervliet JP, Rosseneu M. Diet and essential fatty acid status of term infants. Acta Paediatr 1994; 402(Suppl.):69–74.

36. Innis SM, Nelson CM, Rioux MF, King DJ. Development of visual acuity in relation to plasma and erythrocyte ω-6 and ω-3 fatty acids in healthy term gestation infants. Am J Clin Nutr 1994; 60:347–352.

37. Makrides M, Neumann M, Simmer K, Pater J, Gibson R. Are long-chain polyunsaturated fatty acids essential nutrients in infancy? Lancet 1995; 345:1463–1468.

38. Decsi T, Thiel I, Koletzko B. Essential fatty acids in full term infants fed breast milk or formula. Arch Dis Child 1995; 72:F23–F28.

39. Innis SM, Auestad N, Siegman JS. Blood lipid docosahexaenoic and arachidonic acid in term gestation infants fed formulas with high docosahexaenoic acid, low eicosapentaenoic acid fish oil. Lipids 1996; 31:617–625.

40. Luukkainen P, Salo MK, Visakorpi JK, Räihä NCR, Nikkari T. Impact of solid food on plasma arachidonic and docosahexaenoic acid status of term infants at 8 months of age. J Pediatr Gastroenterol Nutr 1996; 23:229–234.

41. Innis SM, Akrabawi SS, Diersen-Schade DA, Dobson MV, Guy DG. Visual acuity and blood lipids in term infants fed human milk or formulae. Lipids 1997; 32:63–72.

42. Auestad N, Montalto MB, Hall RT, Fitzgerald KM, Wheeler RE, Connor WE, et al. Visual acuity, erythrocyte fatty acid composition, and growth in term infants fed formulas with long chain polyunsaturated fatty acids for one year. Pediatr Res 1997; 41:1–10.

43. Maurage C, Guesnet P, Pinault M, de Lempdes J-BR, Durand G, Antoine J-M, Coutet C. Effect of two types of fish oil supplementation on plasma and erythrocyte phospholipids in formula-fed term infants. Biol Neonate 1998; 74:416–429.

44. Jorgensen MH, Holmer G, Lund P, Hernell O, Fleischer-Michaelsen K. Effect of formula supplemented with docosahexaenoic acid and gamma-linolenic acid on fatty acid status and visual acuity in term infants. J Pediatr Gastroenterol Nutr 1998; 26:412–421.

45. Birch EE, Hoffman DR, Uauy R, Birch DG, Prestidge C. Visual acuity and the essentiality of docosahexaenoic acid and arachidonic acid in the diet of term infants. Pediatr Res 1998; 44:201–209.

46. Decsi T, Kelemen B, Minda H, Burus I. Feeding breast milk or formula influences plasma long-chain polyunsaturated fatty acid values in full-term infants at the age of nine months. J Pediatr Gastroenterol Nutr 1998; 26:A589 (Abstract).

47. Farquharson J, Cockburn F, Patrick WA, Jamieson EC, Logan RW. Infant cerebral cortex phospholipid fatty acid composition and diet. Lancet 1992; 340:810–813.

48. Makrides M, Neumann MA, Byard RW, Simmer K, Gibson RA. Fatty acid composition of brain, retina and erythrocytes in breast- and formula-fed infants. Am J Clin Nutr 1994, 60:189–194.

49. Decsi T, Koletzko B. Growth, fatty acid composition of plasma lipid classes, and plasma retinol and α-tocopherol concentrations in full-term infants fed formula enriched with ω-6 and ω-3 long-chain polyunsaturated fatty acids. Acta Paediatr 1995; 84:725–732.

50. Carlson SE, Ford AJ, Werkman SH, Peeples JM, Koo WWK. Visual acuity and fatty acid status of term infants fed human milk and formulas with and without docosahexaenoate and arachidonate from egg yolk lecithin. Pediatr Res 1996; 39:882–888.

51. Koletzko B, Braun M. Arachidonic acid and early human growth: Is there a relation? Ann Nutr Metab 1991; 35:128–131.

52. Leaf AA, Leighfield MJ, Costeloe KL, Crawford MA. Long chain polyunsaturated fatty acids and fetal growth. Early Hum Dev 1992; 30:183–191.

53. Sellmayer A, Koletzko B. Polyunsaturated fatty acids and eicosanoids in infants: physiological and pathophysiological aspects and open questions. Lipids 1999; 34:199–205.

54. Woltil HA, van Beusekom CM, Schaafsma A, Muskiet FAJ, Okken A. Long-chain polyunsaturated fatty acid status and early growth of low birth weight infants. Eur J Pediatr 1998; 157:146–152.

55. Carlson SE, Werkman SH, Peeples JM, Cooke RJ, Tolley EA. Arachidonic acid status correlates with first year growth in preterm infants. Proc Natl Acad Sci USA 1993; 90:1073–1077.

56. Hansen J, Schade D, Harris C. Dososahexaenoic acid plus arachidonic acid enhance preterm infant growth. Prostaglandins Leukot Essent Fatty Acids 1997; 57:196 (Abstract).

57. Morley R. Nutrition and cognitive development. Nutrition 1998; 14:752–754.

58. Koletzko B, Aggett PJ, Bindels JG, Bung P, Ferre P, Gil A, et al. Growth, development and differentiation: a functional food science approach. Br J Nutr 1998; 80(Suppl. 1):S5–S45.

59. Makrides M, Simmer K, Goggin M, Gibson RA. Erythrocyte docosahexaenoic acid correlates with the visual response of healthy, term infants. Pediatr Res 1993; 34:425–427.

60. Birch E, Birch D, Hoffman D, Everett M, Uauy R. Breast-feeding and optimal visual development. J Pediatr Ophthalmol Strabismus 1993; 30:33–38.

61. Innis SM, Nelson CM, Lwanga D, Rioux FM, Waslen P. Feeding formula without arachidonic acid and docosahexaenoic acid has no effect on preferential looking acuity or recognition memory in healthy full-term infants at 9 mo of age. Am J Clin Nutr 1996; 64:40–46.

62. Agostoni C, Trojan S, Bellu R, Riva E, Giovannini M. Neurodevelopmental quotient of healthy term infants at 4 months and feeding practice: the role of long-chain polyunsaturated fatty acids. Pediatr Res 1995; 38:262–266.

63. Agostoni C, Riva E, Trojan S, Bellu R, Giovannini M. Docosahexaenoic acid status and developmental quotient of healthy term infants. Lancet 1995; 346:638.

64. Agostoni C, Trojan S, Bellu R, Riva E, Bruzesse MG, Giovannini M. Developmental quotient at 24 months and fatty acid composition of diet in early infancy: a follow up study. Arch Dis Child 1997; 76:421–424.

65. Willats P, Forsyth JS, DiModugno MK, Varma S, Colvin M. Effect of long-chain polyunsaturated fatty acids in infant formula on problem solving at 10 months of age. Lancet 1998, 352:688–691.

66. Slater A. Individual differences in infancy and later IQ. J Child Psych Psychiatr 1995; 36:69–112.

67. Carlson SE, Werkman SH, Peeples JM, Wilson WM. Long-chain fatty acids and early visual and cognitive development of preterm infants. Eur J Clin Nutr 1994; 48(Suppl. 2):S27–30.

68. Rodriguez-Palmero M, Koletzko B, Kunz C, Jensen RG. Nutritional and biochemical properties of human milk: II. Lipids, micronutrients, and bioactive factors. Clin Perinatol 1999; 26:335–359.

15 Vitamin A-Related Childhood Blindness, Mortality, and Morbidity
Interventions for Prevention

Barbara A. Underwood

1. INTRODUCTION

1.1. Causes of the Problem

The primary cause of blinding malnutrition and vitamin A-related mortality is a persistent, inadequate dietary intake of absorbable vitamin A, which should be sufficient to meet normal metabolic requirements and the periodically increased need imposed by stress. Protein-energy malnutrition, frequent febrile diseases, and malabsorption are pathophysiological factors contributing to the increased need for the vitamin. Increased need also occurs during physiological periods of rapid growth, such as fetal development and early childhood, and when there is need to replace the maternal vitamin A transferred to breast milk during lactation. As illustrated in Fig. 1, most nonpathophysiological factors contributing to vitamin A deficiency (VAD), in poorly developed countries, are common to the problems associated with overall social, economical, and ecological deprivation *(1)*. VAD in industrialized countries occasionally occurs among malabsorbers of fat who do not receive supplements, those with abnormal liver function *(2)*, and those who may habitually consume cereal-based diets low in vitamin A. Irrespective of age, most people in the United States and other industrialized countries, however, consume diets sufficient in vitamin A to maintain adequate serum levels *(3)*. Dietary and medical interventions that prevent or control conditions causally associated with deficiency are commonly available in the industrialized world, but access to adequate diets or supplements, and disease-control measures are less available in the nonindustrialized world.

1.2. Magnitude and Geographic Distribution of the Problem

1.2.1. CHILDHOOD BLINDNESS

There are no reliable data on the global incidence of childhood blindness. The World Health Organization (WHO), however, estimates that there are about 1.4 million surviving blind children, 15 yr of age and younger, and that nearly 80% are located in Africa, India, and China *(4)*. Childhood blindness, although affecting a much smaller number than those blinded by age-related cataract, causes an estimated 75 million blind years (number blind × average length of life), a close second to years of disablement from cataract *(5)*. It is known that the major cause of childhood blindness in developing

From: *Primary and Secondary Preventive Nutrition*
Edited by: A. Bendich and R. J. Deckelbaum © Humana Press Inc., Totowa, NJ

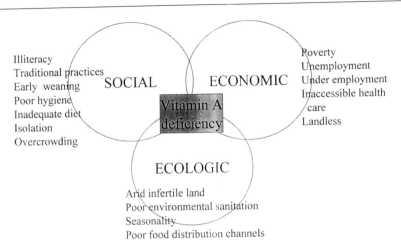

Fig. 1. Conditions associated with social, economic, and ecologic deprivation contribute to VAD.

countries is avoidable: 50–70% of it is caused by VAD, frequently complicated by malabsorption, infection, and protein-calorie malnutrition *(6)*. Most prevalence data, however, come from registries in blind schools, which underestimate the magnitude of the problem, because of the high mortality associated with nutrition-related blindness.

1.2.2. MORTALITY AND MORBIDITY RISK

Children in underprivileged societies who become blind from VAD are said to die at high rates, i.e., 60–70% die within a year of becoming blind *(7)*. Moreover, considering only mortality associated with blindness fails to account for the high mortality from common childhood illnesses, such as diarrhea and measles, in endemically VAD areas, even where eye signs are rare. Reduction in these rates could be expected if vitamin A status were restored *(8)*. Several millions of preschool-age children throughout the world have serum levels of vitamin A below those that are thought to reflect an adequate status *(9)*, and thus are at risk of preventable death when they contract an infection. Meta-analyses indicate that, on average, mortality from common childhood diseases could be reduced by 20–30% by correcting or preventing VAD *(8)*. Indeed, it has been estimated that 1.3–2.5 million of the nearly 8 million late-infancy and preschool-age child deaths (about 15–30%), which occur annually in the highest-risk developing countries, could be averted by improved vitamin A nutriture *(10)*.

2. DIAGNOSIS OF DEFICIENCY

2.1. Ocular Signs and Symptoms: Xerophthalmia

Ocular signs of VAD, i.e., xerophthalmia, are well known and described in textbooks *(11)* and field manuals *(12)*, but they are rare occurrences, thus requiring a large sampling of a suspect population to provide prevalence information *(13)*.

Difficulty seeing in dim light after bright light exposure, i.e., night blindness, is the most common and mild symptom deserving of special mention. This symptom is not observable by routine physical examination. Nonetheless, the symptom among afflicted children is specific, and usually recognized and given a distinctive name in communities where it is common *(14)*. Among adults, other causes of night blindness can confound diagnosis of VAD from only a history. A recently completed study in Nepal, for example, reported that, among pregnant women who reported night blindness, and who were treated with either β-carotene or vitamin A, 83 and 58%, respectively, did not improve *(15)*. Other studies have occasionally misdiagnosed night blindness as reported by history as caused by VAD, when it was caused by retinitis pigmentosa. Dark adaptation time, using electroretinography, is the standard diagnostic procedure in institutional settings *(16)*, but is limited in application in field settings, using currently available instruments, particularly in children under approx 3 yr of age *(14)*. Pupillometric measures of retinal sensitivity is another approach applicable even in infants *(17)*. Pupillary threshold measurements, using a hand-held portable instrument, currently are being evaluated in population surveys, as an index of a population's vitamin A status *(18,19)*.

Clinically evident ocular signs include conjunctiva dryness, i.e., xerosis, often accompanied by Bitot's spots caused by accumulated dead and sloughed epithelial and bacterial cells, and corneal xerosis, which appears as a hazy or milky cornea that may become ulcerated and progress rapidly to irreversible damage and blindness (keratomalacia). All these signs are easily visible to a trained worker, or by using simple instruments. When seen, they require immediate treatment with therapeutic levels of vitamin A supplements, because they signal potential impending and irreversible corneal damage *(20)*. However, early records include experiences in a child malnutrition rehabilitation center in India, in which preulcerative signs responded even to dietary levels of vitamin A *(21)*. This finding should provide encouragement to those who seek to prevent blinding malnutrition when high-dose supplements are not available. Also, cod liver oil has been used for many years in prevention programs before vitamin A capsules were widely available.

2.2. Extraocular Diagnoses

VAD may be present even when ocular symptoms and signs are not present, i.e., subclinical deficiency. However, subclinical deficiency is more difficult to diagnose, even though there are available an array of potentially useful biochemical and histological measurements that relate to vitamin A status. No single indicator, however, is definitive, and it is expensive to perform multiple tests in an effort to balance shortcomings of each *(13,14)*. An urgent search continues for a practical diagnostic methodology with sufficient specificity, sensitivity, and appropriateness for use in young children.

Because of the association of VAD with a series of adverse functional consequences, including mortality, some have suggested using infant mortality rate (IMR) as a surrogate for VAD populations. They suggest that IMR alone justifies vitamin A supplement interventions in the absence of ocular, biochemical, or dietary evidence *(22)*. There are, of course, many nonvitamin A-related contributing factors to infant and under-5-yr mortality rates, and there is currently little agreement on a minimum prevalence level that should trigger broad-based interventions with vitamin A supplements. WHO recommends that diagnosis of VAD, in the absence of ocular signs, preferably should be found using at least two biochemical measures, or one biochemical and a series of indirect indicators, of which infant mortality rates are but one *(13)*. WHO also recommends that, when using indirect indicators, it is also suggested to document at least with qualitative measures the availability as well as the intake of dietary sources of vitamin A-containing foods.

3. CONSEQUENCES OF DEFICIENCY

Although a molecular explanation for vitamin A functioning in vision was among the first described for a vitamin *(23)*, it accounted for only a small portion of the functions the vitamin was known to influence, e.g., growth, reproduction, immunity, and maintenance of cellular integrity. Several years lapsed, with limited progress in elucidating the other molecular functions, until the discovery of nuclear receptors for vitamin A in 1987. This discovery has led to rapid progress in unraveling a fascinating and evolving story, in which retinoids, through their specific nuclear receptors, regulate the expression of a large number of genes critical to normal development and maintenance of a healthy condition *(24)*. The functional effects of deficiency on components of the immune system, growth, reproduction, hematopoiesis, and vision were considered in the first volume of *Preventive Nutrition (25)*. Further elucidation of links between specific molecular events and functional defects are expected over the next few years.

4. EPIDEMIOLOGY OF VAD

The epidemiology of VAD may vary by country, but, overall, bears a similar pattern. It is mostly prevalent amid poverty, environmental deprivation, and social disparity (Fig. 1). The greatest toll is extracted on infants and young children, whose needs are elevated to support rapid growth and to overcome losses resulting from frequent infections. Pregnant and lactating women are also at high risk, because material vitamin A is sacrificed in favor of the fetus, and nursing women lose vitamin A in breast milk during lactation. There are no significant physiological differences in need for vitamin A related to gender, although sociocultural differences in child feeding and care may explain some reported apparent gender disparities (more female children are deficient). The problem tends to cluster within families and communities, which probably reflects common environmental contributing factors. The most pervasive risk factor is poverty, not only because of the limit placed on acquiring relatively expensive bioavailable preformed (animal foods) and provitamin A (plant-based) dietary sources, but also in maintaining sanitary environments to lower disease risk. In addition, poverty often discourages undereducated child caretakers from active participation in community-based social and educational activities in which child-feeding and care are taught *(1,26)*.

5. PREVENTION AND CONTROL PROGRAMS

Providing sufficient dietary sources of vitamin A can prevent childhood blindness, mortality, and morbidity related to VAD. So, why does VAD still prevail as a significant public health problem in many parts of the world, even in tropical countries where provitamin A carotenoids are in abundant supply? Obviously, the answer does not depend only on availability of adequate dietary sources of vitamin A. In many countries, the incidence of infectious disease (enteric and systemic) and severe protein-energy malnutrition contribute to the problem by altering absorption, transport, utilization, and excretion of dietary vitamin A *(26)*. Measles infections are especially devastating to vitamin A metabolism, and, in areas of endemic vitamin A deficits, the infection is associated with blindness, particularly in Africa *(27)*. Where VAD is endemic, elimination of conditions that favor frequent infections would enhance the efficacy of vitamin A provided in existing diets, but, in most situations, a quantitative overall increased intake of vitamin A sources is still needed *(28)*.

5.1. Preventive Dietary Approaches
in which Appropriate Vitamin A-Containing Foods Are Available

5.1.1. ANIMAL FOOD SOURCES

The nature of the available food sources of vitamin A is critical to the amount required to achieve adequacy. Bioavailability from animal products, including breast milk, whole milk and dairy products, eggs, and glandular meats, may be as high as 80–90%; from provitamin A carotenoids, it is much less. Breast milk, even from an undernourished mother, contains sufficient vitamin A, and lipid for its efficient absorption, to prevent deficiency from occurring for at least 4–6 mo postpartum, although the infant and maternal body reserves may be lowered (29). Indeed, breast milk continues to be a very important source of vitamin A for the young child, as long as breast-feeding continues, particularly because most complementary foods available to impoverished families in the developing world, because of expense or tradition, provide few preformed or provitamin A carotenoids (30).

5.1.2. VEGETABLE FOOD SOURCES: BIOAVAILABILITY ISSUES

How much vitamin A-active carotenoids contained in natural foods are absorbed and available for conversion to vitamin A (bioavailable) depends on the provitamin source and how it is prepared and consumed, e.g., raw or cooked, with adequate fat or alone, from cellulose-rich cells found in dark-green leafy vegetables (DGLV), or the crystalline β-carotene found in pigment-containing cells of carrots, or the more soluble dispersion of carotenoids in cells of orange, yellow, and red tubers and fruits (31). A suggested hierarchy (from lowest to highest sources) of bioavailability from natural food sources (Fig. 2) ranks raw DGLV and yellow and orange root vegetables and fruit juices, as least bioavailable, followed by the cooked forms and processed juices, then carotenoids contained in cooked tubers and fruits. All natural carotenoid sources are rendered more bioavailable when taken as part of fat-containing meals. β-carotene-rich red palm oil is highly bioavailable, as well as that from a synthetic oil or water-dispersible carotenoid source (32).

Quantitative differences among food sources in the vitamin A value of dietary carotenoids were recognized long ago. A WHO-sponsored expert subcommittee in 1949 established an international definition for vitamin A equivalencies, based on animal growth studies, setting that for β-carotene on a weight basis as one-half that of retinol, i.e., 0.6 μg β-carotene equivalent is equal to 0.3 μg retinol (33). These weights were each set to be equivalent to an International Unit (IU). Variation in the available vitamin A for metabolism, derived from different vegetable sources of provitamin A carotenoids, was recognized, and various factors, ranging from one-half to as much as one-tenth or less, were arbitrarily suggested, before reaching a compromise of one-sixth retinol equivalence for β-carotene and one-twelfth for other active carotenoids contained in a usual mixed diet (34). These factors assume the average absorption efficiency of β-carotene is one-third, and the efficiency of conversion to vitamin A is one-half (one-fourth for other carotenoids) on a weight basis. Hence, to evaluate the total vitamin A potency of a diet, in IU, necessitated determining the percentage of activity coming from preformed and provitamin sources. In 1967, FAO and WHO proposed the retinol equivalent (RE), defined on a weight basis, to replace IU and thus reduce the confusion generated in evaluating diets by these discrepancies in utilization from foods. A RE, by definition, became equal to 1 μg retinol, or 6 μg β-carotene, or 12 μg other provitamin A carotenoids (34).

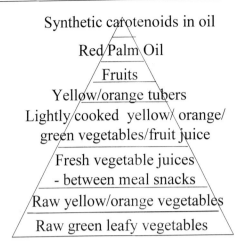

Synthetic carotenoids in oil

Red Palm Oil

Fruits

Yellow/orange tubers

Lightly cooked yellow/orange/
green vegetables/fruit juice

Fresh vegetable juices
- between meal snacks

Raw yellow/orange vegetables

Raw green leafy vegetables

Fig. 2. Suggested hierarchy of bioavailability of carotenoids from natural food sources and synthetic supplements.

Currently, traditional quantitative bioavailability factors are being re-examined for different carotenoid food sources provided as part of meals. Investigators are using several approaches and indicators to establish bioavailability, which vary in their specificity and sensitivity. These approaches include comparative change in serum levels of retinol and/or β-carotene between a control and intervention group *(35,36)*, an indicator that can be influenced by a variety of nonvitamin A-related factors; postprandial retinol/carotenoids in the triglyceride-rich lipoprotein fraction, an indicator that more closely reflects postdosing absorption and bioconversion *(37)*; isotope dilution after feeding stable-isotope-labeled foods *(38)*; and monitoring changes in total body stores following administration of a labeled tracer *(39,40)*. The human studies are further complicated by apparent marked individual differences in absorption efficiency for different carotenoids. Nonetheless, it is highly likely that currently used RE factors (i.e., one-sixth and one-twelfth for β-carotene and other provitamin carotenoids, respectively) will change for various classes of provitamin A food sources, as consistency is reached using intrinsically labeled food sources and newer highly sensitive analytical methodologies. Tang et al. *(40)* reported that Chinese children, habitually consuming primarily fruit and vegetable-based diets, maintained adequate body reserves of vitamin A, even though estimated bioavailability using their methodology was as low as 1:27. This finding underpins the practical importance of promoting provitamin A carotenoids in diets for control of VAD, even though the estimated bioavailability by current methodology is low.

5.1.3. Increasing Consumption by Vulnerable Groups

It seems intuitive that education and social marketing to promote a change in dietary patterns is the intervention that should receive attention where food sources of vitamin A are available, but underutilized. However, there are numerous reports of failed efforts to increase consumption of vitamin A-active foods in the diets of vulnerable groups, even though knowledge and attitudes of food sources improved among those who control household diets. That is, feeding patterns did not change. Currently, educational and social marketing approaches emphasize a process for changing behaviors, not just improving knowledge and attitudes. A critical element in the process is to systemically infuse the desired behavior, through many communication channels, to the community, with reinforcing messages and programs practically suited to the local context *(41,42)*. The process, to be successful, should include participation of community partners, including women from high-risk families and the poor *(43)*.

5.2. Preventive Dietary Approaches in which Natural Food Sources Are Limited

5.2.1. Homestead Gardening

Homestead and/or community gardens can provide sufficient vegetable sources to significantly reduce the risk of household vitamin A inadequacy. This contention is supported by epidemiological studies that consistently associate frequency of consumption of provitamin A sources to reduced risk of VAD *(44,45)*. Unlike controlled intervention trials or distribution of supplements, however, health impacts from gardening projects are difficult to directly attribute to a specific nutrient whose consumption increased through garden products, because food-based interventions provide several essential nutrients simultaneously.

The successful large-scale community gardening program currently implemented in Bangladesh has demonstrated that proximity of the garden to the household, as well as variety in garden sources, are critical to increased consumption by vulnerable groups, including consumption of provitamin A-rich vegetables *(46,47)*. Bangladeshi participants in home gardening reported less night blindness, and experienced slightly higher serum retinol levels, than nonparticipants. In Vietnam, a remarkable reduction in the incidence of respiratory and diarrhea infections occurred in villages participating in a nutrition project based on household food production and nutrition education *(48)*.

Homestead/community gardening also improved the vitamin A status among project communities in Thailand, but the path to achieving success differed from that in Bangladesh. In contrast to the Bangladesh experience, where multiple carotenoid-rich sources were promoted, in Thailand, a single DGLV source that grew easily and was locally acceptable, but socially undervalued (i.e., ivy gourd), served as an entry point. Intensive promotion through multiple community activities and organizations led to adapting homestead gardening, when previously it had not been widely practiced *(49)*. Consumption of ivy gourd and fat (both practices were actively promoted) increased in households, including intake by children and mothers who were the group targeted for benefits. These changed eating behaviors persisted even 10 yr after the promotional period terminated. Further, in the 10-yr period between evaluations, local gardens had expanded to include a variety of provitamin A-containing vegetable *(43)*. The Thai success in establishing homestead gardens through a single entry point, with potential for change coupled to intensive social marketing, built community confidence in adopting self-sufficient practices that provided obvious benefits to households, thereby embedding changed behaviors *(49)*. Thus, multiple vitamin A-active food sources entered local dietary patterns in both Bangladesh and Thailand by processes best suited to the individual local contexts.

5.2.2. Small Animal Production and Fish Farming

Small animal husbandry and fish farming can complement vegetable and fruit gardens in improving household diets, and, in some contexts, potentially generate income. Rabbits, guinea pigs, chickens, ducks, and wild birds (and their eggs), and even snakes, are examples of foods, which, if incorporated even in small amounts, can markedly improve predominantly vegetable-based diets. Because of their market value, however, these micronutrient-rich food sources are often sold, rather than consumed. To retain at least part of the animal products for household use, such programs should be accompanied by practical instructions for economical household use. In southern Thailand, for example, where an outbreak of VAD was reported in a semiurban area, the problem was stemmed initially by distribution of high-dose vitamin A supplements through the Ministry of Public Health (MoPH). Concurrently, the MoPH nutrition division, collaborating with the university's institute of nutrition, identified local inexpensive food sources of vitamin A. Recipes were developed, including liver chips from small animals and poultry *(50,51)*, and a social marketing and demonstration effort was undertaken to prepare for a transition from the medical approach to a food-based approach. Included in the integrated strategy to control VAD, was regulations to ensure that all commercial milk products, which potentially could be used for infant and young child feeding, contained, or were fortified with, vitamin A *(51)*.

In some areas, household/community fishponds and aquaculture, as well as natural water reservoirs and seasonal flooding along rivers, offer a viable dietary source of highly bioavailable preformed vitamin A. Fish, like other animals, concentrate vitamin A in the liver, so that eating small whole fish can provide important amounts of the vitamin, even when the small fish are preserved dry. In some cultures, seasonal flooding into rice paddies brings small fish within household reach, physically and economically, as a dietary adjunct, for short periods of time.

5.2.3. An Approach on the Horizon:
Enhanced Micronutrient Density of Staple Foods Through Plant Breeding

Most national agricultural policies, in food-deficit, poor countries, are guided by farm productivity of energy-dense staples, rather than micronutrient-rich vegetable crops, even though micronutrient deficiency may be common. It is unrealistic to expect significant policy shifts to occur in such countries toward micronutrient-rich, energy-poor crops. In mid-1990, new thinking stimulated research efforts to combine favorable agronomic and nutritional characteristics into cultivars of cereals and other food staples *(52)*. This plant-breeding approach is not expected to replace other interventions needed to rapidly correct existing micronutrient deficiencies. However, a substantial contribution to long-term maintenance of micronutrient adequacy is possible, because of the high portion of the daily diet provided by a staple *(53)*.

Cassava is an example of an inexpensive crop that is easily grown, even in infertile dry soil. The poor consume it because it is inexpensive, and the root is calorie dense, although most varieties are low in essential nutrients. Seventy million people are estimated to obtain more than 500 calories daily from cassava, particularly in Africa and northeast Brazil. Varieties selected to contain high β-carotene content in roots and leaves *(54,55)* can make a substantial contribution to dietary vitamin A sufficiency, as well as calorie adequacy. For example, at the high end (105 mg β-carotene/100 g fresh leaves), as little as 5 g fresh leaves (2 g dry leaf flour) theoretically would supply the daily requirements of vitamin A for an adult male (i.e., 3–4 mg). The comparable figure for carotene-dense cassava roots would be 200 g *(54,55)*. Several years and substantial resources will be needed to complete the breeding, propagation, bioavailability, safety, and consumer acceptability fieldwork, before seeds with optimal agronomic, nutritional, and organoleptic qualities are available to farmers. Once achieved, however, the recurrent expenditure would be low, compared to nonfood-based strategies *(56)*.

5.3. Fortification

5.3.1. CENTRALLY PROCESSED FORTIFIED FOOD PRODUCTS

Vitamin A and other micronutrient deficiencies are no longer public health problems in several industrialized countries, in part, because of central fortification with vitamin A of common items in the food supply, e.g., dairy products and margarine. An educated public in these countries demands the opportunity to buy fortified products, based on the demonstrated or perceived health benefits. This public demand provides a stable market for fortified products without need for government enforcement by regulations or legislation *(57)*.

In recent years, food fortification has been strongly advocated by international agencies and donor groups, as a cost-effective dietary intervention to control VAD. Central fortification becomes an increasingly feasible control strategy as the food industry grows in countries undergoing economic transition, and as markets for commercial products expand to rural areas. Mandatory universal fortification with vitamin A, as widely successful for mandatory iodization of salt, is an attractive intervention to many, because it minimizes the need to alter food habits of undereducated poor populations, among whom deficiencies are most prevalent, a seemingly appealing top-down altruistic approach. However, no low-cost common product comparable to salt has been found to serve as a universal carrier of vitamin A. Most vitamin A-fortifiable products, e.g., oils and margarine, dairy products, flours, and sugar, are consumed in widely variable amounts by age groups and households, for economical and cultural reasons. Furthermore, there are multiple sources of these products, including some that are home-produced. This makes it challenging to implement and enforce a mandatory national fortification policy.

Nonetheless, government mandates for universal vitamin A fortification of a staple product can be effective in some contexts. Such a national directive for sugar fortification was successful in Guatemala *(58)*. However, attempts to replicate the Guatemala sugar success story in Zambia, and to introduce centrally produced vitamin A-fortified mealy meal (a corn-based staple), failed because those most vulnerable to VAD did not consume centrally processed sugar, and, in rural areas, they preferred the traditional home-pounded mealy meal *(59)*. In this context, mandating universal national fortification of a stable is unenforceable and ineffective in reaching those most vulnerable. Government policies that allow a "seal of approval," such as on vitamin A-fortified margarine in the Philippines, coupled to extensive social marketing campaigns *(60)*, are attempts to reinforce market choice for fortified vs unfortified alternatives. Where technical and political elements are favorable for fortification *(61)*, but the distribution infrastructure in rural remote areas is inadequate, fortification could still be effective to reach the majority, if augmented by targeted vitamin A distribution to reach those left out. In the Philippines, for example, efforts are underway to provide a vitamin A-enriched premix to rural households that do not consume centrally fortified rice *(62)*.

A basic conflict between the private sector's profit motivation and the public's willingness to pay for quality is a constraint underlying food fortification as a control measure for VAD. Cost, rather than humanitarian concern or personally experienced health benefits, can be the breaking point that determines choice for producers to fortify, and for poverty-stricken, potential beneficiaries to buy. Removing constraints, therefore, requires changing perceptions and attitudes of both private and public sectors *(62)*. The benefits of fortification must be convincingly sold, both to unsubsidized potential private producers, who risk markets and R&D investment loss, and to local undereducated and undemanding civil society. Thus, it is shortsighted, in free-market economies where public choice remains, to rely on even marginally more expensive fortified products for prevention of VAD, without a substantial education and social marketing investment.

5.3.2. HOUSEHOLD FOOD FORTIFICATION: FOOD-TO-FOOD

There is scope for promoting food-to-food fortification within households. Sun-drying of leaves, vegetables, and fruit is traditional in many cultures. Recent development of simple household solar dryers, which deflect vitamin A-destroying ultraviolet sun rays, provide potential for slight modification to accepted preservation practices that can provide micronutrient-dense products. Such products, e.g., mango, papaya, orange sweet potato, green leaves, and even small, whole fish, could be vitamin sources that can be added to micronutrient-poor, energy-dense staples used for making paps, gruels, and soups for feeding young children and other groups vulnerable to VAD.

5.4. Supplementation

5.4.1. HIGH-DOSE SUPPLEMENTS

The liver's capacity to store large amounts of vitamin A, and to release it under homeostatic control, as needed, is the rationale for periodically administering a concentrated dose of the vitamin for prevention of deficiency. Studies in animals and humans indicate that large oral doses are efficiently absorbed; about 50% of a large dose is retained, and the remainder is excreted as glucoronide conjugates in bile, some of which may be recycled *(63)*. Retained vitamin A is released to supply tissues and maintain a relatively stable level in the circulation, when intake is inadequate until tissues are depleted *(64)*. Hence, concentrated vitamin A supplements are a necessary part of treatment programs, and have a place in some control programs in which: food-based approaches are not feasible within a short time frame; vulnerable populations infrequently contact the health system; and/or subclinical VAD is an established risk.

Safe dosages and frequency of administration for prevention and control programs are age-specific, ranging from 200,000 IU (68,000 µg retinyl acetate) every 4–6 mo beyond infancy, and 50,000 or 100,000 IU for the first and second 6 mo of infancy, respectively *(20)*. Implementing these dosage schedules, through programs with broad coverage of preschool-age children in endemically deficient areas, is associated with substantial reduction in vitamin A-related child blindness, and a reduction in severity and risk of death from some infections *(8,11)*.

High-dose vitamin A supplementation programs require health system monitoring of delivery, because of potential for toxic side effects, including potential teratogenic risks, if very high doses of vitamin A are taken in early pregnancy. It is safe to provide high dosages to fertile women during the 6–8 wk infertile period following a birth *(20,65)*. Supplements containing near-physiological doses of vitamin A (5000–10,000 IU daily) can be safely integrated into community outreach systems without safety concerns, beyond the first postnatal year *(65)*.

Indonesia provides a notable example of a country that implemented a periodic high-dose supplementation program, and progressed from a high prevalence of xerophthalmia to elimination of the clinical problem at a public health level in about 20 yr. Biochemical deficiency (low serum retinol levels), however, persists in half the young child population. The government concluded, therefore, that, to control the problem, vitamin A supplement distribution must continue (66). Persistent low serum retinol levels are common, however, when underlying acute and chronic infections are prevalent (67,68). Thus, persistent low serum concentrations may reflect in part a high prevalence of infections, and, therefore, not be a reliable barometer for evaluation of vitamin A control programs, without confirmation from other indicators.

High-dose vitamin A supplements require controlled periodic distribution through the health system. Historically, this intervention has suffered from low coverage of the vulnerable groups with successive rounds of distribution. Campaign-style twice-yearly distribution days (e.g., national immunization days or micronutrient days) have reduced the continuous contact burden for the health system, and increased coverage among children. After a few years, however, enthusiasm for periodic campaigns often wanes, emphasizing the importance for sustainability of embedding distribution programs into community structures that reach preschool-age children (66).

Recently, a three-country, randomized, controlled trial integrated the delivery of vitamin A (25,000 IU doses) into immunization contacts for breast-fed infants at about 6, 10, and 14 wk of age, and a fourth dose at 9 mo of age. At 9 mo, the placebo group received one dose of 100,000 IU. Vitamin A status on a random subsample was assessed by serum retinol and a modified relative dose-response test (MRDR) at baseline, 6, 9, and 12 mo. Significant excess acute toxic side effects from vitamin A were not encountered. Vitamin A status was maintained above nonsupplemented controls, up to age 6 mo, by 4/wk repeat dosing (Table 1). However, the benefit from the three 25,000 IU doses did not extend during the 22-wk interval from the 14-wk immunization/dosing contact to the 9-mo (about a 36-wk interval) measles immunization/dosing contact (69). However, there was only a 5% difference in vitamin A status at 12 mo between groups given a fourth 25,000 IU dose or 100,000 IU at 9 mo, as measured by MRDR. The data suggest that, for prevention programs, different dosage scenarios are needed to protect the gains from early lower-dose supplementation, and to augment such doses to meet the increasing need documented from about 6 mo through the preschool years. For example, one possible scenario may be to increase the dose from 25,000 to 50 000 IU at 6 mo of age, 100,000 IU at 9 mo of age, and 200,000 IU at any contact for immunization after 12 mo of age, provided the child has not received a high dose through another program within the last month. Other safe scenarios adapted to local contact intervals are possible. These could include contacts made in the process of growth monitoring; through educational programs involving school-aged child to younger siblings (i.e., child-to-child), and similar community-based programs for distribution of physiological doses, when regular immunization contacts no longer apply.

5.4.2. ALTERNATIVE SAFE SUPPLEMENT DOSAGES AND SCHEDULES

Vitamin A supplements (or fortificants), provided frequently at dosages near to physiological needs (e.g., near recommended dietary intakes), appear to provide greatest benefits. For examples, controlled, randomized intervention trials with vitamin A-fortified monosodium glutamate, integrated into daily family diets at one-fourth to one-half the recommended dietary allowance for Indonesian children (70), or supplement doses equivalent to those recommended as adequate, given weekly (8333 IU) (71), provided greater protection from infection-related mortality in children (e.g., 45 and 54% mortality

Table 1
Vitamin A Status of Infants by Visit in Ghana, India, and Peru

Vitamin A indicator	Mean (SD) retinol µmol/L		Retinol % ≤0.35 µmol/L		Retinol % ≤0.70 µmol/L		Ratio A2: retinol % ≤0.06	
	Vit A	Control	Vit A	Control	Vit A	Control	Vit A	Control
First dose	0.67 (0.33)	0.68 (0.32)	6.92[a]	8.34	63.02	62.16	77.95	75.56
6-Mo visit	0.84 (0.29)	0.80 (0.27)	3.60	4.49	29.92	37.15	43.47	52.51
9-Mo visit	0.84 (0.31)	0.82 (0.32)	4.95	8.31	32.57	35.69	37.89	37.42
12-Mo visit	0.85 (0.41)	0.83 (0.47)	10.22	7.18	33.42	31.46	27.51	32.57

[a] % Calculated by a site stratified analysis. Adapted with permission from ref. 69.

reduction, respectively) than was achieved from periodic high doses of 100,000–200,000 IU every 4–6 mo (e.g., about 6–30% mortality reduction *[5]*). Furthermore, all-cause maternal mortality was reduced by 44% with weekly supplements of 23,300 IU *(72)*. Even children acutely ill in hospitals responded best to daily administration of 5000 IU, rather than to a single 200,000 IU dose *(73)*. These findings all support the assumption of greater efficacy from vitamin A supplements provided frequently, e.g., daily, weekly, and perhaps monthly, at dosages close to physiological needs. There have not been large-scale programs in developing countries that have provided access to frequent low-dose supplements to at-risk populations, from which to evaluate program effectiveness. Randomized community trials indicate that such dosing schedules are effective in deficient populations, even where periodic high-dose supplementation programs are also in effect *(74)*.

5.5. Public Health Approaches to Disease Control

Infectious disease prevalence is associated in an iterative downward cycle toward vitamin A depletion *(1,26)*. The effectiveness of an adequate dietary intake for prevention, therefore, may be greatly compromised where disease incidence remains high. Immunization programs can be an important adjunct to prevention efforts that interrupt the downward progression, especially when also combined with programs for promotion of breast-feeding, environmental sanitation, clean water, and personal hygiene. Measles, which usually occurs in children above 6 mo of age, is both a blinder and killer of children that is preventable by immunization *(27)*. Diarrhea and respiratory diseases are major causes of morbidity in unsanitary, congested living conditions, and resident helminth infections characteristic of poor personal hygiene are endemic in unclean environments. Disease control programs contribute to prevention of VAD, but do not replace the need for positive efforts to improve intake of vitamin A *(28)*.

5.6. Socioeconomic and Community Action Programs

Poverty and social disparities are the root cause of most malnutrition, including VAD and other micronutrient deficiencies. Community programs that reduce such disparities have been effective in reducing nutritional deficiencies in several countries, including Thailand, Costa Rica, and Tanzania, as well as in Kerala, South India *(75)*. Social and economic community-action programs that improve the status of women and empower them to make and implement prudent decisions are increasingly recognized as crucial for improved health status of families residing in deprived surroundings *(43)*. A female literacy program in Nepal increased participation in community activities associated with improving family vitamin A status and health *(76)*. In Haiti, income generation through a community-based and female-managed mango-drying enterprise proved efficacious in increasing dietary intake of vitamin A-containing food *(77)*.

6. SUMMARY AND RECOMMENDATIONS

Although the basic cause of VAD as a public health problem is an inadequate dietary intake of bioavailable vitamin A, understanding the context in which this occurs should guide prevention activities. Accessibility to dietary sources for environmental, economic, or sociocultural reasons may be amenable to change in some environments, either directly, by increased local production, or indirectly, through female literacy, income generation, and/or school and community education and awareness programs. These kinds of approaches toward increased accessibility favor community initiatives, management, and support, often with minimum need for external resources. Community-based interventions build local capacity for problem solving, foster community pride and ownership, and decrease dependency. Yet, such projects require investment of time, and frequently must take indirect routes, or meet other priority community needs first, before arriving at the primary goal of increased intake of vitamin A-rich foods. Central or home-based (food-to-food) fortification can be an effective underpinning for dietary control of VAD where feasible and practical. High-dose vitamin A approaches may also contribute, but should not undermine efforts toward attaining dietary adequacy.

As evidenced by the selected material herein, a variety of programs are available for combating immediate and underlying causes of VAD and interrupting the adverse consequences for health and survival. No single vertically implemented intervention is likely to be sustainable. Programs balanced in accord with resources available locally, augmented by external aid as needed, and that are contextually appropriate and affordable, are called for. Local community leaders are best suited to provide a realistic, insightful context for program planners. The concerns of the poor and of women must be considered, and they should be partners in planning, implementing, and monitoring prevention activity *(49)*.

REFERENCES

1. Underwood B. Epidemiology of vitamin A deficiency and depletion (hypovitaminosis A) as a public health problem. In: Retinoids. Progress in Research and Clinical Applications. Livrea MA and Packer L, eds. New York, Marcel Dekker, 1993; 171–183.
2. Underwood BA, Denning CR. Blood and liver concentrations of vitamin A and E in children with cystic fibrosis. Pediatr Res 1972; 6:26–31.
3. National Health and Nutrition Examination Survey III, 1988–1994. CD-ROM Series 11, No. 2A. Centers for Disease Control and Prevention. Hyattsville, MD: April 1998.
4. Report of a Task Force Informal Consultation with WHO. Needs and Priorities for the Control of Blindness in Children, ICEH London, UK: 30–31 March 1998.
5. WHO. Global initiative for the elimination of avoidable blindness. WHO/PBL/97.61. Geneva, Switzerland: World Health Organization, 1997.
6. WHO. Prevention of childhood blindness. Geneva, Switzerland: World Health Organization, 1992.
7. McLaren DS, Shirajian E, Tchalian M, et al. Xerophthalmia in Jordan. Am J Clin Nutr 1965; 17:117–130.
8. Beaton GH, Martorell R, Aronson KJ, et al. Effectiveness of vitamin A supplementation in the control of young child morbidity and mortality in developing countries. ACC/SCN State-of-the-art-series, Nutrition policy discussion paper No. 13. Geneva, Switzerland: Administrative Committee on Coordination, Subcommittee on Nutrition, United Nations, 1993.
9. WHO/UNICEF. Global prevalence of vitamin A deficiency. MDIS Working Paper 2. Geneva, Switzerland: World Health Organization, 1995.
10. Humphrey JH, West KP Jr, Sommer A. Vitamin A deficiency and attributable mortality among under-5-year-olds. Bull WHO, 1992; 70:225–232.
11. Sommer A, West KP Jr. Vitamin A Deficiency Health, Survival, and Vision. New York: Oxford University Press, 1996.
12. Sommer A. Vitamin A Deficiency and Its Consequences: A Field Guide to Their Detection and Control, 3rd ed. Geneva, Switzerland: World Health Organization, 1994.
13. WHO. Indicators of vitamin A deficiency and their use in monitoring intervention programmes. WHO/NU/96.10. Geneva, Switzerland: World Health Organization, 1996.
14. Underwood BA, Olson JA, eds. A Brief Guide to Current Methods of Assessing Vitamin A Status. A report of the International Vitamin A Consultative Group (IVACG), Washington, DC: The Nutrition Foundation, 1993.
15. West KP, Khatry SK, Katz J, et al. Impact of weekly supplementation of women with vitamin A or beta-carotene on fetal, infant and maternal mortality in Nepal. In: Report of the XVIII International Vitamin A Consultative Group Meeting, Cairo, Egypt, 22–26 September 1997; 86.

16. Marmor MF, Arden GB, Nilsson SEG, et al. Standards for clinical electroretinography. Arch Ophthalmol 1989; 107:816–819.

17. Birch EE, Birch DG. Pupillometric measures of retinal sensitivity in infants and adults with retinitis pigmentosa. Vision Res 1987; 27:499–505.

18. Congdon N, Sommer A, Severns M, et al. Pupillary and visual thresholds in young children as an index of population vitamin A status. Am J Clin Nutr 1995; 61:1076–1082.

19. Sanchez AM, Congdon NG, Sommer A, et al. Pupillary threshold as an index of population vitamin A status among children in India. Am J Clin Nutr 1997; 65:61–66.

20. WHO/UNICEF/IVACG. Vitamin A supplements: a guide to their use in the treatment and prevention of vitamin A deficiency and xerophthalmia, 2nd ed. Geneva, Switzerland: World Health Organization, 1997.

21. Venkataswamy G, Krishnamurthy KA, Chandra P, et al. A nutrition rehabilitation centre for children with xerophthalmia. Lancet 1976; 1:1120–1122.

22. Consensus of an Informal Technical Consultation. A strategy for accelerating of progress in combatting vitamin A deficiency. Vitamin A Global Initiative. Washington, DC: USAID, 1998.

23. Wald G. Molecular basis of visual excitation. Science 1968; 162:230–239.

24. Chambon P. A decade of molecular biology of retinoic acid receptors. FASEB J 1996; 10:940–954.

25. Semba RD. Impact of vitamin A on immunity and infection in developing countries. In: Preventive Nutrition. Bendich A, Deckelbaum RJ, eds. Totowa, NJ: Humana, 1997; 337–350.

26. Sommer A, West KP Jr. Epidemiology of deficiency. In: Vitamin A Deficiency: Health, Survival, and Vision. New York: Oxford Press, 1996; 335–354.

27. Foster A, Yorston D. Corneal ulceration in Tanzanian children: relationship between measles and vitamin A deficiency. Trans Royal Soc Trop Med Hyg 1992; 86:454–455.

28. Donnen P, Brasseur D, Dramaix M, et al. Vitamin A supplementation but not deworming improves growth of malnourished preschool children in Eastern Zaire. J Nutr 1998; 128:1320–1327.

29. Underwood BA. Maternal vitamin A status and its importance in infancy and early childhood. Am J Clin Nutr 1994; 59(Suppl.):517S–524S.

30. Zeitlan MFR, Megawangi E, Kramer M, et al. Mothers and children's intakes of vitamin A in rural Bangladesh. Am J Clin Nutr 1992; 56:136–147.

31. Castenmiller JM, West CE. Bioavailability and bioconversion of carotenoids. Ann Rev Nutr 1998; 18:19–38.

32. Boileau TWM, Moore AC, Erdman JW. Carotenoids and vitamin A. In: Antioxidant Status, Diet, Nutrition, and Health. Papas AM, ed. New York: CRC, 1999; 133–158.

33. National Academy Sciences, National Research Council, Food and Nutrition Board. Recommended Dietary Allowances, Revised 1953.

34. FAO. Requirements of vitamin A, thiamine, riboflavin and niacin. FAO Nutr Meet Rep Ser No. 41, WHO Tech Rep Ser No. 362, Rome, Italy, 1967.

35. De Pee S, West CE, Karyadi D, et al. Lack of improvement in vitamin A status with increased consumption of dark-green leafy vegetables. Lancet 1995; 346:75–81.

36. Jalal F, Nesheim MC, Agus Z, et al. Serum retinol concentrations in children are affected by food sources of b-carotene, fat intake, and anthelmintic drug treatment. Am J Clin Nutr 1998; 68:623–629.

37. Vliet T, Schreurs WHP, van den Berg H. Intestinal β-carotene absorption and cleavage in men: β-carotene and retinyl ester response in the triglyceride-rich lipoprotein fraction after a single oral dose of β-carotene. Am J Clin Nutr 1995; 62:110–116.

38. Parker RS, Swanson JE, You C-S, et al. Bioavailability of carotenoids in human subjects. Proc Nutr Soc 1999; 58:1–8.

39. Ribaya-Mercado JD, Mazariegos M, Tang G, et al. Assessment of total body stores of vitamin A in Guatemalan elderly by the deuterated-retinol-dilution method. Am J Clin Nutr 1999; 69:278–284.

40. Tang G, Gu X, Hu S, et al. Green and yellow vegetables can maintain vitamin A body stores of Chinese children. Am J Clin Nutr 1999; 70:1069–1076.

41. Smitasiri S, Attig BA, Dhanamitta S. Participatory actions for nutrition education: social marketing vitamin A-rich foods in Thailand. Ecol Food Nutr 1992; 28:199–210.

42. Underwood B. Prevention of vitamin A deficiency. In: Prevention of Micronutrient Deficiencies. Tools for Policymakers and Public Health Workers. Howsen CP, Kennedy ET, Horwitz A, eds. Washington, DC: National Academy Press, 1998; 103–165.

43. Smitasiri S, Sa-ngobwarchar K, Kongpunya P, et al. Sustaining behavior change to enhance micronutrient status through community and women-based interventions in Northeast Thailand: I. vitamin A. UNU Food Nutr Bull 1999; in press.

44. Mele L, West KP Jr, Kusdiano, et al. Study Group. Nutritional and household risk factors for xerophthalmia in Aceh, Indonesia: a case-control study. Am J Clin Nutr 1991; 53:1460–1465.

45. Christian P, West KP Jr, Khatry SK, et al. Night blindness of pregnancy in rural Nepal: nutritional and health risks. Int J Epidemiol 1998; 27:231–237.

46. Longanathan R, Huq N, Burger S, et al. Consumption of green leafy vegetables among children from households with homestead gardens in rural Bangladesh. In: Sustainable control of vitamin A deficiency. Defining progress through assessment, surveillance, evaluation, Report of the XVIII International Vitamin A Consultative Group Meeting, Cairo, Egypt, Washington, DC: International Life Science Institute, 1997; 51 and 91.

47. Bloem MW, Huq N, Gorstein J, et al. Production of fruits and vegetables on the homestead is an important source of vitamin A among women in rural Bangladesh. Eur J Clin Nutr 1996; 50(Suppl. 3): S62–S67.

48. English RM, Badcock JC, Giay T, et al. Effect of nutrition improvement project on morbidity from infectious diseases in preschool children in Vietnam: comparison with control commune. Br Med J 1997; 315:1122–1125.

49. Underwood BA, Smittasiri S. Micronutrient malnutrition: policies and programs for control and their implications. Ann Rev Nutr 1999; 19: 303–324.

50. South and East Asia Nutrition Research-cum-Action Network. Empowering Vitamin A-rich foods. A food-based process for the Asia and Pacific region. Wasantwisut E, Attig GA, eds. Thailand: Institute of Nutrition, Mahidol University, 1995.

51. Udomkesmalee E. Overview of vitamin A: global situation and the Thai experience. In: Integrating Food and Nutrition into Development: Thailand's Experiences and Future Vision, Winichagoon P, Kachondham Y, Attig GA, Tontisirin K, eds. UNICEF East Asia and the Pacific Regional Office, Bangkok, Thailand, and Institute of Nutrition Mahidol University at Salaya, Thailand, 13:146–152.

52. Graham RD, Senadhira D, Ortiz-Monasterio I. A strategy for breeding staple-food crops with high micronutrient density. Soil Sci Plant Nutr 1997; 43:1153–1157.

53. Ruel MT, Bouis HE. Plant breeding: a long-term strategy for the control of zinc deficiency in vulnerable populations. Am J Clin Nutr 1998; 68(Suppl.):488S–94S.

54. CGIAR Micronutrients Project. Update No. 1, October, 1996; Update No. 2, October. Washington, DC: IFPRI, 1997.

55. Iglesias C, Mayer J, Chavez L, et al. Genetic potential and stability of carotene content in cassava roots. Euphytica 1997; 94:367–373.

56. Bouis H. Enrichment of food staples through plant breeding: a new strategy for fighting micronutrient malnutrition. Nutr Rev 1996; 54:131–137.

57. Mertz W. Food fortification in the United States. Nutr Rev 1997; 55:44–49.

58. Pineda O. Fortification of sugar with vitamin A. UNU Food Nutr Bull 1998; 19:131–136.

59. FAO. Guidelines for national food insecurity and vulnerability information and mapping systems (FIVIMS): Background and principles. Committee on World Food Security, 24th Session. Rome, 2–5 June 1998. CFS:98/5.

60. Solon FS. History of fortification of margarine with vitamin A in the Philippines. UNU Food Nutr Bull 1998; 19:154–158.

61. Darnton-Hill I. Overview: rationale and elements of a successful food-fortification programme. UNU Food Nutr Bull 1998; 19:92–100.

62. Florentino RF, Pedro MRA. Update on rice fortification in the Philippines. UNU Food Nutr Bull 1998; 19:149–153.

63. Ross AC. Vitamin A and retinoids. In: Modern Nutrition in Health and Disease, 9th ed. Shils ME, Olson JA, Shike M, Ross AC, eds. Baltimore, MD: Williams & Wilkins, 1999; 17:305–327.

64. Green MH, Green JB. Dynamics and control of plasma retinol. In: Vitamin A in Health and Disease. Blomhoff R, ed. New York: Marcel Dekker, 1994; 5:119–133.

65. WHO/MI. Safe vitamin A dosage during pregnancy and lactation. Recommendations and report of a consultation. WHO/NUT/98.4. Geneva, Switzerland: World Health Organization, 1998.

66. Underwood BA. Prevention of vitamin A deficiency. In: Prevention of Micronutrient Deficiencies. Tools for Policymakers and Public Health Workers. Howsen CP, Kennedy ET, Horwitz A, eds. Washington, DC: National Academy Press, 1998; 103–165.

67. Filteau SM, Morris SS, Abbott RA, et al. Influence of morbidity on serum retinol of children in a community-based study in northern Ghana. Am J Clin Nutr 1993; 58:192–197.

68. Christian P, Schulze K, Stoltzfus RJ, et al. Hyporetinolemia, illness symptoms, and acute phase protein response in pregnant women with and without night blindness. Am J Clin Nutr 1998; 67:1237–1243.
69. WHO/CHD. Immunisation-Linked Vitamin A Supplementation Study Group. Randomised trial to assess benefits and safety of vitamin A supplementation linked to immunisation in early infancy. Lancet 1998; 352:1257–1263.
70. Muhilal, Permeisih D, Idjradinata YR, et al. Vitamin A-fortified monosodium glutamate and health, growth, and survival of children: a controlled field trial. Am J Clin Nutr 1988; 48:1271–1276.
71. Rahmathulla L, Underwood BA, Thulasiraj T, et al. Reduced mortality among children in southern India receiving a small weekly dose of vitamin A. New Engl J Med 1990; 323:929–935.
72. West KP Jr, Katz J, Khatry SK, et al. Double blind, cluster randomised trial of low dose supplementation with vitamin A or β carotene on mortality related to pregnancy in Nepal. Br Med J 1999; 570–575.
73. Donnen P, Dramaix M, Brasseur D, et al. Randomized placebo-controlled clinical trial of the effect of a single high dose or daily low doses of vitamin A on the morbidity of hospitalized, malnourished children. Am J Clin Nutr 1998; 68:1254–1260.
74. Thu BD, Schultink W, Dillon D, et al. Effect of daily and weekly micronutrient supplementation on micronutrient deficiencies and growth in young Vietnamese children. Am J Clin Nutr 1999; 69:80–86.
75. Commission on the Nutrition Challenges of the 21st Century. Ending malnutrition by 2020: An agenda for change in the millennium. Final report of the ACC/SCN Commission on the Nutrition Challenges of the 21st Century. Geneva, Switzerland, March 1999.
76. Pant CR, Pokharel GP, Curtale F, et al. Impact of nutrition education and mega-dose vitamin A supplementation on the health of children in Nepal. Bull WHO 1996; 74:533–545.
77. Linehan M, Paddack K, Mansour M. Solar drying for vitamin A. Washington, DC: VITAL, USAID Vitamin A Field Support Project, 1993.

.

Polyunsaturated Fatty Acids and Autoimmune Diseases

Andrea Belluzzi

INTRODUCTION

The causes of autoimmune disease (AD) are yet unknown. The hypothesis that there is an abnormal immunological response to an altered antigen, either viral or bacterial, is supported by much scientific evidence. All of the diseases share an immunological pathogenesis, involving mostly T- and B-cells, the cytokine network, and the complement system, resulting in an inflammatory condition that becomes chronic and self-perpetuating.

AD may have pathological and clinical manifestations in any part of the body, and the pathogenesis of the chronic inflammation can be divided in two stages. The first stage is the initiating event of unknown cause that triggers the inflammatory response, which is still unknown. The second stage is the amplification of the inflammatory response, which involves a number of inflammatory cells, including lymphocytes, mast cells, macrophages, and neutrophils. Soluble mediators control the amplification of this inflammatory response; a long list of mediators with putative roles in AD has been enumerated (1), including various eicosanoids, platelet-activating factor, kinins, complement-derived peptides, a long series of cytokines, and bacterial products, neuropeptides, and free radicals.

The second stage, the amplification of the inflammatory response, is important in the pathogenesis of the AD for two reasons. It is more important than the initiating event in causing tissue destruction and histological and functional changes, and is characteristic of AD. Second, those drugs that are effective in the treatment of AD appear to have a therapeutical effect by modulating the production of these soluble mediators. As long as the initiating event remains unknown, it is likely that further advances in medical therapy will result only from pharmacological modulation of these inflammatory mediators.

The rationale for n-3 and n-6 polyunsaturated long chain fatty acid (PUFA) supplementation in the treatment of AD resides in the anti-inflammatory effects of these lipid compounds. Over the past few years, a growing body of evidence has demonstrated that n-3 and n-6 PUFAs alleviate a number of inflammatory diseases. Actually, the first evidence of the importance of dietary intake of these lipids was derived from epidemiological observations about the very low incidence of chronic inflammatory condition in Eskimos.

Dietary eicosapentaenoic acid (EPA) and docosahexaenoic acid (DHA) which are the two major components of fish oil, partially replace arachidonic acid (AA), which is the initiating component of the homonymous metabolic pathway, in a time- and dose-

From: *Primary and Secondary Preventive Nutrition*
Edited by: A. Bendich and R. J. Deckelbaum © Humana Press Inc., Totowa, NJ

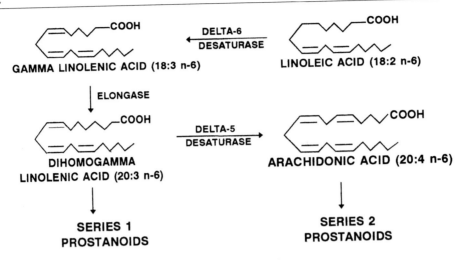

Fig. 1. GLA metabolism.

dependent manner, in plasma and cellular phospholipids (PLs), and, being less readily released upon cell stimulation, reduce substrate availability for eicosanoid generation. In addition, the n-3 PUFAs reduce the production of the 2-series eicosanoids, generated by AA metabolism, which are all proinflammatory, such as leukotriene B4 (LTB[4]), the most potent chemotactic agent, which is responsible for neutrophil recruitment (2), as well as thromboxane A2 (TXA2), which is deeply involved in the inflammatory process by increasing vascular permeability, promoting platelet aggregations, and causing edema (3); n-3 PUFAs serve as a precursor to a class of eicosanoids without inflammatory properties, such as LTB(5) (4). It has also been widely demonstrated that n-3 FAs, such as EPA and DHA, are able to inhibit inflammatory cytokine production (5). Cytokines belong to a class of soluble proteins that influence the immune cell system, resulting in enhancement of production of chronic inflammatory substances, such as interleukin-1 β (IL-1β), IL-2, and IL–6, and tumor necrosis factor (TNF) (6,7). n-3 PUFAs may also be acting as free-radical scavengers (8).

In the same way, γ-linolenic acid (GLA), an n-6 PUFA found in substantial amounts in plants, seems to have anti-inflammatory properties. Its presence in serum and tissue PLs generally results from the metabolic conversion of linoleic acid (LA). The formation of GLA occurs by the action of δ-6-desaturase. This step is considered to be rate-limiting in humans, with only a small proportion of dietary LA being converted to GLA, and further elongated to dihomo-γ-linolenic acid (DGLA) and AA (Fig. 1). Dietary GLA is rapidly converted to DGLA. DGLA may be converted to AA, the substrate for the 2-series of eicosanoids, or may be metabolized to the 1-series eicosanoids, such as prostaglandin E-1 (PGE-1), an eicosanoid with anti-inflammatory and immunoregulating properties that include suppression of diverse T-lymphocyte functions, such as proliferation, cyto-toxicity, and IL-2 production. PGE-1 also suppresses polymorphonuclear leukocyte and monocyte activation (9). Dietary enrichment with GLA and DGLA produces an increase of PGE-1. Different studies in animals have shown the ability of GLA and DGLA to block the inflammatory process, either acute or chronic, mostly by reducing the production of PGE-2 and LTB(4), and suppressing the production of IL-1 and IL2 (10,11). Moreover, DGLA competes with AA for the utilization of the enzymes of the cyclo-oxygenase

(COX) cascade, and also is converted via the anti-inflammatory 15-lipoxygenase, which is known to inhibit the activity of the proinflammatory 5-lipoxygenase *(12)*.

This chapter briefly reviews the literature concerning the use of PUFAs in the treatment of ADs, such as ulcerative colitis, Crohn's disease, psoriasis, immunoglobulin A (IgA) nephropathy, and rheumatoid arthritis (RhA), and to provide recommendations concerning their use.

2. RHEUMATOID ARTHRITIS

2.1. n-6 Trials

RhA is a chronic systemic inflammatory disorder characterized by symmetrical polyarthritis, which affects women 3× more often than men; there is an increase of incidence with age.

Belch et al. *(13)* tested, in a double-blind, placebo-controlled trial, the effectiveness of GLA alone (540 mg/d) or in association with EPA (240 mg/d plus GLA 450 mg/d), in a group of 49 RhA patients on stable nonsteroid, antiinflammatory-drug (NSAIDs) doses, that was tapered throughout the 12-mo study. The results were quite promising, since 73% of patients in GLA alone and 80% in the GLA/EPA arm were able to reduce/stop the NSAIDs intake, compared with 33% in the placebo group *(13)*.

Different results were obtained by Brzeski et al. *(14)*, who treated 40 RhA patients with upper gastrointestinal (GI) side effects caused by chronic consumption of NSAIDs, with GLA 540 mg/d or olive oil as placebo, for 6 mo. Although the patients treated had more severe RhA, the study failed to show NSAID-sparing effects (23% in the GLA group and 18% in olive oil group) *(14)*. It is now well known that olive oil should not be considered a placebo, because there is evidence that it has free-radical scavenger properties, and can inhibit cytokine and eicosanoids synthesis *(15–18)*. Leventhal et al. *(19)* treated 36 RhA patients with stable disease under either NSAID or low dose of steroids with 1.4 g GLA, or with placebo (cotton seed oil), for 24 wk. Treatment with GLA resulted in clinically important reductions of signs and symptoms of disease activity with a beneficial overall clinical response, compared with placebo ($p < 0.05$). No significant changes were observed in acute-phase protein measurements in both groups.

An increased dosage of GLA (2.4 g/d) as free fatty acids (FFAs), was tested either for clinical effects or side effects, in a subsequent double-blind, controlled study in 56 active RhA patients, for 6 mo, then for another 6 mo in a single-blind manner, during which all patients received GLA. Statistically significant improvement and clinical benefits on signs and symptoms was obtained, with also overall meaningful responses (at least 25% improvement in four measures) in the GLA group, compared with placebo. During the second 6 mo, both groups improved, and, in the active group, 16/21 patients showed meaningful improvement at 12 mo. No major side effects were reported, and compliance seemed not to be a problem *(20)*.

It should be emphasized that such high dosage of GLA, i.e., 2.4 g/d, translated into a daily intake of evening primrose oil of 24 g/d, because the GLA content is only 10%. This could affect patients' compliance. One could also speculate that some of the possible benefits of the remaining 90% of FAs in the daily dosage, i.e., n-9 FAs, may also have interfered with the cytokine network, by reducing the production of proinflammatory cytokines *(16)*. It should also be noted that few adverse effects of GLA administration have been observed, such as stool softening, belching, or abdominal bloating.

Other potential problems arising from such a high level of long-chain FA intake are lipid peroxidation and the subsequent need for more antioxidant intake, such as vitamin E, which seem highly suggested. Moreover, the high level of GLA ingested may lead to an unexpected increased accumulation of AA, then of proinflammatory mediators: It has been shown that GLA/DGLA enhances the production of IL-1 from stimulated human monocytes *(21)*.

2.2. n-3 Trials

Few controlled studies were performed in RhA patients with n-3 PUFA supplementation. The overall impression from all these studies seems to indicate good clinical improvement, without impressive modifications in acute-phase proteins. A significant, clinically relevant decrease of NSAID need is demonstrated in many studies.

A meta-analysis, which combined 10 controlled studies involving 395 patients, showed a significant improvement of two important clinical parameters: tender joints and morning stiffness *(22)*. A case–control study in women, by Shapiro et al. *(23)*, comparing 324 incident RhAs with 1245 controls, demonstrated that the consumption of broiled or baked fish was associated with decreased risk of RhA. A Danish, prospective, single-blind study *(24)*, in 109 patients with active RhA, showed, at baseline, that the food habits of RhA patients were very poor in n-3 PUFA intake.

Lau et al. *(25)* treated 64 active RhA patients for 1 yr with 10 g triglyceride with n-3 mixture, and examined the need for NSAIDs. The patients were able to decrease their NSAID need to 50%, compared with placebo, without experiencing any deterioration in clinical and laboratory parameters of RhA activity. This study should be mentioned also for the choice of air-filled placebo capsules, which is a true placebo.

Geunsens et al. *(26)*, in a long-term study (1 yr), supplemented 90 RhA patients with active disease with 2.6 g n-3 PUFA, and was able to demonstrate a significant amelioration of clinical parameters, along with a significant reduction of NSAIDs and/or antirheumatic drugs. Kremer et al. *(27)*, in a similar long-term study, confirmed the n-3 PUFA-sparing effect on NSAIDs (41% of the original dose), by giving 130 mg/kg/d n-3 PUFAs. They also documented the ability of n-3 PUFAs to decrease the serum levels of IL-1β ($p = 0.026$).

In the same way, Faarvang et al. *(28)* were able to demonstrate a small but significant improvement in morning stiffness and joint tenderness, and decreased level of C-reactive protein, by giving 3.6 g n-3 PUFAs, in 51 active RhA patients. Several studies have shown the clinical benefits related to the ingestion of n-3 PUFAs in patients with active RhA. The optimum dosage and the duration of the treatment has still to be determined; higher doses are better associated with clinical improvement *(29)*.

3. PSORIASIS

3.1. n-3 Trials

Psoriasis is a chronic inflammatory disorder of the skin, in which lesions, often infiltrated, scaly, and erythematous, are histologically characterized by hyperplasia, and leucocyte infiltration of dermis and epidermis. As in other autoimmune, chronic inflammatory disorders, it has been demonstrated that there is an increased production of the AA metabolites, such as prostanoids and LTs. For counteracting this overproduction, n-3 PUFA supplementation has been tested in many clinical studies.

Ziboh et al. *(30)*, in an open study, treated 18 patients with stable vulgaris psoriasis, by giving 18 g n-3 PUFAs daily for 2 mo, and obtained mild to moderate improvement in the lesion parameters in 60% of patients. Maurice et al. *(31)* treated 10 psoriasis patients, resistant to conventional topical treatments, with 12 g/d EPA for 6 wk. A significant reduction of LTB(4) production was obtained, but only a mild clinical improvement was demonstrated. Bittiner et al. *(32)*, in the first controlled study against placebo, treated 28 stable, chronic psoriasis patients with 1.8 g/d EPA for 2 mo, with a significant improvement in all patients, compared with placebo.

On the contrary, Soyland et al. *(33)*, in a placebo-controlled, double-blind, multicenter study involving 145 patients with moderate to severe psoriasis, treated with 5 g/d n-3 or n-6 corn oil as placebo, and did not show significant differences between the two regimens. In the corn oil group, there was a significant reduction in some clinical signs of disease. Among the patients taking n-3 PUFAs, it was not possible to correlate the increase concentration of n-3 PUFAs in plasma with clinical improvement; in the corn oil group, the improvement mentioned above was related to an inexplicable increased level in the serum of n-3 PUFAs. These findings are difficult to understand, and, at the same time, many doubts arise from the choice of corn oil as a placebo *(34)*.

Despite this study, some other reports have confirmed the clinical effectiveness of n-3 PUFAs in the treatment of psoriasis *(35–37)*. Two studies administered n-3 PUFAs topically, one by Escobar et al. *(38)*, with positive results, and one by Henneicke-von Zepelin et al. *(39)*, with negative results.

Gupta et al. *(40)* found positive benefits by using n-3 PUFA with UVB, suggesting a synergistic mechanism of action.

3.2. n-6 Trials

Very few data are available on GLA treatment, and, in all these trials, GLA was associated with n-3 PUFAs. In 1989, Kragballe *(41)* treated, in an open manner, 17 psoriatic patients with a mixture of linoleic n-3 PUFA and GLA for 4 mo, with clinical improvement in 14/17 patients. Oliwiecki and Burton *(42)*, in 1994, treated 37 stable psoriasis patients with a combination of n-3 marine oil and n-6 evening primerose oil, in a double-blind parallel trial, without finding significant improvement in clinical severity of the disease.

4. CHRONIC GLOMERULAR DISEASE

4.1. (IgA nephropathy): n-3 Trials

The AA pathway and the eicosanoid products are deeply involved in renal pathophysiologic states. Recent investigations have focused on the role of platelets and neutrophils, which, by enhancing COX expression, significantly affect AA metabolism, and consequently increase renal inflammation. A variety of studies on animals have underlined the importance of PUFAs in modulating the chronic inflammatory responses. More recently, an outstanding study by Donadio et al. *(43)* has highlighted the clinical benefits on n-3 PUFAs in the most common primary glomerulonephritis; IgA nephropathy, which is characterized by a mesangial deposit of IgA, and by a chronic and progressive evolution toward chronic renal insufficiency.

Besides the well-known modes of action of n-3 PUFAs that counteract the chronic inflammatory condition related to eicosanoids and cytokine production, in this particular disease, a specific and positive effect has been claimed: It is suggested that n-3 PUFAs increase red blood cell (RBC) deformability and flexibility *(44)*, which results in improved kidney vascularization and a reduction of proteinuria, perhaps the worst symptom in this chronic inflammatory pathology of the kidney. De Caterina et al. *(45)* showed, first in humans, that dietary supplementation with n-3 PUFAs reduced proteinuria; in 10 patients with chronic glomerular disease, after 6 wk of treatment, it was possible to show a reduction of proteinuria.

Hamazaki et al., in 1984, *(46)*, claimed positive results by using EPA in a small number of IgA nephropathy patients. Two other consecutive small studies, one by Bennet et al. *(47)* and another by Petterson et al. *(48)*, did not confirm these preliminary benefits. It must be pointed out that, because of the slow progression of the disease, a long-term follow-up is mandatory to clarify the potential benefit of any kind of treatment. If the disease it too advanced, with high creatinine levels, the probability of blocking its progression is very low, and patients develop renal failure, despite therapy *(49,50)*.

To clarify the potential benefit of n-3 PUFAs on the progression of the disease, Donadio et al. *(43)* performed a large, multicenter, placebo-controlled, randomized trial involving more than 100 patients, and gave 12 g n-3 PUFAs daily for 2 yr. The primary end point was an increase of 50% or more in the serum creatine concentration at the end of the study. At the end of the study, only three patients (6%) in the fish oil group and 14 patients (33%) in the placebo group (olive oil) reached the expected elevation of serum creatine, with very high protective effect of the fish oil treatment ($p = 0.002$). Proteinuria was slightly reduced and the cumulative percentage of patients who died or had end-stage renal disease was significantly lower in the fish oil group ($p = 0.006$) *(50)*.

Moreover, in an extended observation for 2 yr more, Donadio et al. *(51)* were able to show a beneficial carryover effect in fish oil patients, who showed a reduced rate at which renal function was lost.

The choice of olive oil as the placebo is problematic. It is already well known that olive oil is not an ideal placebo, since it has been shown to have many potential beneficial effects in chronic inflammatory conditions, such as free-radical scavenger properties, blocking cytokines production, and interference with the synthesis of eicosanoids *(15–18)*. For all these reasons, in this study, the benefits of n-3 PUFAs could even have been underestimated.

At present, two more multicenter trials are ongoing in the United States, one *(52)* to test the hypothesis that alternate days of prednisone and fish oil can delay the onset of renal failure in young IgA nephropathy patients, and another *(53)* to determine if even bigger doses of n-3 PUFAs clearly influence the clinical course of the disease.

5. CROHN'S DISEASE AND ULCERATIVE COLITIS

5.1. n-3 Trials

Studies concerning the n-3 PUFA in inflammatory bowel disease (IBD), ulcerative colitis (UC), and Crohn's disease (CD) started at the end of the 1980s. Epidemiological evidence concerning the incidence of IBD in Japan has recently shown that increasing incidence of CD was strongly correlated with, among others, the ratio of n-6 to n-3 FA intake ($r = 0.792$), as demonstrated by Shoda et al. *(54)*, indicating that increased dietary intake of n-6, with less n-3 PUFAs, may contribute to the development of CD. Moreover, multifocal GI infarctions have been suggested as one of the first pathogenic steps in IBD *(55)*, thus suggesting a pivotal role for platelets, and possibly for the powerful platelet aggregator TXA^2 *(4)*; treatment with n-3 PUFAs has been shown to decrease platelet responsiveness in patients with IBD *(56)*.

It has also been demonstrated that fish oil supplementation improves the nutritional state of rats in which a short-bowel syndrome, a clinical condition that may affect also CD patients after multiple surgical bowel resections, was induced. These results were obtained by inducing enterocyte hyperplasia, which markedly increases the mucosal surface area, with a corresponding increase in enteral absorption *(57)*. In this respect, recently it has been shown that increasing dietary polyunsaturated fat intake in IBD patients may enhance, by 65%, the absorption and the utilization of saturated fat, such as palmitic acid, improving the overall nutritional condition *(58)*.

From the clinical point of view, the first evidence of clinical benefit comes from McCall *(59)* who, in an open study, treated six patients with active UC by giving 3–4 g EPA daily (16–24 capsules of fish oil as triacylglycerol [TG]) for 12 wk, and obtained a significant improvement in symptoms and in histological appearance, along with a significant fall in LTB(4) neutrophil production.

In the 1990s, Salomon et al. *(60)*, in another open study, treated 10 UC patients who were refractory to conventional treatment (steroids and salicylates), and obtained a significant improvement of all the activity parameters in 7/10 patients. The first prospective, controlled, and double-blind study was published by Lorenz et al. *(61)*, who treated 39 patients with IBD, of which 29 had CD, in different stages of clinical activity in a 7-mo, controlled, crossover trial. Patients were randomized to receive either 3.2 g/d n-3 PUFAs or olive oil as placebo. Conventional treatment was discontinued whenever possible; otherwise, it was minimized, and kept constant for at least 3 wk before the study, and until completion. Between the two treatments, there was a 1-mo washout period. At the end of the study, in patients with CD, the clinical activity expressed by Crohn's Disease Activity Index (CDAI) *(62)*, was unchanged by n-3 PUFA supplementation. In that study, the crossover design, with a very short washout period between the two treatments, did not allow a complete displacement of the extra n-3 PUFA from cellular membranes, and could have interfered with the final results of the studies, because it has been demonstrated that the biological effect of the n-3 PUFA, i.e., inhibition of cytokine production, lasts for more than 10 wk after the suspension of n-3 PUFA *(5)*.

Hawthorne et al. *(63)* published the first large placebo-controlled study in 1992, in which 96 UC patients in different activity stages were enrolled, and were given 4.5 g/d EPA as TG for 1 yr. The patients in the placebo group received olive oil. In patients with active disease at entry, it was possible to demonstrate a significant steroid-sparing effect, but fish oil failed to prevent clinical relapse in the group of patients enrolled in remission. Remarkably, the LTB(4) production in stimulated neutrophils was reduced by more than 50%.

Stenson et al. *(64)* carried out a randomized, double-blind, placebo-controlled, crossover study with 5.4 g n-3 as TG (18 capsules daily), or olive oil as placebo, in 24 active UC patients.

The patients received treatment for 4 mo, followed by 1 mo of washout. The study demonstrated that fish oil was able to induce a significant gain in body wt, improved significantly the histology score, and reduced by 60% the LTB(4) production in rectal dialysates. No significant steroid-sparing effect, compared to placebo, was found, and the improvement in the endoscopy score did not reach a significant level ($p = 0.06$).

Aslan and Tridafilopoulos *(65)* carried out a similar placebo-controlled crossover trial by giving 4.2 g n-3 PUFAs daily, or corn oil as placebo. Seventeen active UC patients received treatment for 3 mo, followed by 2 mo of washout. In 72% of patients, a steroid-sparing effect was seen; in 56%, the activity score of the disease improved significantly. Improvement of the histology score did not reach statistical significance.

Mate et al. *(66)* reported preliminary data on a group of 38 CD patients in clinical and laboratory remission, characterized by a CDAI < 150. The patients were separated into two groups: group A included 19 patients who were asked not to change their alimentary habits without drug; group B included 19 CD patients who received a diet with high content of fish oil (100–250 g of fish daily) for 2 yr. By the end of the study, six patients in group A and 4 in group B left the trial; among patients who ended the study, 7/13 (54%) relapsed in the placebo group and 3/15 (20%) relapsed in the fish oil group. Thus, those receiving the enriched n-3 PUFA diet seem to have prolonged remission.

More recently, Loeschke et al. *(67)* presented data on a placebo-controlled trial in the prevention of UC relapse. Sixty-four patients in remission were randomized to receive 5.1 g n-3 PUFAs as ethyl-esters or maize oil as placebo for 2 yr. The ongoing treatment with 5-aminosalicylic acid was allowed for 3 mo. After 3 mo of study, the fish oil group had much fewer relapses than the placebo group ($p < 0.02$), but this beneficial effect was lost by the end of the study (2 yr). One can speculate that perhaps fish oil and 5-aminosalicylic acid may have synergetic effects, and also that patient compliance in the fish oil group decreased during the study, and could have affected the clinical outcome.

Lorenz-Meyer et al. *(68)* published data from a large, placebo-controlled trial in 204 CD patients. Patients were included after an acute relapse of their disease, in which remission (CDAI < 150) was obtained under steroid therapy. Patients were randomized to receive either n-3 PUFAs ($n = 70$) (5.1 g/d fish oil as ethyl-esters) or a carbohydrate-reduced diet (72 g/d) ($n = 69$) or placebo (corn oil) ($n = 65$) for 1 yr. Low-dose prednisolone was given to all patients for the first 8 wk of the trial, then discontinued. On an intent-to-treat analysis, none of the treatments were able to prevent clinical flare-up, but the diet poor in carbohydrates, although containing the highest numbers of dropouts (20/69 [35%]), seemed to be effective ($p < 0.05$).

The characteristics of CD population of this study represents a big challenge for gastroenterologists: It is well known that CD patients, treated with steroids for an acute flare-up of the disease, have more than a 60% possibility to relapse in the subsequent 6-mo period after the steroid suspension *(69)*, and that, quite often, these patients become steroid-dependent. Because of the strong side effects of steroids in long-term treatment, most of these patients are shifted to an immunosuppressant treatment, which is the most potent class of drugs available for treating CD.

Some criticisms can be raised on the choice of placebos. In many of these studies, the placebo was olive oil. As mentioned previously, olive oil *(15–18)* may have interfered with the final end point of these trials. Even the used corn oil as a placebo is problematic. Corn oil is a rich source of LA, an essential n-6 PUFA, which is desaturated and elongated to DGLA, a precursor of the 1-series of prostanoids, which have been claimed to have anti-inflammatory properties in many chronic inflammatory disorders *(8)*. The crossover design of most of these studies, with a short washout period between the two treatments, may not allow for complete displacement of the extra n-3-PUFAs from the membrane, and could have interfered with the final results of the studies *(5)*.

Moreover, in many of the studies in which high doses of fish oil have been used, poor patient compliance was registered *(70–72)*. This was induced by poor palatability, and by minor but annoying side effects, such as halitosis, belching, and diarrhea, related to the high daily intake of fish oil preparations necessary for obtaining a satisfactory intestinal absorption and incorporation of n-3 PUFAs into membranes. Moreover, two recent studies have compared the intestinal absorption of three different chemical formulations of fish oil as the TG, ester, or FFA, showing that the absorption of the dose administered was, respectively, 60, 20, or 95%. The better absorption of the FFA formulation may result from its ability to cross the intestinal wall without necessitating the breakdown by lipases, the availability of which could be a limiting factor in the absorption of the other chemical forms *(73,74)*. More recently, it has been shown that even the in vitro lipase-mediated clearance from plasma of the n-3 PUFA emulsions is reduced, in percentage, compared to other long-chain triglyceride emulsions, i.e., soy oil, allowing for much less FFA availability *(75)*.

For all these reasons, in a group of patients with CD, the authors investigated the ability of a new fish oil derivative to modify the PL FA profile in plasma and in RBCs by means of its FA absorption and incorporation *(76)*. This new fish oil formulation had two chief characteristics: It was a FFA mixture of 45% EPA and 20% DHA; and it was coated in three different manners, to minimize the fish-oil side effects. The pills were coated with a special gastroresistant coating, to avoid breaking the capsules in the stomach, and to obtain the delivery of the n-3 PUFAs to the first part of the small intestine. Other control groups of patients were also included: One consumed the new n-3 PUFAs mixture uncoated, and another group was administered a traditional fish oil TG preparation (18% EPA and 10% DHA).

In this study, the authors' chief purpose was to find a product capable of satisfying two main criteria: high incorporation in the PL-membrane, and high tolerability and acceptance by the patients. These two criteria are necessary in order to carry out a long-term controlled trial to test the clinical efficacy of fish oil in patients with IBD. Fifty patients suffering from CD, who were in clinical remission, in accordance to CDAI, were randomized into five groups, and supplemented with four different capsules of this new n-3 PUFAs preparation: uncoated; coated pH 5.5-dependent; coated pH 5.5-/time 60 min-dependent; coated pH 6.9-dependent; and TG fish oil preparation (EPA 18% and DHA 10%). The most effective treatment was the new n-3 PUFA preparation with a pH and time-dependent coating, group C, which showed the best incorporation of the n-3 FAs in the plasma and in the RBC membranes.

Data showed that the FFA mixture seems to be much better absorbed, compared to the traditional TG mixture, and the double mechanism of release allows the best absorption and incorporation. The capsules with the pH 6.9-dependent coating had very poor results. Actually, in this group, 7 patients registered increased bowel motions per day, probably caused by the breakdown of the pills in the lower part of the GI, inducing a cathartic effect. The variability of the intestinal motility can remarkably modify the time of transit of the capsules in the GI tract, and the complete disintegration of the coating, causing the n-3 PUFA delivery to be lower than theoretically supposed.

In contrast, the uncoated new n-3 PUFA preparation delivered its contents in the upper part of the GI tract (stomach–duodenum), and the chief side effect registered in this group was belching. No diarrhea was observed. The triglycerol mixture gave both kinds of side effects, upper (seven patients) and lower (two patients), suggesting poor tolerability.

The authors then investigated the possible beneficial effects of this new n-3 PUFA preparation in the maintenance of remission in patients with CD (77). In the authors' outpatient clinic, patients followed, with a well-established diagnosis of CD in clinical remission, were evaluated for eligibility for this study according to the following criteria: CDAI < 150 for at least 3 mo, but less than 2 yr; at least one of the following: serum α-1 acid glycoprotein > 130 mg/dL (1.3 g/L, reference range < 120 mg/dL), serum α_2-globulin > 0.9 g/dL (9 g/L, reference range < 0.8 g/dL), erythrocyte sedimentation rate > 40 mm/h (reference range < 20 mm/h); no treatment with 5-aminosalicylates, sulfasalazine, or corticosteroids in the previous 3 mo, or with immunosuppressive therapy in the previous 6 mo; in patients with previous resections, documentation of clinical and endoscopic or radiological recurrence, with subsequent remission, after surgery; no previous bowel resection >1 m; and age 18–75 yr.

Seventy-eight patients were enrolled in the 1-yr study. The patients were randomly assigned to receive either three enteric-coated capsules of fish oil 3/d or three enteric-coated capsules of identical appearance containing 500 mg placebo 3/d (the placebo contained a mixed-acid triglyceride of fractionated FAs: 60% caprylic acid and 40% capric acid). The fish oil capsules used contained 500 mg of a new marine lipid concentrate in FFA form (40% EPA and 20% DHA), resulting in daily doses of 1.8 g EPA and 0.9 g DHA. The capsules were specially coated to resist gastric acid for at least 30 min, and to disintegrate within 60 min, thus possibly allowing release of fish oil into the small intestine. There was no difference in odor between fish oil and placebo preparations, if the capsules were not broken. All participants were examined by two physicians on entry to the study, and at 3, 6, 9, and 12 mo, or before, if symptoms worsened. Relapse was defined as an increase in CDAI of at least 100 points over the baseline value, and a score above 150 for more than 2 wk. Compliance was assessed by pill count. At each visit, routine laboratory tests, including blood count, erythrocyte sedimentation rate, serum creatinine, α_1-acid glycoprotein, α_2-globulins, and liver function tests, were performed. Before and at the end of the study, 2 mL packed RBCs were obtained for the determination of the FA PL profile of the cells by gas chromatography.

After 1 yr, in the fish oil group (39 patients), one patient withdrew (moved away), four dropped out because of diarrhea, and 11 relapsed. In the placebo group (39 patients), one patient withdrew (moved away), one dropped out because of diarrhea, and 27 relapsed (intent-to-treat analysis: relapse rate 41% in fish oil group vs 74% in placebo group, difference 33%, 95% confidence interval (CI), 13–54, $p = 0.003$). In the five patients with diarrhea, this began within the first month of treatment, and did not improve when the daily intake of capsules was reduced. There were no other side effects. After 1 yr of treatment, 59% of the patients in the fish oil were still in remission, compared with only 26% in the placebo group ($p = 0.006$) (Fig. 2). Multivariate logistic regression analysis indicated that only fish oil treatment reduced the likelihood of relapse (odds ratio 4.2; 95% CI, 1.6–10.7).

Regarding the laboratory variables of inflammation, there was significant decrease in all these tests in the fish oil group, compared with the placebo group at the end of the study (Table 1).

The analysis of the chief FAs in RBCs in the patients still in remission at the end of the study, indicated incorporation of n-3 FAs in the PL membranes of fish oil patients, almost completely displacing AA.

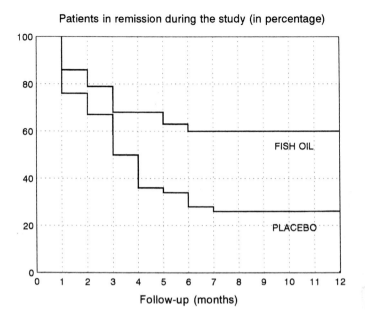

Fig. 2. Life table analysis: percentage of all randomized patients (39/group) remaining in clinical remission in an intent-to-treat analysis. Adapted with permission from ref. 77.

Table 1
Changes of Laboratory Tests During the Trial

		Placebo *n = 39*	*Fish oil* *n = 39*
Erythrocyte-sedimentation rate (mm/h)	Baseline	35 ± 4	36 ± 4
	End of study	42 ± 4.6	28 ± 3.5
	Change	$+ 14 (2,26)$	$-20 (-34,-6)^{a}$
α_2-globulins (g/dL)	Baseline	0.92 ± 0.02	0.96 ± 0.03
	End of study	1.05 ± 0.04	0.85 ± 0.02
	Change	$+ 15 (3,27)$	$-9 (-18,0)^{a}$
α_1-glycoprotein (mg/dL)	Baseline	137 ± 8.7	136 ± 8.5
	End of study	159 ± 10	130 ± 9.4
	Change	$+ 17 (10,24)$	$-4 (2,-10)^{b}$

Values are means $\pm$ SE; changes are % (95% CI). Erythrocyte sedimentation rate (reference range < 20 mm/h); α_2-globulins (reference range < 0.8 g/dL; α_1-glycoprotein (reference range < 120 mg/dL). Mann-Whitney U-test for changes in placebo vs fish oil: [a]p < 0.001; [b]p = 0.02. Adapted with permission from ref. 77.

In the authors' study, patients receiving the fish oil formula had significantly fewer relapses than the patients receiving placebo. Patients were in clinical remission for less than 24 mo before the study, and all had some laboratory evidence of inflammation. Patients of this type have about a 75% greater risk of relapse, compared to patients who are in remission longer and have normal laboratory tests (78). Ten percent of the patients in the fish oil group dropped out because of diarrhea. This may have resulted from the delivery of the capsules' contents into the distal part of the gut. Results indicate that this new fish oil preparation is an effective, well-tolerated, safe treatment for preventing clinical relapses in patients with CD in remission.

A controlled trial should be carried out, which compares directly the effectiveness of this new fish oil preparation with the 5-aminosalicylic acid, which is currently the first choice of treatment in maintenance of remission in CD patients.

Because CD patients frequently require surgery for complications such as strictures, fistulas, and abscesses, the authors recently carried out a new placebo-controlled trial in CD patients who underwent surgical gut resection. The percentage of patients whose ileal region is involved, having undergone surgery within 10 yr after the first symptoms appeared, reaches 86% (79). Unfortunately, resection does not offer cure, and 73–93% of cases show reappearance of new lesions, well documented by endoscopy within 1 yr after surgery, and in 34–86%, subsequent clinical relapse occurs within 3 yr (80,81). However, a recent study (82) seems to minimize this risk, demonstrating that the post-operative endoscopic/radiological recurrences occur later than previously reported, and, furthermore, that many of these patients, especially those with minimal disease, will remain asymptomatic. In a 1-yr, double-blind, placebo-controlled study, 50 patients were treated with nine capsules of this new n-3 preparation, containing a total of 2.7 g FFAs ($n = 26$) or nine placebo capsules ($n = 24$), within 1 mo of ileal resection (83). After 12 mo of treatment, severity of endoscopic lesions was recorded with a five-point score, as suggested by Rutgeerts et al. (84); when it was not possible to reach the anastomosis by endoscopy, a barium enema was performed. The results showed seven clinical relapses (two in the n-3 FAs group) and eight dropouts (four in the n-3 FAs group). After 12 mo, the rate of severe endoscopic recurrences (score 3–4) was 25% (4/16) in the n-3 FAs group vs 53% (8/15) in the placebo group (χ-square 2.6; $p = $ ns); the overall rate of severe recurrence (score 3–4 on endoscopy or radiological documentation) on per-protocol analysis was 23% (5/22) in the n-3 FAs group vs 55% (11/20) in the placebo group (χ-square 4.6; $p = 0.03$ difference 32:95% CI, 7–57) and, on intent-to-treat analysis, was 34% (9/26) in n-3 FAs group vs 62% (15/24) in the placebo group (χ-square 3.8; $p = 0.04$ difference 28%, 95% CI, 2–54). Logistic-regression analysis indicated that, among sex, age, previous surgery, duration of disease, and smoking status, only the n-3 FAs preparation decreased the likelihood of relapse (χ-square 3.75; $p = 0.05$). This novel enteric-coated n-3 FAs preparation seems to be effective in reducing the recurrence after curative surgery for ileal CD, and it is worthy of further, larger studies.

Some UC patients experience persistent symptoms caused by active chronic inflammation, which is resistant to treatment. Chronicity is defined as low-grade symptoms or symptom controlled with low doses of corticosteroids. Immunosuppressants are now the only alternative to long-term steroid therapy. In an open, uncontrolled study, the authors investigated the efficacy of the n-3 preparation in a group of UC steroid-dependent patients (85). Ten patients with chronic active steroid-dependent UC, with a sigmoidoscopic appearance of grade 0–1 and an ongoing treatment of 16 mg prednisolone orally, received nine capsules of this n-3 preparation, containing a total of 2.7 g n-3 FAs, for a period of at least 12 mo (from 12 mo to 24 mo). Steroids were then tapered off by 4 mg every 2 wk, until fully withdrawn over a period of 2 mo. Patients were evaluated clinically and endoscopically every 3 mo, or before, if they became worse. In six patients (6/10; 60%), it was possible to stop steroids without changes in the activity of the disease, one patient was lost to follow-up, one patient stopped the treatment because of cutaneous eruption, and two patients experienced worsening of the disease activity during steroid tapering. This small, uncontrolled experience seems to indicate the possible usefulness of n-3 FAs in steroid-dependent UC, and it is also worthy of further studies.

5.2. n-6 Trials

Only one placebo-controlled study has been performed in UC using GLA. Greenfield et al. *(86)* tested the effectiveness of evening primrose oil, rich in GLA and LA, compared to n-3 or olive oil, in 43 patients with UC in different phases of activity, in addition to their normal treatment. After 6 mo, no beneficial effects were shown, except for an increased stool consistency in the group of patients taking evening primrose oil.

CONCLUSIONS AND RECOMMENDATIONS

Until a few year ago, the n-3 and n-6 PUFAs were considered a nutrition supplement to add to the common drugs' therapy, and few studies were performed, because these FAs were not considered a treatment able, by themselves to obtain clinical benefits. For these reasons, it is currently impossible to draw definitive conclusions on the effectiveness of these substances, and to know what their exact therapeutic role is in the treatment of AD. Recently, clear-cut studies have demonstrated that these FAs may work even better than conventional treatment, especially in the long-term. Now studies are needed in which the current available gold standard regimens are compared to the PUFAs, to obtain clear answers on their clinical effectiveness and for knowing when and how to use them.

Another import question that should be addressed is whether n-3 PUFAs are better than n-6 PUFAs, or, more likely, whether they could be used together, possibly sharing synergetic mechanisms of action.

This review of the literature, concerning the therapeutic use of n-3 and n-6 PUFAs in the ADs discussed, indicates results that are not totally consistent. The reasons for the discrepancies could reside in the different study designs, different treatment regimes, and in the various formulations and dosages used, which could actually lead to results that are difficult to explain. The importance of the formulation in lowering the incidence of side effects, along with a careful selection of patients and experimental design, seems to enhance the therapeutic potential of these lipids in the treatment of AD. It is possible that these FAs act by reducing low-grade active inflammation, rather than by preventing reinitiation of the inflammatory process from a quiescent state. Whether this treatment is applicable to all AD patients has not been fully elucidated. Nevertheless, taken together, all these studies suggest the effectiveness of these new therapeutic approaches, not only when the conventional treatment fails, or when it is not possible to treat chronically, but also, in some instances as first choice. Recommendations follow:

1. RhA. Consistent evidences prove the beneficial effects of n-6 and n-3 PUFAs supplementation in lowering the need of NSAIDs and improving clinical symptoms, mainly in the long term treatment.
2. Psoriasis. The data published, which is very little, is less convincing about a clear benefit of n-3 PUFA supplementation, even if some improvement in symptoms are suggested. No data are available on n-6 PUFAs.
3. IgA nephropathy. Strong evidence supports the positive effects of long term supplementation of n-3 PUFAs as a therapeutic tool for delaying the onset of renal failure. No data are available on n-6 PUFAs.
4. CD. n-3 PUFA supplementation seems to represent an effective regimen for treating patients with low-grade activity, and for keeping the disease in remission. No data on n-6 are available.

5. UC. The best results were obtained in the treatment of chronically active patients, in whom a significant steroid sparing affect has been shown. Again, no data on n-6 are available.

REFERENCES

1. Lauritsen K, Laursen LS, Bukhave K, RaskMadsen J. Inflammatory intermediaries in inflammatory bowel disease. Int J Colorect Dis 1989; 4:75–90.
2. Ford-Hutchinson AW, Leukotriene B. A potent chemokinetic and aggregating substance released from polymorphonuclear leukocytes. Nature 1980; 286:264.
3. Rampton DS, Collins CE. Review article: thromboxanes in inflammatory bowel disease: pathogenic and therapeutic implications. Aliment Pharm Ther 1993; 7:357–367.
4. Lee TH, Hoover RL, Williams D, Sperling RI, Ravalese J 3d, Spur BW, et al. Effect of a dietary enrichment with eicosapentaenoic acid and docosahexaenoic acids on in vitro polymorphonuclear and monocyte leukotriene generation and polymorphonuclear leukocyte function. N Engl J Med 1985; 312:1217–1224.
5. Endres S, Ghorbani R, Kelly VE, Georgilis K, Lonnemann G, van der Meer JW, et al. The effect of dietary supplementation with n-3 fatty acids on the synthesis of interleukin-1 and tumor necrosis factor by mononuclear cells. N Engl J Med 1989; 320:265–270.
6. Calder PC. N-3 polyunsaturated fatty acids and cytokine production in health and disease. Ann Nutr Metab 1997; 41:203–234.
7. Endres S, von Schacky C. N-3 polyunsaturated fatty acids and human cytokine synthesis. Curr Opin Lipidol 1996; 7:48–52.
8. Payan DG, Wong MYS, Chernov-Rogan T, Valone FH, Pickett WC, Blake VA, Gold WM, Goetzl EJ. Alterations in human leukocyte function induced by ingestion of eicosapenatenoic acid. J Clin Immunol 1986; 6:402–410.
9. Horrobin DF. The regulation of prostaglandin biosynthesis by the manipulation of essential fatty acid metabolism. Rev Pure Appl Pharmacol Sci 1983; 4:339–432.
10. Baker DG, Krakauer KA, Tate GA, Laposata M, Zurier RB. Suppression of human synovial cell proliferation by dihomo-y-linolenic acid. Arthritis Rheum 1989; 32:1273–1281.
11. Santoli D, Phillips PD, Colt TL, Zurier RB. Suppression of interleukin 2 dependent human T cell growth by E-series prostaglandins (PGE) and their precursor fatty acids: evidence for a PGE-independent mechanism of inhibition by the fatty acids. J Clin Invest 1990; 35:424–432.
12. Ziboh VA, Chapikin RS. Biologic significance of polyunsaturated fatty acids in the skin. Arch Dermatol 1987; 123:1686–1690.
13. Belch JJ, Ansell D, Madhok R, O'Dowd A, Sturrock RD. Effects of altering dietary essential fatty acids on requirements for non-steroidal anti-inflammatory drugs in patients with rheumatoid arthritis: a double blind placebo controlled study. Ann Rheum Dis 1988; 47:96–104.
14. Brzeski M, Madhok R, Capell HA. Evening primrose oil in patients with rheumatoid arthritis and side-effects of non-steroidal antiinflammatory drugs. Br J Rheumatol 1991; 30:370–372.
15. Budiarso IT. Fish oil versus olive oil. Lancet 1990; 336:1313–1314.
16. Grimble RF. Interaction between nutrient, proinflammatory cytokines and inflammation. Clin Sci 1996; 91:121–129.
17. Petroni A, Blasevich M, Salami M, Papini N, Montedoro GF, Galli C. Inhibition of platelet aggregation and eicosanoids production by phenolic components of olive oil. Thromb Res 1995, 78:151–160.
18. Petroni A, Blasevich M, Papini N, Salami M, Sala A, Galli C. Inhibition of leukocyte leukotriene-B4 production by an olive oil-derived phenol identified by mass-spectrometry. Thromb Res 1997; 87: 315–322.
19. Leventhal LJ, Boyce EG, Zurier RB. Treatment of rheumatoid arthritis with gammalinolenic acid. Ann Intern Med 1993; 119:867–873.
20. Zurier RB, Rossetti RG, Jacobson EJ, DeMarco DM, Liu NY, Temming JE, White BM, Laposata M. Gammalinolenic acid treatment of rheumatoid arthritis: a randomized placebo-controlled trial. Arthritis Rheum 1196; 39:1808–1817.
21. Rothman D, Allen H, Herzog L, Pilapil A, Seiler CM, Zurier RB. Effects of unsaturated fatty acids on interleukin-1beta production by human monocytes. Cytokine 1997; 9:1008–1012.
22. Fortin PR, Lew RA, Liang MH, Wright EA, Beckett LA, Chalmers TC, Sperling RI. Validation of a meta-analysis: the effects of fish oil in rheumatoid arthritis. J Clin Epidemiol 1995; 48:1379–1390.

23. Shapiro JA, Koepsell TD, Voigt LF, Dugowson CE, Kestin M, Nelson JL. Diet and rheumatoid arthritis in women: a possible protective effect of fish consumption. Epidemiology 1996; 7:256–263.

24. Hansen GV, Nielsen L, Kluger E, Thysen M, Emmerstsen H, Stengaard-Pedersen K, et al. Nutritional status of Danish rheumatoid patients and effects of a diet adjusted in energy intake, fish meal, and antioxidants. Scan J Rheumatol 1996; 25:325–330.

25. Lau CS, Morley KD, Belch JJ. Effects of fish oil supplementation on non-steroidal anti-inflammatory drug requirement in patients with mild rheumatoid arthritis: a double blind placebo controlled study. Br J Rheumatol 1993; 32:982–989.

26. Geusens P, Wouters C, Nijs J, Jiang Y, Dequeker J. Long-term effect of omega-3 fatty acid supplementation in active rheumatoid arthritis. A 12-month, double-blind, controlled study. Arthritis Rheum 1994; 37:824–829.

27. Kremer JM, Lawrence DA, Petrillo GF, Litts LL, Mullaly PM, Rynes RI, et al. Effects of high-dose fish oil on rheumatoid arthritis after stopping nonsteroidal anti-inflammatory drugs. Clinical and immune correlates. Arthritis Rheum 1995; 38:1107–1114.

28. Faarvang KL, Nielsen GL, Thomsen BS, Teglbjaerg KL, Lervang HH, Schmidt EB, Dyerberg J, Ernst E. Fish oils and rheumatoid arthritis. A randomized and double blind study. Ugeskr Laeger 1994; 156: 3495–3498.

29. Kremer JM, Lawrence DA, Jubiz W, DiGiacomo R, Rynes R, Bartholomew LE, Sherman M. Dietary fish oil and olive oil supplementation in patients with rheumatoid arthritis . Clinical and immunologic effects. Arthritis Rheum 1990; 33:810–820.

30. Ziboh VA, Cohen Ka, Ellis CN, Miller C, Hamilton TA, Kragballe K, Hydrick CR, Voorhees JJ. Effects of dietary supplementation of fish oil on neutrophil and epidermal fatty acids. Arch Dermatol 1986; 122:1277–1282.

31. Maurice PDL, Allen BR, Barkley ASJ, Cockbill Sr, Stammers J, Bather PC. The effect of dietary supplementation with fish oil in patients with psoriasis. Br J Dermatol 1987; 117:599–606.

32. Bittiner SB, Cartwright I, Tucker WFG, Bleehen SS. A double-blind randomized placebo-controlled trial of fish oil in psoriasis. Lancet 1988; 1:378–380.

33. Soyland E, Funk J, Rajka G, Sandberg M, Thune P, Rustad L, et al. Effect of dietary supplementation with very long chain n-3 fatty acids in patients with psoriasis. N Engl J Med 1993; 328:1812–1816.

34. Kremer JM. Effects of modulation of inflammatory and immune parameters with rheumatic and inflammatory disease receiving dietary supplementation of n-3 and n-6 fatty acids. Lipids 1996; 31: S-243–S-247.

35. Lassus A, Dahlgren AL, Halpern MJ, Santalahti J, Happonen HP. Effects of dietary supplementation with polyunsaturated ethyl ester lipids (Angiosan) in patients with psoriasis and psoriatic arthritis. J Int Med Res 1990; 18:68–73.

36. Kojima T, Terano T, Tanabe E, Okamoto S, Tamura Y, Yoshida S. Long-term administration of highly purified eicosapentaenoic acid provides improvement of psoriasis. Dermatologica 1991; 182:225–230.

37. Collier PM, Ursell A, Zaremba K, Payne CM, Staughton RC, Sanders T. Effect of regular consumption of oily fish compared with white fish on chronic plaque psoriasis. Eur J Clin Nutr 1993; 47:251–254.

38. Escobar SO, Achenbach R, Iannantuono R, Torem V. Topical fish oil in psoriasis: a controlled and blind study. Clin Exp Dermatol 1992; 17:159–162.

39. Henneicke-von Zepelin HH, Mrowietz U, Farber L, Bruck-Borchers K, Schober C, Huber J, et al. Highly purified omega-3-polyunsaturated fatty acids for topical treatment of psoriasis. Results of a double-blind, placebo-controlled multicentre study. Br J Dermatol 1993; 129:713–717.

40. Gupta AK, Ellis CN, Tellner DC, Anderson TF, Voorhees JJ. The role of fish oil in psoriasis. A randomized, double-blind, placebo-controlled study to evaluate the effect of fish oil and topical corticosteroid therapy in psoriasis. Br J Dermatol 1989; 120:801–807.

41. Kragballe K. Dietary supplementation with a combination of n-3 and n-6 fatty acids (super gamma-oil marine) improves psoriasis. Acta Derm Venereol 1989; 69:265–268.

42. Oliwiecki S, Burton JL. Evening primrose oil and marine oil in the treatment of psoriasis. Clin Exp Dermatol 1994; 19:127–129.

43. Donadio JV, Bergstralh EJ, Offord KP, Spencer DC, Holley KE. A controlled trial of fish oil in IgA nephropathy. N Engl J Med 1994; 331:1194–1199.

44. Cartwright IJ, Pockley AG, Galloway JH, Greaves M, Preston FE. The effects of dietary omega-3 polyunsaturated fatty acids on erythrocyte membrane phospholipids, erythrocyte deformability, and blood viscosity in healthy volunteers. Atherosclerosis 1985; 55:267–281.

45. De Caterina R, Caprioli R, Giannessi D, Sicari R, Galli C, Lazzerini G, et al. N-3 fatty acids reduce proteinuria in patients with chronic glomerular disease. Kidney Int 1993; 44:843–850.

46. Hamazaki T, Tateno S, Shishido H. Eicosapentaenoic acid and IgA nephropathy. Lancet 1984; 1:1017–1018.

47. Bennet WM, Walker RG, Kincaid-Smith P. Treatment of IgA nephropathy with eicosapentaenoic acid (EPA): a two year prospective trial. Clin Nephrol 1989; 31:128–131.

48. Petterson EE, Rekola S, Berglund L, Sundqvist KG, Angelin B, Diczfalusy U, Bjorkhem I, Bergstrom J. Treatment of IgA nephropathy with omega-3-polyunsaturated fatty acids: a prospective, double-blind, randomized study.

49. Cheng IKP, Chan PCK, Chan MK. The effect of fish-oil dietary supplement on the progression of mesangial IgA glomerulonephritis. Nephrol Dial Transplant 1990; 5:241–246.

50. Fung SM, Ferril MJ, Norton LL. Fish oil therapy in IgA nephropathy. Ann Pharmacother 1997; 31: 112–113.

51. Donadio JV, Dart RA, Grande JP, Bergstralh EJ, Spencer DC. Long term treatment with fish oil reduces renal progression in patients with IgA nephropathy (IgAN). J Am Soc Nephrol 1997; 8:85A.

52. Hogg RJ. A randomized, placebo controlled, multicenter trial evaluating alternate-day prednisone and fish oil supplements in young patients with IgA nephropathy. Ann Pharmacother 1995; 26:792–796.

53. Donadio JV, Bergstralh EJ, Offord KP, Grande JP, Larson TS, Spencer DC. A prospective comparative study of two doses of Omacor in the treatment of patients with IgA nephropathy. Study in Progress.

54. Shoda R, Matsueda K, Yamato S, Umeda N. Epidemiologic analysis of Crohn disease in Japan: increased dietary intake of n-6 polyunsaturated fatty acids and animal protein relates to the increased incidence of Crohn disease in Japan. Am J Clin Nutr 1996; 63:741–745.

55. Wakefield AJ, Sawyerr AM, Dhillon AP, Pittilo RM, Rowles PM, Lewis AA, Pounder RE. Pathogenesis of Crohn's disease: multifocal gastrointestinal infarction. Lancet 1989; 1:1057–1062.

56. Jaschoenek K, Clemens MR, Scheurlen M. Decreased responsiveness of platelets to a stable prostacyclin analogue in patients with Crohn's disease. Reversal by n-3 polyunsaturated fatty acids. Thromb Res 1991; 63:667–672.

57. Vanderhoof JA, Park JHY, Herrington MK, Adrian TE. Effects of dietary menhaden oil mucosal adaptation after small bowel resection in rats. Gastroenterology 1994; 106:94–99.

58. French MA, Parrot AM, Kielo ES, Rajotte RV, Wang LC, Thomson AB, Clandinin MT. Polyunsaturated fat in the diet may improve intestinal function in patients with CD. Biochim Biophys Acta 1997; 1360:262–270.

59. McCall TB, O'Leary D, Bloomfield J, et al. Therapeutic potential of fish oil in the treatment of ulcerative colitis. Aliment Pharmacol Therap 1989; 3:415–424.

60. Salomon P, Asher A. Kornbluth, Janowitz HD. Treatment of ulcerative colitis with fish oil n-3 fatty acid: an open trial. J Clin Gastroenterol 1990; 12:157–161.

61. Lorenz R, Weber PC, Szimnau P, Heldwein W, Strasser T, Loeschke K. Supplementation with n-3 fatty acids from fish oil in chronic inflammatory bowel disease- a randomized, placebo-controlled, double-blind cross-over trial. J Int Med 1989; 225(Suppl.):225–232.

62. Best WR, Becktel JM, Singleton JW, Kern F. Development of a Crohn's disease activity index. Gastroenterology 1976; 70:439–444.

63. Hawthorne AB, Daneshmend, Hawkey CJ, Belluzzi A, Everitt SJ, Holmes GK, et al. Treatment of ulcerative colitis with fish oil supplementation: a prospective 12 months randomized controlled trial. Gut 1992; 33:922–928.

64. Stenson WF, Cort D, Rodgers J, Burakoff R, DeSchryver-Kecskemeti K, Gramlich TL, Beeken W. Dietary supplementation with fish oil in ulcerative colitis. Ann Intern Med 1992; 116:609–614.

65. Aslan A, Triadafilopoulos G. Fish oil fatty acid supplementation in active ulcerative colitis: a double-blind, placebo-controlled, crossover study. Am J Gastroenterol 1992; 87:432–437.

66. Matè J, Castanos J, Garcia-Samaniego, Pajares JM. Does dietary fish oil maintain the remission of Crohn's disease (CD): a study case control . Gastroenterology 1993; 100:A-228 (Abstract).

67. Loeschke K, Ueberschaer B, Pietsch A, Gruber E, Ewe K, Wiebecke B, Heldwein W, Lorenz R. N-3 fatty acids retard early relapse in ulcerative colitis. Dig Dis Sci 1996; 41:2087–2094.

68. Lorenz-Meyer H, Bauer P, Nicolay C, Schulz B, Purrmann J, Fleig WE, et al. Omega-3 fatty acids and carbohydrate diet for maintenance of remission in Crohn's disease. Scan J Gastroenterol 1996; 31:778–785.

69. Brignola C, De Simone G, Belloli C, Iannone P, Belluzzi A, Gionchetti P, Campieri M, Barbara L. Steroid treatment in active Crohn's disease: a comparison between two regimens of different duration. Aliment Pharmacol Ther 1994; 8:465–468.

70. Appel LJ, Miller ER, Seidler AJ, Whelton PK. Does supplementation of diet with "fish oil" reduce blood pressure? A meta-analysis of controlled following coronary angioplasty. Am J Prev Med 1992; 8:186–192.

71. O'Connors GT, Malenka DJ, Olmstead EM, Johnson PS, Hennekens CH. A meta-analysis of randomized trials of fish oil in prevention of restenosis following coronary angioplasty. Am J Prev Med 1992; 8:186–192.

72. Kunzel U, Bertsch S. Klinsche erfahrungen mit einem standardiserten fischolkonzenntrat. Feldstudie mit 3.958 hyperlipamischen patienten in der praxis des niedergelassenen arztes. Fortschr Med 1990; 108:437–442.

73. El Boustani S, Colette C, Monnier L, Descomps B, Crastes de Paulet A, Mendy F. Enteral absorption in man of eicosapentaenoic acid in different chemical forms. Lipids 1987; 22:711–714.

74. Lawson LD, Hughes BG. Human absorption of fish oil fatty acids as triacylglycerols, free acids, or ethyl esters. Biochem Biophys Res Commun 1988; 152:328–335.

75. Oliveira FL, Rumsey SC, Schlotzer E, Hansen I, Carpentier YA, Deckelbaum RJ. Triglyceride hydrolysis of soy oil vs fish oil emulsions. J Parenter Enteral Nutr 1997; 21:224–229.

76. Belluzzi A, Brignola C, Campieri M, Camporesi EP, Gionchetti P, Rizzello F, et al. Effects of a new fish oil derivative on fatty acid phospholipid-membrane pattern in a group of Crohn's disease patients. Dig Dis Sci 1994; 39:2589–2594.

77. Belluzzi A, Brignola C, Campieri M, Pera A, Boschi S, Miglioli M. Effect of an enteric-coated fish oil preparation on relapses in Crohn's disease. New Engl J Med 1996; 334:1557–1616.

78. Brignola C, Iannone P, Belloli C, De Simone G, Bassein L, Gionchetti P, et al. Prediction of relapse in patients with Crohn's disease in remission: a simplified index using laboratory tests, enhanced by clinical characteristics. Eur J Gastroenterol Hepatol 1994; 6:955–961.

79. Williams JG, Wong WD, Rothenberger DA, Goldberg SM. Recurrence of Crohn's disease after resection. Br J Surg 1991; 78:10–19.

80. Basilisco G, Campanini M, Cesana B, Ranzi T, Bianchi P. Risk factors for first operation in Crohn's disease. Am J Gastroenterol 1989; 84:749–752.

81. Olaison G, Smedh K, Sjodahl R. Natural course of Crohn's disease after ileocolic resection: endoscopically visualised ileal ulcers preceding symptoms. Gut 1992; 33:331–335.

82. Mc Leod RS, Wolff BG, Steinhart AH, Carryer PW, O'Rourke K, Andrews DF, et al. Risk and significance of endoscopic/radiological evidence of recurrent Crohn's disease. Gastroenterology 1997; 113:1823–1827.

83. Belluzzi A, Brignola C, Campieri M, Belloli C, Boschi S, Cottone M, et al. A new enteric coated preparation of omega 3 fatty acids for preventing postsurgical recurrence in Crohn's disease. Gastroenterology 1997; 112:A-930.

84. Rutgeerts P, Geboes K, Vantrappen G, Beyls J, Kerremans R, Hiele M. Predictability of the postoperative course of Crohn's disease. Gastroenterology 1990; 99:956–963.

85. Belluzzi A, Campieri M, Brignola C, et al. A new enteric coated preparation of omega 3 fatty acids for preventing post-surgical recurrence in Crohn's disease. Gastroenterology 1997; 112:A-930.

86. Greenfield SM, Green AT, Teare JP, Jenkins AP, Punchard NA, Ainley CC, Thompson RP. A randomized controlled study of evening primrose oil and fish oil in ulcerative colitis. Aliment Pharmacol Ther 1993; 7:159–166.

V Bone Diseases

17 Osteoarthritis

Role of Nutrition
and Dietary Supplement Interventions

Timothy E. McAlindon

1. INTRODUCTION

1.1. Osteoarthritis

Osteoarthritis (OA) is the most common form of joint disease, and is a leading cause of disability in the elderly. The disease commonly affects the hands, spine, knees, and hips. Multiple joints may be affected in any one individual. The disorder is strongly associated with increasing age, and has been estimated to affect 2–10% of all adults *(1,2)*. It is responsible for approx 68 million work-loss d/yr, and for more than 5% of the annual retirement rate *(3)*. Furthermore, OA is the most frequent reason for joint replacement, at a cost to the community of billions of dollars per year *(4)*.

Focal cartilage damage is the central feature of OA *(5)*. This may range in severity from minor surface roughening to complete cartilage erosion. The process is generally non-inflammatory, and is often described as being degenerative, or caused by wear and tear. The cartilage damage is usually accompanied by some form of reaction in surrounding bone. Osteophytes are an early bony response to cartilage damage, and consist of out-growths of bone from the peripheral margin of the joint. They may confer some protection to an OA joint by reducing instability *(6)*. The trabeculae in the bone adjacent to an area of OA cartilage become thickened, and are susceptible to microscopic fracturing. This gives rise to the appearance of subchondral sclerosis on a radiograph. In severe disease, particularly when full-thickness cartilage has occurred, circumscribed areas of bony necrosis may develop in the subchondral bone. These may be filled with marrow fat, or with synovial fluid that has tracked from the joint space through the cartilage defect into the subchondral bone. They give rise to the radiographic appearance of cysts. Ultimately, the subchondral bone itself may be eroded, or may collapse. In some cases, a low-level synovitis develops as the result of the presence of crystal or other cartilaginous detritus, which may contribute to damage in the joint.

Biochemically, cartilage consists of a network of collagen fibrils (predominantly type II), which constrain an interlocking mesh of proteoglycans (PG) that resist compressive forces through their affinity for water. The tissue is relatively avascular and acellular. Turnover in healthy cartilage is slow, and represents a balance between collagen and PG synthesis and degradation by enzymes, such as metalloproteinases. In early OA, the

From: *Primary and Secondary Preventive Nutrition*
Edited by: A. Bendich and R. J. Deckelbaum © Humana Press Inc., Totowa, NJ

Table 1
Factors Associated with OA

Constitutional factors
    Increased age
    Female gender
    Obesity
Mechanical factors
    Heavy/repetitive occupations
    Heavy physical activity
    Major joint injury
Endocrine factors
    Hemochromatosis
Genetic factors
    Mutations in the type II collagen gene

chondrocytes (cartilage cells) proliferate and become metabolically active. These hypertrophic chondrocytes produce cytokines (e.g., interleukin [IL-1], tumor necrosis factor α [TNF-α]), degradative enzymes (e.g., metalloproteinases), and other growth factors. PG production is increased in early OA, but falls sharply at a later stage, when the chondrocyte fails.

1.1.1. Risk Factors for OA

The striking relationship of OA with increasing age and with heavy physical work has led to its characterization as a degenerative or wear-and-tear disorder (1). In fact, this paradigm is inaccurate, because a variety of mechanical, metabolic, and genetic disorders may lead to OA (7). OA may thus be regarded as a dynamic interaction between destructive and reparative processes within a joint. Established risk factors for OA are listed in Table 1.

1.2. OA and Diet

There is enormous public interest in the relationship between diet and arthritis. Questions about nutrition and supplements are among the most frequently posed by people with OA to their physicians. Speculative lay publications on this subject abound, and health food stores are full of nutritional supplements touted for their putative ability to help arthritis sufferers (8).

In contrast, there has been relatively little focus in traditional scientific studies on the relationship between nutritional factors (other than obesity) and OA. Furthermore, the traditional physician's stance on this question has been to assert the lack of evidence supporting any association between diet and OA. This gulf between the levels of interest among scientists and among the general public is surprising, given the large numbers of studies of osteoporosis, another widespread, age-related skeletal disorder, which have shown widely accepted associations with dietary factors. A more important reason to study the relationship between dietary factors and OA, however, is that there are many mechanisms by which certain micronutrients can be hypothesized to influence OA processes. Furthermore, there have been several recent studies that have shown apparent effects of various micronutrients on the natural history of this disorder.

2. MECHANISMS THROUGH WHICH MICRONUTRIENTS CAN BE HYPOTHESIZED TO INFLUENCE OA PROCESSES

2.1. Antioxidant Effects

There is considerable evidence that continuous exposure to oxidants contributes to the development or exacerbation of many of the common human diseases associated with aging *(9)*. Such oxidative damage accumulates with age, and has been implicated in the pathophysiology of cataract *(10)*, coronary artery disease *(11)*, and certain forms of cancer *(12)*. As the prototypical age-related degenerative disease, OA may also be, in part, a product of oxidative damage to articular tissues.

Reactive oxygen species are chemicals with unpaired electrons. These are formed continuously in tissues by endogenous and some exogenous mechanisms *(9)*. For example, it has been estimated that 1–2% of all electrons, which travel down the mitochondrial respiratory chain, leak, forming a superoxide anion $(O_2{}^{\bullet-})$ *(13)*. Other endogenous sources include release by phagocytes during the oxidative burst, generation by mixed-function oxidase enzymes, and in hypoxia-reperfusion events *(14)*. Reactive oxygen species are capable of causing damage to many macromolecules, including cell membranes, lipoproteins, proteins, and DNA *(15)*. Because these reactive oxygen species are identical to those generated by irradiation of H_2O, living has been likened to being continuously irradiated *(9)*.

Furthermore, there is evidence that cells within joints produce reactive oxygen species, and that oxidative damage is physiologically important *(16)*. In laboratory studies, animal and human chondrocytes have been found to be potent sources of reactive oxygen species *(16,17)*. Hydrogen peroxide production has been demonstrated in aged human chondrocytes after exposure to the proinflammatory cytokines, IL-1 and TNF-α, and has been observed in live cartilage tissue *(18)*. Superoxide anions have been shown to adversely affect collagen structure and integrity in vitro, and appear to be responsible, in vivo, for depolymerization of synovial fluid hyaluronate *(17–20)*.

In fact, the human body has extensive and multilayered antioxidant (AO) defense systems *(9)*. Intracellular defense is provided primarily by AO enzymes, including superoxide dismutase, catalase, and peroxidases. In addition to these enzymes, there are a number of small molecule AOs that play an important role, particularly in the extracellular space, where AO enzymes are sparse *(21)*. These include the micronutrients, α-tocopherol (AT) (vitamin E), β-carotene (a vitamin A precursor), other carotenoids, and ascorbate (vitamin C). The concentrations of these AOs in the blood are primarily determined by dietary intake. The concept that micronutrient AOs may provide further defense against tissue injury, when intracellular enzymes are overwhelmed, has led to the hypothesis that high dietary intake of these micronutrients may protect against age-related disorders. Because higher intake of dietary AOs appears beneficial in respect to outcomes such as cataract extraction and coronary artery disease *(10–12,22)*, it is also plausible that they may confer similar benefits for OA.

2.2. Effects on Collagen Metabolism

In addition to being an AO, vitamin C fulfills several functions in the biosynthesis of cartilage molecules. First, through the vitamin C-dependent enzyme, lysylhydroxylase, vitamin C is required for the posttranslational hydroxylation of specific prolyl and lysyl residues in procollagen, a modification essential for stabilization of the mature collagen, fibril *(10–12,22–24)*. Vitamin C also appears to stimulate collagen biosynthesis by pathways independent of hydroxylation, perhaps through lipid peroxidation *(25)*. In addition, by acting as a carrier of sulfate groups, vitamin C participates in glycosaminoglycan synthesis *(26)*. Thus, relative deficiency of vitamin C may impair not only the production of cartilage, but also its biomechanical quality.

The results of in vitro and in vivo studies are concordant with this possibility. Studies of adult bovine chondrocytes have shown that addition of ascorbate acid to the tissue culture results in decreased levels of degradative enzymes, and increased synthesis of type II collagen and PGs *(26,27)*. Peterkovsky et al. *(28)* observed decreased synthesis of cartilage collagen and PG molecules in guinea pigs deprived of vitamin C. They also reported high levels of insulin-like growth factor 1 binding proteins, which normally inhibit the anabolic effects of insulin-like growth factor 1, a potent growth factor. This suggests that vitamin C may also influence growth factors through pathways that remain to be elucidated.

2.3. Effects on Chondrocyte Metabolism

Vitamin D may have direct effects on chondrocytes in OA cartilage. During bone growth, vitamin D regulates the transition from growth plate cartilage to bone. Normally, chondrocytes in developing bone lose their vitamin D receptors, with the attainment of skeletal maturity. It has recently become apparent, however, that the hypertrophic chondrocytes in OA cartilage can redevelop vitamin D receptors *(29)*. These chondrocytes are metabolically active, and appear to play an important role in the pathophysiology of OA *(30)*. Although this evidence is indirect, it raises the possibility that vitamin D may influence the pathologic processes in OA, through effects on these cells.

2.4. Effects on Bone

Reactive changes in the bone underlying, and adjacent to, damaged cartilage are an integral part of the OA process *(31–37)*. Sclerosis of the underlying bone, trabecular microfracturing, attrition, and cyst formation are all likely to accelerate the degenerative process, as a result of adverse biomechanical changes *(38,39)*. Other phenomena, such as osteophytes (bony spurs), may be attempts to repair or stabilize the process *(6,40)*. It has also been suggested *(41)* that bone mineral density may influence the skeletal expression of the disease, with a more erosive form occurring in individuals with softer bone. Although some cross-sectional studies have suggested a modest inverse relationship between OA and osteoporosis, recent prospective studies *(42)* have suggested that individuals with lower bone mineral density are at increased risk for OA incidence and progression. The idea that the nature of bony response in OA may determine outcome has been further advanced by the recent demonstration *(43)* that patients, with bone scan abnormalities adjacent to an OA knee, have a higher rate of progression than those without such changes.

Normal bone metabolism is contingent on the presence of vitamin D, a compound that is derived largely from the diet or from cutaneous exposure to ultraviolet light. Suboptimal vitamin D levels may have adverse effects on calcium metabolism, osteoblast activity, matrix ossification, and bone density *(44,45)*. Low tissue levels of vitamin D may, therefore, impair the ability of bone to respond optimally to pathophysiological processes in OA, and predispose to disease progression.

2.5. Anti-Inflammatory Properties

Vitamin E has diverse influences on the metabolism of arachadonic acid, an anti-inflammatory fatty acid found in all cell membranes. Vitamin E blocks formation of arachidonic acid from phospholipids, and inhibits lipoxygenase activity, although it has little effect on cyclo-oxygenase *(46)*. It is, therefore, possible that vitamin E reduces the modest synovial inflammation that may accompany OA.

3. STUDIES OF EFFECTS OF NUTRIENTS IN OA

3.1. Obesity and OA

Overweight people are at considerably increased risk for the development of OA in their knees, and may also be more susceptible to both hip and hand joint involvement *(47)*. Since overweight individuals do not necessarily have increased load across their hand joints, investigators have wondered whether systemic factors, such as diet or other metabolic consequences of obesity, may mediate some of this association. Indeed, early laboratory studies, using strains of mice and rats, appeared to suggest an interaction among body wt, genetic factors, and diet, although attempts to demonstrate a direct effect of dietary fat intake proved inconclusive *(48,49)*.

3.2. The Case for Vitamin C and Other Antioxidant Micronutrients

3.2.1. ANIMAL STUDIES

OA can be induced in animals by various surgical procedures. Schwartz et al. *(50)* treated guinea pigs, prior to such surgery, with either a high (150 mg/d) or low (2.4 mg/d) dose of vitamin C. Guinea pigs treated with the higher dose of vitamin C (which would correspond to vitamin C in humans of at least 500 mg/d) showed "consistently less severe joint damage than animals on the low level of the vitamin" *(50)*. Features of OA were significantly less frequent in animals treated with the high dose of vitamin C. Similar findings were reported by Meacock et al. *(50)* in another surgically induced guinea pig model of OA. That study supplemented the feeds of half of the animals with vitamin C after the surgical procedure *(51)*. They reported, "Extra ascorbic acid appeared to have some protective effect ($p = 0.008$) on the development of spontaneous (OA) lesions..." *(51)*.

3.2.2. EPIDEMIOLOGIC STUDIES

The author investigated the association of self-reported dietary intake of AO micronutrients among participants followed longitudinally in the Framingham Knee OA Cohort Study *(52)*, a population-based group derived from the Framingham Heart Study Cohort. Participants had knee X-rays taken at a baseline examination performed during 1983–1985, and had follow-up X-rays approx 8 yr later, during 1992–1993. Knee OA was classified using the Kellgren and Lawrence grading system (ref. *34*). Knees without OA at baseline (Kellgren and Lawrence grade ≤ 1) were classified as incident OA, if they had developed grade 2 or greater changes by follow-up. Knees with OA at baseline were classified as progressive OA, if their score increased by 1 or more.

Nutrient intake, including supplement use, was calculated from dietary habits reported at the midpoint of the study, using a food frequency questionnaire. The author's analyses ranked micronutrient intake into sex-specific tertiles, and looked specifically to see if higher intakes of vitamin C, vitamin E, and β-carotene, compared with a panel of non-

AO control micronutrients, were associated with reduced incidence and reduced progression of knee OA. The lowest tertile for each dietary exposure was used as the reference category. Odds ratios (ORs) were adjusted for age, sex, body mass index, weight change, knee injury, physical activity, energy intake, and health status.

Six hundred forty participants (mean age 70.3 yr) had complete assessments. Incident and progressive knee OA occurred in 81 and 68 knees, respectively. The author found no significant association of incident radiographic knee OA with any micronutrient (e.g., adjusted OR for highest vs lowest tertile of vitamin C intake = 1.1; 95% confidence limits, 0.6–2.2). On the other hand, for progression of radiographic knee OA, the author found a threefold reduction in risk for those in the middle and highest tertiles of vitamin C intake (adjusted OR for highest vs lowest tertile = 0.3; 95% confidence limits 0.1–0.6). Those in the highest tertile for vitamin C intake also had reduced risk of developing knee pain during the course of the study (OR = 0.3; 0.1–0.8). Reduction in risk of progression was also seen for β-carotene (OR = 0.4; 0.2–0.9) and vitamin E, but was less consistent, in that the β-carotene association diminished substantially after adjustment for vitamin C, and the vitamin E effect was seen only in men (OR = 0.07; 0.01–0.6). No significant associations were observed for any of the micronutrients among the non-AO panel.

Thus, this study does not support the hypothesis that diets high in AO micronutrients reduce the risk of incident knee OA. On the other hand, the data suggest that some of these micronutrients, particularly vitamin C, may reduce the risk of OA progression among those who already have some radiographic changes.

If AOs are, indeed, protective for individuals with OA, one is left with questions about why the effect appears to be confined to those with existing radiographic changes. One possible explanation relates to differences in the intra-articular environment between healthy and OA knees. For example, several pathologic mechanisms, including raised intra-articular pressure *(15)*, low-grade inflammation *(53)*, and increased metabolic activity *(14)*, increase the opportunity for oxidative damage in an OA knee. Therefore, AOs could have a greater role in preventing progression rather than incidence, which can result from a variety of nonmetabolic insults, such as knee injury *(54)*.

Another important observation in this study was that the effect of vitamin C was stronger and more consistent than those for β-carotene and vitamin E. Vitamin C is a water-soluble compound with a broad spectrum of AO activity, because of its ability to react with numerous aqueous free-radicals and reactive oxygen species *(9)*. The extracellular nature of reactive oxygen species-mediated damage in joints, and the aqueous intra-articular environment, may favor a role for a water-soluble agent, such as vitamin C, rather than fat-soluble molecules, such as β-carotene or vitamin E. In addition, it has been suggested that vitamin C may regenerate vitamin E at the water–lipid interface by reducing AT radical back to AT. Whether this occurs in vivo, however, appears controversial. An alternative explanation is that the protective effects of vitamin C relate to its biochemical participation in the biosynthesis of cartilage collagen fibrils and PG molecules, rather than its AO properties.

3.2.3. CLINICAL TRIALS

Benefit from vitamin E therapy has been suggested by several small studies of human OA *(55–58)*, of which the most rigorous was a company-sponsored 6-wk, double-blind, placebo-controlled trial of 400 mg AT (vitamin E) in 56 OA patients in Germany *(59)*. Vitamin E-treated patients experienced greater improvement in every efficacy measure, including pain at rest (69% better in vitamin E vs 34% better in placebo, $p < 0.05$), pain on movement (62% better on vitamin E vs 27% on placebo, $p < 0.01$), and use of analgesics (52% less on vitamin E; 24% less on placebo, $p < 0.01$). The rapid response in symptoms observed in this study precludes a structural effect in this disorder, and suggests that the beneficial effect may result from some metabolic action, such as inhibition of arachidonic acid metabolism.

Selenium (Se) has also been tested in a clinical trial as a therapy for OA symptoms *(60)*. Hill and Bird conducted a 6-mo, double-blind, placebo-controlled study of Selenium-ACE, a proprietary nutritional supplement in the UK, among 30 patients with unspecified OA. The active treatment contained, on average, 144 µg Se, and contained unspecified quantities of vitamins A, C, and E. In fact, the placebo also contained 2.9 µg Se. Pain and stiffness scores remained similar for the two groups at all time-points. The authors concluded that their data did not support efficacy for selenium-ACE in relieving OA symptoms.

3.3. Studies of Vitamin D

In a separate investigation, the author tested the association of vitamin D status on the incidence and progression of knee OA among the cohort of participants in the Framingham OA Cohort Study described above *(61)*. The methodology for this investigation was essentially identical, except that the analysis was confined to the subset of individuals who both participated in the dietary assessment and provided serum for assay of 25-hydroxy vitamin D (25-OH-D) ($n = 556$). Dietary intake of vitamin D and serum 25-OH-D levels were modestly correlated in this sample ($r = 0.24$), and, as in the previous study, were unrelated to OA incidence. Risk of progression, however, increased threefold for participants in the middle and lower tertiles of both vitamin D intake (OR for lowest vs highest tertile = 4.0, 95% CI, 1.4–11.6) and serum level (OR = 2.9, 95% CI, 1.0–8.2). Low serum vitamin D level also predicted cartilage loss, assessed by loss of joint space (OR = 2.3, 95% CI, 0.9–5.5) and osteophyte growth (OR = 3.1, 95% CI, 1.3–7.5). The author concluded that low serum level, and low intake, of vitamin D were each associated with a highly significant increase in the risk of knee OA progression.

Lane et al. *(62)* subsequently examined the relationship of serum 25- and 1,25-OH-D with the development of radiographic hip OA among Caucasian women aged over 65 yr, who were participating in the Study of Osteoporotic Fractures. They measured serum vitamin D levels in 237 subjects randomly selected from 6051 women who had pelvic radiographs taken at the baseline examination, and after 8 yr of follow-up. Radiographs in this study were graded using a validated scoring system for hip OA, based on individual radiographic features (osteophytes and joint space narrowing). The investigators analyzed the association of vitamin D levels (ranked in tertiles) with the occurrence of joint space narrowing and development of osteophytosis, and with changes in the mean joint space width and individual radiographic feature scores (treated as continuous variables) during the study period. Multivariate analyses were adjusted for age, clinic, weight at age 50 yr, and health status. They found a significantly increased risk for development of joint space narrowing among those in the lowest tertile for 25-OH-D (OR = 2.5, 95% confidence limits 1.1, 5.3), as well as associations with continuous measures of progression ($\beta = -0.1$, 95% confidence limits –0.2, –0.02). An increased risk for development of joint space narrowing, among those in the middle tertile for 25-OH-D, was also apparent, but did not reach statistical significance.

Table 2
Epidemiologic Studies of Nutritional Factors and OA

Author (ref.)	Nutritional factors studied	Outcome variables	Summary
McAlindon et al. (52)	Dietary AO intake	Knee OA incidence and progression	Vitamin C appeared protective for OA progression (but not incidence).
McAlindon et al. (61)	Vitamin D: dietary and serum	Knee OA incidence and progression	Vitamin D appeared protective for progression (but not incidence).
Lane et al. (62)	Vitamin D: serum	Hip OA incidence and progression	Vitamin D appeared protective for hip OA incidence and progression.

There are, therefore, two independent epidemiologic studies demonstrating an inverse association of vitamin D status with risk for OA. Both of these studies used a prospective design, and included relatively robust measures of vitamin D status. The findings of Lane et al. (62) are of considerable importance, because of their remarkable similarity to those found for knee OA in the Framingham Study, and because they additionally suggest that vitamin D may be protective in respect to OA incidence, at least at the hip. Taken together, these studies provide the most compelling evidence for the role of any nutritional factor in the development of OA (Table 2). One important implication of these findings is that individuals with the lowest risk were in the highest tertile for 25-OH-D, corresponding to levels of over 30 ng/mL.

3.4. Folic Acid and Cobalamin

Flynn et al. (63) performed a 2-mo, double-blind, randomized, three-arm crossover clinical trial of 6400 µg folate vs 6400 µg folate with 20 µg cyanocobalamin vs a placebo, among 30 individuals with symptomatic hand OA. Participants were assessed for tender joints, grip strength, symptoms, and analgesic use. In their analyses, the authors stratified the participants according to their baseline grip strength. Ultimately, some benefits were found among some strata for certain measures of grip strength and tender joints, favoring the folate/cyanocobalamin arm. Few differences, however, were noted in respect to pain scores, global assessments, or analgesic use, suggesting that this intervention had limited, if any, efficacy.

Dietary intake of folate was also tested as a non-AO control micronutrient in the Framingham Osteoarthritis Study described above. In this observational study, the author found no convincing effect of this micronutrient on knee OA incidence or progression.

3.5. Se and Iodine: Studies of Kashin-Beck Disease

Kashin-Beck disease (KB) is an osteoarthropathy of children and adolescents, which occurs in geographic areas of China in which deficiencies of both Se and iodine (I) are endemic. Strong epidemiologic evidence exists (64) supporting the environmental nature of this disease. Although the clinical and radiologic characteristics of KB differ from OA, its existence raises the possibility that environmental factors also play a role in the occurrence of this disorder.

Se deficiency, together with pro-oxidative products of organic matter in drinking water (mostly fulvic acid) and contamination of grain by fungi, have been proposed as environmental causes for KB. The efficacy of Se supplementation in preventing the disorder, however, is controversial. Because Se is an integral component of iodothyronine deiodinase, as well as glutathione peroxidase, Moreno-Reyes et al. *(65)* studied Io and Se metabolism in 11 villages in Tibet in which KB was endemic and one village in which it was not. They found Io deficiency to be the main determinant of KB in these villages, although it should be noted that Se levels were very low in all the subgroups examined. In an accompanying editorial, Utiger inferred that KB probably results from a combination of deficiencies of both of these elements, and speculated that growth plate cartilage is dependent on locally produced triiodothyronine and also sensitive to oxidative damage.

It should be noted that there is little evidence, if any, to suggest that KB has any similarities with OA. Further, the single published clinical trial of supplemental Se (Selenium-ACE) *(60)*, in the treatment of symptoms associated with OA, demonstrated no efficacy from this product.

4. STUDIES OF OTHER NUTRIENTS IN OA

4.1. Glucosamine and Chondroitin Sulfate

The idea that administration of glucosamine or chondroitin sulfate (CS) may have therapeutic effects in treating OA, by providing substrate for reparative processes in cartilage, has been around since at least the 1960s. These compounds occur naturally in the body, and may be involved in the repair and maintenance of normal cartilage. They have been used for many years in veterinary medicine for the symptomatic relief of arthritis. Recently, health and nutrition stores, and numerous news shows and popular books, have promoted the use of glucosamine and CS for the treatment of arthritis. On the basis of anecdotal evidence, the products appear to be gaining popularity among consumers. Different formulations of glucosamine are available in nutrition stores, which sell these products as dietary supplements.

Although there has been continuing interest in these compounds, this appears to have been tempered by lack of a plausible mechanism to explain how they may achieve a therapeutic effect. In fact, recent laboratory studies *(66)* have indicated that glucosamine is absorbed through the gastrointestinal tract, then rapidly distributed throughout the body, with selective uptake by articular cartilage *(67,68)*, in which it stimulates both glycosaminoglycan and PG synthesis *(69–71)*. The biologic fate of orally administered CS is less clear, but some evidence exists to suggest that the compound may be absorbed following oral administration, possibly as a result of pinocytosis *(72)*. CS is able to cause an increase in RNA synthesis by chondrocytes *(73)*, which appears to correlate with an increase in the production of PGs and collagens *(74–77)*. In addition, there is evidence that CS partially inhibits leukocyte elastase, and may, therefore, reduce the degradation of cartilage collagen and PGs, which is prominent in the OA process *(78–81)*.

Glucosamine and CS have been the subject of numerous clinical trials in Europe and Asia, all of which have demonstrated favorable effects from these compounds *(82–96)*. The author performed a meta-analysis and quality assessment of double-blind, placebo-controlled clinical trials of glucosamine and chondroitin compounds, to evaluate their likely efficacy for OA *(97)*. Thirteen trials met eligibility criteria. Quality scores were substantially lower for abstracts, compared with manuscripts, with major deficiencies apparent in descriptions of randomization, blinding, and completion rates. Most, if not all, were sponsored by a manufacturer of the product. No negative studies were found. All studies were classified as positive, and demonstrated large effects, with a mean score reduction, compared to placebo, of 39.5% for glucosamine, and 40.2% for chondroitin.

The author concludes that clinical trials of glucosamine and chondroitin show substantial benefits in the treatment of OA symptoms, but provide insufficient information about study design and conduct to allow definitive evaluation. Another difficulty that arises, when the vast majority of the published trials are industry-supported, as here, is the potential for publication bias (i.e., censure of trials with negative results). Also, it should be noted that the trials the author analyzed measured symptoms only. One cannot draw any inferences, therefore, in respect to the potential of these compounds to have any effect on the pathologic progression of OA. Further, high-quality, independent studies are, therefore, needed to test the efficacy of glucosamine and CS.

4.2. Other Nutritional Products

A large number of nutritional products are touted for their purported benefits in arthritis, and it is encouraging that some of these are now being scientifically evaluated. Blotman et al. *(98)* recently tested the efficacy and safety of avocado/soybean unsaponifiables among 164 individuals with symptomatic OA of the knee or hip. The primary outcome measure in this 3-mo randomized, controlled trial was requirement for analgesics. The treated arm fared modestly better, with reduced analgesic requirement (43 vs 67%), and slightly greater improvement on a composite measure of pain and function.

An ayurdevic remedy, prepared from certain herbs and roots, has also been tested in an industry-sponsored, placebo-controlled, clinical trial, presented recently as abstract *(99)*. This 32-wk study of 90 participants appeared to show a greater rate of improvement in many of the outcomes tested, including a validated OA assessment instrument.

5. CONCLUSIONS/RECOMMENDATIONS

The idea that nutritional factors may influence the occurrence or course of OA is relatively new to the scientific community (although not to the general public). As a result, research in this field is at an early stage, and few definitive conclusions can be reached. Nevertheless, it is clear that there are many plausible mechanisms through which various nutritional factors may influence the occurrence and course of this major public health problem. Furthermore, preliminary findings do suggest a role in reducing OA progression for vitamin C, and particularly vitamin D. Of all the data available so far, the results for vitamin D are, perhaps, the most robust, in that these have been replicated using a serum measure in two large epidemiologic studies for two different joint sites. The results of clinical trials of glucosamine and CS for OA symptoms also appear promising, although it remains to be established whether these compounds have any effect on the disease process (Table 3).

The question arises as to what might be reasonable nutritional advice for an individual with OA, given the incomplete state of current knowledge. From a pragmatic standpoint, the data suggest interventions that are mostly concordant with general advice about healthy eating, particularly increasing consumption of fresh fruit and vegetables, and optimizing vitamin D status. It is notable in the Framingham Osteoarthritis Study, that

Table 3
Clinical Trials of Nutritional Products in Osteoarthritis

Author (ref.)	Compound tested	Comparator	Study N	Route of administration	Outcome
Flynn (63)	Folic acid and cyanocobalamin	Placebo	30	Oral	No consistent difference between groups
Hill (60)	Selenium-ACE	Placebo	30	Oral	No effect observed
Blankenhorn (59)	Vitamin E	Placebo	56	Oral	Favored vitamin E
Reichelt (87)	Glucosamine	Placebo	155	Oral	Favored glucosamine
Vajaradul (89)	Glucosamine	Placebo	54	Intra-articular	Favored glucosamine
Drovanti (84)	Glucosamine	Placebo	80	Oral	Favored glucosamine
Pujalte (86)	Glucosamine	Placebo	20	Oral	Favored glucosamine
Muller (96)	Glucosamine	Ibuprofen	200	Oral	Ibuprofen initially more efficacious; similar effects by wk 4
Vaz (88)	Glucosamine	Ibuprofen	40	Oral	Ibuprofen initially more efficacious; similar effects after wk 4
L'hirondel (92)	Chondroitin	Placebo	125	Oral	Favored chondroitin
Kerzberg (93)	Chondroitin	Placebo	17	Intramuscular	Favored chondroitin
Mazieres (94)	Chondroitin	Placebo	120	Oral	Favored chondroitin
Conrozier (100)	Chondroitin	Placebo	129	Oral	Favored chondroitin
Rovetta (95)	Chondroitin	Placebo	40	Intramuscular	Favored chondroitin
Morreale (101)	Chondroitin	Diclofenac	146	Oral	Favored chondroitin

an individual could move out of the high-risk tertile for vitamin C intake, by increasing consumption by as little as an orange per day. For vitamin D, an intake of 400 IU/d, or serum levels of greater than approx 30 ng/mL, appear to confer maximum benefit. Vitamin D is derived from a number of sources, and there is a small risk of toxicity for individuals consuming large daily doses. Supplementation with 400–800 IU/d appears to be safe. For instances in which there are concerns about adequate supplementation, or toxicity, the author would recommend an estimation of serum 25-OH-D levels.

There appear to be no compelling reasons to discourage the use of glucosamine and CS. These products are substantially safer than many drugs prescribed in the treatment of OA symptoms; however, they are often expensive, lack pharmaceutical-level manufacturing standard controls, and may not work.

REFERENCES

1. Lawrence JS, Bremner JM, Bier F. Osteo-arthrosis. Prevalence in the population and relationship between symptoms and x-ray changes. Ann Rheum Dis 1966; 25:1–24.
2. Cooper C. Osteoarthritis: epidemiology. In: Rheumatology. Klippel JH, Dieppe PA, eds. London: Mosby, 1994; 7.3.1–5.
3. Mankin HJ. Clinical features of osteoarthritis. In: Textbook of Rheumatology, 4th ed. Kelly WN, Harris EDJ, Ruddy S, Sledge CB, eds. Philadelphia: Saunders, 1993; 1374–1384.
4. The Incidence and Prevalence Database for Procedures. Sunnyvale, CA: Timely Data Resources, 1995.
5. Hough AJJ, Sokoloff L. Pathology of osteoarthritis. In: Arthritis and Allied Conditions, 11th ed. McCarty DJ, ed. Philadelphia: Lea and Febiger, 1989; 1945–1968.
6. Pottenger LA, Philips FM, Draganich LF. The effect of marginal osteophytes on reduction of varus-valgus instability in osteoarthritis knees. Arthritis Rheum 1990; 33:853–858.
7. Creamer P, Hochberg MC. Osteoarthritis. Lancet 1997; 350:503–508.
8. Theodosakis J, Adderly B, Fox B. The Arthritis Cure. New York: St. Martin's Press, 1997.
9. Frei B. Reactive oxygen species and antioxidant vitamins: mechanisms of action. Am J Med 1994; 97(Suppl. 3A):5S–13S.
10. Jacques PF, Chylack LT, Taylor A. Relationships between natural antioxidants and cataract formation. 1994; 515–533.
11. Gaziano JM. Antioxidant vitamins and coronary artery disease risk. Am J Med 1994; 97(Suppl. 3A): 18S–21S.
12. Hennekens CH. Antioxidant vitamins and cancer. Am J Med 1994; 97(Suppl. 3A):2S–4S.
13. Boveris A, Oshino N, Chance B. The cellular production of hydrogen peroxide. Biochem J 1972; 128:617–630.
14. Blake DR, Unsworth J, Outhwaite JM, Morris CJ, Merry P, Kido BL, et al. Hypoxic-reperfusion injury in the inflamed human. Lancet 1989; 11:290–293.
15. Ames BN, Shigenaga MK, Hagen TM. Oxidants, antioxidants and the degenerative diseases of aging. Proc Natl Acad Sci USA 1993; 90:7915–7922.
16. Henrotin Y, Deby-Dupont G, Deby C, Franchimont P, Emerit I. Active oxygen species, articular inflammation, and cartilage damage. Exs 1992; 62:308–322.
17. Henrotin Y, Deby-Dupont G, Deby C, Debruin M, Lamy M, Franchimont P. Production of active oxygen species by isolated human chondrocytes. Br J Rheumatol 1993; 32.
18. Rathakrishnan C, Tiku K, Raghavan A, Tiku ML. Release of oxygen radicals by articular chondrocytes: a study of luminol-dependent chemoluminescence and hydrogen peroxide secretion. J Bone Miner Res 1992; 7:1139–1148.
19. Greenwald RA, Moy WW. Inhibition of collagen gelation by action of the superoxide radical. Arthritis Rheum 1979; 22.
20. McCord JM. Free radicals and inflammation: protection of synovial fluid by superoxide dismutase. Science 1974; 185:529–530.
21. Briviba K, Seis H. Non-enzymatic antioxidant defense systems. In: Natural Antioxidants in Human Health and Disease, Frei B eds. San Diego: Academic; 1994; 107–128.

22. Hankinson SE, Stampfer MJ, Seddon JM, et al. Nutrient intake and cataract extraction in women: a prospective study. Br Med J 1992; 305:335–339.
23. Peterkofsky B. Ascorbate requirement for hydroxylation and secretion of procollagen: relationship to inhibition of collagen synthesis in scurvy. Am J Clin Nutr 1991; 54:1135S–1140S.
24. Spanheimer RG, Bird TA, Peterkofsky B. Regulation of collagen synthesis and mRNA levels in articular cartilage of scorbutic guinea pigs. Arch Biochem Biophys 1986; 246:33–41.
25. Houglum KP, Brenner DA, Chijkier M. Ascorbic acid stimulation of collagen biosynthesis independent of hydroxylation. Am J Clin Nutr 1991; 54:1141S–1143S.
26. Schwartz ER, Adamy L. Effect of ascorbic acid on arylsulfatase activities and sulfated proteoglycan metabolism in chondrocyte cultures. J Clin Invest 1977; 60.
27. Sandell LJ, Daniel LC. Effects of ascorbic acid on collagen mRNA levels in short-term chondrocyte cultures. Connect Tissue Res 1988; 17:11–22.
28. Peterkofsky B, Palka J, Wilson S, Takeda K, Shah V. Elevated activity of low molecular weight insulin-like growth factor binding proteins in sera of vitamin C deficient and fasted guinea pigs. Endocrinology 1991; 128:1769–1779.
29. Bhalla AK, Wojno WC, Goldring MB. Human articular chondrocytes acquire AU1,25(OH)2 vitamin D-3 receptors. Biochim Biophys Acta 1987; 931:26–32.
30. Poole RA. Imbalances of anabolism and catabolism of cartilage matrix components in osteoarthritis. Amer Acad Orthop Surgeons 1995; 247–260.
31. Radin EL, Paul IL, Tolkoff MJ. Subchondral changes in patients with early degenerative joint disease. Arthritis Rheum 1970; 13:400–405.
32. Layton MV, Golstein SA, Goulet RW, Feldkamp LA, Kubinski DJ, Bole GG. Examination of subchondral bone architecture in experimental osteoarthritis by microscopic computed axial tomography. Arthritis Rheum 1988; 31.
33. Milgram JW. Morphological alterations of the subchondral bone in advanced degenerative arthritis. Clin Orthop Rel Res 1983; 173:293–312.
34. Kellgren JH, Lawrence JS. The Epidemiology of Chronic Rheumatism: Atlas of Standard Radiographs, Vol. 2 Oxford, UK: Blackwell Science; 1962.
35. Anonymous. Cartilage and bone in osteoarthrosis. Br Med J 1976; 2:4–5.
36. Dequecker J, Mokassa L, Aerssens J. Bone density and osteoarthritis. J Rheumatol 1995; 22(Suppl. 43): 98–100.
37. Dedrick DK, Goldstein SA, Brandt KD, O'Connor BL, Goulet RW, Albrecht M. A longitudinal study of subchondral plate and trabecular bone in cruciate-deficient dogs with osteoarthritis followed up for 54 months. Arthritis Rheum 1993; 36:1460–1467.
38. Ledingham J, Dawson S, Preston B, Milligan G, Doherty M. Radiographic progression of hospital-referred osteoarthritis of the hip. Ann Rheum Dis 1993; 52:263–267.
39. Radin EL, Rose RM. Role of subchondral bone in the initiation and progression of cartilage damage. Clin Orthop Rel Res 1986; 213:34–40.
40. Perry GH, Smith MJG, Whiteside CG. Spontaneous recovery of the joint space in degenerative hip disease. Ann Rheum Dis 1972; 31:440–448.
41. Smythe SA. Osteoarthritis, insulin and bone density. J Rheumatol 1987; 14(Suppl.):91–93.
42. Zhang Y, Hannan M, Chaisson C, McAlindon T, Evans S, Felson D. Low bone mineral density (BMD) increases the risk of progressive knee osteoarthritis (OA) in women. Arthritis Rheum 1997; 40:1798.
43. Dieppe P, Cushnaghan J, Young P, Kirwan J. Prediction of the progression of joint space narrowing in osteoarthritis of the knee by bone scintigraphy. Ann Rheum Dis 1993; 52:557–563.
44. Kiel DP. Vitamin D, calcium and bone: descriptive epidemiology, 1995; 277–290.
45. Parfitt AM, Gallagher JC, Heaney RP, Neer R, Whedon GD. Vitamin D and bone health in the elderly. Am J Clin Nutr 1982; 36:1014–1031.
46. Pangamala RV, Cornwell DG. The effects of vitamin E on arachidonic acid metabolism. Ann NY Acad Sci 1982.
47. Felson DT. Weight and osteoarthritis. J Rheumatol 1995; 22(Suppl. 43):7–9.
48. Sokoloff L, Mickelsen O. Dietary fat supplements, body weight and osteoarthritis in DBA/2JN mice. J Nutr 1965; 85:117–121.
49. Sokoloff L, Mickelsen O, Silverstein E, Jay GE Jr, Yamamoto RS. Experimental obesity and osteoarthritis. Am J Physiol 1960; 198:765–770.

50. Schwartz ER, Leveille C, Oh WH. Experimentally induced osteoarthritis in guinea pigs: effect of surgical procedure and dietary intake of vitamin C. Lab Animal Sci 1981; 31:683–687.
51. Meacock SCR, Bodmer JL, Billingham MEJ. Experimental OA in guinea pigs. J Exp Pathol 1990; 71:279–293.
52. McAlindon TE, Jacques P, Zhang Y, Hannan MT, Aliabadi P, Weissman B, et al. Do antioxidant micronutrients protect against the development and progression of knee osteoarthritis? Arthritis Rheum 1996; 39:648–656.
53. Schumacher HR Jr. Synovial inflammation, crystals and osteoarthritis. J Rheumatol 1995; 22(Suppl. 43): 101–103.
54. McAlindon TE, Hannan MT, Naimark A, Weissman B, Felson DT. Comparison of risk factors for tibiofemoral and patellofemoral osteoarthritis. Arthritis Rheum 1994; 37(Suppl.):1254.
55. Hirohata K, Yao S, Imura S, Harada H. Treatment of osteoarthritis of the knee joint at the state of hydroarthrosis. Kobe Med Sci 1965; 11(Suppl.):65–66.
56. Doumerg C. Etude clinique experimentale de l'alpha-tocopheryle-quinone en rheumatologie et en reeducation. Therapeutique 1969; 45:676–678.
57. Machetey I, Quaknine L. Tocopherol in osteoarthritis: a controlled pilot study. J Am Ger Soc 1978; 26:328–330.
58. Scherak O, Kolarz G, Schodl C, Blankenhorn G. Hochdosierte vitamin-E-therapie bei patienten mit aktivierter arthrose. Z Rheumatol 1990; 49:369–373.
59. Blankenhorn G. Clinical efficacy of spondyvit (vitamin E) in activated arthroses. A multicenter, placebo-controlled, double-blind study. Z Orthop 1986; 124:340–343.
60. Hill J, Bird HA. Failure of selenium-ace to improve osteoarthritis. Br J Rheumatol 1990; 29: 211–213.
61. McAlindon TE, Felson DT, Zhang Y, Hannan MT, Aliabadi P, Weissman B, et al. Relation of dietary intake and serum levels of vitamin D to progression of osteoarthritis of the knee among participants in the Framingham Study. Ann Intern Med 1996; 125:353–359.
62. Lane NE, Nevitt MC, Gore LR, Cummings SR, Hochberg MC, Scott J. Serum levels of vitamin D and hip osteoarthritis in elderly women: a longitudinal study. Arthritis Rheum 1997; 40(Suppl.):S1243.
63. Flynn MA, Irvin W, Krause G. The effect of folate and cobalamin on osteoarthritic hands. J Am Coll Nutr 1994; 13:351–356.
64. Utiger RD. Kashin-Beck disease: expanding the spectrum of iodine-deficiency disorders. N Engl J Med 1998; 339:1156–1158.
65. Moreno-Reyes R, Suetens C, Mathieu F, Begaux F, Zhu D, Rivera MT, et al. Kashin-Beck osteoarthropathy in rural Tibet in relation to selenium and iodine status. N Engl J Med 1998; 339:1112–1120.
66. Dones F, Tesoriere G. Intestinal absorption of glucosamine and N-acetyl-glucosamine. Experientia 1972; 28:770.
67. Setnikar I, Giachetti C, Zanolo G. Absorption, distribution and excretion of radioactivity after a single I.V. or oral administration of [^{14}C]glucosamine to the rat. Pharmatherapeutica 1984; 3:358.
68. Setnikar I, Giachetti C, Zanolo G. Distribution of glucosamine in animal tissues. Arzneimittel forschung/Drug Res 1986; 36:729.
69. Karzal K, Domenjoz R. Effects of hexosamine derivatives on glycosaminoglycan metabolism of fibroblast cultures. Pharmacology 1971; 5:337.
70. Vidal Y, Plana RR, Karzal K. Glucosamine: its role in articular cartilage metabolism studies on rat and human articular cartilage. Fostscher Med 1980; 98:801–806.
71. Vidal Y, Plana RR, Bizzarri D, Rovati AL. Articular cartilage pharmacology: in vitro studies on glucosamine and NSAIDs. Pharmacol Res Commun 1978; 10:557.
72. Theodore G. Untrsuchung von 35 arhrosefallen, behandelt mit chondroitin schwefelsaure. Schweiz Rundschaue Med Praxis 1977; 66.
73. Vach J, Pesakova V, Krajickova J, Adam M. Effect of glycosaminoglycan polysulfate on the metabolism of cartilage RNA. Arzneim Forsch/Drur Res 1984; 34:607–609.
74. Ali SY. The degradation of cartilage matrix by an intracellular protease. Biochem J 1964; 93:611.
75. Hamerman D, Smith C, Keiser HD, Craig R. Glycosaminoglycans produced by human synovial cell cultures collagen. Rel Res 1982; 2:313.
76. Lilja S, Barrach HJ. Normally sulfated and highly sulfated glycosaminoglycans affecting fibrillogenesis on type I and type II collage in vitro. Exp Pathol 1983; 23:173–181.
77. Knanfelt A. Synthesis of articular cartilage proteoglycans by isolated bovine chondrocytes. Agents Actions 1984; 14:58–62.

78. Baici A, Salgam P, Fehr K, Boni A. Inhibition of human elastase from polymorphonuclear leucocytes by a GAG-polysulfate. Biochem Pharmacol 1979; 29:1723–1727.

79. Baici A. Interactions between human leucocytes elastase and chondroitin sulfate. Chem Biol Interact 1984; 51:11.

80. Marossy K. Interaction of the antitrypsin and elastase-like enzyme of the human granulocyte with glycosaminoglycans. Biochim Biophys Acta 1981; 659:351–361.

81. De Gennaro F, Piccioni PD, Caporali R, Luisetti M, Contecucco C. Effet du traitement par le sulfate de galactosaminoglucuronoglycane sur l'estase granulocytaire synovial de patients atteints d'osteoarthrose. Liter Rhumatol 1992; 14:53–60.

82. D'Ambrosio E, Casa B, Bompani R, Scali G, Scali M. Glucosamine sulphate: a controlled clinical investigation in arthrosis. Pharmatherapeutica 1981; 2:504–508.

83. Crolle G, D'Este E. Glucosamine sulphate for the management of arthrosis: a controlled clinical investigation. Curr Med Res Opin 1980; 7:104–109.

84. Drovanti A, Bignamini AA, Rovati AL. Therapeutic activity of oral glucosamine sulfate in osteoarthrosis: a placebo-controlled double-blind investigation. Clin Ther 1980; 3:260–272.

85. Noack W, Fsicher M, Forster KK, Rovatis LC, Senikar I. Glucosamine sulfate in osteoarthritis of the knee. Osteoarthritis Cart 1994; 2:51–59.

86. Pujalte JM, Llavore EP, Ylescupidez FR. Double-blind clinical evaluation of oral glucosamine sulphate in the basic treatment of osteoarthrosis. Curr Med Res Opin 1980; 7:110–114.

87. Reichelt A, Forster KK, Fischer M, Rovati LC, Setnikar I. Efficacy and safety of intramuscular glucosamine sulfate in osteoarthritis of the knee: a randomized, placebo-controlled, double-blind study. Drug Res 1994; 44:75–80.

88. Vaz AL. Double-blind clinical evaluation of the relative efficacy of ibuprofen and glucosamine sulphate in the management of osteoarthrosis of the knee in out-patients. Curr Med Res Opin 1982; 8:145–149.

89. Vajaradul Y. Double-blind clinical evaluation of intra-articular glucosamine in outpatients with gonarthrosis. Clin Ther 1981; 3:336–343.

90. Tapadinhas MJ, Rivera IC, Bignamini AA. Oral glucosamine sulphate in the management of arthrosis: report on a multi-centre open investigation in Portugal. Pharmatherapeutica 1982; 3:157–168.

91. Vetter VG. Glukosamine in der therapie des degenerativen rheumatismus. Duet Med J 1965; 16:446–449.

92. L'Hirondel JL. Klinische doppelblind-studie mit oral verabreichtem chondroitinsulfat gegen placebo bei der tibiofemoralen gonarthrose (125 patienten). Litera Rhumatol 1992; 14:77–84.

93. Kerzberg EM, Roldan EJ, Castelli G, Huberman ED. Combination of glycosaminoglycans and acetyl-salicylic acid in knee osteoarthrosis. Scand J Rheumatol 1987; 16:377–380.

94. Mazieres B, Loyau G, Menkes CJ, Valat JP, Dreiser RL, Charlot J, et al. [Chondroitin sulfate in the treatment of gonarthrosis and coxarthrosis. 5-months result of a multicenter double-blind controlled prospective study using placebo]. Rev Rhum Mal Osteoartic 1992; 59:466–472.

95. Rovetta G. Galactosaminoglycuronoglycan sulfate (matrix) in therapy of tibiofibular osteoarthritis of the knee. Drugs Exp Clin Res 1991; 17:53–57.

96. Muller-Fassbender H, Bach GL, Haase W, Rovato LC, Setnikar I. Glucosamine sulfate compared to ibuprofen in osteoarthritis of the knee. Osteoarthritis Cartilage 1994; 2:61–69.

97. Mcalindon TE, Gulin J, Felson DT. Glucosamine and chondroitin treatment for osteoarthritis of the knee or hip: meta-analysis and quality assessment of clinical trials. Arthritis Rheum 1998; 41(Suppl.):S994.

98. Blotman F, Maheu E, Wulwik A, Caspard H, Lopez A. Efficacy and safety of avocado/soybean unsaponifiables in the treatment of symptomatic osteoarthritis of the knee and hip. A prospective, multicenter, three-month, randomized, double-blind, placebo-controlled trial. Rev Rhum Engl Ed 1997; 64:825–834.

99. Chopra A, Lavin P, Chitre D, Patwardhan B, Polisson R. A clinical study of an ayurvedic medicine (Asian medicine) in OA knees. Arthritis Rheum 1998; 41:S992.

100. Conrozier T, Vignon E. Die Wirkung von Chondroitinsulfat bei der Behandlung der Huftgelenksarthrose Eine Doppelblindstudie gegen Placebo. Litera Reumatol 1992; 14:69–75.

101. Morreale P, Manopulo R, Galati M, Boccanera L, Saponati G, Bocchi L. Comparison of the antiinflammatory efficacy of chondroitin sulfate and diclofenac sodium in patients with knee osteoarthritis. J Rheumatol 1996; 23:1385–1391.

18

Calcium Requirements During Treatment of Osteoporosis in Women

Calcium Supplements Alone and in Association with Antiresorptive Drugs in Osteoporosis

Claudia A. Pereda and Richard Eastell

1. INTRODUCTION

There is accumulating evidence that calcium (Ca) supplementation of the diet may be useful, under certain circumstances, for the prevention of osteoporosis (OP) in postmenopausal women. This chapter reviews this evidence, and considers whether Ca supplementation should also be considered in women taking other treatment for postmenopausal OP.

1.1. Effect of Ca Supplementation

Ca intake is an important determinant of bone health. Several clinical trials of Ca supplementation in the prevention and treatment of OP have shown that Ca can decrease the rate of bone loss and risk of fracture in postmenopausal women. This effect is more clearly seen after the first 5 yr of menopause, rather than in early menopause. As an example, Dawson-Hughes et al. (1), in a longitudinal, controlled trial, investigated the effect of Ca supplementation on bone loss from spine, and femoral neck and radius, in early and late postmenopausal women. They observed a significant decline in bone mineral density (BMD) from the spine, in the group of women who had undergone menopause ≤5 yr earlier. This was not affected by Ca supplementation. Conversely, among women who had been postmenopausal for ≥6 yr, and who were given placebo, bone loss was less rapid. In the matched group, Ca supplementation proved to be of benefit. It is likely that, during the first few years after menopause, there is high bone resorption. Parathyroid hormone (PTH) may be partially suppressed, because of a slight increase in serum Ca level. Consequently, Ca supplements may be ineffective in retarding this phase of menopausal bone loss, because it is essentially mediated by estrogen deficiency (2).

Ca nutrition depends on Ca absorption efficiency, as well as on intake. There is good evidence to suggest that Ca absorption and renal Ca conservation are less efficient in the elderly, and, therefore, there is an increased requirement for dietary Ca (3). There may,

From: *Primary and Secondary Preventive Nutrition*
Edited by: A. Bendich and R. J. Deckelbaum © Humana Press Inc., Totowa, NJ

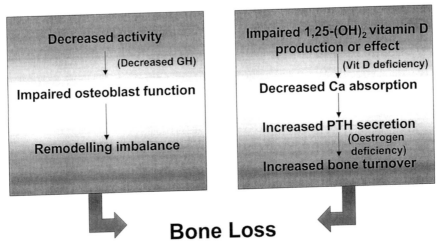

Fig. 1. Model for age-related bone loss. In this model, bone loss results from a combination of increased bone turnover and remodeling balance.

therefore, be an increasing imbalance between absorption and excretion of Ca with age, particularly at the menopause (Fig. 1). In an early study, Heaney et al. *(4)* studied the menopausal changes in Ca balance in 16 postmenopausal women who went through the menopause during the study. This group exhibited a statistically significant negative balance when evaluated against a theoretical Ca mean change of zero. Subsequently, the group was compared to premenopausal women and estrogen-treated postmenopausal women who were in Ca balance. The mean intake required for zero Ca balance (absorption = excretion), in the postmenopausal untreated group, was estimated to be approx 1504 mg/d. However, in premenopausal women and estrogen-repleted postmenopausal women, mean Ca intakes for zero balance was approx 990 mg/d. The increase in Ca intake required to meet the extra loss during the menopause is about 5.0 mmol (200 mg), which raises the mean requirement to 26 mmol (1040 mg), after allowing for skin losses. The optimal Ca intake in postmenopausal women, up to 65 yr or older, is about 1500 mg/d, in the absence of estrogen replacement (5; Table 1). However, Ca intake of less than 600 mg/d at this stage is common. This deficit may increase PTH secretion, and result in bone resorption. Cross-sectional studies *(6)* have shown that Ca intake declines about 10% in men and women between 35 and 75 yr of age. Moreover, the redress of Ca nutritional deficiency (in the form of diet or Ca supplements) had beneficial effect in patients with low Ca intake. For example, Dawson-Hughes et al. *(1,7)* showed that postmenopausal women, with a Ca intake below 400 mg/d, had a better response to Ca therapy than those with an intake of 400–650 mg/d. In other words, the lower the habitual Ca intake, the greater the benefit of Ca supplementation. Most studies suggest that this beneficial effect is achieved during the first 6–12 mo of therapy, with little added BMD benefit thereafter *(8)*.

Two recent long-term studies *(9,10)* found a decrease in the rate of bone loss after 4 yr of treatment with Ca. However, the chief benefit was observed more during the first year of therapy. A recent analysis of the 20 major Ca trials in postmenopausal women, reported in the last 20 yr, yielded a mean rate of bone loss of 1.00%/yr in the controls and 0.014%/yr in Ca-treated subjects *(11)*. The beneficial effect on BMD has been observed

Table 1

Optimal Ca Intake in Postmenopausal Women

Postmenopausal women up to 65 yr (not receiving HRT)	1000 mg/d
Postmenopausal women up to 65 yr (receiving HRT)	1500 mg/d
Postmenopausal women older than 65 yr	1500 mg/d

Adapted with permission from ref. 5.

Table 2

Vertebral Fracture Incidence in Ca-Treated Elderly Women,
with and without Pre-Existing Fractures

	Number of patients	
Fracture status and outcome	Placebo	Ca
With pre-existing fractures (n = 94)		
New fractures	21	15[a]
No new fractures	20	38[a]
Without pre-existing fractures (n = 103)		
New fractures	13	12
No new fractures	48	30

[a]p = 0.023 compared to placebo.
Adapted with permission from ref. 10.

mostly in cortical bone (12–13). However, the effect on trabecular bone is less well defined (14–15). Among elderly women with low Ca intake, there was also a reduction in the rate of vertebral fractures (10; Table 2). In that study, Ca supplementation, in 94 late-postmenopausal women with pre-existing vertebral fractures, resulted in a 2.8× reduction in the incidence of new fractures than those without treatment. But, in 103 women without pre-existing fractures, Ca had no effect. Chevalley et al. (12) also found a decrease in vertebral fracture rates in 82 postmenopausal women receiving Ca supplements. In addition, there was a reduction in femoral BMD, but hip fracture rate was not reported (12). A later report from a Swedish prospective study (16) found no correlation between Ca intake and hip fracture risk.

A recent study investigated the response of six markers of bone resorption to Ca supplementation (1200 mg/d) over 2 mo (17; Fig. 2). Ca supplementation led to a significant decrease in all resorption markers, except for free deoxypyridinoline. Nevertheless, the decline of resorption markers, although being significant, never exceeded 30%. This response could be considered weak, when compared with other antiresorptive agents, such as bisphosphonates or estrogen, in which the average reduction ranges from 30 to 80%. Indeed, these results are reinforced by a study by Riggs et al. (13), in which free pyridinoline, a marker of bone resorption, and osteocalcin, a marker of bone formation, were reduced by 32.2 and 11.9% respectively, after 4 yr of Ca treatment.

It seems clear that Ca supplementation can prevent bone loss in postmenopausal women. However, the greatest benefits seem to be obtained in those subjects whose basal Ca intake is low.

Ca's effect, alone, on bone is considerably less, compared to antiresorptive drugs (Table 3). Yet, most studies with these drugs include Ca supplements in both arms (active

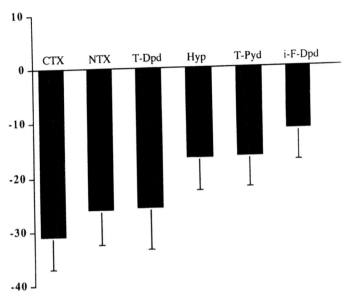

Fig. 2. Response of bone resorption markers in postmenopausal women with low Ca intake (<800 mg/d), after 2 mo of Ca supplementation. Data is expressed as mean % change and SE from baseline values. Adapted with permission from ref. *17*.

Table 3
Antiresorptive Drugs

"Therapeutic agents that slow the loss
of bone mass by primarily decreasing bone resorption"

⇒
They comprise   ⇒ Estrogens
                                 ⇒ Bisphosphonates
                                 ⇒ CALC
                                 ⇒ Congeners of vitamin D

and placebo). Dawson-Hughes et al. *(18)* also suggested that Ca supplementation reduces the rate of bone loss by about 30%, compared to untreated women.

The mechanism of action of Ca on bones seems to differ from that of antiresorptive drugs. It is likely that the beneficial effect could result from the correction of, or reduction in, negative Ca balance mediated by PTH. Previous studies *(19)* have shown modest, but significant decreases in fasting serum PTH levels after dietary Ca supplementation. Recently, McKane et al. *(20)* studied this effect in elderly women, with 3 yr of controlled high and usual Ca intakes on PTH secretion and bone resorption. The mean 24-h serum PTH and deoxypyridinoline were 40 and 35% lower in the higher-intake group, respectively, at the third year of the trial. Riggs et al. *(13)* demonstrated that postmenopausal women receiving a dose of elemental Ca of 1600 mg/d had a 19% decrease in PTH levels after 4 yr of treatment. Osteocalcin and free pyridinoline, a marker of bone resorption, were reduced by 12 and 32%, respectively, in this same study.

More conventional drugs used in the prevention and treatment of OP, such as hormone replacement therapy (HRT), bisphosphonates, or calcitonin (CALC), act on bone by decreasing the rate of bone resorption. This reduction in remodeling space may result, however, in a decrease in serum Ca levels, and therefore an increase in PTH levels. For example, HRT is thought to act on bone through a series of complex mechanisms involving the modulation of cytokines *(21,22)* and growth factors, leading possibly to inhibition of osteoclastic function and, consequently, apoptosis *(23)*. Bisphosphonates have direct effect on osteoclasts and osteoclast precursors, by inhibiting adenosine triphosphate activity, and it has been shown to inhibit the mevalonate pathway in myeloma cells, resulting in osteoclast apoptosis *(24)*. CALC also acts on osteoclasts, modifying their morphology and decreasing motility.

Ca may act by decreasing PTH secretion, and by a permissive effect on mineralization, particularly secondary mineralization. Additional Ca, given in conjunction with antiresorptive therapy, prevents the increase in PTH induced by these treatments, and so could result in a synergetic effect on bone *(25)*.

2. CLINICAL TRIALS OF ANTIRESORPTIVE THERAPY

2.1. HRT and Ca

HRT has proven to be effective in the prevention and treatment of OP in women. Indeed, it acts not only by preventing bone loss, but also by increasing bone density and decreasing the risk of OP fractures. For example, bone density has been shown to increase by up to 10% in postmenopausal women treated for 1 yr with HRT, and fracture risk was reduced by as much as 60% when HRT is taken for 6 yr or longer, following menopause *(26)*.

Several clinical trials have compared the effectiveness of HRT vs Ca supplementation in postmenopausal OP. In an early study, Recker et al. *(27)* compared the effect of estrogen and calcium carbonate ($CaCO_3$) on bone loss. Sixty postmenopausal women were assigned to one of three groups: control, $CaCO_3$, 2600 mg/d (representing 1040 mg/d of elemental Ca), or HRT; they were followed for 2 yr. In all cases, both Ca supplements and HRT reduced the rate of bone loss, compared to controls. However, the former was clearly less effective. Because Ca supplements have a minor but measurable effect on bone loss in postmenopausal women, it has been suggested that there could be a synergistic or modifying effect on bone, when co-administered with estrogens. However, few studies have investigated this possibility. The synergism was first implied in a nonrandomized study *(28)* that compared changes in bone density in two groups. One was given conjugated equine estrogen (CEE), 0.3 mg, plus Ca supplementation, to a total elemental Ca intake of at least 1500 mg/d, and was compared to a group given Ca alone *(28)*. Using quantitative computerized tomography to measure spine density, the low-dose estrogen–Ca group had an increase in spine density of 2.3%, compared to a decrease of 9.0% in the Ca-only group, after 2 yr of treatment.

On average, postmenopausal women have a daily Ca intake lower than 600 mg/d, which is well below the 1500 mg suggested by the National Institutes of Health Consensus. Although HRT increases Ca absorption, this effect is probably not enough to overcome the chronic Ca deficit. Consequently, these patients may perhaps not obtain full benefit from estrogen alone.

In another study by the same group (29), a small but positive interaction between estradiol, 1 mg, and total elemental Ca intake, above 1000 mg/d, was seen in spine density. Aloia et al. (30), in a three-arm, placebo-controlled, randomized trial, investigated whether augmentation of dietary Ca was effective in the prevention of early postmenopausal bone loss. One hundred and eighteen postmenopausal women were allocated to daily intake of 1700 mg elemental Ca, placebo, or 0.625 mg/d CEE plus 10 mg progesterone (d 18–25) and 1700 mg elemental Ca as $CaCO_3$. As a result, estrogen-progesterone with Ca supplement exerted a beneficial effect in preventing bone loss, especially from the hip. The response to Ca alone was once more intermediate between responses to placebo and estrogen-progesterone–Ca.

More recent studies investigated the synergistic effect between Ca and HRT, compared to HRT alone. Mizunuma et al. (31) administered 600–800 mg elemental Ca, in the form of Ca lactate, to postmenopausal women who had been undergoing unopposed estrogen therapy for 2 yr, and whose serum Ca level was suppressed to below the normal range. To patients whose serum Ca levels had been within normal range, the same dose of estrogen alone was continued. Changes in lumbar spine (LS) BMD, before and after Ca supplementation, was measured by dual-energy X-ray absorptiometry. LS BMD decreased by –0.4% for 2 yr in women treated with estrogen alone. The BMD of those women treated with estrogen plus Ca increased by 2.7% ($p < 0.01$). However, in a different study, two groups of menopausal women were allocated to receive estrogen alone or in conjunction with 1000 mg/d elemental, supplemental Ca. Women in this last group had a significant increase in BMD at the femoral neck ($p < 0.05$), but not in other areas of the femur, nor in the lumbar spine (32).

This interaction was also investigated among a cohort of Japanese-American women in the late menopause (33). All women had a median dietary Ca intake of 384 mg/d. During a 3-yr follow-up, 188 patients received the equivalent of 0.6 mg/d conjugated estrogen, 195 received a daily supplement of 355 mg/d elemental Ca, and 364 patients combined both therapies. Bone loss decreased at the calcaneus by 0.5%/yr during estrogen use alone, 0.25%/yr with Ca supplements, and 1%/yr during combined therapy.

Recently, Nieves et al. (25) reviewed the published clinical studies that measured bone mass of postmenopausal women from at least one skeletal site, to evaluate whether Ca supplementation influenced the efficacy of estrogen on bone mass change. Of the 31 published estrogen trials investigated, 20 involved modification of diet, or included Ca supplements (total 1183 mg/d), and 11 did not. The mean increase in bone mass of LS, when estrogen was given alone, was 1.3%, compared with 3.3% when given in conjunction with Ca. Femoral neck BMD increased 0.9% with estrogen alone; combined with Ca, the increment was about 2.4%. Similarly, forearm bone mass increased 0.4% with estrogen, compared with 2.1% when given with Ca.

These results raise the possibility that a high Ca intake potentiates the positive effect of estrogen on bone mass, possibly in either or both the cortical and trabecular bone. It is also possible that elderly women with low dietary Ca intake may not obtain full benefits from estrogen without Ca supplementation.

2.2. CALC and Ca

CALC is a hormonal factor produced by the C-cells of the thyroid. CALC lowers plasma Ca concentrations; its main target is the skeleton, where it inhibits bone resorption by a direct action on osteoclasts (34). Preparations of CALC from four different species have been developed for use in humans, i.e., porcine, human, salmon, and eel. Currently, salmon CALC is the most widely used in the prevention and treatment of postmenopausal bone loss, especially in those women in whom estrogen therapy is not advisable. Intranasal salmon CALC has become a more accepted mode of administration. Although studies involved different doses and various routes of administration, based on Nieves et al. *(25)*, the authors have focused in those studies in which patients were treated with at least 200 IU intranasal salmon CALC.

Unlike HRT, the vast majority of trials involve CALC and Ca being compared to Ca alone. For instance, Overgaard et al. *(35)* examined the effect of intranasal CALC therapy on bone mass and bone turnover in early postmenopausal women, at different doses. All patients received 500 mg elemental Ca in conjunction with CALC. The groups receiving 200 and 400 IU exhibit prevention of bone loss (0.2 to –0.6%), compared to placebo.

The effect of CALC in the prevention of bone loss seems to be more pronounced in trabecular bone, with little or no impact in cortical bone *(36)*. In one study, 41 healthy postmenopausal women with low bone density, but no fractures, received the mentioned dose of nasal CALC plus 500 mg Ca. They were followed for 2 yr. Bone mineral content in the LS increased by 3%, compared to controls, but decreased in distal forearm by nearly 1%. Thamsborg et al. *(37)*, using a similar study design, also detected significant increments in bone density of postmenopausal women, with Colles' fractures only at the spine, with no effect at the distal radius.

Ellerington et al. *(38)* compared intranasal CALC alone vs placebo. That study was randomized, double-blind, and controlled. Data indicated that daily CALC, administered intranasally, was effective in preventing postmenopausal bone loss. However, this response was restricted to those women more than 5 yr postmenopause. The increase in BMD in the LS was 3.1% after 2 yr. However, there was no significant change in BMD in the femoral neck during that period.

In a recent study, Nieves et al. *(25)* analyzed seven studies related to intranasal CALC. Of those, six used a Ca supplement in conjunction with CALC. The populations were similar regarding age (55 yr, compared to 59 yr), and years since menopause (5 yr, compared to 8 yr). These data showed that the bone-sparing benefit of CALC on the spine appears to be enhanced when Ca intake is adequate. Intranasal CALC in a population of postmenopausal women, with a mean dietary Ca intake of 627 mg/d, was only able to halt bone loss. Moreover, when elemental Ca intakes were around 1500 mg/d, there was an increment in bone mass in LS of approx 2.1%. It has been proposed that the apparent synergistic effect of CALC and Ca, compared to Ca alone, in LS, could result from a suboptimal dose of CALC, i.e., more than 200 IU intranasal salmon CALC may be needed to produce gain in bone mass.

Unfortunately, there are very few data available on the effect of CALC treatment on fracture incidence in osteoporotic patients. The difficulty in demonstrating the therapeutic effect of CALC on fracture incidence may be the result of the small number of patients and relatively short periods of observation.

2.3. Bisphosphonates and Ca

The bisphosphonates form a new class of drugs that have been developed during the past two decades. Chemically, they are analogs of endogenous pyrophosphate, and possess high-binding affinity for hydroxyapatite crystals. They are poorly absorbed from the intestine (between 1 and 10%), probably because of their low lipophilicity *(39)*, and should not be taken with food *(40)*. The mode of action of these compounds is still not completely elucidated. However, there is a general consensus that the bisphosphonates act by inhibiting the activity of osteoclasts or their precursors *(41)*, resulting in an inhibition of bone remodeling, particularly bone resorption. The skeletal half-life of bisphosphonates is on the order of several years, but this appears to be of little consequence, since the pharmacological effect is of relatively short duration. Several compounds of this family have been used, in clinical practice or research studies, for the prevention of bone loss, e.g., etidronate, clodronate, pamidronate, alendronate, tiludronate, risedronate, ibandronate, and olpadronate, and new ones are in the process of being developed. Data on prevention of bone loss and vertebral fractures are available for etidronate and alendronate.

For etidronate, a first-generation bisphosphonate, the dose that inhibits resorption is very close to that which impairs normal mineralization, when given continuously. This can be avoided by low-dose intermittent therapy, in combination with Ca. The drug is usually given at a dose of 400 mg/d for 2 wk, followed by 500 mg elemental Ca for 11 wk. Ca is always given with etidronate to prevent any impairment of mineralization, and so it is not possible to evaluate the separate effect of Ca and etidronate. This combination increased LS BMD by 2.1% and femoral neck by 1.8%, after 2 yr, in 135 postmenopausal women *(42)*. In a previous study, Harris et al. *(43)* demonstrated an increment in LS BMD of more than 4.0%, and of 2.0% in femoral neck, as well as a decrease in vertebral fracture rate, after 3 yr of treatment. Markers of bone turnover are also influenced by this therapy. Bettica et al. *(44)* showed a decrease in bone resorption markers between 20 and 40% within 2–4 wk of treatment.

Alendronate, a second-generation bisphosphonate, is given orally at a dose of 10 mg/d. Unlike the previous compound, no impairment in bone quality and mineralization has been observed in the long-term, when used continuously *(45)*. Several multicenter studies have evaluated the effect of alendronate in conjunction with Ca vs Ca alone *(46)*. The first one involved 994 postmenopausal women with idiopathic OP, who were randomized to receive 5, 10, or 20 mg alendronate daily, plus a daily supplement of $CaCO_3$ providing 500 mg elemental Ca, or only the Ca supplement, for a period of 3 yr. The largest increase in BMD in the alendronate-treated group was seen in the 10-mg group. The increment was about 8.8% at LS and 5.9% in the femoral neck *(46)*. The control group showed no increase, and thus no loss in BMD. The investigators also examined the effect of alendronate on vertebral and nonvertebral fractures. A reduction in the number of fractures was observed, in addition to a reduction in the number of patients experiencing a fracture at the end of the 3-yr treatment with 10 mg alendronate.

The fracture intervention trial consisted of 2027 women with postmenopausal OP *(47)*. They were randomly assigned to alendronate (initially 5 mg/d), and later increased to 10 mg/d, or placebo. However, total Ca intake in all participants was estimated to be about 1000 mg/d. If this level was not achieved, 500 mg elemental Ca and 250 IU vitamin D was provided. Treatment with alendronate significantly increased bone mass at LS by 6.2%, femoral neck by 4.1%, and total hip by 4.7%, compared to controls. There was a 28% reduction in risk of incident clinical fractures in the treatment group.

Ensrud et al. *(48)* using data from this study, showed that there was a 47% significant reduction in risk of new vertebral fractures in the alendronate group, compared with the control group. The reduction in risk of new vertebral fractures was consistent across fracture-risk categories, including age, BMD, and number of pre-existing vertebral fractures. In another study, 19 centers enrolled 516 postmenopausal women, aged 45–80 yr, with spine BMD 2.5 SD below the mean for premenopausal women, in a 3-yr study. The treatment group received alendronate plus 500 mg elemental Ca as $CaCO_3$; the control group received only the Ca supplement. BMD increased in the treated group by 5.4% LS and 7.4% in femoral neck. Nonsignificant decreases in BMD occurred in the control group (49).

Recently, a meta-analysis (five trials) (50) evaluated the effect of alendronate plus 500 mg Ca in postmenopausal women with LS BMD, 2 SD below the mean, for young adult women. The control group received the same amount of Ca supplement. Once more, the concurrent use of an antiresorptive drug plus Ca was more effective than Ca alone. Indeed, the cumulative incidence of nonvertebral fractures was 12.6% in the Ca group and 9% in the alendronate–Ca group.

The authors found one study in which a single 6-wk course of alendronate therapy was compared to placebo in 65 postmenopausal women, without Ca supplementation (51). Median percent changes in integral BMD were –2.3, +0.7, and +1.2, after treatment with placebo, and 20 and 40 mg alendronate, respectively.

Strong evidence suggests that a combination of bisphosphonates and Ca is beneficial in the prevention of bone loss after the menopause. However, there is scarce documentation in the use of bisphosphonates alone. Because of the small number of patients and the short period of follow-up, it is difficult to arrive to a definitive conclusion in the comparison between the use of bisphosphonates alone and in combination with Ca.

2.4. Vitamin D and Ca

Vitamin D plays a significant role in the prevention of OP, because the active metabolite (1,25-OH_2-D), increases the absorption of Ca through the intestinal mucosa (52) and stimulates bone formation (53). Vitamin D is synthesized in the skin from the precursor 7-dehydrocholesterol, after exposure to ultraviolet radiation. The product of the irradiation is known as cholecalciferol, or vitamin D_3. However, ergocalciferol, or vitamin D_2, is produced by UV irradiation of the plant sterol, ergosterol, and is also used as a vitamin D supplement (54). Several metabolites of cholecalciferol, e.g., calcifediol (25-OH-D), alphacalcidiol (1 α-OH-D), and calcitriol (1,25-OH_2-D), are used as therapies in the prevention of OP. Vitamin D is actively synthesized by sun exposure during the spring and summer seasons, and synthesis decrease during autumn and winter. This variation is especially seen in populations from extreme latitudes, which are deprived of sunlight during several months of the year. Serum levels of vitamin D also differ according to the usual daily intake in different countries.

It has been suggested that up to 50% of all OP patients are Ca deficient. Burnell et al. (55) studied a large cohort of OP women, and detected two chief abnormalities in chemical composition of bone in approx 25% of cases. The irregularities consisted of a decrease in the mineral content of bone (reflecting Ca deficiency) and a decrease in hydroxyproline in bone and in matrix (reflecting increased bone resorption). When women with low mineral content were treated with Ca and vitamin D for 2 yr, there was a 12% increase in BMD. There was also a 5% increment in BMD in the women with normal bone mineral content (56).

Most studies have shown that plasma levels of 25-OH-D decrease with age by about 50% in both men and women (57,58). Blumsohn and Eastell (59) proposed several

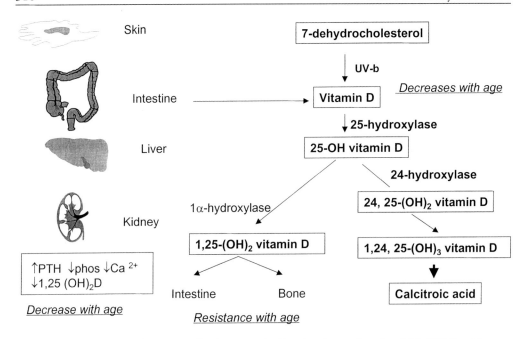

Fig. 3. Possible mechanisms contributing to a decline in plasma levels of 25-OH-D with age. Adapted with permission from Blunshn et al. ref *59*.

possible factors contributing to this decline associated with a decrease in 25-OH-D or 1,25-OH-$_2$-D, and involve different organs, i.e., intestine, skin, liver, and kidneys (*see* Fig. 3). Factors responsible for a decrease in 25-OH-D levels include a decrease in sunshine exposure and/or intestinal vitamin D absorption. Other possible mechanisms may involve decreased dietary intake of vitamin D and reduced capacity of the skin to produce vitamin D in response to UV light. Likely causes for this response include 25-OH-D substrate deficiency and reduced 1α-hydroxylase activity. However, other studies *(60)* did not find this decrease, and assumed that there could be a resistance in vitamin D action in the elderly.

The principal action of vitamin D and its metabolites is to increase intestinal absorption of Ca, and, by that means, to increase serum Ca and suppress PTH, therefore decreasing bone turnover and reducing bone loss. Dawson-Hughes et al. *(61)* examined 246 healthy late-postmenopausal women who consumed a mean 118 IU vitamin D and 800 mg elemental Ca daily. A daily 400 IU dose of supplemental vitamin D prevented the winter decrease in 25-OH-D and the increase in PTH that occurred in the control group.

Several studies have reported the effects of vitamin D intake on bone mass and rate of fractures. In almost every one, the diet was adjusted for a fixed daily amount of Ca or Ca supplements were given in conjunction with vitamin D, and adjusted for serum Ca. The chief reason for this kind of study design probably results from the narrow therapeutic window of the active metabolites of vitamin D. Hypercalcemia is possibly the primary side effect of this therapy, which could lead to impaired renal function or nephrocalcinosis. Consequently the use of these agents demands frequent surveillance of serum and urine Ca.

In a middle-aged population of British women, Khaw et al. *(62)* found a positive relationship between bone mass in the spine and femoral neck and serum 25-OH-D concentrations.

However, the effect of vitamin D on bone mass has been found to differ considerably between studies. Aloia et al. *(63)* studied postmenopausal women, with OP between the ages of 50 and 80 yr, who received 400 IU vitamin D/d and were instructed to maintain an intake of 1000 mg Ca/d. After 24 mo, there was an increase in bone mineral content of the radius, for the vitamin D–Ca group, of 1.26%, compared to a change of –1.63%/yr for the Ca group.

In the study by Chapuy et al. *(64)*, in which 18 mo treatment with 800 IU vitamin D_3 and the equivalent of 1.2 g elemental Ca was compared to placebo (no Ca and no vitamin D) in elderly women living in sheltered accommodation, bone density in the proximal femur showed an increase of 2.7% in the treated group, compared with a decrease of 4.6% in the placebo group. After 18 mo, there was a 43% decrease in the risk in of hip fractures, and a 32% decrease in the risk of all nonvertebral fractures.

Tilyard et al. *(65)* undertook a prospective, randomized 3-yr study with 622 post-menopausal women. They received either 0.5 µg calcitriol or 1000 mg elemental Ca daily. This study was confined to the assessment of new vertebral fractures, and there were no data on BMD. The women who received calcitriol had a significant reduction in the rate of new vertebral fractures during the second and third years of treatment, compared to Ca alone (second year, 9.3 vs 25.0 fractures/100 patient-yr; third year, 9.9 vs 31.5 fractures/100 patient-yr).

Results are still controversial on the effect of vitamin D on fracture rates. In a study with 2578 postmenopausal women in the Netherlands *(66)*, who were treated with vitamin D (400 IU/d) or placebo for 3.5 yr, with no supplemental Ca, the rate of hip fractures in the two groups was similar. Other authors did not find any beneficial effect of vitamin D on fractures *(67,68)*.

In a recent study, late postmenopausal women received either 500 mg elemental Ca plus 700 IU vitamin D_3/d or placebo, for a period of 3 yr. The difference in BMD between the Ca–vitamin D and placebo groups was significant at femoral neck and LS for all 3 yr, but was significant for total body BMD only in the second and third years. However, the incidence of nonvertebral fractures in the treatment group was significantly reduced *(69)*.

Although there is some evidence to suggest that a combination of vitamin D plus Ca may prevent bone loss in postmenopausal women, the data do not permit any conclusion as to the optimum dose or length of administration. Dawson-Hughes et al. *(52)* suggested that in healthy, Ca-supplemented postmenopausal women residing at latitude 42° N, an intake between 200 and 800 IU vitamin D may reduce bone loss, not only from LS, but also from femoral neck. Thus, the value of vitamin D supplementation may depend on latitude, as well as lifestyle.

There is no study that evaluates the bone effects of vitamin D without Ca. However, Heikinheimo et al. *(70)* examined the results of a single annual high-dose intramuscular injection of ergocalciferol, with no Ca supplementation, in two groups of elderly people. The fracture rate was reduced in the vitamin D recipients in females, and especially in the upper limbs and ribs. The rate of fractures in lower limbs did not change in both groups, and no deleterious effects of vitamin D were seen. The results suggested an antifracture effect of vitamin D in this population, which possibly predominated over the patients' Ca status.

3. MECHANISM OF INTERACTION
BETWEEN CA AND ANTIRESORPTIVE THERAPY

The mechanism of action by which Ca seems to interact with antiresorptive drugs appears to be complex. Ca is thought to induce an initial increase in bone density through the closure of remodeling space. However, one might expect that the reduction in remodeling space induced by antiresorptive compounds would prevail over the probably weaker antiresorptive effect of Ca.

Nieves et al. proposed several possible explanations *(25)*. In relation to HRT, additional Ca, superimposed on an estrogen effect, may allow an increase in mineral deposition density (secondary mineralization) of newly formed or even previously formed bone. Consequently, the size of newly formed bone packets or wall width would not be increased, but each packet would be hypermineralized. This could possibly result in apparent increase in bone mass and bone strength.

The synergistic effect cannot be explained as a simple result of filling in of remodeling sites, because, if this was the case, one would expect the results to be achieved mostly in the short term, and only transiently. In other words, once the remodeling sites were filled, one would not expect to see further increases in BMD. However, some of the studies presented in this review were longer than 2 yr, and BMD continue to increase.

4. CONCLUSIONS AND RECOMMENDATIONS

The chapter has displayed evidence suggesting that the effect of supplemental Ca on bone in postmenopausal women is clearly less than seen with antiresorptive drugs (estrogen, bisphosphonates, and CALC). It has also shown evidence indicating a synergetic effect when Ca is associated with either HRT or CALC, and Ca also seems beneficial when given in conjunction with bisphosphonates and vitamin D.

The authors strongly recommend a daily Ca intake between 1000 and 1500 mg/d in postmenopausal women receiving antiresorptive drugs. Ca intake in postmenopausal women is well below this target. The most important source of Ca is milk and other dairy products. It is also possible to reach the recommended level of intake by including one of many Ca supplements as part of the daily Ca intake.

REFERENCES

1. Dawson Hughes B, Dallal GE, Krall EA, Sadowski L, Sahyoun N, Tannenbaum S. A controlled trial of the effect of calcium supplementation on bone density in postmenopausal women. N Engl J Med 1990; 323:878–883.
2. Recker RR. Prevention of osteoporosis: calcium nutrition. Osteoporosis Int 1993; 1(Suppl.):163S–165S.
3. Eastell R, Riggs BL. Vitamin D and osteoporosis. In: Vitamin D. Feldman D, Glorieux FH, Pike JW, eds. London: Academic, 1997:695–711.
4. Heaney RP, Recker RR, Saville PD. Menopausal changes in calcium balance performance. J Lab Clin Med 1978; 92:953–963.
5. NIH Consensus. Optimal calcium intake. JAMA 1994; 272:1942–1948.
6. Carroll MD, Abraham S, Dresser CM. Dietary intake source data: United States, 1976–80. Vital and health statistics. Series 11, No. 231. DHHS Publ. (PHS) 83-1681, 1983.
7. Dawson-Hughes B, Jacques P, Shipp C. Dietary calcium intake and bone loss from the spine in healthy postmenopausal women. Am J Clin Nutr 1987; 46:685–687.
8. Dawson-Hughes B. The role of calcium in the treatment of osteoporosis. In: Osteoporosis. Marcus R, Feldman D, Kelsey J, eds. Academic, London, 1996; 1159–1168.

9. Devine A, Dick M, Heal SJ, Criddle RA, Prince RL. A 4-year follow-up study of the effects of calcium supplementation on bone density in elderly postmenopausal women. Osteoporosis Int 1997; 7:23–28.

10. Recker RR, Hinders S, Davies M, Heaney RP, Stegman MR, Lappe JM, et al. Correcting calcium nutritional deficiency prevents spine fractures in elderly women. J Bone Miner Res 1996; 11: 1961–1966.

11. Nordin C. Calcium and osteoporosis. Nutrition 1997; 13:664–686.

12. Chevalley T, Rizzoli R, Nydegger V, Slosman D, Rapin CH, Michel JP, et al. Effects of calcium supplements on femoral bone mineral density and vertebral fracture rate in vitamin-D-replete elderly women. Osteoporosis Int 1994; 4:245–252.

13. Riggs BL, O'Fallon WM, Muhs J, O'Connor MK, Kumar R, Melton LJ III. Long-term effects of calcium supplementation on serum parathyroid hormone level, bone turnover, and bone loss in elderly women. J Bone Miner Res 1998; 13:168–174.

14. Reid IR, Ames RW, Evans M, Gamble GD, Sharpe S. Effect of calcium supplementation on bone loss in postmenopausal women. N Engl J Med 1993; 328:460–464.

15. Riis B, Thomsen K, Christiansen C. Does calcium supplementation prevent postmenopausal bone loss? N Engl J Med 1987; 316:173–177.

16. Michaelsson K, Holmberg L, Mallmin H. Diet and hip fracture risk: a case-control study. Int J Epidemiol 1995; 24:771.

17. Kamel S, Fardellone P, Meddah B, Lorget-Gondelmann F, Sebert JL, Brazier M. Response of several markers of bone collagen degradation to calcium supplementation in postmenopausal women with low calcium intake. Clin Chem 1998; 44:1437–1442.

18. Dawson-Hughes B. Calcium supplementation and bone loss: a review of controlled clinical trials. Am J Clin Nutr 1991; 54(Suppl.):274S–280S.

19. Kochersberger G, Bales C, Lobaugh B, Lyles KW. Calcium supplementation lowers serum parathyroid hormone levels in elderly subjects. J Geront 1990; 45:M159–M162.

20. McKane WR, Khosla S, Egan KS, Robins SP, Burritt MF, Riggs BL. Role of calcium intake in modulating age-related increases in parathyroid function and bone resorption. J Clin Endocrinol Metab 1996; 81:1699–1703.

21. Pacifici R. Cytokines, estrogen and postmenopausal osteoporosis-the second decade. Endocrinology 1998; 139:2659–2661.

22. Horowitz MC. Cytokines and estrogen in bone: anti-osteoporotic effects. Science 1993; 260:626–627.

23. Hughes DE, Wright KR, Uy HL. Bisphosphonates promote apoptosis in murine osteoclasts in vitro and in vivo. J Bone Miner Res 1995; 10:1478–1487.

24. Shipman CM, Croucher PI, Russell RGG, Helfrich M, Rogers MJ. Bisphosphonates cause apoptosis in human myeloma cells in vitro by inhibiting the mevalonate pathway. Bone 1998; 23:S213.

25. Nieves JW, Komar L, Cosman F, Lindsay R. Calcium potentiates the effect of estrogen and calcitonin on bone mass: review and analysis. Am J Clin Nutr 1998; 67:18–24.

26. Spencer CP, Stevenson JC. Oestrogens and anti-oestrogens for the prevention and treatment of osteoporosis. In: Osteoporosis: Diagnosis and Management. Meunier PJ, ed. Martin Dunitz, London, 1998; 111–122.

27. Recker RR, Saville PD, Heaney RP. Effect of estrogens and calcium carbonate on bone loss in postmenopausal women. Ann Intern Med 1977; 87:649–655.

28. Ettinger B, Genant HK, Cann CE. Postmenopausal bone loss is prevented by treatment with low-dosage estrogen with calcium. Ann Intern Med 1987; 106:40–45.

29. Ettinger B, Genant HK, Steiger P, Madvig P. Low-dosage micronized 17 β estradiol prevents bone loss in postmenopausal women. Am J Obstet Gynecol 1992; 166:479–488.

30. Aloia JF, Vaswani A, Yeh JK, Ross PL, Flaster E, Dilmanian FA. Calcium supplementation with and without hormone replacement therapy to prevent postmenopausal bone loss. Ann Intern Med 1994; 120:97–103.

31. Mizunuma H, Okano H, Soda M, Tokizawa S, Kagami I, Miyamoto S, et al. Calcium supplements increase bone mineral density in women with low serum calcium levels during long-term estrogen therapy. Endocr J 1996; 43:411–415.

32. Haines CJ, Chung KH, Leung PC, Hsu SYC, Leung DH. Calcium supplementation and bone mineral density in postmenopausal women using estrogen replacement therapy. Bone 1995; 16:529–531.

33. Davis JW, Ross PD, Johnson NE, Wasnich RD. Estrogen and calcium supplement use among Japanese-American women: effects upon bone loss when used singly and in combination. Bone 1995; 17:369–373.

34. Singer FR, Melvin KEW, Mills BG. Acute effects of calcitonin on osteoclasts in man. Clin Endocrinol (Oxf) 1976; 5:333–340.

35. Overgaard K. Effect of intranasal salmon calcitonin therapy on bone mass and bone-turnover in early postmenopausal women: a dose-response study. Calcif Tissue Int 1994; 55:82–86.

36. Overgaard K, Hansen MA, Jensen SB, Christiansen C. Effect of salcatonin given intranasally on bone mass and fracture rates in established osteoporosis: a dose-response study. Br Med J 1992; 305:556–561.

37. Thamsborg G, Storm TL, Sykulski R, Brinch E, Nielsen HK, Sorensen OH. Effect of different doses of nasal salmon calcitonin on bone mass. Calcif Tissue Int 1991; 48:302–307.

38. Ellerington MC, Hillard TC, Whitcroft SIJ, Marsh MS, Lees B, Banks LM, et al. Intranasal salmon calcitonin for the prevention and treatment of postmenopausal osteoporosis. Calcif Tissue Int 1996; 59:6–11.

39. Fleisch H, ed. Bisphosphonates in Bone Disease. Parthenon, Carnfurth Lanes, 1997.

40. Eastell R. Treatment of postmenopausal osteoporosis. N Engl J Med 1998; 338:736–746.

41. Hughes DE, MacDonald BR, Russell RGG, Gowen M. Inhibition of osteoclast-like cell formation by bisphosphonates in long-term cultures of human bone marrow. J Clin Invest 1989; 83:1939–1935.

42. Herd RJM, Blake JM, Ryan P, Fogelman I. Regional DXA studies in a double blind placebo controlled trial of cyclical etidronate therapy for the prevention of early post-menopausal bone loss. Bone 1995; 17:611.

43. Harris ST, Watts NB, Jackson RD. Four-year study of intermittent cyclic etidronate treatment of post-menopausal osteoporosis: three years of blinded therapy followed by one year of open therapy. Am J Med 1993; 95:557–567.

44. Bettica P, Bevilaqua M, Vago T, Masino M, Cucinotta E, Norbiato G. Short-term variations in bone remodelling biochemical markers: cyclical etidronate and alendronate effects compared. J Clin Endocrinol Metab 1997; 82:3034–3039.

45. Chavassieux P, Arlot ME, Reda C, Wei L, Yates AJ, Meunier PJ. Histomorphometric assessment of the long-term effects of alendronate on bone quality and remodelling in patients with osteoporosis. J Clin Invest 1997; 100:1475–1480.

46. Liberman UA, Weiss SR, Broll J, Minne HW, Quan H, Bell NH, et al. Effect of oral alendronate on bone mineral density and the incidence of fractures in postmenopausal osteoporosis. N Engl J Med 1995; 333:1437–1443.

47. Black DM, Cummings SR, Karpf DB, Cauley JA, Thompson D, Nevitt MC, et al. Randomised trial of effect of alendronate on risk of fracture in women with existing vertebral fractures. Lancet 1996; 348:1535–1541.

48. Ensrud KE, Black DM, Palermo L, Bauer DC, Barrett-Connor E, Quandt S, et al. Treatment with alendronate prevents fractures in women at higher risk. Arch Intern Med 1997; 157:2617–2624.

49. Devogelaer JP, Broll H, Correa-Rotter R, Cumming DC, Nagant De Deuxchaisnes C, et al. Oral alendronate induces progressive increases in bone mass of the spine, hip, and total body over 3 years in postmenopausal women with osteoporosis. Bone 1996; 18:141–150.

50. Karpf DB, Shapiro DR, Seeman E, Ensrud KE, Johnston CC, Adami S, et al. Prevention of nonvertebral fractures by alendronate. JAMA 1997; 277:1159–1164.

51. Harris ST, Gertz BJ, Genant HK, Eyre DR, Survill TT, Ventura JN, et al. The effect of short-term treatment with alendronate on vertebral density and biochemical markers of bone remodelling in early postmenopausal women. J Clin Endocrinol Metab 1993; 76:1399–1406.

52. Dawson-Hughes B, Harris SS, Krall EA, Dallal GE, Falconer G, Green CL. Rates of bone loss in postmenopausal women randomly assigned to one or two dosages of vitamin D. Am J Clin Nutr 1995; 61:1140–1145.

53. Seino Y, Ishizuka S, Shima M, Tanaka H. Vitamin D in bone formation. Osteoporosis Int 1993; 1(Suppl.):196S–198S.

54. Reid IR. Vitamin D and its metabolites in management of osteoporosis. In: Osteoporosis. Marcus R, Feldman D, Kelsey J, eds. Academic, New York 1996; 1169–1190.

55. Burnell JM, Baylink DJ, Chestnut CH, Mathews MW, Teubner EJ. Bone matrix and mineral abnormalities in postmenopausal osteoporosis. Metabolism 1982; 31:1113–1120.

56. Burnell JM, Baylink DJ, Chestnut CH, Teubner EJ. The role of skeletal calcium deficiency in postmenopausal osteoporosis. Calcif Tissue Int 1986; 38:187–192.

57. Baker MR, Peacock M, Nordin BEC. The decline in vitamin D status with age. Age Ageing 1980; 9:249–252.

58. Lund B, Sorensen OH. Measurement of 25-hydroxyvitamin D in serum and its relation to sunshine, age and vitamin D. Scand J Clin Lab Invest 1979; 39:23–30.

59. Blumsohn A, Eastell R. Age-related factors. In: Osteoporosis. Riggs BL, Melton LJ III, eds. Lippincott-Raven, Philadelphia 1996; 161–182.

60. Francis RM, Peacock M, Taylor GA, Stoner JH, Nordin BEC. Calcium malabsorption in elderly women with vertebral fracture: evidence for resistance to the action of vitamin D metabolites on the bowel. Clin Sci 1984; 66:103–107.

61. Dawson-Hughes B, Dallal GE, Krall EA, Harris S, Sokoll LJ, Falconer G. Effect of vitamin D supplementation on wintertime and overall bone loss in healthy postmenopausal women. Ann Intern Med 1991; 115:505–512.

62. Khaw KT, Sneyd ML, Compston J. Bone density, parathyroid hormone and 25-hydroxyvitamin D concentrations in middle aged women. Br Med J 1992; 305:273–277.

63. Aloia JF, Vaswani A, Yeh JK, Ellis K, Yasumura S, Cohn SH. Calcitriol in the treatment of postmenopausal osteoporosis. Am J Med 1988; 84:401–408.

64. Chapuy MC, Areot M, Duboece F, Brun J, Crouzel B, Arnaud S. Vitamin D_3 and calcium to prevent hip fractures in elderly women. N Engl J Med 1992; 327:1637–1642.

65. Tilyard MW, Spears GFS, Thomson J, Dovey S. Treatment of postmenopausal osteoporosis with calcitriol or calcium. N Engl J Med 1992; 326:357–362.

66. Lips P, Graafmans WC, Ooms ME, Bezemer PD, Bouter LM. Vitamin D supplementation and fracture incidence in elderly persons. Ann Intern Med 1996; 124:400–406.

67. Ott SM, Chestnut CH. Calcitriol treatment is not effective in postmenopausal osteoporosis. Ann Intern Med 1989; 110:267–274.

68. Christiansen C, Christiansen MS, McNair P, Hagen C, Stocklund E, Transbol IB. Prevention of early postmenopausal bone loss: controlled 2-year study in 315 normal females. Eur J Clin Invest 1980; 10:273–279.

69. Dawson-Hughes B, Harris SS, Krall EA, Dallal GE. Effect of calcium and vitamin D supplementation on bone density in men and women 65 years of age or older. N Engl J Med 1997; 337:670–676.

70. Heikinheimo RJ, Inkovaara JA, Harju EJ, Haavisto MV, Kaarela RH, Kataja JM, et al. Annual injection of vitamin D and fractures of aged bones. Calcif Tissue Int 1992; 51:105–110.

VI

CRITICAL ISSUES
FOR THE 21ST CENTURY

19 Preventive Nutrition Issues in Ethnic and Socioeconomic Groups in the United States

Shiriki K. Kumanyika
and Susan M. Krebs-Smith

1. INTRODUCTION

Comparisons of dietary patterns across populations or demographic groups with different disease patterns have provided numerous insights about diet as it relates to disease (1–4). Now that there is substantial consensus about the specific aspects of an optimal diet (5), the social epidemiology of dietary risk factors, within and across populations, becomes an increasingly important focus of such comparisons: How do dietary intakes of various populations adhere to or deviate from guidelines for healthful eating patterns? What factors are influencing current dietary patterns and dietary changes over time? Are there populations or subgroups where improvements in dietary profiles are occurring, or where new patterns of diet-related diseases are emerging?

Within the U.S. population, ethnicity and socioeconomic status (SES) are associated with major health disparities (6,7), and it is critical to examine whether and how dietary changes can help in reducing these disparities. This chapter highlights variation in food and nutrient intakes among U.S. ethnic minority populations and by SES. Issues addressed include the nature of apparent differences in food intake, evidence that these differences have a net impact on nutrient intakes, and dietary quality in relation to dietary guidelines. Whenever possible, data presented are based on recent national or other population-based surveys. The scope of this chapter is limited to data on adults in the U.S. population, although the findings clearly have implications for children who live in the same households.

2. BACKGROUND

2.1. Demographics

In the United States, "minority" populations are those racial or ethnic groups comprising less than 50% of the U.S. population (6). The U.S. Census Bureau approach to racial and ethnic classifications has typically used four "racial" categories (i.e., categories that imply different genetic origins): white or Caucasian, black or African American, American Indian or Alaskan Native, and Asian or Pacific Islander. A recent change in the Asian/Pacific

From: *Primary and Secondary Preventive Nutrition*
Edited by: A. Bendich and R. J. Deckelbaum © Humana Press Inc., Totowa, NJ

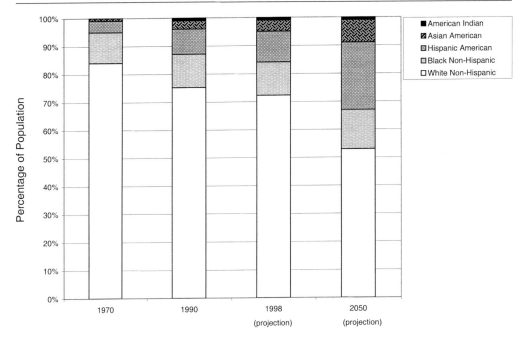

Fig. 1. Racial/ethnic composition of the U.S. population, 1970–2050. Changing America. Indicators of social and economic well-being by race and Hispanic origin. Source: ref. 6.

Islander classification allows for a separate categorization of "Native Hawaiians and Other Pacific Islanders." In addition, one "ethnic" category: "Hispanic" or "Latino," has been used to classify all persons with origins in Spanish-speaking countries, regardless of the racial classification, leading to the five "racial/ethnic" populations shown in Fig. 1 *(6,8)*. As shown in Fig. 1, the proportion of minorities in the U.S. population was estimated at less than 20% in 1970, but had increased to more than 25% by 1998, and will approach 50% by the year 2050.

The five commonly used racial/ethnic classifications are very general with respect to describing subpopulations with different cultural origins and food habits *(8)*. The classification of all persons who do not fit any of the minority classifications as "white" (e.g., persons with origins in various European countries) clearly creates a very diverse category with respect to ethnic origins. Hispanic Americans—projected to be the largest minority group in the U.S. by the year 2005—include Mexican Americans, Puerto Ricans, Cuban Americans, Central Americans, as well as people from Spain. Asian Americans and Pacific Islanders include persons with ancestry from any part of Asia (e.g., including China, Japan, Korea, the Indian subcontinent, and Southeast Asia), along with a small percent (5% of the Asian/Pacific Islander population in 1990) from the Pacific Islands (e.g., Filipinos and Samoans) and Native Hawaiians. American Indians and Alaskan Natives include people from more than 500 different ethnic groups.

The term "ethnic," rather than racial/ethnic, is used here to emphasize that the topic being addressed—dietary patterns—generally relates to the cultural, rather than the presumed genetic, differences among different populations and subpopulations. Moreover, ethnicity is usually based on the individual's self-identification, which also sometimes involves more than one category. In addition to ethnic origins, many demographic factors

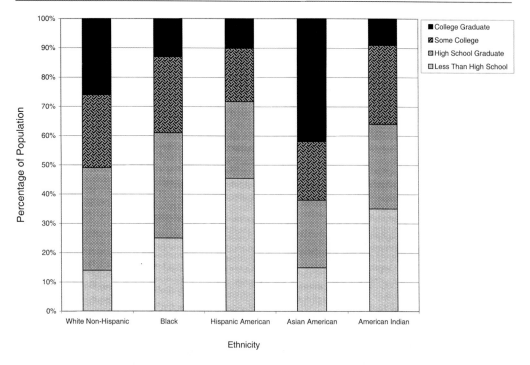

Fig. 2. Educational attainment of U.S. adults, aged 25 yr and over, by ethnicity, 1997. Changing America. Indicators of social and economic well-being by race and Hispanic origin. Source: ref. 6.

that may influence food intake and lifestyle vary within minority populations: region of residence, urban vs rural residence, nativity or duration of residence in the United States, income and wealth, educational attainment, occupation, and household composition (e.g., the percent of single parent families) *(6,8)*. For example, more than half of black non-Hispanics live in the South, and about half of Hispanic Americans, Asian Americans, and American Indians live in the West. Residence in central cities of urban areas is more common among minority populations than among whites, with the exception of American Indians, who are more likely to live outside of metropolitan areas. In addition, segregation (defined here as living in a neighborhood with members of the same ethnic group) is much more common among minorities than among whites. With respect to variation in duration of U.S. residence, in 1997, the percent foreign born was 61% for Asian Americans, 38% for Hispanic Americans, 8% for whites, and 6% for blacks and American Indians *(8)*. More than 50% of American Indians have a spouse of a different ethnic group, but this occurs among only a small percentage of whites and blacks, and among only 15–30% of Hispanic or Asian American men and women.

The generally lower SES of ethnic minority populations is evident from a variety of indicators *(6,8)*. Differences in educational attainment by ethnicity are shown in Fig. 2. White and Asian Americans have the smallest proportion of nonhigh school graduates; Hispanic Americans and American Indians have the highest; Asian Americans have the highest percent of college graduates. The Asian American population also has a higher median income, compared to all other ethnic groups, but is extremely diverse with respect to SES. As shown in Fig. 3, all minority populations, including Asian Americans, have

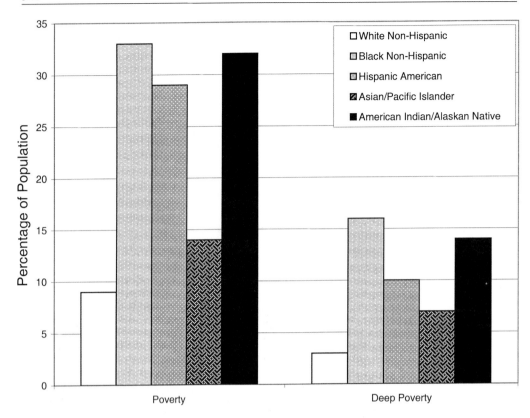

Fig. 3. Percentage of U.S. adults in poverty and deep poverty, by ethnicity, 1991. "Poverty" refers to household income at or below the federal poverty threshold for a given household size. "Deep poverty" refers to household income at or below 50% of the federal poverty threshold. Source: ref. *8*.

a higher percent of persons living in poverty, compared to whites. Beyond the superficial indicators of current income, discretionary income and economic security are also worse among minority populations. Minority populations have a higher percent of persons whose housing costs are more than one-third of their income *(8)*. Net worth, a measure of net savings or accumulated or inherited assets, of blacks and Hispanic Americans is only one-tenth that of whites: a median of $44,000 among white households, and $3800 and $5500, respectively, in black and Hispanic American households *(8)*. For female-headed households, median net worth is even more disparate: $25,000 for whites and $700 and $500, respectively, for blacks and Hispanic Americans.

2.2. Health Status

The major markers of diet-related health risks in U.S. ethnic minority and low SES populations are the disproportionate occurrence of obesity, diabetes, cardiovascular disease (CVD) and certain cancers (e.g., lung, prostate, cervical, gallbladder, stomach, and liver cancers) *(9–17)*. Within minority populations, as among whites, CVD and cancer are among the two or three leading causes of death *(18)*. As shown in Fig. 4, blacks have overall higher mortality from CVD and cancer than whites and other minority populations *(6)*. Among the other ethnic groups, the aggregate may hide subpopulations with very high risks. For example, unusually high CVD mortality (twice as high as the

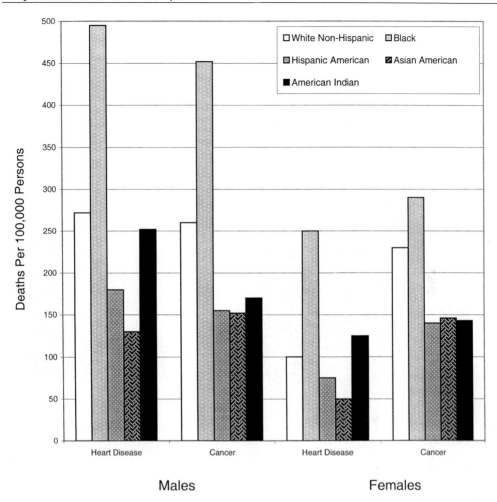

Fig. 4. U.S. death rates by cause and ethnicity, for persons aged 45 to 65 yr, 1995. Changing America. Indicators of social and economic well-being by race and Hispanic origin. Rates are age-adjusted. Source: ref. *6.*

U.S. average) has been observed among 45–64-yr-old American Indians in North Dakota (ND) and South Dakota (SD); CVD mortality in this age group was close to the U.S. average for Indians in Oklahoma (OK) and Arizona (AZ) *(19)*. Minority populations generally have higher rates of diabetes than whites, and all except Asian Americans have a higher prevalence of obesity *(11,14)*.

Although reducing health disparities between ethnic minorities and whites has been a focus of the U.S. Public Health Service since 1985 *(20)*, the additional importance of disparities defined by SES has received increasing attention *(7)*. Chronic disease death rates among those with less than a high school education are more than double the rates for those with 13 or more years of education: 531 vs 212/100,000, respectively, among men; and 318 vs 148/100,000, respectively, for women *(7)*. The gradient of diabetes mortality on SES gives a similar picture. The 1979–1989 average annual diabetes mortality, among men aged 45 yr and older, was 21/100,000 among those with annual incomes of $25,000 and above, compared with 55/100,000 among those with annual incomes

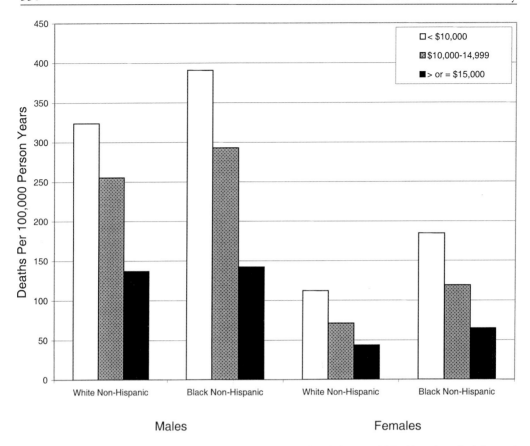

Fig. 5. Average annual heart-disease mortality among U.S. adults, aged 25–64 yr, by ethnicity and income, 1979–1989. Rates are age-adjusted. Source: ref. *7.*

below $10,000. For women, the rates in high- and low-income groups were 14/100,000 and 43/100,000, respectively. Figure 5 shows the income gradient in heart disease mortality (1979–1989 average annual rates) separately, for blacks and whites. Although there is some overlap between the effects of ethnicity and SES on the health status of minority populations, not all ethnic disparities are readily explained by adjustment for, or stratification on, conventional SES variables, such as income or education *(7,21).* Whether the residual differences can be explained on the basis of a more in-depth consideration of demographic or SES differences, or are attributable to cultural factors that may be present regardless of demographic or SES variation, has not been adequately studied.

SES gradients in risk factors, such as current cigarette smoking and sedentary behavior, are parallel to gradients in chronic disease outcomes, i.e., more common in the lower SES strata (Table 1). Variation in levels of overweight or obesity with SES are less consistent *(22),* and differs for men and women. The relationship between obesity and SES tends to be inverse in women, but is sometimes not present in men, or shows increasing obesity with increasing income. In addition, although not directly observable in cross-sectional data, the association of SES with weight status also differs across generations, as economic and societal conditions change *(11,23).* Obesity tends to affect the affluent in poor societies, e.g., as they are able to avoid undernutrition and wasting diseases.

Table 1

Prevalence of Cigarette Smoking, Overweight, and Sedentary Behavior Among U.S. Adult Males and Females, by Ethnicity and Income

Income[a] and ethnicity	Cigarette smoking[b]	Overweight[c] % ± SE	Sedentary behavior[d]
Males			
Poor			
White non-Hispanic	42.3 ± 3.5	26.8 ± 3.2	33.7 ± 2.1
Black non-Hispanic	41.3 ± 4.4	29.4 ± 1.8	35.0 ± 3.4
Hispanic Americans[e]	26.3 ± 3.3	36.2 ± 1.8	46.7 ± 5.0
Near poor			
White non-Hispanic	37.5 ± 2.0	38.7 ± 2.7	29.1 ± 1.7
Black non-Hispanic	40.1 ± 4.5	31.4 ± 2.1	29.5 ± 3.2
Hispanic Americans[e]	19.7 ± 2.5	40.8 ± 2.0	42.4 ± 3.9
Middle income[f]			
White non-Hispanic	24.6 ± 0.9	33.3 ± 1.3	20.1 ± 0.8
Black non-Hispanic	20.9 ± 2.6	38.6 ± 1.7	23.2 ± 2.3
Hispanic Americans[e]	16.3 ± 2.0	38.2 ± 2.2	23.3 ± 3.2
High income			
White non-Hispanic	—[f]	—[f]	13.1 ± 0.9
Black non-Hispanic	—[f]	—[f]	11.2 ± 3.0
Hispanic Americans[e]	—[f]	—[f]	19.1 ± 5.3
Females			
Poor			
White non-Hispanic	38.6 ± 2.5	42.0 ± 3.2	35.5 ± 1.7
Black non-Hispanic	29.3 ± 2.7	55.0 ± 2.3	39.0 ± 2.5
Hispanic Americans[e]	16.6 ± 2.4	54.9 ± 2.4	47.8 ± 2.8
Near poor			
White non-Hispanic	31.6 ± 1.7	36.6 ± 2.4	30.6 ± 1.2
Black non-Hispanic	24.9 ± 3.0	51.0 ± 1.9	36.4 ± 2.6
Hispanic Americans[e]	14.7 ± 1.9	48.7 ± 2.2	45.3 ± 4.5
Middle income[f]			
White non-Hispanic	22.2 ± 0.8	30.0 ± 1.2	22.6 ± 0.8
Black non-Hispanic	15.7 ± 2.0	52.4 ± 2.4	32.6 ± 2.1
Hispanic Americans[e]	13.9 ± 1.8	45.3 ± 2.2	32.2 ± 3.0
High income			
White non-Hispanic	—[f]	—[f]	17.1 ± 1.0
Black non-Hispanic	—[f]	—[f]	24.7 ± 4.0
Hispanic Americans[e]	—[f]	—[f]	21.1 ± 4.3

All percentages are age-adjusted.

[a]Income categories defined as follows: poor, below federal poverty level; near poor, between 100 and 199% of federal poverty level; middle income, at least 200% of the federal poverty level, but less than $50,000; high income, at least $50,000.

[b]Data are for adults age 18 yr and over. 1995 prevalence of current smokers, which includes persons who smoke only on "some days."

[c]Data are for persons aged 20 yr and over. 1988–1994 prevalence of overweight, defined as body mass index ≥ 27.8 for men and ≥ 27.3 for women. Pregnant women are excluded.

[d]Data are for persons aged 18 yr and over. 1991 prevalence of sedentary behavior, defined as no self-reported leisure time physical activity during the past 2 wk.

[e]"Hispanic American" represents only Mexican American in the data on overweight.

[f]For data on cigarette smoking and overweight, the figures for middle income represent both middle- and high-income groups.

Source: ref. 7.

In contrast, obesity tends to affect the poor in affluent societies, because they have more lifestyle constraints that render them vulnerable to the obesity-promoting forces in the environment *(11,23,24)*. As described in the next subheading, data for U.S. minority populations may reflect a mixture of such effects.

2.3. Changing Patterns of Diet-Related Risks

Dissimilarities in health profiles of ethnic groups reflect differences in both current and past exposures, and in the trajectories of both risk development and risk reduction *(25,26)*. Therefore, current data indicating low risk in minority relative to white populations (e.g., as in Fig. 4 for American Indians, Asian Americans, and Hispanic Americans) cannot necessarily be interpreted as evidence that these populations will always have lower risk. In fact, because of social and economic transitions, minority populations (and some low SES white populations) may show stable or increasing morbidity or mortality rates from chronic diseases, while rates are decreasing among whites in the majority U.S. population. Crossovers have been observed, in which, over time, a once lower-risk group becomes a higher-risk group *(25)*.

The concept of the epidemiologic transition is highly relevant to an understanding of how the dietary changes of different ethnic or SES groups influence current and future disease risks, and why different approaches to prevention may be needed in different populations *(27)*. Populations in transition, from economic circumstances in which food supplies, especially animal products, have been limited, and in which obligatory daily physical activity has been high, tend to show relatively rapid development of obesity when economic conditions improve. Key features of improved economic conditions are increased and more consistent availability of food, and changes in the type of food available (e.g., more processed and refined-carbohydrate food) and progressive decreases in obligatory physical activity (e.g., activity needed to obtain food, perform work, or for transportation) *(23,27)*. Ironically, perhaps, the comfortable lifestyle characterized by overconsumption and sedentariness (e.g., the "all-you-can-eat/why-walk-when-you-can-ride?" syndrome) is symbolic of high social status, and may be actively sought out by the upwardly mobile, but, among those who have attained high social status, these behaviors have been identified as undesirable and unhealthy. Nevertheless, even in societies or social strata in which the consequences of overconsumption and sedentariness are recognized, the culture of voluntary risk-reduction behaviors, such as deliberate avoidance of high-fat foods or adoption of leisure time physical activity that has no function other than health maintenance, develops slowly and variably, over generations *(25,26)*. Among some ethnic groups, the effects of the time lag before protective lifestyle behaviors become established may be offset by the persistence of certain lower-risk traditional practices, such as continued high consumption of plant-based staple foods, or by culturally influenced resistance to the adoption of adverse behaviors, such as smoking or alcohol abuse.

2.4. Dietary Factors as Mediators of Ethnic or SES Effects on Health

Although the revolution in the ability to identify genes is occurring now, it is unlikely that identifying or manipulating genes alone can stem the tide of chronic diseases. Dietary and other environmental factors explain more of the variation between populations in chronic disease patterns among racial or ethnic groups than do genetic differences *(1,2,23)*. The genetic similarities among racial or ethnic groups are greater than the genetic differences *(28)*. In addition, genetic predisposition may be a necessary condition for the expression of chronic diseases, but is not a sufficient one. Although the genetic predisposition to chronic disease has changed little in recent history, there have been dramatic upward trends in the prevalence of these diseases in parallel with environmental and lifestyle changes. As summarized by Davies: "It is reasonable to consider patients as individuals of the species Homo sapiens sapiens, whose genetic make-up is that of hunter-gatherers, but who have been transposed into the modern 20th century environment" *(29)*.

Dietary risks related to ethnicity and SES may be mediated through cultural or economic factors that influence individual food selection, food preparation practices, and/or activity patterns, and by social structure factors that influence the context for food choices and activity patterns (e.g., targeted food and beverage advertising and marketing, and neighborhood differences in food availability and food prices) *(30–33)*. By definition, SES variation in diet-related disease risks is environmentally mediated and, although not entirely under the control of the individual, potentially modifiable by some type of behavioral or social intervention.

3. FOOD AND NUTRIENT INTAKES AMONG ETHNIC AND SES GROUPS

3.1. Data Sources

Data on food and nutrient intakes are obtained from surveys of individuals. These surveys principally use 24-h recalls, in which respondents are asked to recount the foods they ate on the previous day, as the primary method of gathering such information. Among the major surveys in the U.S. National Nutrition Monitoring and Related Research Program (NNMRRP) are the Third National Health and Nutrition Examination Survey (NHANES III) and Hispanic Health and Nutrition Examination Survey (HHANES), conducted by the Department of Health and Human Services National Center for Health Statistics (DHHS, NCHS), and the 1994–1996 Continuing Surveys of Food Intakes by Individuals (CSFII), conducted by the U.S. Department of Agriculture (USDA). The dates covered, populations studied, and data collected in each are summarized in Table 2.

Other than the HHANES, the surveys in the NNMRRP were designed primarily to provide nationally representative estimates, and therefore are limited in their ability to provide useful data regarding selected subgroups. The proportions of many minority groups within the general population are so small that drawing a sufficient number of sample persons from each of these groups, in order to make valid estimates, is difficult, without using purposeful sampling. Some of the surveys have included oversamples of blacks, Hispanic Americans, and/or persons from low-income households, but not of other groups. The HHANES was designed to provide representative samples of three different Hispanic American groups in specific geographic pockets of the country where their numbers are concentrated: Mexican Americans in the Southwest, Puerto Ricans in metropolitan New York City, and Cuban Americans in Dade County, FL.

Data from food consumption surveys are subject to the limitations of reporting. Subjects are asked to provide detailed information about the quantities and types of foods eaten, which is a tedious task that requires a basic level of literacy and other cognitive skills. If there is differential reporting bias among the segments of the population under study, then comparisons will be affected accordingly. One source of such bias is

Table 2
Selected U.S. Surveys of Food and Nutrient Consumption

Survey	Sponsoring agency (department)	Date	Population	Data collected
Hispanic Health and Nutrition Examination Survey (HHANES)	NCHS[a] (DHHS)	1982–1984	Civilian, noninstitutionalized Mexican Americans in five Southwestern states, Cuban Americans in Dade County, FL, and Puerto Ricans in metropolitan New York City aged 6 mo–74 yr	Dietary intake (one 24-h recall). socioeconomic and demographic information, biochemical analyses of blood and urine, physical examination, and body measurements.
Third National Health and Nutrition Examination Survey (NHANES III)	NCHS[a] (DHHS)	1988–1991	Civilian, noninstitutionalized population 2 mo of age and older. Oversampling of Black non-Hispanics and Mexican Americans, children < 6 yr of age, and adults aged ≥ 60 yr.	Dietary intake (one 24-h recall and one food frequency questionnaire), socioeconomic and demographic information, biochemical analyses of blood and urine, physical examination, body measurements, blood pressure measurements, bone densitometry, dietary and health behaviors, and health conditions. Two additional 24-h recalls for participants aged ≥50 yr.
Continuing Survey of Food Intakes by Individuals (CSFII)	ARS[b] (USDA)	1994–1996	Individuals of all ages in households in the 48 conterminous States. The survey was composed of two separate samples: households with incomes at any level (basic sample) and households with income ≤130% of the poverty thresholds (low-income sample).	Dietary intake (two nonconsecutive 24-h recalls), socioeconomic and demographic information. Intakes available for 28 nutrients and food components and in terms of servings from food guide pyramid groups.

[a]National Center for Health Statistics, U.S. Department of Health and Human Services.
[b]Agriculture Research Service, U.S. Department of Agriculture.
Source: ref. *13*.

underreporting of food intakes, which can be substantial when using 24-h recalls *(34,35)*. More recent surveys are employing methods to correct for this, but studies suggest that certain subgroups, including women, black non-Hispanics, persons from low-income households, and those with less education, are more likely to underreport than are other groups *(35)*.

Results obtained are also affected by the nutrient databases used to translate foods reported into data on nutrients obtained from those foods. If the databases used are not sufficiently attuned to cultural variations in the makeup of foods, resulting nutrient values may not reflect the actual foods eaten. For example, a burrito prepared by an immigrant from Mexico may have different proportions of meat, beans, cheese, and so on, than the Americanized version available in fast food restaurants. Efforts are being made to allow for specific changes to default characterizations of different foods, through the use of recipe-modification databases *(36)*.

3.2. Food and Nutrient Intake Variables

With the above caveats in mind, food and nutrient intakes can be examined in a number of ways. Foods reported in a survey can be grouped with like foods, to summarize intakes, but the fact that some foods are reported as individual items and others as mixtures, such as bread consumed separately and bread consumed as part of a sandwich, may lead to misinterpretation. Another method, developed recently, disaggregates the components of food mixtures, combines them with similar items, and summarizes food intakes in terms of servings of the Food Guide Pyramid groups *(36)*. The advantages of this method are that intakes are directly comparable to the recommendations in current food guidance, and that all fruits, vegetables, and so on, are accounted for in their appropriate groups.

Nutrient intakes, derived by assigning a specific nutrient profile to each food reported in a survey and, summing these across all foods for each person, can be compared in terms of absolute intakes, nutrient density, or relative to current recommendations. Absolute intakes are the total nutrient intakes, reported on a per day basis, and they can be compared to recommendations such as the Recommended Dietary Allowances (RDAs) *(37)*. Nutrient densities are intakes expressed on a per-1000-kcal basis; because they control for the total energy consumed, they give a sense of the qualitative differences in diets among various groups. Nutrient densities from the energy-yielding macronutrients can be expressed another way, as the percentage of energy from the macronutrients. This allows comparisons with recommendations for total fat and the various fatty acids, which are often given in terms of percentages of energy.

3.3. Dietary Pattern Indices

Variables that summarize the overall dietary pattern, such as the USDA Healthy Eating Index (HEI) *(38)*, have also been created. Such indices convert the multidimensional nature of diet into a single scale, in order to simplify dietary comparisons among subpopulations. Although summary indices can mask differences regarding certain aspects of the diet, they are useful in evaluating the overall dietary quality of one group relative to another. Examination of component scores for specific food groups and other aspects of the diet is helpful for obtaining insights into differences in dietary intake across population groups with similar overall scores, and for identifying factors that contribute to particularly low or high scores on the overall index.

Table 3
Components of the Healthy Eating Index and Scoring System

Component	Criteria for maximum score of 10[a]	Criteria for minimum score of 0[a]
Grain consumption	6–11 servings[b]	0 servings
Vegetable consumption	3–5 servings[b]	0 servings
Fruit consumption	2–4 servings[b]	0 servings
Milk consumption	2–3 servings[b]	0 servings
Meat consumption	2–3 servings[b]	0 servings
Total fat intake	30% or less energy	45% or more energy
Saturated fat intake	Less than 10% energy	15% or more energy
Cholesterol intake	300 mg or less	450 mg or more
Sodium intake	2400 mg or less	4800 mg or more
Food variety	8 or more different items in a day	3 or fewer different items in a day

[a]People with consumption or intakes between the maximum and minimum ranges or amounts were assigned scores proportionately.
[b]Number of servings depends on recommended energy allowance for all groups except milk consumption, which depends on age and gender. All amounts are on a per day basis. Source: ref. *38*.

The HEI was developed by the USDA to assess diet quality relative to the Dietary Guidelines for Americans. It is composed of 10 components (Table 3), each evaluating a different aspect of diet: grains, vegetables, fruits, milk, and meat intakes; fat and saturated fat intakes as a percentage of energy; cholesterol and sodium intakes; and dietary variety. Each of the components has a maximum score of 10, indicating complete compliance with recommendations, for a total possible index score of 100.

3.4. Food and Nutrient Intakes of White Non-Hispanics, Blacks, and Mexican Americans

The following review examines selected aspects of food and nutrient intakes among three ethnic groups for which there are sufficient samples to make such estimates (black non-Hispanics, white non-Hispanics, and Mexican Americans), using the most recent survey data available: the 1994–1996 CSFII *(36)*. One-d dietary recall data are weighted to adjust for differential rates of selection and nonresponse, and to calibrate the sample to match a range of characteristics in the population. Thus, the age distribution of each ethnic group is not necessarily the same as that of other ethnic groups. SUDAAN, statistical software designed to account for the complex sample in estimating the standard errors, was used *(39)*. Results are presented in terms of absolute levels of nutrients, nutrient densities, and pyramid food group servings.

3.4.1. NUTRIENT INTAKES

Table 4 shows the mean nutrient and food intakes for black non-Hispanic, white non-Hispanic, and Mexican American males and females aged 20 yr and older. Reported energy intakes were not substantially different among the ethnic groups for men or women. However, as indicated previously, real differences may be masked if there is a differential level of underreporting among the groups.

The Dietary Guidelines for Americans suggest limiting total fat intakes to 30% or less of energy, and saturated fat intakes to less than 10% *(40)*. Mean intakes for none of the groups met these criteria. The guidelines also recommend that daily average cholesterol

Table 4
Food and Nutrient Intakes of Male and Female Adults, by Ethnicity, 1994–1996

Nutrient/food	Males (20 yr and older)			Females (20 yr and older)		
	White non-Hispanic (n = 3930)	Black non-Hispanic (n = 500)	Mexican American (n = 213)	White non-Hispanic (n = 3619)	Black non-Hispanic (n = 605)	Mexican American (n = 192)
	Mean kcal ± SE, 1 d					
Energy	2472 ± 30	2414 ± 138	2475 ± 104	1649 ± 13	1630 ± 29	1588 ± 44
	Mean g ± SE, 1 d					
Protein	94.6 ± 1.2	94.5 ± 4.0	95.8 ± 4.8	62.7 ± 0.5	63.3 ± 1.3	63.1 ± 1.8
Total fat	93.4 ± 1.4	96.5 ± 6.2	91.6 ± 4.1	60.4 ± 0.7	62.9 ± 1.5	60.0 ± 2.3
Saturated fatty acids	31.7 ± 0.6	32.3 ± 2.9	30.2 ± 1.6	20.1 ± 0.2	20.5 ± 0.5	20.0 ± 0.8
Monounsaturated fatty acids	36.1 ± 0.5	37.8 ± 2.1	35.2 ± 1.7	22.9 ± 0.3	24.5 ± 0.6	23.0 ± 1.0
Polyunsaturated fatty acids	18.4 ± 0.2	18.8 ± 1.1	18.8 ± 0.8	12.8 ± 0.2	12.9 ± 0.5	12.0 ± 0.6
Total carbohydrate	300.5 ± 3.9	284.3 ± 18.0	309.4 ± 13.7	212.9 ± 1.8	201.9 ± 4.6	203.7 ± 6.0
Dietary fiber	18.8 ± 0.3	15.8 ± 0.5	23.7 ± 1.2	14.2 ± 0.2	11.3 ± 0.4	15.1 ± 0.7
	Mean % kcal ± SE, 1 d					
Protein	15.8 ± 0.1	16.3 ± 0.3	15.6 ± 0.2	15.7 ± 0.1	15.8 ± 0.3	16.5 ± 0.4
Total fat	33.5 ± 0.2	34.4 ± 0.5	32.4 ± 0.6	32.3 ± 0.2	34.1 ± 0.5	33.5 ± 0.6
Saturated fatty acids	11.3 ± 0.1	11.3 ± 0.2	10.6 ± 0.3	10.8 ± 0.1	11.1 ± 0.2	11.2 ± 0.3
Monounsaturated fatty acids	12.9 ± 0.1	13.5 ± 0.3	12.4 ± 0.3	12.2 ± 0.1	13.2 ± 0.2	12.8 ± 0.2
Polyunsaturated fatty acids	6.6 ± 0.1	6.8 ± 0.2	6.6 ± 0.2	6.8 ± 0.1	7.0 ± 0.2	6.6 ± 0.2
Total carbohydrate	49.2 ± 0.2	48.4 ± 0.8	51.0 ± 0.9	52.1 ± 0.2	50.3 ± 0.6	51.4 ± 0.8
Alcohol	2.8 ± 0.2	1.9 ± 0.3	2.2 ± 0.3	1.6 ± 0.1	0.9 ± 0.2	0.2 ± 0.1

(continued)

Table 4 (continued)

Nutrient/food	Males (20 yr and older)			Females (20 yr and older)		
	White non-Hispanic (n = 3930)	Black non-Hispanic (n = 500)	Mexican American (n = 213)	White non-Hispanic (n = 3619)	Black non-Hispanic (n = 605)	Mexican American (n = 192)
	Mean $\mu g \pm SE$, 1 d					
Vitamin A (retinol equivalents)	1147 ± 25	1263 ± 262	865 ± 121	944 ± 23	867 ± 78	874 ± 104
Carotenes (retinol equivalents)	552 ± 20	485 ± 30	454 ± 70	508 ± 18	446 ± 30	506 ± 92
Folate	307 ± 5	266 ± 11	324 ± 25	229 ± 3	195 ± 9	241 ± 15
Vitamin B_{12}	6.54 ± 0.32	9.82 ± 2.76	5.07 ± 0.46	4.14 ± 0.14	4.53 ± 0.63	3.99 ± 0.38
	Mean $mg \pm SE$, 1 d					
Vitamin E (α-tocopherol equivalents)	10.1 ± 0.2	9.1 ± 0.4	10.1 ± 0.7	7.2 ± 0.1	6.3 ± 0.2	7.9 ± 0.9
Vitamin C	106 ± 2	118 ± 12	127 ± 11	87 ± 2	97 ± 6	102 ± 10
Thiamin	1.92 ± 0.02	1.79 ± 0.09	1.83 ± 0.11	1.34 ± 0.01	1.21 ± 0.03	1.31 ± 0.07
Riboflavin	2.29 ± 0.03	2.06 ± 0.13	2.06 ± 0.15	1.62 ± 0.02	1.39 ± 0.05	1.54 ± 0.09
Niacin	28.3 ± 0.4	25.7 ± 0.8	25.0 ± 1.4	18.9 ± 0.2	18.0 ± 0.4	17.1 ± 1.0
Vitamin B_6	2.19 ± 0.03	2.03 ± 0.06	2.19 ± 0.14	1.51 ± 0.02	1.42 ± 0.05	1.62 ± 0.09
Calcium	924 ± 15	706 ± 59	890 ± 58	668 ± 8	525 ± 20	621 ± 25
Phosphorus	1499 ± 19	1345 ± 83	1527 ± 76	1037 ± 8	904 ± 30	1017 ± 28
Magnesium	335 ± 5	274 ± 11	337 ± 18	239 ± 2	194 ± 6	225 ± 7
Iron	18.7 ± 0.3	18.1 ± 1.5	17.5 ± 1.0	13.2 ± 0.1	11.4 ± 0.3	12.9 ± 0.9
Zinc	14.0 ± 0.2	13.8 ± 1.0	13.6 ± 0.8	9.2 ± 0.1	8.6 ± 0.2	10.0 ± 0.6
Copper	1.5 ± 0.0	1.4 ± 0.1	1.5 ± 0.1	1.1 ± 0.0	0.9 ± 0.0	1.0 ± 0.0
Sodium	4129 ± 57	3889 ± 154	3834 ± 189	2764 ± 29	2667 ± 69	2541 ± 87
Potassium	3262 ± 42	2886 ± 151	3248 ± 172	2371 ± 18	2009 ± 51	2281 ± 82
Cholesterol	319 ± 5	395 ± 21	378 ± 28	204 ± 3	246 ± 11	256 ± 19

Mean servings ± SE, 1 d

Total grain products	8.1 ± 0.1	7.0 ± 0.4	8.3 ± 0.4	5.7 ± 0.1	4.9 ± 0.1	5.2 ± 0.2
Whole grains	1.3 ± 0.1	0.8 ± 0.1	0.7 ± 0.2	1.0 ± 0.0	0.6 ± 0.1	0.7 ± 0.1
Total vegetables	4.3 ± 0.1	3.9 ± 0.2	4.9 ± 0.3	3.1 ± 0.0	2.9 ± 0.1	3.3 ± 0.2
Green/yellow	0.4 ± 0.0	0.5 ± 0.1	0.2 ± 0.0	0.4 ± 0.0	0.5 ± 0.0	0.4 ± 0.1
White potatoes	1.5 ± 0.2	1.5 ± 0.2	1.3 ± 0.2	0.8 ± 0.0	0.9 ± 0.1	0.9 ± 0.1
Dried beans/peas	0.2 ± 0.0	0.3 ± 0.1	1.0 ± 0.1	0.1 ± 0.0	0.1 ± 0.0	0.4 ± 0.1
Other starchy	0.3 ± 0.0	0.3 ± 0.1	0.1 ± 0.0	0.2 ± 0.0	0.1 ± 0.0	0.1 ± 0.0
Tomatoes	0.6 ± 0.0	0.5 ± 0.0	0.8 ± 0.1	0.4 ± 0.0	0.2 ± 0.0	0.5 ± 0.0
Other vegetables	1.3 ± 0.0	0.9 ± 0.1	1.5 ± 0.1	1.2 ± 0.0	0.4 ± 0.0	0.5 ± 0.0
Fruits	1.5 ± 0.0	1.4 ± 0.1	1.7 ± 0.3	1.5 ± 0.0	0.8 ± 0.0	1.0 ± 0.1
Milk, cheese or yogurt	1.7 ± 0.0	1.0 ± 0.1	1.4 ± 0.1	1.2 ± 0.0	1.3 ± 0.1	1.6 ± 0.2
Meat/meat alternates	6.2 ± 0.1	7.3 ± 0.2	6.2 ± 0.3	3.7 ± 0.0	0.8 ± 0.1	1.1 ± 0.1
Meat, poultry, fish	5.6 ± 0.1	6.6 ± 0.2	5.4 ± 0.3	3.3 ± 0.0	4.7 ± 0.2	4.0 ± 0.1
						3.5 ± 0.1

Mean % of kcal ± SE, 1 d

Discretionary fat	25.1 ± 0.2	25.3 ± 0.5	23.8 ± 0.5	24.6 ± 0.2	25.4 ± 0.4	24.8 ± 0.6
Added sugars	14.4 ± 0.2	16.4 ± 0.9	15.1 ± 0.7	15.0 ± 0.3	17.9 ± 0.5	14.2 ± 0.7

Source: ref. 36.

intakes be kept to under 300 mg. Mean intakes for females among all groups examined were below this level; intakes for all groups of males, especially black non-Hispanics, were above.

Fiber and the antioxidants, carotene and vitamin C, are supplied principally by plant-based foods, and are thought to be possibly protective against cancer *(2)*. Fiber intakes for only Mexican American adult males met the 20–30 gm recommended by the National Cancer Institute *(41)*. In general, black non-Hispanics consumed less fiber than either of the other ethnic groups, and females consumed less than males, though the gender differences nearly disappeared when examined as nutrient density (data not shown). Intakes of carotene, which is concentrated in relatively few foods, varied widely, but seemed to be generally higher for white non-Hispanics than for other groups; vitamin C intakes were generally lower.

A recent report on Dietary Reference Intakes for folate and other B-vitamins recommended intakes of 400 mcg/d of folacin, for all adults, with additional allowances for pregnant and lactating women *(42)*. Mean intakes by all groups fell considerably short of this and, among the ethnic groups studied, were lowest for black non-Hispanics. Although intakes below the recommendation do not necessarily indicate a deficiency, the likelihood of deficiency increases as intakes move further from recommendations. Mean intakes of the B-vitamins, other than folate, were closer to recommendations, with the exception of B_{12}, and did not vary among the ethnic groups as widely.

Recent guidelines for adequate intakes of calcium (Ca) are 1000–1200 mg/d *(43)*, but intakes among all groups, especially women, were considerably lower. Women of all ethnic groups have more Ca-dense diets than do men (data not shown), but because of their generally lower energy intakes, they consume less Ca overall. Intakes were especially low for black non-Hispanics, compared to other groups. Iron is another mineral for which women's intakes, especially black women's, are below their recommendation (15 mg) *(37)*.

The minimal dietary requirement for sodium (Na) is very small, about 500 mg for adults, and high intakes may lead to hypertension among susceptible individuals. For this reason, the Dietary Guidelines suggest that intakes be limited to 2400 mg or less *(40)*. Average intakes shown in Table 4, which reflect only the Na occurring naturally in foods and that added in food preparation (i.e., not salt added at the table), are well above that level for all groups.

3.4.2. FOOD GROUP INTAKES

It is a maxim within the nutrition community that dietary advice should be based on the fact that "people eat foods, not nutrients." For this reason, the nutrition principles in the Dietary Guidelines were translated into suggestions regarding what foods to eat in the Food Guide Pyramid *(44)*. This publication provides recommended intakes for each of five major food groups, and for the pyramid tip, which includes discretionary fats, added sugars, and alcohol; recommendations are given as a range of servings to cover the energy needs in the population and differing nutrient needs based on age and physiological status.

The pyramid recommends 6–11 servings of grains daily, and suggests that several of those servings be whole grain. Women's grain intakes fell short of even the minimum recommendation; men's intakes averaged around 7–8 servings, but a more appropriate level would have been closer to 11, considering their relatively high energy intakes. Black non-Hispanics had the lowest intakes of grains, among men and women. None of the groups had whole grain intakes that averaged close to several per day; white non-Hispanics, with the highest intakes, averaged just over one serving.

The recommended range of servings for vegetables is 3–5/d, including several servings per week of both dark green vegetables and dried beans and peas. Total intakes were generally in the recommended range; black non-Hispanics had slightly higher intakes of green and yellow vegetables; Mexican Americans had greater intakes of tomatoes and much higher intakes of dried beans and peas.

Fruit intakes for all groups examined were below the recommended 2–4 daily servings, with little difference among the ethnic groups. Total dairy intakes (i.e., servings of milk, yogurt, and cheese) were also below recommendations (2–3 servings/d, depending on age and physiological status). Black non-Hispanics had the lowest intakes of dairy products, a finding that is common among non-Caucasian populations, and is often attributed to lactose intolerance *(45)*.

The meat group includes not only red meat, fish, and poultry, but eggs, nuts, and seeds; recommendations for this group, in terms of lean meat equivalents, are 5–7 oz. Black non-Hispanics consumed greater amounts than either of the other groups, with black non-Hispanic men consuming slightly more than the recommendation. These differences were driven largely by differences in the intake of meat, fish, and poultry.

The tip of the Food Guide Pyramid conveys the relatively small role fats and sweets should play in the diet, and suggests that they be used sparingly. However, for all ethnic groups, intakes were high for both discretionary fat (i.e., fats and oils added to foods, and incidental fat from fattier choices within the meat, milk, vegetable, fruit, and grain groups) and added sugars (caloric sweeteners added to foods), totaling about 40% of total energy intakes. Black non-Hispanics consumed relatively more discretionary fat and added sugars, relative to recommendations or other groups.

3.4.3. SUMMARY

Black non-Hispanics, compared to the other ethnic groups, tended to have fewer servings from the grain and milk groups and more from the meat group. These food consumption differences are consistent with their relatively high intakes of cholesterol and their low intakes of folate, fiber, and calcium. Iron intakes of black non-Hispanic women were lower than those of white non-Hispanic women, despite their relatively high intakes of meat, fish, and poultry, which are rich sources of bioavailable iron, probably because their grain intakes were limiting. Mexican Americans seemed to have slightly higher intakes of fruits and vegetables, especially dried beans and peas. This pattern of eating resulted in relatively high intakes of fiber.

3.5. Comparisons of Food and Nutrient Intakes Among Groups Defined by SES

SES can be gaged in several ways, but is generally measured in terms of income and/or education. Tables 5 and 6, respectively, show nutrient and food intakes by these two variables. Income is assessed as the percentage of the federal poverty threshold for a given household's size, and education as years of education. Within each income and education category, results are shown for males and females separately for persons aged 20 yr and older.

Grain, fruit, vegetable, and milk intakes are generally highest for the high income and high education groups, among both men and women; servings from the meat group

Table 5
Food and Nutrient Intakes of Male and Female Adults, by Income, 1994–1996

Nutrient/food	Males (20 yr and older)			Females (20 yr and older)		
	<131% Poverty	131–350% Poverty	>350% Poverty	<131% Poverty	131–350% Poverty	>350% Poverty
	Mean kcal ± SE, 1 d					
Energy	2595 ± 145	2421 ± 32	2448 ± 31	1593 ± 28	1631 ± 22	1686 ± 18
	Mean g ± SE, 1 d					
Protein	99.8 ± 4.6	93.0 ± 1.4	95.2 ± 1.3	61.9 ± 1.1	62.1 ± 0.8	65.0 ± 0.8
Total fat	99.2 ± 6.1	91.7 ± 1.4	91.8 ± 1.4	59.2 ± 1.4	60.6 ± 1.0	61.0 ± 0.9
Saturated fatty acids	34.3 ± 2.6	30.9 ± 0.5	30.7 ± 0.6	19.9 ± 0.5	20.3 ± 0.4	19.8 ± 0.4
Monounsaturated fatty acids	38.3 ± 2.1	35.7 ± 0.6	35.2 ± 0.6	22.7 ± 0.6	23.1 ± 0.4	23.0 ± 0.4
Polyunsaturated fatty acids	18.8 ± 1.2	17.9 ± 0.4	18.7 ± 0.3	11.9 ± 0.4	12.5 ± 0.2	13.4 ± 0.3
Total carbohydrate	311.3 ± 18.0	295.6 ± 4.2	298.1 ± 4.1	204.7 ± 3.7	210.2 ± 2.8	216.6 ± 2.2
Dietary fiber	18.4 ± 0.7	18.0 ± 0.3	19.1 ± 0.4	12.3 ± 0.2	13.5 ± 0.3	15.0 ± 0.3
	Mean % of kcal ± SE, 1 d					
Protein	16.3 ± 0.3	15.8 ± 0.1	16.0 ± 0.1	16.0 ± 0.2	15.7 ± 0.1	16.0 ± 0.1
Total fat	33.7 ± 0.4	33.5 ± 0.3	33.0 ± 0.3	32.8 ± 0.3	32.8 ± 0.3	31.7 ± 0.2
Saturated fatty acids	11.6 ± 0.1	11.2 ± 0.1	11.0 ± 0.1	11.1 ± 0.2	11.0 ± 0.1	10.3 ± 0.1
Monounsaturated fatty acids	13.0 ± 0.2	13.1 ± 0.1	12.6 ± 0.1	12.5 ± 0.1	12.5 ± 0.1	11.9 ± 0.1
Polyunsaturated fatty acids	6.4 ± 0.1	6.5 ± 0.1	6.8 ± 0.1	6.6 ± 0.1	6.8 ± 0.1	7.0 ± 0.1
Total carbohydrate	48.6 ± 0.6	49.4 ± 0.3	49.4 ± 0.3	51.9 ± 0.4	52.1 ± 0.3	51.8 ± 0.3
Alcohol	2.3 ± 0.5	2.5 ± 0.2	2.9 ± 0.2	0.5 ± 0.1	1.0 ± 0.1	2.2 ± 0.1
	Mean µg ± SE, 1 d					
Vitamin A (retinol equivalents)	1034 ± 64	1125 ± 64	1168 ± 31	824 ± 35	911 ± 31	999 ± 42
Carotenes (retinol equivalents)	447 ± 29	518 ± 24	594 ± 25	442 ± 27	459 ± 17	588 ± 34
Folate	296 ± 12	293 ± 6	310 ± 6	208 ± 5	217 ± 4	243 ± 5
Vitamin B$_{12}$	8.35 ± 1.97	6.19 ± 0.37	6.68 ± 0.57	3.85 ± 0.25	4.30 ± 0.27	4.20 ± 0.25

		Mean mg ± SE, 1 d			
Vitamin E (α-tocopherol equivalents)	9.3 ± 0.5	9.6 ± 0.3	10.3 ± 0.2	6.2 ± 0.2	6.9 ± 0.2	7.7 ± 0.2
Vitamin C	111 ± 10	103 ± 3	114 ± 3	88 ± 4	86 ± 1	97 ± 3
Thiamin	1.93 ± 0.09	1.87 ± 0.02	1.92 ± 0.03	1.28 ± 0.03	1.29 ± 0.02	1.38 ± 0.02
Riboflavin	2.30 ± 0.11	2.19 ± 0.04	2.23 ± 0.03	1.48 ± 0.03	1.56 ± 0.03	1.64 ± 0.02
Niacin	27.8 ± 1.2	27.1 ± 0.5	28.5 ± 0.4	17.5 ± 0.4	18.2 ± 0.3	19.7 ± 0.3
Vitamin B_6	2.13 ± 0.09	2.11 ± 0.04	2.23 ± 0.03	1.41 ± 0.03	1.48 ± 0.02	1.59 ± 0.03
Calcium	917 ± 56	869 ± 17	893 ± 16	593 ± 13	639 ± 15	670 ± 11
Phosphorus	1531 ± 78	1446 ± 20	1485 ± 20	967 ± 17	1005 ± 18	1058 ± 12
Magnesium	322 ± 13	316 ± 6	336 ± 5	214 ± 4	227 ± 4	249 ± 3
Iron	18.6 ± 1.3	18.1 ± 0.3	18.6 ± 0.3	12.2 ± 0.3	12.5 ± 0.2	13.6 ± 0.2
Zinc	14.3 ± 0.9	13.8 ± 0.3	13.7 ± 0.2	8.9 ± 0.2	9 ± 0.2	9.4 ± 0.2
Copper	1.5 ± 0.1	1.4 ± 0.0	1.5 ± 0.0	1.0 ± 0.0	1.0 ± 0.0	1.1 ± 0.0
Sodium	4261 ± 191	4067 ± 64	4028 ± 52	2693 ± 51	2714 ± 47	2819 ± 33
Potassium	3186 ± 138	3110 ± 43	3280 ± 47	2162 ± 32	2293 ± 33	2451 ± 35
Cholesterol	390 ± 19	330 ± 8	316 ± 7	233 ± 6	216 ± 5	202 ± 4
		Mean servings ± SE, 1 d			
Total grain products	8.4 ± 0.4	7.9 ± 0.1	8.0 ± 0.1	5.2 ± 0.1	5.4 ± 0.1	5.9 ± 0.1
Whole grains	0.9 ± 0.1	1.1 ± 0.1	1.3 ± 0.1	0.7 ± 0.1	0.8 ± 0.0	1.0 ± 0.0
Total vegetables	4.2 ± 0.2	4.1 ± 0.1	4.4 ± 0.1	2.8 ± 0.1	3.1 ± 0.1	3.3 ± 0.1
Green/yellow	0.3 ± 0.1	0.4 ± 0.0	0.4 ± 0.0	0.3 ± 0.0	0.4 ± 0.0	0.5 ± 0.0
White potatoes	1.5 ± 0.1	1.4 ± 0.1	1.4 ± 0.1	0.8 ± 0.0	0.9 ± 0.0	0.8 ± 0.0
Dried beans/peas	0.4 ± 0.1	0.3 ± 0.0	0.2 ± 0.0	0.2 ± 0.0	0.2 ± 0.0	0.1 ± 0.0
Other starchy	0.2 ± 0.0	0.3 ± 0.0	0.3 ± 0.0	0.2 ± 0.0	0.2 ± 0.0	0.2 ± 0.0
Tomatoes	0.6 ± 0.0	0.6 ± 0.0	0.6 ± 0.0	0.4 ± 0.0	0.4 ± 0.0	0.5 ± 0.0
Other vegetables	1.2 ± 0.1	1.2 ± 0.0	1.4 ± 0.0	0.9 ± 0.0	1.1 ± 0.0	1.3 ± 0.0
Fruits	1.2 ± 0.1	1.4 ± 0.1	1.7 ± 0.1	1.3 ± 0.1	1.4 ± 0.0	1.6 ± 0.1
Milk, cheese or yogurt	1.6 ± 0.1	1.5 ± 0.0	1.6 ± 0.0	1.0 ± 0.0	1.2 ± 0.0	1.2 ± 0.0
Meat/meat alternates	6.8 ± 0.3	6.3 ± 0.1	6.3 ± 0.1	4.2 ± 0.1	3.9 ± 0.1	3.9 ± 0.1
Meat, poultry, fish	6.0 ± 0.3	5.6 ± 0.1	5.7 ± 0.1	3.6 ± 0.1	3.4 ± 0.1	3.5 ± 0.1
		Mean % of kcal ± SE, 1 d			
Discretionary fat	24.7 ± 0.3	25.0 ± 0.2	24.7 ± 0.3	24.4 ± 0.3	24.8 ± 0.2	24.1 ± 0.2
Added sugars	15.1 ± 0.8	14.9 ± 0.3	14.0 ± 0.3	16.2 ± 0.5	15.7 ± 0.4	13.8 ± 0.4

Source: ref. 36.

Table 6
Food and Nutrient Intakes of Male and Female Adults, by Education, 1994–1996

Nutrient/food	Males (20 yr and older)			Females (20 yr and older)		
	<High school	High school	>High school	<High school	High school	>High school
	Mean kcal l ± SE, 1 d					
Energy	2285 ± 114	2426 ± 46	2515 ± 30	1471 ± 22	1632 ± 18	1724 ± 18
	Mean g ± SE, 1 d					
Protein	91.0 ± 3.2	93.4 ± 1.8	96.6 ± 1.1	58.9 ± 1.1	62.9 ± 0.9	65.1 ± 0.6
Total fat	90.5 ± 5.3	93.0 ± 1.9	92.8 ± 1.4	55.9 ± 1.2	61.1 ± 1.1	61.7 ± 0.9
Saturated fatty acids	30.9 ± 2.3	31.5 ± 0.7	31.0 ± 0.6	18.6 ± 0.4	20.5 ± 0.4	20.2 ± 0.3
Monounsaturated fatty acids	34.8 ± 1.8	36.2 ± 0.8	35.7 ± 0.6	21.6 ± 0.5	23.4 ± 0.4	23.2 ± 0.3
Polyunsaturated fatty acids	17.7 ± 1.0	18.0 ± 0.4	18.8 ± 0.3	11.2 ± 0.3	12.4 ± 0.3	13.6 ± 0.2
Total carbohydrate	268.2 ± 14.3	292.0 ± 5.8	310.6 ± 3.9	186.2 ± 2.9	207.8 ± 2.2	224.8 ± 2.8
Dietary fiber	17.2 ± 0.6	17.2 ± 0.3	19.8 ± 0.4	12.5 ± 0.3	12.8 ± 0.2	15.2 ± 0.2
	Mean % of kcal ± SE, 1 d					
Protein	16.5 ± 0.2	15.9 ± 0.1	15.8 ± 0.1	16.6 ± 0.2	15.8 ± 0.1	15.6 ± 0.2
Total fat	34.6 ± 0.4	33.9 ± 0.3	32.5 ± 0.3	33.4 ± 0.4	32.8 ± 0.3	31.6 ± 0.2
Saturated fatty acids	11.7 ± 0.2	11.4 ± 0.1	10.8 ± 0.1	11.2 ± 0.2	11.0 ± 0.1	10.3 ± 0.1
Monounsaturated fatty acids	13.4 ± 0.2	13.1 ± 0.1	12.5 ± 0.1	12.9 ± 0.2	12.5 ± 0.1	11.8 ± 0.1
Polyunsaturated fatty acids	6.7 ± 0.1	6.6 ± 0.1	6.7 ± 0.1	6.7 ± 0.1	6.7 ± 0.1	7.0 ± 0.1
Total carbohydrate	47.8 ± 0.5	48.8 ± 0.3	50.0 ± 0.3	50.9 ± 0.4	51.7 ± 0.3	52.6 ± 0.3
Alcohol	2.0 ± 0.2	2.5 ± 0.2	2.9 ± 0.2	0.4 ± 0.1	1.2 ± 0.1	2.0 ± 0.2
	Mean µg ± SE, 1 d					
Vitamin A (retinol equivalents)	984 ± 56	1108 ± 83	1199 ± 36	772 ± 31	867 ± 31	1039 ± 37
Carotenes (retinol equivalents)	451 ± 33	499 ± 25	604 ± 24	413 ± 25	433 ± 16	600 ± 29
Folate	262 ± 10	283 ± 9	325 ± 7	196 ± 5	209 ± 5	250 ± 4
Vitamin B_{12}	8.35 ± 2.00	6.65 ± 0.53	6.29 ± 0.35	3.71 ± 0.20	4.31 ± 0.26	4.27 ± 0.22

Mean mg ± SE, 1 d

Vitamin E (α-tocopherol equivalents)	8.5 ± 0.4	9.5 ± 0.3	10.5 ± 0.2	6.1 ± 0.2	6.7 ± 0.2	7.7 ± 0.2
Vitamin C	88 ± 7	98 ± 4	122 ± 3	80 ± 3	80 ± 2	102 ± 3
Thiamin	1.73 ± 0.06	1.87 ± 0.04	1.97 ± 0.03	1.19 ± 0.02	1.30 ± 0.02	1.40 ± 0.02
Riboflavin	2.06 ± 0.09	2.17 ± 0.05	2.31 ± 0.03	1.40 ± 0.03	1.54 ± 0.03	1.66 ± 0.02
Niacin	24.8 ± 0.8	27.2 ± 0.7	29.0 ± 0.4	16.7 ± 0.4	18.5 ± 0.3	19.6 ± 0.2
Vitamin B_6	1.93 ± 0.06	2.09 ± 0.05	2.28 ± 0.04	1.36 ± 0.03	1.44 ± 0.03	1.62 ± 0.02
Calcium	803 ± 43	839 ± 24	941 ± 14	565 ± 14	621 ± 13	686 ± 10
Phosphorus	1378 ± 63	1430 ± 28	1528 ± 18	920 ± 16	994 ± 15	1074 ± 10
Magnesium	293 ± 9	310 ± 7	346 ± 5	206 ± 3	222 ± 3	253 ± 3
Iron	17.0 ± 1.2	17.6 ± 0.4	19.4 ± 0.3	11.5 ± 0.2	12.4 ± 0.2	13.8 ± 0.2
Zinc	13.5 ± 0.8	13.8 ± 0.4	14.0 ± 0.2	8.4 ± 0.3	9.0 ± 0.1	9.5 ± 0.1
Copper	1.3 ± 0.0	1.4 ± 0.0	1.6 ± 0.0	0.9 ± 0.0	1.0 ± 0.0	1.1 ± 0.0
Sodium	3766 ± 116	4053 ± 83	4177 ± 57	2486 ± 48	2769 ± 40	2843 ± 30
Potassium	2932 ± 124	3108 ± 56	3332 ± 43	2100 ± 30	2250 ± 30	2478 ± 31
Cholesterol	375 ± 16	340 ± 8	311 ± 6	219 ± 6	222 ± 6	204 ± 4
Mean servings ± SE, 1 d						
Total grain products	7.4 ± 0.3	7.7 ± 0.2	8.4 ± 0.1	4.9 ± 0.1	5.4 ± 0.1	6.0 ± 0.1
Whole grains	0.8 ± 0.1	1.0 ± 0.1	1.4 ± 0.1	0.6 ± 0.0	0.7 ± 0.0	1.1 ± 0.0
Total vegetables	3.9 ± 0.2	4.1 ± 0.1	4.4 ± 0.1	2.8 ± 0.1	3.0 ± 0.1	3.4 ± 0.1
Green/yellow	0.3 ± 0.1	0.3 ± 0.0	0.5 ± 0.0	0.3 ± 0.0	0.3 ± 0.0	0.5 ± 0.0
White potatoes	1.2 ± 0.1	1.6 ± 0.1	1.4 ± 0.1	0.8 ± 0.0	0.9 ± 0.0	0.8 ± 0.0
Dried beans/peas	0.5 ± 0.1	0.2 ± 0.0	0.2 ± 0.0	0.2 ± 0.0	0.1 ± 0.0	0.2 ± 0.0
Other starchy	0.3 ± 0.0	0.3 ± 0.0	0.2 ± 0.0	0.2 ± 0.0	0.2 ± 0.0	0.2 ± 0.0
Tomatoes	0.5 ± 0.0	0.6 ± 0.0	0.7 ± 0.0	0.4 ± 0.0	0.4 ± 0.0	0.5 ± 0.0
Other vegetables	1.1 ± 0.1	1.1 ± 0.0	1.5 ± 0.0	0.9 ± 0.1	1.0 ± 0.0	1.3 ± 0.0
Fruits	1.2 ± 0.1	1.3 ± 0.1	1.8 ± 0.1	1.3 ± 0.1	1.3 ± 0.1	1.7 ± 0.1
Milk, cheese or yogurt	1.3 ± 0.1	1.5 ± 0.1	1.7 ± 0.0	1.0 ± 0.0	1.1 ± 0.0	1.2 ± 0.0
Meat/meat alternates	6.4 ± 0.2	6.5 ± 0.2	6.2 ± 0.1	3.9 ± 0.1	4.1 ± 0.1	3.8 ± 0.1
Meat, poultry, fish	5.7 ± 0.2	5.8 ± 0.1	5.6 ± 0.1	3.5 ± 0.1	3.6 ± 0.1	3.4 ± 0.1
Mean % of kcal ± SE, 1 d						
Discretionary fat	25.3 ± 0.4	25.3 ± 0.3	24.5 ± 0.2	24.8 ± 0.4	24.8 ± 0.3	24.0 ± 0.2
Added sugars	13.8 ± 0.5	15.5 ± 0.4	14.0 ± 0.3	14.4 ± 0.4	16.1 ± 0.3	14.5 ± 0.4

Source: ref. 36.

Table 7
Prevalence of Food Insufficiency Among U.S. Adults, by Ethnicity, Income, and Education,
1994–1996

Population subgroup	Enough food	Sometimes not enough food	Often not enough food
Ethnicity			
White non-Hispanic	98.4	1.5	0.2
Black non-Hispanic	97.4	2.3	0.3
Mexican Americans	87.0	11.3	1.7
Income			
<131% Poverty	91.1	7.2	1.7
131–350% Poverty	98.8	1.1	0.1
>350% Poverty	99.8	0.2	0.0
Education			
<High school	94.1	4.7	1.2
High school	98.2	1.7	0.1
>High school	99.1	0.8	0.1

Source: ref. 36.

tended to be lower. There was little difference among the income and education groups
in their intakes of discretionary fat; added sugars were highest as a percentage of energy
among middle-income groups, and seemed to decline with education. For women,
intakes of fat and saturated fat are lowest in the upper income and education groups;
among both men and women, intakes of fiber, vitamin A, and folate are highest in the
upper-income group.

Food insufficiency has been defined as "inadequate food intake due to lack of money
or resources" (13). Table 7 shows the estimated prevalence of food insufficiency among
several groups, determined through the use of the question, "Which of these statements
best describes the food eaten in your household in the last three months: enough of the
kinds of food we want to eat; enough but not always the kinds of food we want to eat;
sometimes not enough to eat; or often not enough to eat?" Mexican American households
were far less likely than those of other ethnic groups to indicate their food supplies were
sufficient, and there appears to be both an income and an education gradient: The percentage of households indicating they had enough food in the last 3 mo was lower for households with incomes below 131% of the federal poverty level, and for those with less
than a high school education. Within each group, results were consistent between males
and females.

3.6. Food and Nutrient Intakes of American Indians, Alaskan Natives, Asian Americans, and Pacific Islanders

3.6.1. DATA SOURCES

As previously indicated, African Americans and Hispanic Americans are the only
ethnic minority populations included in national nutrition surveys in numbers that are
sufficiently large to support subgroup-specific tabulations of food and nutrient intakes.
Furthermore, the diversity of cultural backgrounds, demographic characteristics, and
health profiles among subgroups, within the American Indian/Alaskan Native and
Asian/Pacific Islander populations, makes it especially difficult to use the broad Census

Bureau categories. Some attempts have been made to summarize available studies of American Indian/Alaskan Natives, and to identify, indirectly, the apparent influence of the qualitative dietary changes that have taken place in these populations, on the observed increases in the occurrence of chronic diseases and cancer (14,46). Much of this is intuitive, e.g., increasing westernization of the diet is observed to parallel increasing rates of CVD and cancer. However, ecological associations between the extent of westernization and of chronic disease over time further strengthen the inference that dietary changes are among the factors responsible for the observed changes in disease patterns. The next two subheadings review the limited data available on dietary intakes of American Indians/Alaskan Natives and Asian/Pacific Islanders.

3.6.2. INTAKES AMONG AMERICAN INDIAN/ALASKAN NATIVES POPULATIONS

Nobmann et al. (46) reported dietary intakes of 351 Alaskan Native adults, ages 21–60 yr, from 11 communities, in a population-based survey conducted in 1987–1988. Respondents were 53% Eskimos, 34% Indians, and 13% Aleuts, representative of the ethnic distribution in the relevant 1980 Census data, and balanced across age and sex. Data were collected with 24-h recalls taken in-person, and repeated up to five times across seasons, when possible, and were analyzed from a special data base that included values for 210 Alaskan Native foods. NHANES II data were used as reference data on average intakes in the United States. Among the key findings, with respect to food and beverage intakes, were high consumption of coffee and table sugar (about twice the U.S. average), and the very high consumption of fish and shellfish (e.g., mean daily intake of 109 g, compared with 17 g as a U.S. average). Consumption of beef, milk, salad, vegetable, orange juice, and alcoholic beverages was reported less frequently among the Alaskan Natives than in the U.S. general population. Energy intakes and both total nutrient intakes and nutrient density were higher than the U.S. average for other nutrients, with the exception of Ca, for which the Alaskan Native diets were significantly lower overall and per kcal (68–69% of average U.S. intakes). Seasonal variation was noted, e.g., lower energy intakes in the Spring. Sources of certain nutrients were very different from those in the NHANES sample, e.g., orange-flavored breakfast drinks were a major source of vitamin C in the diets of the Alaskan natives (contributing 35 vs 2% in the NHANES sample); fruit and vegetable consumption was relatively low, and high fish consumption, with consequent difference in the types of fatty acids. Comparison of the 1987–1988 data with surveys of Alaskan Natives, approx 30 yr prior, suggested that the percent fat was relatively stable, at around 35–39% of kcal, that adequacy of the diet for vitamins A and C and for Ca and iron (men only) had improved substantially, and that there were noteworthy declines in the adequacy of B-vitamin intake. Energy intake did not appear to have declined, despite clear declines in energy expenditure resulting from the increased use of labor-saving devices. Taken together, the findings were consistent with the interpretation that some protection from chronic diseases was provided by the continued high use of traditional foods, and possibly by seasonal variation, which lowered the average annual exposure to potential atherogenic dietary constituents. However, elements of the dietary patterns (e.g., persistent high energy intake in the face of decreasing expenditure, high refined sugar consumption, and low fiber intake) were consistent with the observation of increased prevalence of chronic diseases over time, so that the relatively lower rates of most chronic diseases among Alaskan Natives, compared to general U.S. population, would not persist indefinitely. A high prevalence of hip fracture among Eskimo women was noted in relation to their low Ca intakes, possibly in conjunction with high protein intakes.

The review by Bell et al. *(14)* focused on 12 studies published between 1959 and 1996, which reported nutrient intakes of Pima Indians in AZ, Seminole Indians in FL, Standing Rock Sioux in ND and SD, Omaha and Sioux Indians in Nebraska, Navajo Indians in New Mexico (NM), AZ, and Utah, Hualapai in AZ, Waccamaw-Siouan Indians in North Carolina (NC), Pueblo and Navajo Indians in NM, Lumbee Indians in NC, and included the Nobmann et al. report *(46)* on Alaskan Natives. With the caveat that the data are sparse and of uncertain validity, these authors advanced the overall impression that the dietary patterns reported for these populations were moderately high in fat and saturated fat, and low in fiber, with relatively adequate intakes of antioxidant vitamins. The authors noted co-variation in dietary patterns and disease patterns within American Indian/Alaskan Native populations, and recommended paying particular attention to the Indian Health Service regions where CVD and cancer mortality are high, compared to average rates for other American Indian/Alaskan Native populations.

The 1995 nutrition monitoring report *(13)* incorporated nutrient intake data from a federally funded study of American Indians, aged 45–74 yr, in AZ, OK, and SD. Data were based on 1 d dietary intake as reported in 1990–1991. Mean energy intakes were somewhat below the RDAs for males and females, and lower for those 60–74 yr old, compared to 45–49 yr old. With respect to fat and fiber intake, the diets of the younger group of men in AZ were more favorable than for any other subgroups: a total fat intake of 32% of kcal and fiber intake of 23 g/d. However, cholesterol intake was highest in AZ (range 361–447 mg/d). Mean vitamin C intake was substantially above the RDA (range 75–142 mg/d), and mean iron was also at or substantially above the RDA, except for the older group of women in OK. Mean vitamin A intake in AZ was lower than the recommended 1000 :g retinol equivalents/day for men and women in both age groups (778–954 :g RE/d), and for the older women in OK, but was otherwise at or slightly above recommended levels.

An extensive monograph related to cancer research in American Indians/Alaskan Natives explores traditional and contemporary consumption practices of Native Americans and the influence of policies and programs, such as commodity foods (the Food Distribution Program on Indian Reservations) and Food Stamps, on current nutrient intakes *(15)*. The primary conclusion of this review is that there are tremendous gaps in knowledge of dietary intakes of American Indians and Alaskan Natives and how they relate to disease patterns. Food availability "which may be limited to commodities or to the types of snack foods or convenience foods found in local grocery stores or vending machines" *(15)* may be a major problem for native people who live in remote areas. Although certain improvements may have been made in recent years, the mix of commodities usually available, although perhaps compliant with policy guidelines, has not necessarily promoted diets that would adhere to the U.S. Dietary Guidelines. In part, this may reflect the relatively recent shift in priorities of food programs, such as the Indian Health Service Nutrition Program, from addressing malnutrition to addressing optimal nutrition in a way that would include reduction of obesity, diabetes, and other chronic disease factors. Burhansstipanov and Dresser *(15)* cite the requests included in a 1986 report to the USDA from the Navajo Tribal Food and Nutrition Service, to improve the quality of certain commodities, specifically: lower the fat content of pork, beef, and meatball stew, provide chicken and turkey on a regular basis, omit luncheon meats, and reduce the Na content of canned meats and vegetables.

3.6.3. INTAKES AMONG ASIAN/PACIFIC ISLANDER POPULATIONS

As noted previously, there are varied diet and disease concerns for Asian/Pacific Islander subpopulations *(10)*. Diabetes is a generalized problem in conjunction with a sometimes extremely high prevalence of obesity in minority populations *(11)*, but also is associated with abdominal obesity in populations such as Japanese Americans or Asian Indians, who may have average or even below-average levels of overall obesity. Coronary heart disease mortality, although lower than average in Chinese and Japanese Americans, is higher among Asian Indians than in whites *(47)*. Hypertension is particularly common in Filipino Americans, compared to other Asian/Pacific Islander populations, and stroke mortality is high in Japanese Americans *(10)*. Thus, on this basis, as well as given differences in the traditional diets of these different Asian/Pacific Islander subpopulations *(30)*, it would be desirable to have separate population-based data sources, in order not to overgeneralize about dietary patterns, or to miss important aspects of risk that might affect a particular group. Unfortunately, nutrition data sources for Asian/Pacific Islander populations are limited, and comments about dietary issues are, therefore, limited to some general themes.

The nature of many traditional Asian foods, and a limited amount of data, suggest that sodium intake is higher than average in Asian/Pacific Islander populations. For example, a cross-cultural comparison of urinary Na and potassium excretion among young adults in Hawaii indicated consistently higher Na excretion and, in men, lower potassium excretion, in all Asian/Pacific Islander subgroups, compared to the Caucasian sample; these differences were not statistically significant, however *(48)*. Other themes in the literature on diet-related risks in Asian/Pacific Islander populations relate to low Ca intake *(49)*, although typical dietary assessments may not capture all of the available Ca in Asian foods. Because of the observed lower hip fracture rates in Asian American and other minority populations *(9,50)*, the possibility that low Ca intake may be less associated with risk than in white populations must be considered, e.g., because of adaptations that occur in Ca absorption under different dietary intake conditions, or because of genetic differences *(10)*. For Pacific Islanders, the high prevalence of obesity and diabetes is indirect evidence of an imbalance in the ration of energy intake to energy output. For Asian Indians who migrate to the United States, or their children, the dietary issues of interest include changes in the overall eating pattern that might increase risk, e.g., when those who were initially vegetarian become nonvegetarian, as well as changes that may decrease risk (e.g., reduced consumption of ghee) *(51)*. Substituting common U.S. foods for traditional cultural foods may also lead to reduced salt intake among Asian/Pacific Islander populations. Each of these dietary variables would be important to track in nutrition surveys, with appropriately designed methods of ascertainment, to determine the mix of dietary practices that results from the type of original dietary pattern (e.g., in the country of origin for migrants) and the type of new dietary habits adopted over time. Dietary assessments by age cohort may be especially important in populations in which the older generation is more traditional in their way of eating than the younger generation *(52–54)*. The influence of SES on eating patterns within the Asian/Pacific Islander populations has not been described, but may be relevant, given the bipolarity of the Asian/Pacific Islander SES distribution.

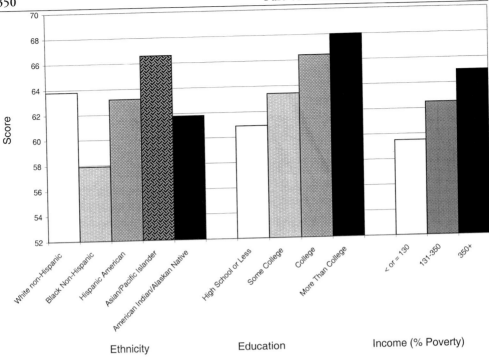

Fig. 6. Mean healthy eating index (HEI) composite scores for U.S. adults aged 20 yr and over, by ethnicity, education, and income, 1994–1996. The overall HEI score ranges from 0 to 100. An HEI score over 80 implies a "good" diet, and HEI score between 51 and 80 implies a diet that "needs improvement," and an HEI score less than 51 implies a "poor" diet. Adapted from refs. *38* and *55*.

3.7. Overview of Dietary Patterns by Ethnicity and SES

The 1994–1996 CSFII data have been analyzed by ethnicity, education, and income, using the gage of the HEI (Fig. 6) and its individual component scores (Table 8; 55). Data are provided for all five broad ethnic groups (white non-Hispanic, black non-Hispanic, Hispanic American, Asian/Pacific Islander, and American Indian/Alaskan Native), although the sample sizes for the latter group are particularly small.

Developers of the HEI have suggested that scores over 80 represent good diets, those between 51 and 80 need improvement, and those of 51 and under are poor diets. According to these criteria, diets of all subgroups are in need of improvement, but those of some groups are healthier than those of others. HEI scores for Asian/Pacific Islanders were highest, and those for black non-Hispanics lowest, among the ethnic categories, and scores increased with increasing levels of education and income.

Differences in the overall HEI among these subpopulations can be traced to differences in its various components. Asian/Pacific Islanders had particularly good scores (8 or greater) for fat, saturated fat, and variety; no other ethnic group had average scores that high for any of the individual components. Black non-Hispanics had the lowest scores for several of the food group components (grains, vegetables, fruits, and milk), and, consequently, for the variety component as well. All groups, however, tended to have low scores for fruits and milks. Scores for nearly all components seemed to increase with education and income, but only at the uppermost levels did any of the individual

Table 8
Mean Healthy Eating Index Component Scores for U.S. Adults Aged 20 Yr and Over, by Ethnicity, Education, and Income, 1994–1996

Population subgroup (n)	Healthy Eating Index Component									
	Grains	Vegetables	Fruits	Milk	Meat	Total fat	Saturated fatty acids	Cholesterol	Sodium	Variety
Ethnicity										
White non-Hispanic (7549)	6.6	6.6	3.7	5.4	6.6	6.7	6.5	7.8	6.1	7.8
Black non-Hispanics (1105)	5.6	5.8	3.3	3.5	7.2	6.2	6.3	7.1	6.6	6.3
Hispanic Americans (865)[a]	6.2	6.2	3.8	4.9	7.1	7.0	6.7	7.1	6.5	7.6
American Indians/ Alaskan Natives (59)[b]	5.8	6.6	4.4	4.6	7.0	6.6	6.4	7.2	6.1	7.0
Asian American and Pacific Islanders (233)[b]	7.3	7.0	4.1	3.5	7.3	8.3	8.3	7.2	5.5	8.1
Education										
<4 Yr high school (5427)	6.2	6.2	3.2	4.7	6.8	6.5	6.3	7.5	6.4	7.1
Some college (2025)	6.5	6.6	3.7	5.2	6.7	6.7	6.6	7.6	5.9	7.7
4 Yr college (1100)	6.8	6.8	4.2	5.6	6.7	7.1	7.0	8.1	6.0	8.3
>4 Yr college (1161)	6.9	6.9	5.1	5.6	6.7	7.3	7.2	8.2	5.7	8.5
Income										
<131% Poverty (2279)	6.1	5.8	3.2	4.5	6.7	6.5	6.3	7.1	6.5	6.7
131–350% Poverty (3911)	6.3	6.5	3.6	5.0	6.7	6.6	6.4	7.6	6.2	7.5
>350% Poverty (3682)	6.7	6.7	4.0	5.3	6.8	6.9	6.8	7.9	6.0	8.0

[a]Includes Mexican Americans, Puerto Ricans, Chicanos, Cuban Americans, and other Spanish/Hispanic Americans.
[b]Excludes Hispanic Americans.
Source: ref. 55.

scores reach 8 or more (the cholesterol and variety scores for those with a college education or greater, and the variety score only for those in the upper-income bracket).

4. SUMMARY AND IMPLICATIONS

The traditional dietary patterns of different ethnic groups can be readily described according to the nature of the foods, food preparation methods, flavoring principles, and food usage patterns associated with a particular cuisine (30). However, to characterize the net effects of cultural food patterns on current nutrient intakes of ethnic groups in the U.S. populations and, further, to identify the implications for preventive health, are much more difficult. Ethnic subpopulations are difficult to define meaningfully; the available data use broad classifications that understate within-group cultural diversity. There is tremendous individual variation in how cultural factors influence dietary practices, and it must, therefore, be considered that the differences within ethnic groups may be greater than the differences among them. This is particularly so when considering the net effects of food choices on nutrient intakes, rather than possible differences in food sources of various nutrients.

Furthermore, there are serious gaps in the completeness of dietary intake data. Targeted sampling among a larger number of minority groups than are currently included in the NNMRRP surveys is needed. The estimates reported here for Mexican Americans were based on relatively small numbers, which made the estimates less precise and, consequently, the differences more difficult to interpret. HHANES included larger samples of Mexican Americans, as well as targeted samples of Puerto Ricans and Cuban Americans, but those data are now 15 yr old. Furthermore, there are many more Hispanic American and Asian American subgroups, each with their own distinctive cuisine, for which estimates are needed. Similarly, a more systematic and coordinated approach to identifying and surveying American Indians and Alaskan Natives, also with attention to subethnic variation, is needed. This could be accomplished either through oversampling within large, nationally representative surveys, or through targeted surveys of these groups. In either case, sample sizes should be sufficiently large to allow examination of ethnicity in a multivariate context, together with sex, age, and SES. SES, in turn, should be examined in a broader context, considering not only income, but other individual characteristics, such as education, wealth, occupation, and social status, as well as environmental factors.

The political sensitivity of this topic should also be acknowledged, because it affects how questions are asked of the available nutrition data, and how the results are interpreted. The suggestion that a particular ethnic minority population has a poor-quality diet, particularly if the reference for the comparison is middle-class U.S. whites, carries an implicit risk of ethnocentrism i.e., devaluing the culture of others because it is different. Cultures throughout the world are able to meet their nutritional health needs through a variety of food choices, and no particular dietary pattern is inherently superior to any other. In addition, pointing to differences in the diets of ethnic groups may imply that one still sees the melting pot concept of American society, in which everyone renounces his or her ethnicity, as the ideal. On the other hand, there is a striking similarity between the dietary pattern currently recommended for the U.S. population (i.e., emphasizing grain and cereal products and fruits and vegetables products, and de-emphasizing animal foods) and the diets of low-income and economically developing nations, in which chronic diseases have not fully emerged. In this sense, movement toward the typical American diet is usually viewed as nutritionally harmful. Political sensitivity arises from what may be viewed as romanticizing traditional lifestyles that signify less-than-full participation in American society. Should one actively discourage adoption of mainstream culture by individuals in ethnic minority populations, or deprive minority populations of the type of lifestyle that has been available to whites? The issue of stereotyping arises from the suggestion that minority populations and whites do not eat from a common table, when in fact there is an obvious, high degree of overlap in the types of foods eaten by people living in American society, including a variety of ethnic foods. Therefore, the observer cannot know to what extent a person's ethnic cuisine impacts overall eating pattern.

Overall, there is a consistent impression that improvements are needed in the diets of all ethnic groups, in order to better align them with current preventive nutrition recommendations. In this sense, the commonalities among ethnic groups are more evident than the differences. Nevertheless, the number of indicators on which the diets of African Americans were less favorable than for whites or Mexican Americans (low intakes of fiber, folate, grains, vegetables, and fruit; high intakes of cholesterol and meat; and a lower overall HEI score) is both noteworthy and consistent with the fact that African Americans have the least-favorable CVD and cancer mortality.

The issue of low Ca and dairy product intake in African Americans deserves special mention, because this is one aspect of ethnic differences in dietary practices for which the interpretation does require consideration of gene–environment interactions. Some assert that higher dairy product intake is inappropriate or unnecessary for African Americans (56), and it is unclear that the long-term health implications of low dairy product consumption are as unfavorable for African Americans as for whites. As noted previously, lower dairy product consumption is a consistent finding among black and other minority populations (45,57), and is probably related in part to population differences in the genetic predisposition to lactose intolerance. Genetic factors may also partly explain why African Americans have a lower incidence, on average, of osteoporotic fractures than whites, despite having lower Ca intake (13,58). Lower fat intake from dairy sources may partly explain the similar fat intake of African Americans and whites, despite the higher intakes of meat and poultry among African Americans.

The analyses by SES were consistent in demonstrating less favorable dietary profiles among those with less education and less income. Whether this holds within each minority population cannot be determined; nor can the contribution of SES to the nutritional problems in African Americans be identified. Assuming that this applies generally, it is also consistent with the large SES disparities in mortality from chronic diseases, and suggests that SES is as, or more, important than ethnicity as a basis for targeting interventions to improve dietary quality of U.S. adults. It would seem imperative to give more detailed consideration to the underlying reasons for these SES differentials, in order to close these gaps over time.

REFERENCES

1. Committee on Diet and Health, Food and Nutrition Board, Commission on Life Sciences, National Research Council. Diet and Health: Implications for reducing chronic disease risk. Washington, DC: National Academy Press, 1989.
2. World Cancer Research Fund/American Institute for Cancer Research. Food, nutrition and the prevention of cancer: a global perspective. Menasha, WI: Bantam, 1997.
3. Labarthe DR. Epidemiology and prevention of cardiovascular diseases. A global challenge. Gaithersburg, MD: Aspen, 1998.

4. Bendich A, Deckelbaum R. Preventive Nutrition. The Comprehensive Guide for Health Professionals. Totowa, NJ: Humana, 1997.
5. Deckelbaum RJ, Fisher EA, Winston M, Kumanyika S, Lauer RM, Pi-Sunyer FX, et al. Summary of a scientific conference on preventive nutrition: pediatrics to geriatrics. Circulation 1999; 100:450–456.
6. Council on Economic Advisers for the President's Initiative on Race. Changing America. Indicators of social and economic well-being by race and Hispanic origin. http://www.access.gpo.gov/eop/ca/index.html, September 1998.
7. Pamuk E, Makuc D, Heck K, Reuben C, Lochner K. Socioeconomic Status and Health Chartbook. Health, United States, 1998. Hyattsville, MD: National Center for Health Statistics, 1998.
8. O'Hare WP. America's minorities: the demographics of diversity. Population Bulletin. Washington, DC: Population Reference Bureau, 1992; 47:1–45.
9. Kumanyika SK. Diet and disease issues for minority populations. J Nutr Ed 1990; 22:89–96.
10. Kumanyika S. Diet and nutrition as influences on the morbidity/mortality gap. Ann Epidemiol 1993; 3:154–158.
11. Kumanyika SK. Obesity in minority populations. An epidemiologic assessment. Obes Res 1994; 2:166–178.
12. Kumanyika SK. Racial and ethnic issues in diet and cancer epidemiology. In: Diet and Cancer: Markers, Prevention, and Treatment, Advances in Experimental Medicine and Biology. Jacobs M, ed. 1994; 354:59–70.
13. Federation of American Societies for Experimental Biology, Life Sciences Research Office. Prepared for the Interagency Board for Nutrition Monitoring and Related Research. Third Report on Nutrition Monitoring in the United States, Vol. 1. Washington, DC: Government Printing Office, 1995.
14. Bell R, Mayer-Davis E, Jackson Y, Dresser C. An epidemiologic review of dietary intake studies among American Indians and Alaskan Natives: implications for heart disease and cancer risk. Ann Epidemiol 1997; 7:229–240.
15. Burhansstipanov L, Dresser C. Documentation of the cancer research needs of American Indians and Alaska Natives. Native American Monograph No. 1. U.S. Department of Health and Human Services. Public Health Service. NIH. Cancer Control Science Program. Division of Cancer Prevention and Control. Bethesda, MD: National Cancer Institute, 1993; 7-1–7-41.
16. National Diabetes Data Group. Diabetes in America, 2nd ed. Bethesda, MD: NIH. National Institute of Diabetes and Digestive and Kidney Diseases. NIH Publication No. 95-1468, 1995.
17. Miller BA, Kolonel LN, Bernstein L, Young JL Jr, Swanson GM, West D, et al., eds. Racial/Ethnic Patterns of Cancer in the United States 1988–92, Bethesda, MD: National Cancer Institute. NIH Pub. No. 96-4104, 1996.
18. American Heart Association. 1999 Heart and Stroke Facts. Statistical Update. Dallas, TX: American Heart Association, 1999.
19. Lee ET, Cowan LD, Welty TK, Wievers M, Howard WJ, Oopik A, et al. All-cause mortality and cardiovascular disease mortality in three American Indian Populations, aged 45–74, 1984–1988. Am J Epidemiol 1998; 147:995–1008.
20. Nickens HW. The role of race/ethnicity and social class in minority health status. Health Serv Res 1995; 30:151–162.
21. Winkleby MA, Kraemer HC, Ahn DK, Varady AN. Ethnic and socioeconomic differences in cardiovascular risk factors. Findings for women from the Third National Health and Nutrition Examination Survey, 1988–1994. JAMA 1998; 280:356–362.
22. Sobal J, Stunkard AJ. Socioeconomic status and obesity. A review of the literature. Psychol Bull 1989; 105:260–275.
23. World Health Organization. Obesity. Preventing and managing the global epidemic. Report of a WHO consultation on obesity. Geneva, Switzerland: WHO, 1998.
24. Cockerham WC, Rütten A, Abel T. Conceptualizing Contemporary Health Lifestyles. Moving Beyond Weber. Sociol Q 1997; 38:321–341.
25. Kumanyika SK, Golden PM. Cross-sectional differences in health status in U.S. racial/ethnic minority groups. Potential influence of temporal changes, disease, and lifestyle transitions. Ethn Dis 1991; 1:50–59.
26. Gillum RF. The epidemiology of cardiovascular disease in black Americans. N Engl J Med 1996; 335:1597–1599.
27. Drewnowski A, Popkin BM. The nutrition transition: new trends in the global diet. Nutr Rev 1997; 55:31–43.
28. Chakraborty R, Kamboh MI, Ferrell RE. 'Unique' alleles in admixed populations: a strategy for determining 'hereditary' population differences of disease frequencies. Ethn Dis 1991; 1:245–256.

29. Davies S. Scientific and ethical foundations of nutritional and environmental medicine. Part II. Further glimpses of 'the Higher Medicine.' J Nutr Environ Med 1995; 5:5–11.

30. Kittler PG, Sucher KP. Food and Culture in America. A Nutrition Handbook, 2nd ed. Washington, DC: West/Wadsworth, 1998.

31. Wallendorf M, Reilly MD. Ethnic migration, assimilation, and consumption. J Consumer Res 1983; 10:292–302.

32. Freedman AM. Habit forming. Fast-food chains central role in diet of the inner-city poor. Wall Street J, Dec 19, 1990; 1, A6.

33. Cheadle A, Psaty BM, Curry S, Wagner E, Diehr P, Koepsell T, Kristal A. Community-level comparisons between the grocery store environment and individual dietary practices. Prev Med 1991; 20:250–261.

34. Bingham SA. The use of 24-hour urine samples and energy expenditure to validate dietary assessments. Am J Clin Nutr 1994; 59:227–231.

35. Briefel RR, Sempos CT, McDowell MA, Chien SC, Alaimo K. Dietary methods research in the third National Health and Nutrition Examination Survey: underreporting of energy intake. Am J Clin Nutr 1997; 65:1203–1209.

36. Tippett KS, Tasmin SC, eds. Design and operation: the continuing survey of food intakes by individuals and the diet and health knowledge survey, 1994–96. U.S. Department of Agriculture, Agricultural Research Service, Nationwide Food Surveys Report No. 96-1. Riverdale, MD: Agricultural Research Service, 1998.

37. Subcommittee on the Tenth Edition of the RDAs, Food and Nutrition Board, Commission on Life Sciences, National Research Council. Recommended dietary allowances, 10th ed. Washington, DC: National Academy Press, 1989.

38. Bowman SA, Lino M, Gerrior SA, Basiotis PP. The Healthy Eating Index: 1994–96. Washington, DC: U.S. Department of Agriculture, Center for Nutrition Policy and Promotion, CNPP-5, 1998.

39. SUDAAN: Survey Data Analysis Software, release 6.34. Research Triangle Institute, Research Triangle Park, NC, September, 1993.

40. U.S. Department of Agriculture and U.S. Department of Health and Human Services. Nutrition and your health: Dietary guidelines for Americans, 4th ed. Home and Garden Bulletin No 232. Washington, DC: U.S. Government Printing Office, 1995.

41. Butrum RV, Clifford CK, Lanza E. NCI dietary guidelines: rationale. Am J Clin Nutr 1988; 48:888–895.

42. Standing Committee on the Scientific Evaluation of Dietary Reference Intakes, Food and Nutrition Board. Dietary reference intakes for thiamin, riboflavin, niacin, vitamin B6, folate, vitamin B12, pantothenic acid, biotin, and choline. Institute of Medicine. Washington, DC: National Academy Press, 1999.

43. Standing Committee on the Scientific Evaluation of Dietary Reference Intakes, Food and Nutrition Board. Dietary reference intakes for calcium, phosphorus, magnesium, vitamin D, and fluoride. Institute of Medicine. Washington, DC: National Academy Press, 1999.

44. U.S. Department of Agriculture, U.S. Department of Health and Human Services. The Food Guide Pyramid. Home and Garden Bulletin No. 252. Washington, DC: U.S. Government Printing Office, 1992.

45. Scrimshaw NS, Murray EB. The acceptability of milk and milk products in populations with a high prevalence of lactose intolerance. Am J Clin Nutr 1988; 48:1079–1159.

46. Nobmann ED, Byers T, Lanier AP, Hankin JH, Jackson MY. The diet of Alaska Native adults: 1987–1988. Am J Clin Nutr 1992; 55:1024–1032.

47. Wild SH, Laws A, Fortmann SP, Varady AN, Byrne CD. Mortality from coronary heart disease and stroke for six ethnic groups in California 1985–1990. Ann Epidemiol 1995; 5:432–439.

48. Young F, Lichton IJ, Hamilton RM, Dorrough SA, Alford EJ. Body weight, blood pressure, and electrolyte excretion of young adults from six ethnic groups in Hawaii. Am J Clin Nutr 1987; 45:126–130.

49. Kim KK, Yu ES, Liu WT, Kim J, Kohrs MB. Nutritional status of Chinese-, Korean-, and Japanese-American elderly. J Am Diet Assoc 1993; 93:1416–1422.

50. Lauderdale DS, Jacobsen SJ, Furner SE, Levy PS, Brody JA, Goldberg J. Hip fracture incidence among elderly Asian-American populations. Am J Epidemiol 1997; 146:502–509.

51. Karim N, Bloch DS, Falciglia G, Murthy L. Modifications in food consumption patterns reported by people from India, living in Cincinnati, Ohio. Ecology Food Nutr 1986; 19:11–18.

52. Netland PA. Acculturation and the diet of Asian-American elderly. J Nutr Elderly 1984; 3:37–56.

53. Wu-Tso P, Yey I-Li, Tam CF. Comparisons of dietary intake in young and old Asian Americans: a two-generation study. Nutr Res 1995; 15:1445–1462.

54. Pan YL, Dixon Z, Himburg S, Huffman F. Asian students change their eating patterns after living in the United States. J Am Diet Assoc 1999; 99:54–57.

55. Personal communications from Shanthy Bowman, USDA/ARS/BHNRC, Beltsville, MD.
56. Bertron P, Barnard ND, Mills M. Racial bias in federal nutrition policy, Part I: The public health implications of variations in lactase persistence. J Natl Med Assoc 1999; 91:151–157.
57. Kumanyika SK, Helitzer DL. Nutritional status and dietary patterns of racial minorities in the United States. In: Report of the Secretary's Task Force on Black and Minority Health. Vol II: Crosscutting Issues in Minority Health. U.S. Department of Health and Human Services. Washington, DC: Public Health Service, 1985; 118–190.
58. Weinstein RS, Bell NH. Diminished rates of bone formation in normal black adults. N Engl J Med 1988; 319:1698–1701.

20 Micronutrient Deficiencies

First Link in a Chain of Nutritional and Health Events in Economic Crises

Martin W. Bloem and Ian Darnton-Hill

1. INTRODUCTION

The scale of crises affecting populations has moved from the local level, in hunter-gatherer societies, to subcontinental epidemics and famines (e.g., the Black Death in medieval Europe), to world wars. These were clear disasters for those involved, both individuals and nations, and this has been reflected in high mortality levels and, usually, malnutrition. In the latter half of the twentieth century, crises often became more subtle, such as those caused by differing economic systems.

It is now well recognized that restructuring in the early 1980s had measurable impacts on malnutrition levels and national health, particularly among those most vulnerable *(1)*. However, this most recent crisis is yet again different, and has devastated the economies and social structures of several Asian societies, with repercussions being felt throughout the world, in Brazil, the Russian Federation, and even economies such as Australia. This is resulting not only in an immediate impact, but it will also result in a "lost generation." Further, this chapter shows that this crisis is best characterized and tracked by using micronutrient malnutrition and maternal malnutrition as indicators, instead of childhood malnutrition, and that these types of crises are felt more among the urban poor than among the rural population. The global significance of these findings is then discussed.

In 1996, Lester Thurow wrote about "the future of capitalism" *(2)*. In the summer of 1994, Mexico was a country that had a bright economic future: the budget was balanced, more than 1000 state-owned companies had been privatized, government regulations were slashed, and tariffs and quotas were dramatically reduced. Private capital was pouring in. However, by April 1995, Mexico's economy had collapsed, the average purchasing power declined by 30%, and 500,000 Mexicans had lost their jobs. Mexico had implemented all the policies that economists had recommended. Clearly, the nature of economic crises was changing.

Thurow borrowed two concepts from the physical sciences: the punctuated equilibrium theory of evolution from biology, and plate tectonics from geology. Punctuated equilibrium is the phenomenon in which the dominant species dies out rapidly as the environment suddenly changes. Earthquakes and volcanic explosions are a result of the invisible movement of the continental plates beneath the economic surface of the earth. In his book, Thurow recognized five economic "plates": the end of communism;

From: *Primary and Secondary Preventive Nutrition*
Edited by: A. Bendich and R. J. Deckelbaum © Humana Press Inc., Totowa, NJ

a technological shift to an era dominated by man-made brainpower industries; a demography never seen before; a truly global economy; and an era in which there is no dominant economic, political, or military power. He concluded from this conjunction that, as the "second world" collapsed, the third world had splintered. Within it, there were clear winners (the little tigers of Hong Kong, Singapore, South Korea, and Taiwan), potential winners (Malaysia and Thailand), those rapidly integrating with global capitalism (China), and the losers (most African countries). The third world is gone just as much as the second world is gone, he contended *(2)*.

One year later, the Asian economic crisis began. Not only had the predicted economic instability happened earlier than predicted, it also hit hardest among the so-called "clear winners." Once again, the health and well being of the common people were the victims of the global response to this new crisis. The International Monetary Fund (IMF) recommended a tight monetary policy, stringent fiscal policy, and structural and banking reforms, in exchange for multibillion dollar bailout schemes. Not only were these prescriptions relatively unsuccessful in the short term, but the effects on health (as measured by the impact on malnutrition, among other things) were seriously underestimated, and, to some extent, continued to be for some time into the crisis (World Bank Report 1999). As the economic recession spreads out to other countries of Asia and adjoining regions, there is a fear of a much larger meltdown in Eastern Europe and Latin America. It is important that lessons be learned from these events, not only from the political and economic points of view, but also how to predict, judge, and track their effects on the health and nutrition of populations.

2. THE INDONESIAN CRISIS

Indonesia is the world's fourth most populous country, with an estimated population of 203 million in 1998. It is a geographically vast country extending for more than 4800 km from west to east and 2000 km from north to south, between the Asian mainland and Australia. It has a highly diverse archipelagic structure, consisting of some 17,000 islands, of which 6000 are inhabited. About 55% of Indonesia's total population lives on Java, the most densely populated region. Java itself is divided into five provinces: West Java, Central Java, Yogyakarta, East Java, and the capital, Jakarta.

The country is endowed with substantial agricultural potential, as a result of which agriculture, including forestry and fisheries, is the most important sector of the economy in terms of employment. In addition, there is a vast range of mineral resources, including petroleum. Since the mid-1980s, the manufacturing sector has expanded dramatically, and its share in gross domestic product (GDP) exceeded that of agriculture in 1996.

In the past 30 yr, Indonesia was frequently hailed as a leading economic success story. Real GDP growth averaged over 7%/yr for the decade since 1987. In 1996, GDP per capita surpassed $1000 US, compared with $70 US in 1965. The rupiah was stable. Annual inflation was reported in the single digits, and foreign capital was pouring in. As a result, the prevalence of poverty, measured against the official poverty line, declined from about 40% in 1976 to 11.3% in 1996, a remarkable decline, given that the population increased from 120 to 195 million. Over the same period, the infant mortality rate declined, from an estimated 145 infant deaths per thousand live births, to 52, and the under-five mortality rate declined from about 217 to 75. Indonesia was one of the first developing countries to identify that its high levels of severe vitamin A deficiency (VAD) constituted a serious public health problem. Over the past 30 yr, the country has come a long way in reducing the levels of severe VAD, and, prior to the crisis, it was no longer considered a public health problem, except in three provinces *(3)* *(see* Chapter 15).

However, in 1997, Indonesia experienced a severe drought (El Nino), massive forest fires in Sumatra and Kalimantan, low world petroleum prices, and regional financial instability, domestic social unrest, and ultimately, a change of government. Total rice production in 1997 fell by 4%, but some provinces in the country registered sharper declines.

At the beginning of the Asia-wide economic crisis, Indonesia was an unaffected bystander as the economic events started in Thailand. However, by August 1997, the Indonesian rupiah began to come under pressure, and rapidly depreciated in the following months. The rupiah, which was trading 2450 to the dollar in July 1997, plunged to a low of 17,000 in January 1998, before strengthening to around 8000 in October 1998. The United States was in a strong cyclical upswing during the Mexican crisis, and was able to bail Mexico out, but the weakness of Japan's economy in 1997 exacerbated the Asian crisis, and worsened the unfolding of the currency crisis. Exchange rate volatility made planning almost impossible for many businesses. Annual inflation was running at an estimated 80%. Foreign capital had fled, closing off access to new foreign lending. Between 1992 and July 1997, about 85% of the increase in external debt resulted from private sector borrowing from private foreign resources attracted by the previous apparently continuous economic growth. However, with the increasingly unfavorable exchange rates, businesses struggled to service existing foreign debts.

The IMF moved quickly to play a role in encouraging Indonesia to formulate reform programs aimed at tackling the perceived roots of the problems and restoring investor confidence. The Indonesian government signed its first letter of intent to the IMF on October 31, 1997. However, the economic situation only worsened, and Indonesia's agreement with the IMF was revised several times in the following months. In May 1998, after fuel prices were increased and demonstrating students were shot, riots and looting swept across Jakarta and other cities, leading to the May 21 resignation of President Soeharto, who was replaced by his Vice President, B. J. Habibie.

3. HELEN KELLER INTERNATIONAL NUTRITIONAL SURVEILLANCE

In 1998, in reaction to the Indonesian economic crisis, Helen Keller International started out a nutritional surveillance project, which had commenced in December 1995, originally to monitor a social marketing campaign promoting the consumption of eggs and vegetables to improve the vitamin status of the target population. Subsequently, the crisis nutritional surveillance project expanded to six provinces, including four urban areas.

The impact of macroeconomic adjustment programs or economic crises on food security and the nutritional status of the poor is not well documented *(4)*. Helen Keller International had extensive experience in natural disaster impact assessment in Bangladesh *(5)*. The agency was in the unique position of having a nutritional surveillance system in place in the Central Java province since December 1995. Data have been collected every 3 mo since then, for four rounds over 1 yr, until January 1997 *(6,7)*. The original purpose of that surveillance system was to assess the impact of a large-scale social marketing program promoting the consumption of vitamin A-rich foods. As a response to the crisis, the surveillance system was revived in June 1998, and expanded to five more provinces:

the provincial and national capital of Jakarta, rural West Java, East Java (with a special focus on its capital, Surabaya), West Nusa Tenggara (specifically, the island of Lombok), and South Sulawesi (specifically, its capital city, Ujung Pandang). The rural data presented in this chapter were collected between June 1996 and January 1997, June 1998, and January 1999. The comparisons between the different levels of urbanization were collected between January and March 1999.

It is shown that measuring protein-energy malnutrition is not the most appropriate indicator to use in such a crisis; levels of iron deficiency anemia (IDA) and VAD, and food intake of animal products, are all more sensitive measures that can also be detected earlier. As has been seen in Asia, large numbers of people in affected countries have, or will have, less purchasing power because of the crisis. What will be the impact on the health and nutritional status of these segments of the population?

4. CHARACTERIZING UNDERLYING MALNUTRITION USING THE UNITED NATIONS CHILDREN'S FUND CONCEPTUAL FRAMEWORK

In 1990, UNICEF applied a conceptual framework to determine the most likely causes of malnutrition (8). The framework has proven to be a very useful concept, and consists of the following key elements:

- Nutritional status is identified as an outcome of processes in society.
- Malnutrition is a result of immediate, underlying, and basic causes in a hierarchical manner.
- Delivery of services, e.g., feeding programs, oral rehydration therapy, vitamin A supplementation, expanded programs of immunization, and so on, primarily addresses the immediate causes.
- Access to food, adequate care of children and women, and access to basic health services, together with a healthy environment, are necessary conditions for nutritional security. Inadequate access to food may include macro- (energy, protein) and micronutrients (vitamins and minerals).
- The basic causes are defined by the economic, political, and ideological environment in which the malnutrition is occurring.

Using the UNICEF conceptual framework to better understand the coping strategies of the Indonesian population, it has also been possible to identify which indicators are the most crisis-sensitive.

4.1. Basic Causes

As mentioned previously, two fundamental causes of the apparent increase in malnutrition in Indonesia were the drought resulting from El Nino and the recent Asian economic crisis.

Although the two phenomena were distinct, both have had the same effect of a decrease in the real income of virtually all sectors of the society. The prices of most food items increased dramatically in the period between January and July 1998, with an inflation rate of 78% during that year. The economic crisis had serious, adverse social impacts. The National Socioeconomic Survey (SUSSENAS), conducted in February 1998, showed that 10% of the urban population and 5% of the rural population were unemployed. The unemployment rate for the whole country was estimated at 7% in February 1998.

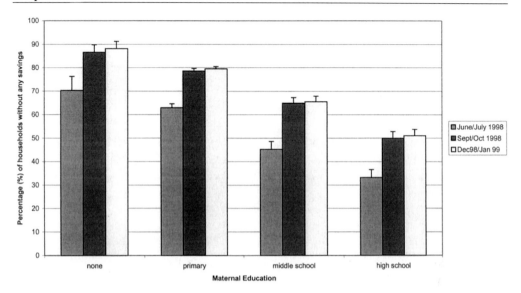

Fig. 1. Percentage of households without any savings by socioeconomic status (using maternal education as proxy).

High inflation and the increased unemployment rates resulted in a sharp decline in real earnings, and a consequent rise in the incidence of poverty. Figure 1 shows the percentage of households without any savings by socioeconomic group (using maternal education as a proxy) between June 1998 and January 1999. Unfortunately, these data were not collected before the crisis. Although, proportionally, the poor were more affected than the middle class, the crisis affected all socioeconomic strata. These data, and a World Bank report, indicated an increase in the incidence of poverty, and that the social impact has been very unequally distributed across sectors and regions. Urban and periurban areas were hardest hit, mostly because of massive contraction in the manufacturing and construction sectors, in particular. Among the regions, Java was the worst affected.

4.2. Underlying Causes

Inadequate access to food, inadequate care for mothers and children, insufficient health services, and unhealthy environments are the underlying causes of malnutrition. What was the impact of increased poverty on access to food? Although rice prices had increased considerably, rice consumption did not change; the poorer households in fact consumed more rice per capita than the higher socioeconomic groups.

However, the consumption of the more expensive food items, such as animal products, was also surveyed and found to be affected. In 1996, the government of Indonesia, in close collaboration with Helen Keller International and UNICEF, had carried out a social marketing campaign to promote the consumption of eggs as an important food source for vitamin A. Based on formative research, it was determined that eggs were the most affordable animal source of micronutrients in Central Java. The program was very successful, and serum retinol levels increased as a result of the campaign (7). Figure 2 shows the households with mothers consuming no eggs, i.e., more households were including eggs in their diets. After the start of the program, there was a decrease in the number of

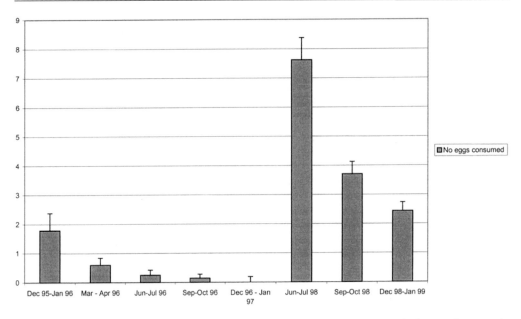

Fig. 2. Percentage of households in which mothers did not consume any eggs in the previous week.

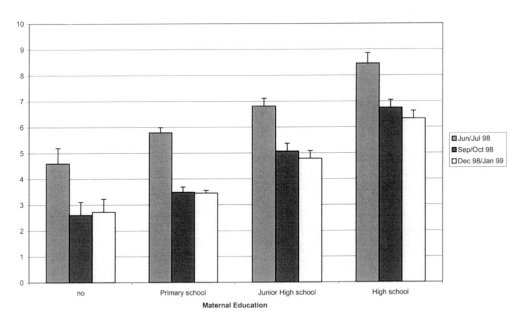

Fig. 3. Percentage of households in which mothers did not consume any eggs in the previous week by socioeconomic status.

households consuming no eggs. However, 1 yr after the start of the economic crisis, this percentage almost 8%. Although the percentage of households with women not consuming any eggs in the previous week improved in the following 6 mo, Fig. 3 clearly shows that there was a decline in the number of eggs consumed in all socioeconomic groups, but most dramatically among the poorest stratum. The difference between June/June and September/October is statistically significant ($p < 0.00$).

Given the inflation and rising unemployment, the economic crisis resulted in a decrease in the real income of large segments of the society. As a result, those affected had to increase their expenditure on food as a percentage of their total expenditure. Although the expenditure on staple foods remained the same, expenditure on more expensive animal products declined.

5. EFFECT OF THE CRISIS ON MALNUTRITION

5.1. Effect of the Crisis on Micronutrient Deficiencies

It is well established that, without fortification or supplementation, communication strategies for dietary behavior change are unlikely to be adequate, in themselves, in either treating or preventing iron (Fe) deficiency and anemia in developing countries. Meats (beef, pork, lamb, fowl, fish, and so on) and liver, which are rich in heme-Fe, are the best sources of Fe, but are also relatively expensive and unaffordable for poor segments of societies (9). Moreover, recent research from Indonesia has shown that plant sources of vitamin A (those more eaten by the poor) are about 5× less effective in improving the vitamin A status than was previously thought (10,11). Animal products, such as eggs and liver, are high in micronutrients, not only Fe and vitamin A, but also zinc and B-vitamins. As mentioned previously, the economic crisis showed a decline in the consumption of animal products, including eggs; but the consumption of the staple food, rice, remained the same. Based on these data, it was expected that an increase of micronutrient deficiencies would be observed. The authors used iron deficiency anemia (IDA) as a proxy for micronutrient status in general, and the first sign of clinical Vitamin A deficiency (VAD), night blindness, as a proxy for severe forms of micronutrient deficiencies.

5.1.1. IRON DEFICIENCY ANEMIA

Although more than 22 countries have adopted public health policies calling for Fe supplementation of infants and preschool children, the effectiveness of those programs is still very low (9). Infants born of mothers with IDA are more likely to have low Fe stores. Birth weight is also an important determinant of an infant's Fe status at the time of birth. That is why low-birth-weight infants need Fe supplementation from 2 mo up to at least 18 mo of age. Those infants born with lower Fe stores also require more Fe than can be supplied by breast milk at a younger age (12). Although breast-feeding remains a key to the health and nutrition of infants, after 6 mo, even infants with normal Fe stores will have used the Fe stores they had at birth, and breast milk will not provide the amount needed as they continue to grow and develop rapidly. So the high prevalence of Fe deficiency is largely the result of inadequate dietary intake to meet the relatively high Fe requirements of early childhood (13).

There is an array of evidence showing that moderate to severe anemia in infancy has a lasting impact on mental development; Fe deficiency at any age has adverse effects on cognitive performance (14–17). Fe deficiency has also been shown to reduce immunocompetence and resistance to infection, and to affect child development and growth.

Figure 4 shows that there was an increase in the levels of childhood IDA between June–July 1996 and June–July 1998. In the same time period, there were no changes in child-

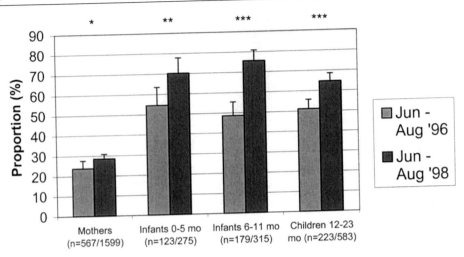

Fig. 4. Proportion of infants, children, and mothers as a percentage with iron deficiency anemia (using WHO cut-off points for hemoglobin levels).

hood malnutrition, except in one of the poorest ecological zones. In the following months, the situation improved, and, by January 1999, the prevalence of anemia was similar to precrisis levels (50%). However, it is recommended that, if the prevalence of anemia is greater than 40%, all children should be supplemented daily until 18 mo of age *(18)*. In 1996, the distribution of Fe syrup to children under 5 yr, in less-developed villages in Eastern Indonesia was started, but the prevalence rates reported showed that the program is far from being effective, and there is a great need to improve the effectiveness of this program.

Figure 5 shows that the prevalence of anemia increases by level of urbanization. The urban poor also have greater exposure to contaminants such as lead (Pb). Pb is very toxic during the fetal stage of life and early childhood, and causes long-term damage to the neural system *(19,20)*. Children who are Fe-deficient have a greater susceptibility to toxicity from heavy metals (including Pb) *(9)*. Jakarta has a high level of Pb pollution, and these children live in the poorest areas of urban Jakarta, close to the roads. Although we have no data on the prevalence of Pb poisoning, it can be assumed that this will be high among these Fe-deficient infants.

The prevalence of anemia among pregnant women and women of reproductive age showed a similar pattern to that of the infants (Fig. 4). Levels increased in four of the six ecological zones of Central Java, markedly so in Central North, Central South, and the Northeast.

5.1.2. Vitamin A Deficiency

Vitamin A is required for the proper maintenance and functioning of the immune system, and is essential to ensure the integrity of the respiratory and digestive epithelia that protect people from acute infections. Vitamin A supplementation among children reduces the risk of mortality by 23%. A recent study also showed that vitamin A supplementation may reduce maternal mortality by 40–50% *(21)*.

The first national vitamin A survey in Indonesia in 1978 showed that xerophthalmia was a public health problem. Indonesia became one of the first developing countries to recognize that its high levels of severe VAD constituted a serious public health problem, and to begin implementing programs to eliminate the problem. Over the past 30 yr, the

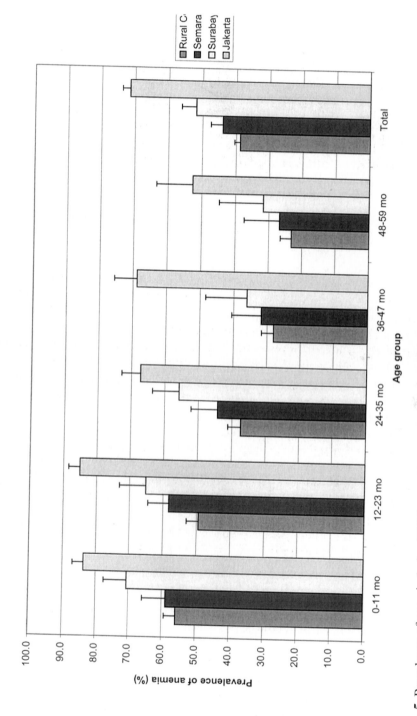

Fig. 5. Prevalence of anemia (using WHO cut-off points for hemoglobin levels) for infants and children according to degree of urbanization.

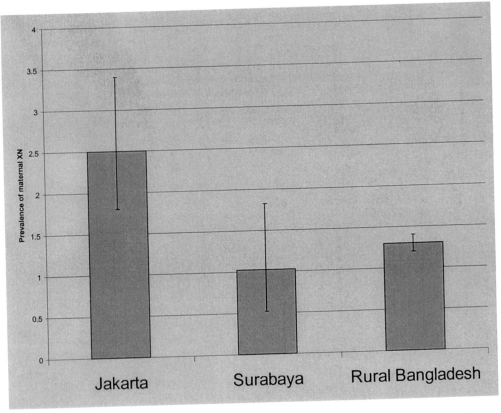

Fig. 6. Prevalence of night blindness from two urban sites in Indonesia compared with rural Bangladesh.

country has been considered a major success story in reducing the level of severe VAD, and, prior to the crisis, xerophthalmia was no longer considered a public health problem, although subclinical VAD was still prevalent in rural areas.

A dramatically decreased intake of micronutrient-rich foods following the advent of the crisis, caused by the increased prices of commodities and reduced purchasing power, was identified by the Indonesian Department of Health, University of Diponegoro, and Helen Keller International. This decrease has been correlated with an increase in the prevalence of night blindness among children aged 0–35 mo, and an increase in the prevalence of night blindness among women of reproductive age. Figure 6 shows the high prevalence of maternal night blindness from two urban sites in Indonesia, compared with the level found in rural Bangladesh. There was a dramatic increase in clinical VAD among women in urban areas.

5.2. Effect of the Crisis on Undernutrition

Since the start of the crisis in August 1997, until December 1998, more than 600 new cases of marasmus and kwashiorkor have been detected by the Indonesian government's health information system.

The Central Java surveillance system did not, however, reveal any overall effect of the Indonesian crisis on the prevalence of stunting, underweight, or wasting in rural Central

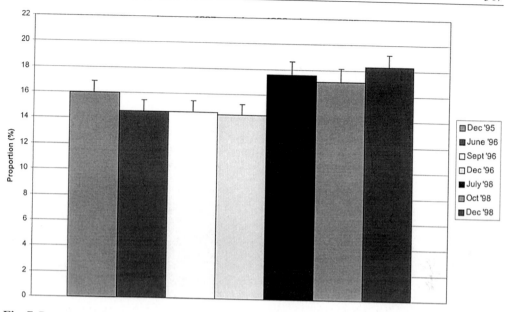

Fig. 7. Prevalence of maternal malnutrition as determined by body mass index (BMI) using FAO cut-off points.

Java. When stratified for the various ecological zones, there was an increase of wasting in northeast Central Java, which is one of the poorest areas in Central Java. Urbanization was found to be an important factor, with the level of stunting lowest in Jakarta and highest in the rural areas of Central Java; the level of acute malnutrition (wasting) was highest in Jakarta.

Figure 7 shows the prevalence of maternal malnutrition in rural Indonesia as determined by a low body mass index (BMI). Maternal malnutrition, as indicated by the prevalence of low BMI, is a good and early indicator of the population's food security (Table 1), because a woman often reduces her own food intake before reducing that of her children and/or husband, as, e.g., was observed with egg consumption. Although an increase of acute childhood malnutrition was only seen in pocket areas, maternal malnutrition increased significantly in all sites.

Recent research by Pelletier and Rahn (22), based on a compilation and analysis of mean BMI in 1432 published samples from developing countries, has shown that average BMI among women in South and Southeast Asian countries had increased from 20.9 kg/m^2 in 1960 to 21.4 kg/m^2 in 1990. The average BMI among women from rural Java had dropped by 0.45 kg/m^2, almost equivalent to the 0.5 kg/m^2 increase achieved since the early 1960s. This raises the question of whether 30 yr of nutritional improvement in Southeast Asia has disappeared in 1 yr of crisis? The further question is what will be the intergenerational impact of this on subsequent generations?

Although there are no baseline data in the urban areas, the level of malnutrition was higher in the urban areas, compared with rural Central Java, and reached almost 20%. According to the World Health Organization, a prevalence of 20–39% of the population with a low BMI constitutes a very serious food insecurity problem (23). Because chronic malnutrition among the children was lowest in the urban areas and acute malnutrition

Table 1
Underlying Causes of Malnutrition Using the UNICEF Framework and Their
Contribution to Undernutrition, Anemia, and Night Blindness for Women and Children

Indicator	Access to food (Macro-and micronutrients)	Inadequate care	Health services/ unhealthy environment
Childhood malnutrition	++	++	++
Maternal Malnutrition	++	±	-
Childhood anemia	+	±	- (No supplementation program)
Maternal anemia	+	±	+ - (Supplementation programs for pregnant women and factory workers)
Childhood night blindness	+	±	++ (VAC-supplementation program)
Maternal night blindness	+	±	± (Post partum VAC-supplementation program)

highest, it can be assumed that the high level of maternal malnutrition was also an effect of the economic crisis.

6. EFFECT OF THE CRISIS ON URBAN VS RURAL POPULATIONS

The economic crisis had different effects in the urban and in the rural areas. For this differential analysis of urban and rural, the data from both rural and urban Central Java, (Semarang), Surabaya (urban East Java, second largest city of Indonesia), and Jakarta (urban West Java) were used. Figure 8 shows the prevalence of stunting among children aged 12–24 mo, stratified by urbanization level. The level of stunting is lowest in Jakarta and highest in the rural areas of Central Java. Since the level of chronic malnutrition was lowest in the more urbanized areas, it is very likely that the quality of the food was more optimal in the urban areas before the crisis.

It is well documented globally that, as populations move from rural to urban areas, their diets change from being rich in complex carbohydrates and fiber to more varied diets with a higher proportion of fat, refined sugars, and meat products. However, it is more complex than just changing dietary patterns, and there is increasing understanding that the causes of malnutrition and food insecurity in urban and rural areas are different, because of factors that are unique to, or exacerbated by, urban living (24). Findings consistently show that both childhood mortality rates and the prevalence of stunting and underweight are generally lower in urban, compared with rural, areas (25). The authors' findings from the Indonesian situation, showing that the prevalence of stunting is generally lower in urban than in rural areas, are consistent with several recent reviews (25–27).

The urban population in Indonesia is mostly dependent on the market as the main source of food. Food prices and the ability to earn a cash income are, in general, crucial to the achievement of food security in urban areas (25). However, the prices of many food

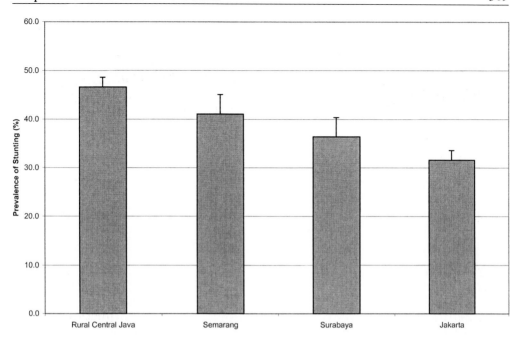

Fig. 8. Prevalence of stunting (height for age) among children 12–23 months by levels of urbanization.

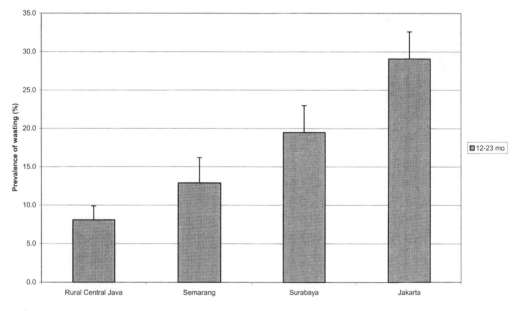

Fig. 9. Prevalence of wasting (weight for height) among children 12–23 months by level of urbanization.

items became 2–3× more expensive, and the urban poor had hardly any coping mechanisms. Furthermore, despite the fact that this was recognized in September 1998, the safety net programs of the government focused mostly on the rural areas. Figure 9 shows the level of wasting, by urbanization level (collected in January–March 1999), showing the level of acute malnutrition was the highest in Jakarta. This suggests that there is more acute, and infection-related, malnutrition in the urban areas, which would be consistent with other findings in the rest of the world *(25)*. The data on the urban areas were collected from households in the poorest neighborhoods and slums, where most of the people had jobs in the construction industry.

The chapter has already shown that there is also a high prevalence of micronutrient malnutrition among women and children in the urban areas. Micronutrient deficiencies lead to greater susceptibility to infections, and this may have exacerbated infection rates. However, the prevalence of underweight showed a similar pattern to the prevalence of wasting; there was a higher prevalence of underweight by level of urbanization. This suggests that, previously, there had been relative food security in the urban areas in Indonesia, and also that, for the urban poor, nutrition safety nets are less secure than in rural areas.

7. OUTCOME INDICATORS

The UNICEF conceptual framework can also be used to analyze the most crisis-sensitive indicators. As explained earlier, the greatest immediate effect of the crisis was a drop in the real income of the population, caused by rising prices of several commodities, and by increased unemployment. This is likely to result in a reduced consumption of expensive food items in particular. Furthermore, the IMF program included measures to reduce government spending on food subsidies and other social programs.

Although the underlying causes of malnutrition consist of inadequate access to food, inadequate care for mothers and children, insufficient health services, and unhealthy environments, the importance of each component differs for the various outcome indicators. Table 1 shows that it can be argued that maternal malnutrition, childhood anemia, and maternal night blindness are the best indicators to follow the effect of the crisis on food insecurity in Indonesia, because the health services and environmental components have little effect on the underlying changes reflected in these indicators. Conversely, the reduced access to food, especially more nutrient-rich foods, will be quickly reflected in changing prevalences of childhood anemia, maternal night blindness, and maternal malnutrition.

What impact the crisis would have on the other underlying causes of malnutrition (inadequate care, insufficient health services, and unhealthy environments) is still unclear. The vitamin A capsule distribution program, for children aged 1–5 yr, is a program that has been in place since the early 1970s. The capsule distribution, evaluated between June 1998 and January 1999, showed only a slight decline in its coverage (Fig. 10). The distribution was only 10% lower than 2 yr before the crisis. This suggests an important lesson in terms of sustainability of this mode of delivering vitamin A, and suggests that health services are not yet being seriously compromised.

Monitoring of food intake gives useful further information, in terms of reduced accessibility to more expensive foods, leading to increased chances of micronutrient deficiencies, and thus greater exposure to the impact of infectious diseases. For planning, some indication of the limits to which coping mechanisms are being stretched is necessary to give a more complete picture.

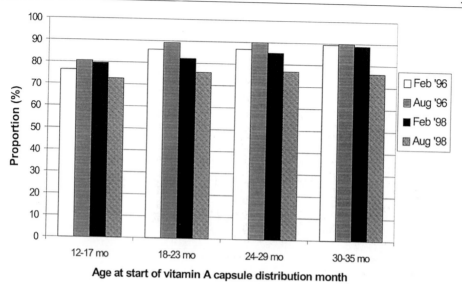

Fig. 10. Proportion of children as a percentage receiving a routine vitamin A capsule stratified by 6 monthly age group.

8. CONCLUSIONS AND RECOMMENDATIONS

The first effect of the Indonesian economic crisis on the food intake was a decrease in the consumption of animal products; the consumption of rice remained the same. This resulted in a dramatic increase in the prevalence of childhood anemia in both urban and rural Indonesia. Since animal products are rich in other micronutrients, as well, these data suggest that these children would probably also be deficient in other micronutrients. IDA in children in areas without extensive Fe fortification efforts, and/or Fe supplementation programs, is likely to be a very sensitive indicator to measure the potential impact of structural adjustment programs or economic crises similar to the Indonesian economic crisis. In June/July of the crisis, the authors found a significant increase of IDA among infants, young children, and women, and a slight increase of VAD. In the following 6 mo, the situation appeared to improve enough, so that the prevalence decreased to the still high, precrisis level.

However, the vitamin A capsule distribution system remained mostly intact, which presumably accounts for the fact there was only a slight increase in childhood night blindness detected. Mothers do not have access to vitamin A capsules, in general, which is why a change in the prevalence of maternal night blindness is likely to be a more useful indicator in such situations.

Between June–July 1998 (1 yr after the beginning of the crisis) and December 1998–January 1999, there was no increase of stunting and underweight in rural Central Java. The data did not show an overall increase in the prevalence of wasting, except in one of the poorest ecological zones. The effect of these types of crises on protein energy malnutrition appears, therefore, to be secondary. Although there was no dramatic increase in childhood malnutrition, the data did show a significant increase of maternal malnutrition (low BMI), suggesting that this is a more immediate indicator.

The urban areas were more affected by the Indonesian crisis than the rural areas. The Indonesian economic crisis resulted in collapse of the construction sector and increase of food prices. Because the urban poor were dependent on food prices and the ability to earn cash income, an increase in malnutrition rates could be predicted. Although the level of chronic childhood malnutrition (stunting) was significantly negatively associated with the level of urbanization, the prevalence of underweight (weight-for-age) and acute malnutrition (weight-for-length) was significantly positively associated with the level of urbanization. Furthermore, the prevalence of micronutrient deficiencies (IDA and VAD) was significantly higher in the urban areas than in the rural areas.

These data suggest that the urban poor were hit significantly harder by the crisis, which resulted both in low macronutrient and micronutrient intakes. About 30% of Jakarta's urban poor are not officially registered as citizens of Indonesia's capital city. Even when this is acknowledged, it complicates the official response, and is presumably one of the reasons why safety-net programs did not prevent the most vulnerable urban groups, detected in this Helen Keller International-led surveillance system, from falling into poverty.

8.1. Recommendations

The Indonesian crisis had specific effects on the nutritional and health status of its population. There are many lessons to be learned from these data. From all the above, it is recommended, in such economic crises, that the most efficient way of detecting nutrition distress, and, hence, likely increased morbidity and impaired development, is to track the following indicators: child anemia levels, maternal night blindness, and maternal undernutrition. It is less useful to rely on signs of protein-energy malnutrition, as has been customarily done in other forms of emergencies.

In 1993, the World Bank came out with the report, *Investing in Health (28)*. The report highlighted to what extent health interventions were cost-effective, in economic terms. Besides the fact that micronutrient deficiencies may result in an increased risk of both childhood and maternal mortality, these deficiencies also have a proven longer-term impact on poor development of children as future human resources. This is often forgotten in economic adjustment programs, and the authors would argue for more emphasis on micronutrient deficiency control as part of safety net programs. Countries cannot afford to lose a generation. Fe deficiency has a massive, but until recently almost totally unrecognized, economic cost. Indonesia will eventually recover from the economic crisis, and again have to compete economically with other countries in the region, and globally. This will depend, to a large extent, on human resources, and the adequacy of their health and nutrition.

REFERENCES

1. Editorial. Structural adjustment too painful? Lancet 1994; 344:1377–1378.
2. Thurow LC. The Future of Capitalism: How Today's Economic Forces Shape Tomorrow's World. New York: Penguin, 1996.
3. Sommer A, West KP Jr. Vitamin A deficiency, health, survival, and vision. New York: Oxford University Press, 1996.
4. Pinstrup-Andersen P. Assuring food security and adequate nutrition for the poor. Health, nutrition and economic crises: approaches to policy in the Third World. Can J Dev Stud 1998; 19:special issue, 147–175.

5. Bloem MW, Hye A, Gorstein J, Wijnroks M, Hall G, Matzger H, Sommer A. Nutrition surveillance in Bangladesh: a useful tool for policy planning at the local and national levels. Food Nutr Bull 1995; 16:131–138.

6. de Pee S, Bloem MW, Gorstein J, Sari M, Satoto, Yip R, Shrimpton R, Muhilal. Re-appraisal of the role of vegetables in the vitamin A status of mothers in Central Java, Indonesia. Am J Clin Nutr 1998; 68:1068–1074.

7. de Pee S, Bloem MW, Satoto, Yip R, Sukaton A, Tjiong R, et al. Impact of a social marketing campaign promoting dark-green leafy vegetables and eggs in Central Java, Indonesia. Int J Vit Nutr Res 1998; 68:389–398.

8. Jonsson U. Towards an improved strategy for nutrition surveillance. Food Nutr Bull 1995; 16:102–111.

9. UNU/UNICEF/WHO/MI. Preventing iron deficiency in women and children: consensus on key technical issues. Ottawa: Micronutrient Initiative, 1999.

10. de Pee S, West CE, Permaesih D, Martuti S, Muhilal, Hautvast JGAJ. Orange fruit is more effective than are dark-green, leafy vegetables in increasing serum concentrations of retinol and B-carotene in school children in Indonesia. Am J Clin Nutr 1998; 68:1058–1067.

11. de Pee S, Bloem MW, Gorstein J, Sari M, Satoto, Yip R, Shrimpton R, Muhilal. Reappraisal of the role of vegetables for vitamin A status of mothers in Central Java, Indonesia. Am J Clin Nutr 1998; 68: 1068–1074.

12. UNICEF/WHO. The World Summit for Children: strategy for reducing iron deficiency anaemia in children. UNICEF-WHO Joint Committee on Health Policy, JCHP30/95/4.5, December 1994.

13. Yip R. The challenge of improving iron nutrition: limitations and potentials of major intervention approaches. Eur J Clin Nutr 1997; 51:S16–S24.

14. Pollitt E, Gorman KS, Engle PL, Martorell R, Rivera J. Early supplementary feeding and cognition. Monograph of the Society for Research and Child Development. Ser 235. 1993; 58:7.

15. Lozoff B, Jiminez E, Wolf AW. Long-term developmental outcome of infants with iron deficiency. N Engl J Med 1991; 325:687–695.

16. Holst M. Nutrition and the life cycle: developmental and behavioral effects on iron deficiency anemia in infants. Nutr Today 1998; 13:27–36.

17. Scrimshaw NS. Malnutrition, brain development, learning, and behavior. Nutr Res 1998; 18:351–379.

18. INACG/WHO/UNICEF (Stoltzfus RJ, Dreyfuss ML). Guidelines for the use of iron supplements to prevent and treat iron deficiency anemia. Washington, DC: ILSI Press, 1998.

19. Goyer RA. Nutrition and metal toxicity. Am J Clin Nutr 1995; 61(Suppl.):646S–650S.

20. Peraza MA, Rael LT, Casarez E, Barbaer DS, Ayala-Fierra F. Effects of micronutrients on metal toxicity. Environ Health Pers 1998; 106(Suppl.):203–216.

21. West KP, Katz J, Khatry SK, LeClerq SC, Pradhan EK, Shrestha SR, et al., on behalf of the NIPPS-2 Study Group. Double blind, cluster randomized trial of low dose supplementation with vitamin A or beta-carotene on mortality related to pregnancy in Nepal. Br Med J 1999; 318:570–575.

22. Pelletier DL, Rahn M. Trends in body mass index in developing countries. Food Nutr Bull 1998; 19:223–229.

23. WHO. Physical status: the use and interpretation of anthropometry. Report of a WHO Expert Committee. Geneva: World Health Organization, 1995.

24. Ruel MT, Haddad L, Garrett JL. Some urban facts of life: implications for research and policy. IFPRI Discussion Paper 64 (Discussion Paper Brief). Food Consumption and Nutrition Division of the International Food Policy Research Institute. Washington, DC: IFPRI, 1999.

25. Haddad L, Ruel MT, Garrett JL. Are urban poverty and undernutrition growing? Some newly assembled evidence. IFPRI Discussion Paper 63 (Discussion Paper Brief). Food Consumption and Nutrition Division of the International Food Policy Research Institute. Washington, DC: IFPRI, 1999.

26. Hussain AM, Lunven P. Urbanization and hunger in the cities. Food Nutr Bull 1987; 9:50–61.

27. von Braun J, McComb J, Fred-Mensah B, Pandya-Lorch R. Urban food insecurity and malnutrition in developing countries: trends, policies, and research implications. Washington, DC: International Food Policy Research Institute, 1993.

28. World Bank. Investing in Health. World Development Report 1993. The International Bank for Reconstruction and Development/The World Bank. New York: Oxford University Press, 1993.

21

Alcohol
The Balancing Act

William E. M. Lands

1. OVERVIEW

Intakes of nutrients by individuals are customarily described with broad areas of acceptable choice between some average lower limit of needed supply and an average safe upper limit. Safe upper limits of average alcohol consumption by individuals have been a principal focus of national dialog for 200 yr. The *Dietary Guidelines for Americans (1)* recommend no more than 1 drink/d for women or 2 drinks/d for men (with a standard drink being either 12 oz regular beer, 5 oz wine, or 1.5 oz distilled spirits, each containing about 14 g [100 calories] of ethanol). At this time, no major scientific body recognizes a nutritional need for alcohol, or recommends that those who do not drink should begin doing so.

A recent hypothesis that moderate alcohol may decrease cardiovascular (CV) death rates prompted review of the information that can place possible future preventive nutrition advice in the context of what has been learned from past advice. A useful context for balancing benefits and risks in drinking alcohol comes from weighing the possible benefits of drinking alcohol against the effectiveness of treating those at risk for developing alcohol use disorders, individuals whom we are still unable to identify *a priori*. The possible benefit of less CV mortality remains uncertain, and the risk of more alcohol disorders has a long history of inadequate intervention. Insufficient evidence on definite mechanisms of how cardiovascular disease (CVD) processes operate is paralleled by insufficient evidence on how alcohol acts to diminish those processes, and even whether or not alcohol does diminish CVD. Readers interested in designing preventive nutrition interventions, or in making personal decisions based on a fully informed choice, may find that the slow rate of acquiring conclusive evidence on causes and effects makes policy-setting seem premature at this time. The information assembled below does not form a smooth, solid series of proofs, but instead represents key concepts arrayed as beads on a string for the reader's contemplation.

2. BALANCING CAUSES AND CONSEQUENCES

2.1. Importance of Contexts

Causes and consequences are the stuff of science. They are the way that scientists interpret events by converting instinctive questions of purpose, i.e., "Why?", into the dimensions of "How come?" and "So what?" By balancing new information about things

From: *Primary and Secondary Preventive Nutrition*
Edited by: A. Bendich and R. J. Deckelbaum © Humana Press Inc., Totowa, NJ

and events with previously accumulated associations and memories, people learn to understand life and their surroundings. Experience provides each person with a new balance of combined positive and negative associations from which the mind produces conscious and subconscious outcomes that shape interpretations, emotions, and actions. It is the context within which new evidence is assimilated that strongly influences the cognitive and emotional significance of that information for each individual. Each of us believes that we know some things with certainty, and that we can use that knowledge to choose a rational course of action. This review examines some of that knowledge in a context that can aid informed choices.

Scientific procedures are designed to maintain an overall context, while systematically assembling the evidence needed to convert conjectures into conclusions. When possible, we controlled interventions are designed in a given context to gain certainty about how an event can directly cause a consequence. There is a constant challenge in such experiments to recognize which evidence proves direct cause–effect links, which reflects secondary consequences, and which comes from unrelated associated events. All three types of information occur in an uncertain balance, as the observational science of epidemiology collects and records diverse events associated with alcohol drinking. The strength of epidemiology is in its ability to define boundaries of a problem and to prompt new hypotheses about causes. However, testing those hypotheses requires interventions with well-designed positive and negative controls that are often hard to achieve with human subjects. In balancing information on the possible benefits and risks of drinking beverage alcohol in the context of preventive nutrition, one needs to recognize whether the information is from an association suitable for suggesting a hypothetical cause, or whether it is from a controlled intervention that can prove a causal relationship. Such recognition is difficult, because of two ways that diversity among individuals in a society inevitably confounds measurements of risk, as well as attempts at collective agreement about what those risks are.

2.2. Individuals Within Populations

First, human life is the complex consequence of 100,000 genes producing products in different amounts at different times in response to gene–gene and gene–environment interactions. Although the genomic sequence for each individual is finite, the adaptations produced from the interactions of a given set of 100,000 genes include such a vast number of possible outcomes as to be completely unpredictable in detail, even though general trends may be predicted. Imprecision is further assured by the action of another layer of inherent complexity: that of neuronal adaptation during learning and memory storage, fixing associations of interactions with the environment into cognitive and emotional memories that then influence future behaviors and preferences. Each thing learned is through neural associations that involve thousands of synaptic links, and "learning from experience" inevitably differs for each individual. As a result, the combined associative memories that link events together have a different balance of cognitive and emotional valence for each individual, leading to diverse interpretations, when attempting to answer complex questions, such as "Is drinking alcohol beneficial or harmful?" and "Why do some people drink so much?" Such diverse interpretations and priorities can confound efforts at consensus on the possible causes of events, and they need open evaluation in the process of scientific dialog (discussed further in Subheading 6.). In fact, consensus may be further confounded because the questions truly have different answers for different individuals.

Second, above and beyond the complex adaptive systems of the living body and the collective memories and emotions of the mind is the added level of complexity of societal adaptations. Consensus among individuals is difficult when democratic societies struggle to balance the preferences and priorities of diverse individuals with those of the collective society. Efforts in preventive nutrition to maximize the number of people free from any harm, or to minimize the degree of overall harm to the community, inevitably develop conflicts in balancing each individual's free choice with the effort to decrease perceived risk to the group. To develop a consensus for interventions, precision is needed in defining the physiological condition to be prevented and the causal mediators to be targeted. However, precise statistical descriptions of an aggregate community cannot precisely describe any individual within the community for which a balanced consensus is desired. As epidemiologists gather more information on larger numbers of subjects to increase the certainty of an average association, they also increase the number of people who are not precisely described by the population mean values. Thus, a struggle for balance is evident in efforts to develop scientifically credible targets for acceptable community intervention that could also be credibly sound advice for individuals. The resultant compromise about possible causes of good and bad health find expression in a nation's guidelines for healthy lifestyles. For example, the *Surgeon General's Report on Nutrition and Health (2)* described a situation and state of knowledge in 1988 similar to that today: "Excessive alcohol intake is a prominent contributor to 4/10 leading causes of death in the United States." Subsequently, the *Dietary Guidelines for Americans (1)*, provided in 1995, were intended to meet nationwide nutrient requirements, promote health, support active lives, and reduce chronic disease risks, by combining available, affordable, and enjoyable foods to make healthful diets that fit appropriate physical activity. That report recommends that "if you drink alcoholic beverages, do so in moderation" *(1)*.

In a broader approach, a healthy diet indicator was developed from World Health Organization's dietary recommendations, to evaluate dietary patterns and mortality in different cultures *(3)*. For different regions (in Finland, Italy, and the Netherlands), the 20-yr mortality was lowest in men with the highest healthy diet indicator. The indicator had a strong inverse association with mortality from CVDs, and it was positively associated with alcohol intake. The association between these two factors makes it important to decide what evidence can define how much benefit is to be allocated to each factor. Can the existing data assign healthiness to the diet or to the alcohol? An ironic uncertainty comes from the knowledge that, in assembling the data, energy provided by alcohol was segregated and not included in calculations for macronutrients as a percentage of energy intake *(3)*. In developing social policy, do alcohol calories count or not? Such a question echoes the long-standing uncertainty about how to interpret alcohol calories *(4)*, which is described further in Subheading 4.

2.3. Lifestyle Choices

A 6-yr longitudinal study of 43,757 male health professionals gave useful insight into patterns of voluntary food choice made by well-informed individuals *(5)*. When individuals were ranked by increasing quintiles of mean saturated fat intake (g/d), there were corresponding progressive increasing gradients for mean saturated fat and total fat

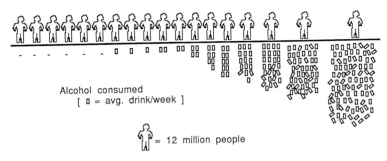

Fig. 1. Is alcohol everybody's problem? The figure represents results reported in the *Surgeon General's Report on Nutrition and Health*, 1988. Each small rectangular symbol represents one standard alcoholic beverage (14 g ethanol) consumed per week, and each human figure represents 12 million Americans aged 14 yr or older. The population in July, 1988, was about 270 million, of whom about 80% were 14 yr and older.

intake as percent of energy, servings of high-fat dairy food, and servings of red meat; there were progressively decreasing gradients for servings of fruits, vegetables, and fish. The percent of individuals who smoked increased with higher quintiles of saturated fat intake; mean physical activity and mean alcohol consumption decreased. The coupled lifestyle choices of these well-informed individuals illustrate a difficulty in unraveling the web of factors that contribute to the overall health status of each individual. If clusters of choices go together in a healthy lifestyle that accompanies eating less saturated fats, what evidence will indicate the degree to which each variable was a risk factor for CV mortality? Could the current evidence attribute a lower relative risk to more alcohol intake, rather than to parallel choices favoring exercise, fruits, vegetables, and fish, or to inverse choices of high-fat dairy, total fat, or smoking? In this regard, an earlier report on these subjects *(6)* noted that increased alcohol intake was also associated with an increased percent of individuals regularly using aspirin, an agent well-known to decrease thrombotic mechanisms in CV mortality, which illustrates another lifestyle feature that may have an impact on interpretation. Finally, the earlier report *(6)* is instructive in showing a rise in the percent of individuals smoking that parallels higher alcohol intakes, but Ascherio et al. *(5)* reported opposing smoking and drinking gradients when subjects were stratified by saturated fat intake. Such apparently divergent attributes illustrate the well-known need for caution in interpreting associative relationships in epidemiologic data *(7,8)* for which many variables differ simultaneously among individuals, and no controlled interventions provide conclusive proof of cause.

3. BALANCING DIVERSITY AND COLLECTIVITY

3.1. Medians vs Means

Diversity among individuals is frequently reflected in measures of variance, such as standard deviations around a mean value, which is commonly observed in Gaussian bell-shaped distributions. Such distributions accompany the concept of average attributes of average people. Familiarity with such curves can lead easily to the use of that paradigm as a first approximation in discussing new, unfamiliar situations. However, published patterns of alcohol consumption in many different communities approximate a skewed distribution similar to the pattern shown in Fig. 1, which schematically indicates that

33% of Americans drink 95% of the beverage alcohol *(2)*, and about 33% abstain. Also, the average (mean) weekly intake of 10 drinks/wk is much greater than the middle person's (median) value of 1–2, and much less than that for individuals in the upper 5% of alcohol intake, who may account for almost 50% of total alcohol consumption *(2)*. Thus, a tendency to think of alcohol intakes in terms of a Gaussian distribution produces dissonance among people evaluating aggregate information on benefits and risks for a population of individuals. In this situation, concepts about average behavior or average consequences need careful and patient description, to avoid misrepresenting the actual evidence. Although people may assume Gaussian distributions and regard the mean value as that of an average person, the median value is probably closer to that intent. Social policy in a democratic society may be expected to develop more from median values than mean values.

3.2. Aspects of Collectivity

The skewed relationship of median and mean values creates another important public health question: "Will the incidence of heavy problem drinking in a community be greater when the mean value is greater?" This question about collectivity acquires importance as communities consider implementing preventive nutrition tactics based on possible benefits of light drinking on the risk of CVD. Encouraging this tactic may cause median and mean alcohol consumption to rise as some abstainers feel encouraged to begin drinking alcohol. Past reports of an almost log-normal distribution of alcohol consumption among adults in France *(9)* led to suggestions that some collective social mechanism may influence drinking patterns within a population, possibly linking an increase in heavy drinking with an increase in mean consumption. Many subsequent studies confirmed a close relationship between mean and heavy consumption in alcohol for diverse populations *(10)*. Even though the positively skewed distribution of consumption is not exactly log-normal, Ledermann's hypothesis *(9)* provides a useful predictive rough estimate. A recent report used health surveys for 32,333 adults from 14 separate regions in England, and found a strong positive association between mean regional consumption and the prevalence of heavy drinking *(11)*. The associations were similar for men and women, and they were of similar magnitude when the analysis was restricted to those under age 65 yr, and when abstainers were excluded. Values for mean alcohol consumption by men in the different regions ranged from 15 to 22.7 U/wk, with an English alcohol beverage unit equivalent to 8 g ethanol (contrasting with 14 g for the standard in the U.S. Dietary Guidelines). A difference in mean consumption of alcohol of 1 U/wk was associated with 6.3% more men drinking above 21 U/wk. A serious implication for public health is that heavy drinkers may not be indifferent to the acceptability of drinking in their culture. Further analysis suggested that the social determinants for abstention may differ from determinants for heavy drinking *(11)* in ways that do not permit assuming that adverse consequences of more heavy drinking will be offset by beneficial CV effects from a decrease in abstention.

An alternate study of the aspect of collectivity used data from the U.S. National Longitudinal Alcohol Epidemiologic Survey (NLAES), with a sophisticated multiple linear logistic regression model fitted to major significant predictive variables to project possible outcomes of different public policies *(12)*. Different prevention strategies were compared, to test their possible effect upon the predicted prevalence of alcohol abuse and dependence in the population, and predictions were comparable for either the collective population or the high-risk individual strategy. A 25% reduction in average daily intake of all current drinkers reduced the predicted prevalence of alcohol use disorders from 16.7 to 13%. Alternatively, a 28% reduction in average daily intakes of all drinkers, who occasionally or usually exceeded the moderate drinking cut point, lowered the predicted prevalence to 12.6%. Finally, reducing the consumption of usually immoderate drinkers by 41% resulted in a 13% predicted prevalence of alcohol abuse and dependence within the drinking population. The authors concluded that neither reducing overall consumption nor high-risk consumption appeared to be superior in reducing the prevalence of alcohol abuse and dependence.

Another important finding from NLAES, which has implications for prevention policies, is that more than 40% of respondents who initiated drinking before 15 yr of age were classified with alcohol dependence at some time in their lives *(13)*. Furthermore, the odds of lifetime alcohol dependence were 14% lower with each increasing year of age at first use. Efforts to prevent auto accidents, by limiting access to alcohol for adolescents newly introduced to driving skills and judgments, may also be evaluated as a possible strategy to decrease the prevalence of alcohol-use disorders. Is early onset a potentially modifiable risk factor in development of disorders, or is it only a marker of an inevitable, possibly unmodifiable development of alcohol-use disorders? More controlled evidence will need to be evaluated to resolve these alternatives, and they must be resolved if preventive strategies are to be based on proved causal factors.

Another indication of a possible collective population influence derives from the strong positive association of mean apparent alcohol consumption in the 50 States in the United States with two indices of heavy drinking: the prevalence of total ethanol-related disease and chronic liver disease in each state *(14,15)*. Like the results from England, these results suggest that the heavy drinkers may be a predictable portion of a population. Collectivity was also evident in the standardized data from the Intersalt study, an international, multicenter study of adults representing 52 populations in 32 countries, which showed close and independent associations between the population mean and the prevalence of deviance for each of the variables examined: Correlation coefficients were 0.85 for blood pressure (BP), 0.94 for body mass index, 0.97 for alcohol intake, and 0.78 for sodium intake *(16)*. These findings imply that distributions of health-related characteristics move up and down as a whole. As a result, an increase in average alcohol intake intended for the health and well-being of the general population could be responsible for increased harm to deviant subgroups.

3.3. Temporal Variance in Intakes

Another feature of diversity in alcohol drinking that impacts upon health outcomes is the pattern of intake within the period of time being used for comparisons. The biological impact of one drink/d for 7 d is clearly different from that of seven drinks on 1 d/wk, even though both lifestyles have mean intakes of one drink/d. Unfortunately, few epidemiological reports allow recognition of such temporal variances in intake, placing serious limits on interpretations of the aggregate means. Because aggregate data fail to give clear insight into the daily or weekly intensities of alcohol exposure that occur in individual cases, the credibility of general interpretations made from aggregate data may be compromised by that failure. To avoid that weakness, careful, systematic records of average daily intake were obtained from 50 male volunteers enrolled at the Vermont Alcohol

Research Center, who reported daily their alcohol intake for 112 d, using a computer-automated interactive voice simulation system, accessed by touch-tone telephone, through a dedicated 800 number (17). Results from the 5151 self-reports of daily drinking documented a wide variance, with somewhat greater drinking on weekends than weekdays (Fri. = 5.7 ± 5; Sat. = 5.7 ± 4; Sun. = 4.2 ± 4; Mon. = 3.6 ± 3; Tue. = 3.5 ± 3; Wed. = 4.2 ± 4; Thur. = 4.2 ± 3). Other data, collected immediately after the study by traditional methods, confirmed the expectation that heavier-drinking subjects retrospectively underreported their consumption significantly more than lighter-drinking subjects. A more detailed analysis of individual daily alcohol intake (18) was made for 12 subjects with comparable quantity and frequency of alcohol consumption, six lighter-drinking alcohol-dependent and six heavy-drinking nondependent subjects. Alcohol consumption by nondependent heavy drinkers had long-term variations (weeks or months, perhaps reflecting social occasions); the dependent subjects had stable, characteristic 7-d drinking cycles. These studies show that weekend drinking may be a form of collective social influence, and they illustrate more clearly than most the inability of mean aggregate values to describe the level of alcohol consumption of an individual at a given time.

Each person metabolizes alcohol in a fairly reproducible and consistent manner, with characteristic rising and falling curves of tissue alcohol levels (19), and most ingested alcohol is apparently converted to CO_2 within 24 h. The intervening transitory period of elevated tissue alcohol levels constitutes a controversial period within which scientists attempt to interpret the ways in which alcohol has its impact. With one drink during a day, blood alcohol will probably be very low for 22 of the 24 h of the day. Are the benefits and risks of alcohol drinking linked to the alcohol levels attained in tissues, or are they linked to some unknown associated aspect of metabolizing alcohol? Such questions are difficult to answer with existing information (20), but they need to be addressed in developing explanations for how the drinking of alcohol can cause the effects attributed to it. Although many hypotheses interpret impaired functions and health risks of alcohol, few rationales or mechanisms for benefits caused by alcohol have much supporting evidence from controlled experimental interventions. One example is in preventing physiologic signs of alcohol withdrawal, for which alcohol was infused intravenously (nearly equivalent to 7 standard drinks of alcohol over a 24-h period), without elevating blood alcohol levels beyond that regarded as nondetectable (21). Apparently, very low levels of alcohol can influence human physiology in ways not widely recognized, discussed, or even carefully documented. One may well wonder when (and by what mechanism), during the variations in tissue alcohol levels, could people obtain the putative benefits or risks associated with and attributed to the beverage alcohol. Instinctive questions of why associative phenomena occur with nondetectable alcohol levels call for some causal mechanism by which the effect could be interpreted or understood.

3.4. Considering the Disease Concept

During the eighteenth century, the balance in attitudes toward chronic drunkenness gradually shifted away from a voluntary choice that people made, toward the concept of alcoholism as a progressive, addictive disease for which total abstinence was offered as the only remedy (reviewed in ref. 22). In 1785, Benjamin Rush (reviewed in ref. 23) described alcoholism as an addictive disease associated with toxic consequences of alcohol. Linked with the disease concept was another concept that reappeared in teachings by the temperance movement in the nineteenth century, and by Alcoholics Anonymous and Jellinek in the twentieth century: Total abstinence was needed once a drinker became helpless with the appetite for alcohol. Although the need for abstinence by vulnerable individuals acquired many proponents for more than a century, much optimism about moderate, controlled drinking seems prevalent among the majority of the population that has not experienced alcohol dependency. However, it may not be possible for individuals in the majority to use their own personal experience to balance successfully the benefits and risks of moderate alcohol intake for the 5–10% of individuals who are vulnerable.

A broad look at mean alcohol consumption shows more similarity than might be expected for people in different countries and cultural periods. For example, Batel *(24)* noted that aggregate average annual per capita intake of alcohol in France is now about 3 gal, and the prevalence of alcohol dependence may be about 6%. Average intake by the U.S. population in 1994 was about 2.2 gal, and the prevalence of alcohol abuse and dependence was about 7.4% *(25)*. Such values are similar to those in other developed countries, for which alcohol is second only to tobacco as a risk factor for disability-adjusted life years *(26;* and *see* Subheading 5.). In addition, the current average annual per capita consumption in the United States of about 2–2.5 gal ethanol *(14)* has been at a similar level in the face of major cultural and lifestyle changes from the time preceding the Civil War (1850–1870; 2.2 gal) into the twentieth century. During the period 1881–1910, with its waves of immigration, the advent of the automobile, and the use of electric power, consumption was also about 2.2 gal. Then, after limited access to alcohol during two World Wars, Prohibition, and the Depression, per capita consumption continued during widespread social change that accompanied a shift from trains, radio, and movies (1945–1950, 2.1 gal) to air travel, television (1960–1969, 2.2 gal), space exploration, and changing roles for women (1970–1989, 2.6 gal), home computers, and the internet (1990–1994, 2.3 gal). The consistency of intake is striking. One may wonder if the characteristics 5–10% risk of alcohol use disorders was also constant during these times.

The concept of collectivity may be extended to consider it an average phenotypic expression of disease resulting from an average of multiple polygenic interactions common to the general human genotype. In that sense, aggregate data from different populations around the world with open access to alcohol may tend to have similar aggregate alcohol intakes, with about 5–10% vulnerable to heavy drinking as a collective result of multiple combined gene–environment interactions. Such an approximate average outcome may occur from collective interactions, reflecting the heterogeneous mixtures of alleles among the diverse individuals of the population. For example, the prevalence, incidence, and lifetime risk of schizophrenia has been remarkably consistent across various populations and geographic areas during the past century *(27)*. Clear evidence for the heritable nature of alcohol dependency *(28)* has prompted an extensive genomic search to identify genes that contribute to the risk of the alcohol dependency disease that appears in about 5–10% of the population. The study found suggestive evidence for genes increasing susceptibility to alcoholism on chromosomes 1, 2, and 7, and the possibility of a gene decreasing the risk on chromosome 4 *(29)*. Also, other studies indicate that variant alleles, for some dehydrogenases involved in alcohol metabolism, are associated with reduced risk of developing alcoholism *(30)*. Clearly, not all individuals are the same.

4. BALANCING NUTRIENTS AND TOXINS

4.1. A Useful Nutrient?

Although biochemistry and physiology began to develop insight into the three principal uses of alcohol during the nineteenth century (medical, nutritional, and recreational), attitudes about alcohol shifted widely, ranging from it being a useful nutrient to harmful toxin. As new information developed, an instructive situation occurred in the balance between academic theory and clinical practice. Physiological theories changed rapidly in the mid-century, with scientific reports postulating a nutritive value for alcohol, then regarding it worthless as nourishment, because of being eliminated unchanged from the body, and, still later, promoting its ability to lower body temperature (31). However, most physicians continued unchanged in their clinical use of alcohol, balancing a continued belief in prior practice with the changing contradictory theories. Research results were accepted in constructing medical theories of how alcohol works, but they were mostly irrelevant in the balance of opinions formulating therapeutic practice. It may be humbling for scientists to realize that, however much scientific research results may change theories of alcohol action, theories may not be the basis upon which clinicians recommend alcohol use or the basis upon which the public uses alcohol. Alcohol remained a widely prescribed therapeutic agent through the end of the nineteenth century, even though there was uncertainty about its nutritive value (which still remains today). A low public awareness of that uncertainty contrasts with widespread speculation about a possible therapeutic role in preventing heart attacks.

By the end of the nineteenth century, an intense polarization had developed in the balance of attitudes between nutrient and toxin status of alcohol. The balance of power shifted during an unusual human tragedy involving Mary Hunt, National Superintendent of the Scientific Department of the Woman's Christian Temperance Union (WCTU), and Wilbur Atwater, first head of the U.S. Department of Agriculture (USDA) Experimental Stations (23). Publishers of public school textbooks were under intense political pressure, led by Mary Hunt, to include information on "hygienic physiology," which presented the temperance movement viewpoint. It characterized alcohol as a dangerous and seductive poison of no useful value that could create an addictive appetite apt to become an uncontrollable disease. Alcohol addicts were regarded to have lost control and required complete abstinence from alcohol, renewing the concepts from Benjamin Rush a century earlier, and preceding the positions by Jellinek and Alcoholics Anonymous in the next century (22). For a generation of school children, these concepts were presented in textbooks as proven findings of science.

However, by 1895, the political struggle for a new balance in power over alcohol physiology moved to include Atwater's unique calorimetric research on human alcohol metabolism (32). Atwater campaigned vigorously for regarding alcohol as a valuable nutrient (while agreeing that it was not a food), and he attempted to reduce extremism in the teaching about alcohol in the public schools. He reported that alcohol was almost fully oxidized, and replaced the caloric equivalent of either fat or carbohydrate, i.e., it acted as a food (33). Although Atwater (in concert with academic physiologists) succeeded in removing from the schools the polarized teaching about alcohol's toxicity, the political struggle led the Secretary of Agriculture to remove support for further alcohol experiments, or for publishing the results in USDA bulletins. Eventually, limited support from the Carnegie Institution of Washington and the National Academy of Sciences assisted in distributing the experimental research results (*32*; reviewed in ref. *23*). Atwater was joined by a committee of 50 academic physiologists, who claimed to focus on scientific studies of physical and social facts "without reference to the conclusions to which they might lead" (*34*). The committee was an expression of the nineteenth century liberal movement, and it attempted to integrate concepts of rational reform from four sub-committees: physiological aspects, legislative aspects, economic aspects, and substitutes for the saloons. Ironically, events combined to create a paradox in which, insisting on their lack of knowledge, the academicians "eliminated physiology from school curricula, and who, in the course of asserting their expertise over alcohol, made themselves irrelevant to the one American constitutional question with a substantial physiological component" (*23*). The intense public struggle of Hunt and Atwater came to an abrupt end in 1904, as Hunt lost power within the WCTU, and died in 1906; Atwater died in 1907, after being incapacitated since 1904 by a possible series of strokes.

The harsh conditions of obtaining support may have diminished enthusiasm for alcohol research for many years, and the advent of Prohibition in 1918 removed much motivation for academics to pursue curiosity further. The absence of organized continuing research led Mitchell to note (*35*), in 1935, that the physiologic value of alcohol was in a state of "utmost confusion," and World et al. (*4*) later suggested that alcohol-derived calories perhaps should be disregarded completely as an energy source in predicting dietary-induced changes in weight. Results from 89,538 women in the Nurses Health Study, and from 48,493 men in the Health Professionals Follow-up Study, showed that alcohol intake appeared not to contribute to overall body mass of women or men (*36*). In fact, women had a clear inverse relation between total energy intake or alcohol consumption and body mass index. This counterintuitive situation was supported by other studies (*37*), and by cumulative evidence of 31 separate surveys, which showed that reduced alcohol consumption would not likely help achieve or maintain a lower body wt (*38*). The balance of information about alcohol as a nutrient remains uncertain to the present time (*39,40*), with the nutritive value of alcohol calories still the subject of much debate and research experimentation. Somehow, all of the scientific research effort has still not provided a convincing resolution of the uncertainty. The debate, at the Sixth European Congress on Obesity, by Schutz (*41*) and Westererp (*42*), helped the scientific community become familiar with a topic that has remained unsettled throughout the past century (*43,44*). Whether alcohol is a useful nutrient, whose calories count the same as other calories, seems likely to remain uncertain and controversial among scientists for some time.

Although calorimetric results, since Atwater (*32*), have been interpreted to indicate that the energy of alcohol is handled similarly to that of other macronutrients, caloric compensation (in which one nutrient satiates appetite for other nutrients) does not seem to occur with alcohol (*44–50*). For example, men reported no decreased intake of average food energy (7555 kJ/d) or amounts of various macronutrients, irrespective of an alcohol-altered average total energy intake, which ranged from 7576 to 9822 kJ/d (*36*). Similarly, Rose et al. (*51*) reported that drinkers added alcohol energy to their diet, rather than displacing food with alcohol, and there was no increase in BMI for women, despite increased total energy intake with increased alcohol consumption. Alternatively, recent USDA results, nearly 100 yr after Atwater, described alcohol being metabolized like other foods (*52*). Clearly, epidemiologic surveys seem to contradict laboratory calorimetric studies, and one of the methods will eventually prove to give a correct interpretation.

A hundred years of research still does not provide concurrence on alcohol's value as a nutrient, and serious questions about the consequences of alcohol intake perturbing metabolism and fuel selection need explanation.

4.2. A Toxic Substance?

The rational suggestion 100 yr ago, to assign the controversy over alcohol's toxic status to university professors' scientific examination, diminished the flow of temperance-oriented information on alcohol as a toxin, but has not provided needed alternative explanations, as researchers lost interest in the questions *(23)*. The balance of information on alcohol as a toxin shifted over the years, with attention to the dose and conditional toxic states in which nutrient balances influence toxic actions of alcohol or to how alcohol causes a deficit of important nutrients. When arguing for maintenance or repeal of Prohibition, different applications of scientific measurements were used on both sides of the debate over intoxicating effects of alcohol *(53)*. The experimental psychologist, Walter Miles, urged maximizing human efficiency in measures of impaired performance; Carlson effectively used the null hypothesis with low doses in which low signal-to-noise ratios prevent statistical proof of any alcohol effect. Further support for ending Prohibition was espoused by the chemical physiologist, Yarnell Henderson, who focused on minimum performance necessary for the smooth operation of society. That view prevailed in the end, in part because its perspective on intoxication and the degree of hazard it represented was consistent with the personal experience of a majority of Americans (rather than the much smaller proportion that suffers from alcohol use disorders). Ironically, although repeal won in 1933, maximum accepted exposures of toxicants are now appreciably below the levels accepted at that time, as modern scientists urge policies minimizing exposure to any known deleterious substance, as much as possible *(53)*.

Subsequent efforts to interpret toxic actions of alcohol have been confounded for decades by controversy over whether alcohol is toxic *per se*, or whether it has a conditional toxicity dependent on interaction with other nutrients. Academic arguments continue over whether or not the diet during a given study was adequate in certain nutrients, such as choline, methionine, folic acid, thiamine, zinc, antioxidant vitamins, or carbohydrate *(54)*. For example, animal models of alcohol toxicity seemed more severe with high fat, low carbohydrate diets *(55–57)*, and molecular mechanisms for impaired growth and liver pathology with alcohol remain the subject of controversy *(58)*. Unfortunately, development of documented mechanisms by which alcohol and its metabolite, acetate, perturb normal carbohydrate and fat metabolism has been slow *(20)*. Alternatively, progress in recognizing the complex network of cellular mediators involved in alcohol-induced liver injury *(59)* was recently extended by detection of significant isoprostane formation, a marker of tissue oxidant stress, during conditions similar to social drinking *(60)*. The results with such biomarkers are alerting the biomedical community to previously unsuspected tissue injury during conditions regarded as benign by many people.

5. BALANCING RISK FACTORS AND CAUSES

5.1. Death and Disease Burdens

Death is generally accepted as a precise condition, although the complexity of life makes it inevitable that there are a near infinite number of ways in which the complex adaptive living system arrives at death. Nevertheless, despite the multiple factors involved, each fatality is conventionally characterized by a single cause of death. Statistical analyses associate diverse risk factors with the listed cause of death, but the predictive association is not proof of a causal role, and interpretations about associated risk factors need to be made with caution. For example, the risk factor most powerfully associated with all deaths is age, and tables of vital statistics are careful to stratify information by age groups, to permit more meaningful age-adjusted interpretations. Nevertheless, age itself is usually not the direct cause of a fatal event, and health experts assign other causes of premature deaths as useful information, to begin designing appropriate public health interventions. In the same sense, gender and socioeconomic status are important risk factors strongly associated with health outcomes for an individual. Epidemiologists carefully examine the balance among risk factors, to find evidence that may help identify more direct causal factors for which interventions could be arranged. Knowing more mechanisms in the causal chain of events provides alternate targets for successful intervention, and ensures the likelihood of a credible and generalizable eventual solution.

Social values and preferences need careful and prominent inclusion when discussing health problems and priorities linked to a possibly successful intervention. To facilitate this, one recent study *(61)* developed a standard unit, the disability-adjusted life year (DALY), to aid comparisons in a standardized approach to epidemiological assessment (reviewed in ref. *26*), and DALYs were estimated for each age–sex group, to designate leading risk factors for death and disability in each major socioeconomic region. In this analysis, alcohol was a major risk factor, tied with unsafe sex as the third-ranked worldwide risk factor (3.5%), behind malnutrition (15.9%) and poor water, sanitation, and hygiene (6.8%). In established market economies, alcohol was second only to tobacco as a risk factor for DALY. In these economies, a possible protective effect of alcohol may have averted as many deaths as its harmful effects caused, but worldwide alcohol caused 750,000 more deaths than it averted *(26)*.

Although age is strongly associated with mortality, it role as a risk factor involves many important variations in interaction with alcohol at different stages of life, which involve different social values and preferences.

1. Relatively low levels of alcohol disturb cellular signals in the developing fetus, causing serious life-long physical and mental abnormalities for the individual (that led to national requirements for warning labels on alcoholic beverages). Late nineteenth-century reports showed that offspring of dogs fed alcohol died young or were deformed, and inebriated inmates had more miscarriages and defective children than nonalcoholic inmates *(83)*. Following this, researchers developed controlled alcohol fume chambers to demonstrate that alcohol impaired rat pup viability, with offspring of alcoholized guinea pigs having lower fertility and higher death rates than their grandparents or parents. Despite such evidence of alcohol-impaired reproduction, the research ceased, and subsequent experts asserted a lack of evidence for alcohol causing any abnormality in the offspring *(83)*. Research on this topic apparently remained uninteresting for decades, until Jones *(84)* described fetal alcohol syndrome, and the newly formed National Institute on Alcohol Abuse and Alcoholism shifted the balance of interest toward understanding this important problem. Now the scientific community is fully aware of fetal alcohol risks, but the information seems not uniformly transmitted or not perceived by the public in ways that sufficiently change behavior.

2. Additionally, alcohol is known to be transferred to nursing infants, and low levels of alcohol in mother's milk may decrease the infant's sleep *(62)*. Further research may

clarify whether or not a preference for the flavor of alcohol may develop in infants obtaining detectable alcohol levels during nursing.

3. Early access to alcohol in adolescence is strongly associated with the eventual acquisition of alcohol dependence *(13)*, with associated high social costs. Age restrictions on access to alcoholic beverages have been regarded as a useful preventive nutrition strategy. The very high DALYs and loss of life in road-traffic accidents (ninth ranked cause of world-wide DALYs) led to U.S. adoption of a nationwide uniform legal 21-yr age limit, to restrict access to alcohol.

4. On the other hand, changes in personal priorities during life seem evident in the finding that 22% of heavy drinkers, who previously met criteria for DSM-IV alcohol dependence, subsequently achieved total abstinence *(63)*, and an additional 50% reduced their consumption to a level matching that of persons who had never been classified as dependent. Most reduction occurred in individuals not participating in any type of alcohol treatment program, suggesting that individual current heavy drinkers may someday voluntarily curtail their drinking. In this case, an eventual reduction in the proportion of heavy drinkers in the population may be achieved by continued prevention of new individuals from becoming heavy drinkers. Unfortunately, the worldwide history of collective attempts to diminish heavy alcohol drinking provides few encouraging examples of successful long-term tactics to achieve this, beyond that obtained with social support for total abstinence, an approach long-espoused by the 12-step facilitation therapy of Alcoholics Anonymous. A recent large-scale clinical trial, comparing outcomes from well-controlled therapeutic interventions, showed sustained, modest success rates, but gave little indication of succeeding better, with matching treatment modality to different subtypes of patient, than was obtained with the 12-step facilitation therapy *(64)*.

5.2. Associated Risks

An important confounding factor in interpreting results from epidemiological studies is the clustering of variables in patterns that reflect linked voluntary lifestyle choices, preventing the variables from being treated as independent variables. This phenomenon was evident in the recent report on health professionals noted earlier *(5)*. With linked lifestyle choices being common, one might wonder when (and by what mechanism), during the wide variations in tissue alcohol levels, could people obtain the putative benefits or risks associated with and attributed to beverage alcohol. Instinctive questions about why the associative phenomenon occurs will need some causal mechanism identified, before the effect can be truly understood. In approaching such questions, more precision in defining the attributes that are used in the statistical comparisons can greatly aid the interpretations. Clustering all cancer deaths or all CV deaths together fails to handle the diversity involved, and it interferes with attempts to discuss preventive nutritional interventions that may decrease the prevalence of selected types of tumor or CV process. Hypotheses for benefits and risks of drinking alcoholic beverages need to be examined, by considering the precision with which current epidemiologic information outlines possible causal mechanisms. The following examples illustrate some current knowledge about risks and possible benefits.

5.2.1. CIRRHOSIS

Alcohol drinking shows a dose-related risk of cirrhosis that progressively increases to dramatically high rates with heavier drinking levels, with relatively little associated with moderate drinking *(65)*. Mechanisms by which alcohol can cause liver injury have been extensively studied, possible therapeutic targets have been suggested *(59)*, and recent evidence of oxidant stress at moderate drinking levels (60) points to a need for more detailed examination of underlying mechanisms (66).

5.2.2. CANCER

Alcohol drinking has a clear association with cancer of the oral cavity, pharynx, larynx, esophagus, and liver, and a suggestive association with cancer of the large bowel and breast (67). Mortality from breast cancer (BC) is 30% higher among women reporting at least one drink daily, compared to nondrinkers (68). The finding that moderate intake of beer or spirits was associated with considerable risk among Danes, but wine was not (69), may reflect an effect of different components of the beverages (rather than alcohol per se), or it may reflect associated lifestyle events that affected the risk of cancer. The similar finding of a lower risk for stroke among Danes drinking wine, but not beer or spirits (70), seems provocative regarding possible lifestyle interactions. In contrast, a progressively increased relative risk for BC was described for a different set of people (65). With 3% of all cancers attributed to alcohol consumption (71), there is a need to identify mechanisms whereby alcohol acts to increase or decrease the risk. One mechanism explored recently is that alcohol may increase risk of BC by causing elevated plasma estrogen levels (72) in two ways: decreased clearance of plasma estrogen (73) and increased absorption during hormone replacement therapy (74). If these mechanisms cause increased BCs, a prevention program aimed at women who are at high risk for BC must be weighed against the possible CV benefits for moderate drinkers.

5.2.3. HYPERTENSION, STROKE, AND HEART ATTACKS

Reducing these major causes of death in the United States motivates a careful look at all possible alternatives. Of 48 centers worldwide in which some people reported consuming at least 300 mL/wk of alcohol, 35 centers had positive regression coefficients linking heavy alcohol consumption to BP (75). Overall, alcohol consumption was directly associated with BP, especially at the highest intake. The significant relation of heavy drinking (3–4 or more drinks/d) to BP, observed in both men and women, and in younger and older men, was independent of, and added to, the effect on BP of body mass index and urinary excretion of sodium and potassium. Thus, hypertension (HT) appears to have many alternative causal factors as targets for preventive nutrition tactics, of which one is to decrease alcohol intake for some individuals. Different factors may be pivotal for different individuals, and each HT patient must discern which factor is causal in their life.

Chronic alcohol intakes also seems linked with cardiac arrhythmias and atrial fibrillation in sudden cardiac death (76), although no mechanism is known. Alternatively, among 22,071 men in the Physicians Health Study, using those who consumed less than one alcoholic drink/wk for comparison, the relative risk of all-cause mortality for those who consumed 2–4 drinks/wk was 0.72; for 5–6/wk, 0.79; for 7/wk, 0.98; and 14 or more/wk, 1.51 (77). A similar 30–40% lower CVD death rate associated with moderate drinking was seen in a large cancer prevention study (68). Additionally, a population-based case-control study concluded that the relative risk of a major coronary event was lowest among men who report 1–4 drinks/d on 5–6 d/wk, and among women who report 1–2 drinks/d 5–6 d/wk (78). However, a much more cautious position was provided by Svarsudd (79), who noted concerns over selection bias and limits in transferring conclusions from small subgroups to the general population.

Interventions for targeted individuals or situations, in the form of therapeutic steps for clearly demonstrated pathology, probably will have more overall support than general preventive interventions, for which the small minority at risk is unidentified and uncertain. In this case, individuals among the majority not at risk can easily lose confidence in the credibility of using preventive tactics that succeed only for a minority. Credibility is further strained when the mechanism of the disease or the intervention is not clear or has multiple alternatives, a situation encountered in balancing CV death and alcohol drinking. Interpreting CV death must overcome differences in understanding about whether blood cholesterol level is only a predictive risk marker associated with dietary and metabolic imbalance, or whether it has a causal role in mediating the disease processes (2,80; see also Subheading 6.).

The certainty of diminishing thrombosis with low-dose aspirin has no counterpart for low-dose alcohol. Preventive nutrition approaches to decrease CV mortality have long been thought to involve reducing calories as total fat and saturated fat (2), and molecular mediators of thrombosis, arrhythmia, and atherogenesis have been identified (81). In fact, decreasing the formation and function of the n-6 eicosanoid, thromboxane, with low-dose aspirin inhibition of platelet cyclo-oxygenase, is a strikingly effective tactic. This known mechanism has a parallel nutrition intervention in elevating the ratio of dietary n-3/n-6 essential fatty acids. Mechanisms whereby alcohol may diminish fatal CV events remain unknown.

In considering the often-discussed "French paradox" of low CV death rates, relative to average blood cholesterol values, it is instructive to know that, for subgroups of men aged 40–44 yr, in 1960, 34% in France had died before reaching the age of 70–74 yr, compared with 37% in the United States, and 36% in England and Wales (82). Although these overall rates seem similar, there was a dramatic difference in death rates caused by ischemic heart disease: 4.5, 14.1, and 15.2%, respectively. However, if all men who died early of alcohol-associated causes had died of ischemic heart disease, the rates would have been 21, 26, and 25%. Even though the small unexplained residual difference in the three populations needs explanation, it is evident that the large portion of French men who die early from the serious negative impacts of alcohol tends to balance the low ischemic heart disease death rate in the French population. Such a balanced trade off is not consistently emphasized in discussing possible protective effects of moderate drinking, and more information on causal mechanisms is needed. Many different sources of information need to be compared, when balancing benefits and risks for complex multivariant situations.

6. BALANCING IGNORANCE AND KNOWLEDGE

The history of handling the totality of evidence on alcohol-related physiology provides interesting and sometimes perplexing examples of waxing and waning attention to evidence that presumably reflects changing attitudes and priorities. As a result, developing wide-scale recommendations and social policies involves much more than scientific information, although such information can make the decision process more rational (85). The information needed to alter behavior often is more than a statement of risk, and the ways by which behavior-modifying information moves within society needs deeper analysis. For example, people initially believed that warning labels would alter behavior, but a post-policy analysis of the value of the labels showed little effect *(86)*. The labels seemed to increase public awareness without appearing to have a major influence on changing drinking behavior (reminiscent of physicians' use of alcohol in the late nineteenth century). In contrast to uncertain results with labels, restricting access to alcohol by changing the minimum legal drinking age from 18 to 21 dropped alcohol-related auto crashes significantly *(87)*. In addition, young people then continued to drink less through their early twenties.

Expectations about possible personal benefits of moderate drinking, by the majority, not particularly vulnerable to alcohol use disorder, will rest on a balance with information about personal risk of moderate drinking. A thorough analysis of the risks and protective effects of alcohol on the individual was recently provided at a state-of-the-art conference sponsored by the Swedish Medical Research Council *(88)*. The organizers noted that each community or professional group must examine the scientific literature to make policies that fit their own perceptions and priorities. The assembled reports of the conference facilitate such an examination. One overview balancing risks and benefits of alcohol consumption *(65)* concluded by noting that younger and elderly adults are now advised to drink less than other adults, and that men below 35 yr of age, premenopausal women, and older persons not in good health are not likely to benefit from light-to-moderate drinking. A similar view of risks and benefits over the life-span *(89)* noted the limited portion of the population likely to achieve demonstrable benefit from alcohol drinking, concluding with a reminder that priorities other than health will likely continue to motivate alcohol drinking.

With Atwater's calorimetry, moderate alcohol intake was presented as scientifically proved to have beneficial effects on health (similar to some attitudes regarding CV risks today). Hindsight permits recognition of the struggle to balance highly inflexible attitudes over positions now regarded as common knowledge: Many people can drink moderately, even though alcohol causes major problems for some people *(22,23)*. The current awareness of genetic diversity, and a shift away from the melting-pot concept of creating a uniform, homogeneous American society, make it likely that revisiting the struggle between the liberal movement and the temperance movement may avoid the overpolarized positions that created historic weaknesses and lack of credibility. At this time, society still has no sure way to identify and assist the 5–10% of the population that is vulnerable to alcohol use disorders, and health benefits of alcohol remain unproved. The scope of the problem and the chronic lack of a solution may spur researchers to put sharper attention on causal factors and mediators for the disorders, so that targets for successful preventive interventions can be selected. With no certain answers, individuals remain free to choose their own accommodation to a risk for vulnerability.

Two recent large-scale public education efforts at preventive nutrition illustrate the challenge of advising a diverse population about heterogeneous disorders, for which mechanisms are mostly not known, and the minority (albeit large) of the population at risk cannot be identified prior to disease initiation. The first effort is noted in a lengthy analysis of the National High Blood Pressure Education Program. Taubes *(90)* noted a philosophical clash between the public health policy need to act and the requirement of good science for institutionalized skepticism. Limiting the flow of information about alternative explanations to advance a single option may decrease some distractions, but it intensifies the risk of impaired credibility. Although some factors for various aspects of HT are recognized, controversy continues over general public health interventions that seem to oversimplify a complex issue in which many different factors act in different individuals. The decades-long debate *(90,91)* about salt intake and population-wide BP involves situations instructive for people contemplating preventive nutrition with alcohol. The second effort, even more relevant to alcohol decreasing CV deaths, is the National Cholesterol Education Program *(92)*. In this effort, the clinical measure of elevated blood cholesterol associated with increased risk became a target for intervention *(93)*; considerable controversy continued *(80)* over whether the elevated level caused the disease, or was merely an associated marker. At issue is whether physicians were treating the cause of the disease or only a symptom of it. With multiple mechanisms involved, CVD, like HT, should not be oversimplified when designing credible interventions. Some causal mechanisms for various aspects of CV mortality (inflammatory atherogenesis, myocardial arrhythmia, platelet thrombosis) are recognized and are targets for intervention *(81)*, but there is still no accepted hypothesis or mechanism by which drinking alcohol decreases risk. Rather, decreasing dietary saturated fats *(2,94)* and increasing dietary n-3 fats *(95)*, or using low-dose aspirin *(96)*, seem to be effective preventive alternatives for decreasing the causal mechanisms.

7. RECOMMENDATIONS

Exercising informed choice about foods from the wide range of acceptable options requires careful assessment of the context within which information about them was obtained, and will be applied. Because a risk–benefit ratio for using alcohol in a preventive nutrition tactic involves balancing risks for developing one or more diseases against risks for developing alcohol use disorders, the following points should be considered.

A majority of individuals seem not at risk for alcohol use disorders, but current insight into human genetic diversity allows recognition and acceptance that the effect of alcohol differs greatly among individuals. Thus, the risk of increased average drinking of alcohol involves a vulnerability to consume high levels that is not uniformly distributed among individuals, and generalizations from population medians or means do not reliably describe individuals in the vulnerable minority.

The median intake of alcohol in the United States may be about 1–2 drinks/wk, much less than the proposed preventive level of 1–2/d, which is currently consumed by a small fraction of the population.

Each person not yet exposed to beverage alcohol is unable to predict with certainty whether or not they are among the 5–10% at risk for developing alcohol use disorders. Thus, their election to drink can never be a fully informed choice between benefits and risks. The best guess about risk comes from an imprecise extrapolation from a family history of alcohol use disorder. As a result, acceptance of a restrictive alcohol policy for young people seems likely to continue as a primary prevention policy by the majority, because of concern for the unidentifiable vulnerable minority.

Once genetic vulnerability collides with environmental facilitation, efforts at primary prevention end for that individual, and attention shifts to treatment and secondary prevention, for which total abstinence remains the principal successful option.

Risks associated with high levels of drinking are clearly evident for cancer, cirrhosis, and HT. However, the variance in those risks is wide enough for the results at lower levels of alcohol to permit many hypotheses to apply, including the null hypothesis. As a result, uncertain logic could alter the balance between designating alcohol as harmful or harmless, because what appears true for the complete general set may not be true for a specific subset.

Information that describes an associative relationship is suitable for hypothesizing possible causes, but interventions with positive and negative controls are needed to prove a causal mechanism. Lifestyle choices of multiple variables confound associative relationships, decreasing the likelihood of assigning any one variable as the apparent cause. At this time, a causal role for alcohol in decreasing CV mortality has not been proved by controlled intervention studies.

Fully informed choice regarding the use of moderate drinking to prevent CVD requires weighing evidence of possible benefits and risks, much of which is indirect and imprecise at this time. Health benefits of drinking have been hypothesized from associative data, but no hypothetical mechanism is generally accepted for alcohol's actions, and no results from a well-controlled intervention have proved that alcohol causes the apparent benefit. To lower CV risks, alternative preventive nutrition tactics other than alcohol drinking are available.

ACKNOWLEDGMENT

The author gratefully acknowledges helpful advice and conversations about this review with Loren Archer, Deborah Dawson, Mary Dufour, Michael Eckardt, Richard Fuller, Brenda Hewitt, and Robert Karp.

REFERENCES

1. Nutrition and Your Health: Dietary Guidelines for Americans, 4th ed., USDA Home and Garden Bulletin No. 232, Washington, DC: U.S. Department Agriculture, 1995.
2. Surgeon General's Report on Nutrition and Health. DHHS (PHS) Publication No. 88-50210. Washington, DC: U.S. Government Printing Office, 1988.
3. Huijbregts P, Feskens E, Rasanen L, Fidanza F, Nissinen A, Menoti A, Kromhout D. Dietary pattern and 20 year mortality in elderly men in Finland, Italy, and the Netherlands: longitudinal cohort. Br Med J 1997; 315:13–17.
4. World MJ, Ryle PR, Pratt OE, Thomson AD. Alcohol and body weight. Alcohol Alcoholism 1984; 19:1–6.
5. Ascherio A, Rimm EB, Giovannucci EL, Spiegelman D, Stampfer M, Willett WC. Dietary fat and risk of coronary heart disease in men: cohort follow up study in the United States. Br Med J 1996; 313:84–90.
6. Rimm EB, Giovannucci EL, Willett WC, Colditz GA, Ascherio A, Rosner B, Stampfer M. Prospective study of alcohol consumption and risk of coronary disease in men. Lancet 1991; 338:464–468.
7. Taubes G. Epidemiology faces its limits. Science 1995; 269:164–169.
8. Willett W, Greenland S, MacMahon B, Trichopoulos D, Rothman K, Thomas D, Thun M, Weiss N. The discipline of epidemiology. Science 1995; 269:1325–1326.
9. Ledermann S. Alcohol, Alcoholism, Alcoholization, Vol. I, PUF, Paris (1956), as described by M. Bresard. In: International Encyclopedia of Pharmacology and Therapeutics, Vol. II, Oxford: Pergamon, 1970; 352–355.
10. Schmidt W, Popham RE. Discussion of a paper by Parker and Harman. In: Normative Approaches to the Prevention of Alcohol Abuse and Alcoholism. Harford TC, Parker DA, Light L, eds. NIAAA Research Monograph 3. Washington, DC: DHEW Publication No. (ADM) 79–847, 1980; 89–105.
11. Colhoun H, Ben-Schlomo Y, Dong W, Bost L, Marmot M. Ecological analysis of collectivity of alcohol consumption in England: importance of average drinker. Br Med J 1997; 314:1164–1168.
12. Dawson DA, Archer LD, Grant BF. Reducing alcohol-use disorders via decreased consumption: a comparison of population and high-risk strategies. Drug Alcohol Depend 1996; 42:39–47.
13. Grant BF, Dawson DA. Age at onset of alcohol use and its association with DSM-IV alcohol abuse and dependence: results from the National Alcohol Epidemiologic Survey. J Substance Abuse 1997; 9: 103–110.

14. Williams GD, Stinson FS, Lane JD, Tunson SL, Dufour MC. Surveillance Report 39. Apparent per capita alcohol consumption: National, state, and regional trends, 1977–94. National Institute on Alcohol Abuse and Alcoholism, December, 1996.

15. State trends in alcohol-related mortality, 1979–92. NIH Publication No. 96-4174, National Institute on Alcohol Abuse and Alcoholism, September, 1996.

16. Rose G, Day S. The population mean predicts the number of deviant individuals. Br Med J 1990; 301:1031–1034.

17. Searles JS, Perrine MW, Mundt JC, Helzer JE. Self-report of drinking using touch-tone telephone: Extending the limits of reliable daily contact. J Stud Alcohol 1995; 56:375–382.

18. Mundt JC, Searles JS, Perrine MW, Helzer JE. Cycles of alcohol dependence: Frequency-domain analyses of daily drinking logs for matched alcohol-dependent and nondependent subjects. J Stud Alcohol 1995; 56:491–499.

19. Wilkinson PK, Sedman AJ, Sakmar E, Kay DR, Wagner JG. Pharmacokinetics of ethanol after oral administration in the fasting state. J Pharmacokinet Biopharmocol 1977; 5:207–224.

20. Lands WEM. A review of alcohol clearance in humans. Alcohol 1998; 15:147–160.

21. Craft PP, Foil MB, Cunningham PRG, Patselas PC, Long-Snyder BM, Collier MS. Intravenous ethanol for alcohol detoxification in trauma patients. South Med J 1994; 87:47–54.

22. Levine HG. The discovery of addiction: changing conceptions of habitual drunkenness in America. J Stud Alcohol 1978; 39:143–174.

23. Pauly PJ. The struggle for ignorance about alcohol: American physiologists, Wilbur Olin Atwater, and the Woman's Christian Temperance Union. Bull Hist Med 1990; 64:366–392.

24. Batel P. The treatment of alcoholism in France. Drug Alcohol Depend 1995; 39(Suppl. 1):S15–S21.

25. Grant BF, Harford TH, Dawson DA, Chou SP, Dufour M, Pickering R. Prevalence of DSM-IV alcohol abuse and dependence, United States, 1992. Alcohol Health Res World 1994; 18:243–248.

26. Murray CJL, Lopez AD. Global mortality, disability, and the contribution of risk factors: Global Burden of Disease Study. Lancet 1997; 349:1436–1442.

27. Jablensky A. The 100-year epidemiology of schizophrenia. Schizophr Res 1997; 28:111–125.

28. Heath AC, Bucholz KK, Madden PAF, Dinwiddie SH, Slutske WS, Bierut LJ, et al. Psychol Med 1997; 27:1381–1396.

29. Reich T, Edenberg HJ, Goate A, Williams JT, Rice JP, Van Eerdewegh P, et al. Genome-wide search for genes affecting the risk for alcohol dependence. Am J Med Genet (Neuropsych Genet) 1998; 81: 207–215.

30. Whitfield JB. Meta-analysis of the effects of alcohol dehydrogenase genotype on alcohol dependence and alcoholic liver disease. Alcohol Alcoholism 1997; 32:613–619.

31. Warner JH. Physiological theory and therapeutic explanation in the 1860s: the British debate on the medical use of alcohol. Bull Hist Med 1980; 54:235–257.

32. Atwater WO, Benedict FG. An experimental inquiry regarding the nutritive value of alcohol. Mem Natl Acad Sci 1902; 8:231–397.

33. Carpenter KJ. The life and times of Atwater, W.O. (1844–1907). J Nutr 1994; 124:S1707–S1714.

34. Billings JS, Eliot CW, Farnam HW, Greene JL, Peabody FG. The Liquor Problem: A Summary of Investigations Conducted by the Committee of Fifty, 1893–1903. Boston: Houghton Mifflin, 1905.

35. Mitchell HH. The food value of ethyl alcohol. J Nutr 1935; 10:311–335.

36. Colditz GA, Giovannucci E, Rimm EB, Stampfer MJ, Rosner B, Speizer FE, Gordis E, Willett WC. Alcohol intake in relation to diet and obesity in women and men. Am J Clin Nutr 1991; 54:49–55.

37. Williamson DF, Forman MR, Binkin NJ, Gentry EM, Remington PL, Trowbridge FL. Alcohol and body weight in United States adults. Am J Public Health 1987; 77:1324–1330.

38. Hellerstedt WL, Jeffery RW, Murray DM. The association between alcohol intake and adiposity in the general population. Am J Epidemiol 1990; 132:594–611.

39. Pirola RC, Lieber CS. The energy cost of the metabolism of drugs, including ethanol. Pharmacology 1972; 7:185–196. (*See also*: Hypothesis: energy wastage in alcoholism and drug abuse: possible role of hepatic microsomal system. Am J Clin Nutr 1976; 29:90–93).

40. Suter PM, Hasler E, Vetter W. Effects of alcohol on energy metabolism and body weight regulation: Is alcohol a risk factor for obesity? Nutr Rev 1997; 55:157–171.

41. Schutz Y. Alcohol calories count the same as other calories. Int J Obes 1995; 19(Suppl. 2):12–13.

42. Westerterp KR. Alcohol calories do not count the same as other calories. Int J Obes 1995; 19(Suppl. 2): 14–15.

43. Lands WEM. Alcohol and energy intake. Am J Clin Nutr 1995; 62(Suppl.):1101S–1106S.

44. Lands WEM. Alcohol, calories, and appetite. Vitamins Hormones 1998; 54:31–49.
45. Camargo CA, Vranizan KM, Dreon DM, Frey-Hewitt B, Wood PD. Alcohol, calorie intake, and adiposity in overweight men. J Am College Nutr 1987; 6:271–278.
46. deCastro JM, Orozco S. Moderate alcohol intake and spontaneous eating patterns of humans: evidence of unregulated supplementation. Am J Clin Nutr 1990; 52:246–253.
47. Jaques PF, Sulsky S, Hartz SC, Russell RM. Moderate alcohol intake and nutritional status in nonalcoholic elderly subjects. Am J Clin Nutr 1989; 50:875–883.
48. Jones BR, Barrett-Connor E, Criqui MH, Holdbrook MJ. A community study of calorie and nutrient intake in drinkers and nondrinkers of alcohol. Am J Clin Nutr 1982; 35:135–139.
49. Tremblay A, St-Pierre S. The hyperphagic effect of a high-fat diet and alcohol intake persists after control for energy density. Am J Clin Nutr 1996; 63:479–482.
50. Mattes RD. Dietary compensation by humans for supplemental energy provided as ethanol or carbohydrate in fluids. Physiol Behav 1996; 59:179–187.
51. Rose D, Murphy SP, Hudes M, Viteri FE. Food energy remains constant with increasing alcohol intake. J Am Diet Assoc 1995; 95:698–700.
52. Rumpler WV, Rhodes DG, Baer DJ, Conway JM, Seale JL. Energy value of moderate alcohol consumption by humans. Am J Clin Nutr 1996; 64:108–114.
53. Pauly PJ. Is liquor intoxicating? Scientists, prohibition, and the normalization of drinking. Am J Public Health 1994; 84:304–313.
54. Lieber CS. Alcohol, liver and nutrition. J Am Coll Nutr 1991; 10:602–603.
55. Derr RF. The quantities of nutrients recommended by the NRC abate the effects of a toxic alcohol dose administered to rats. J Nutr 1989; 119:1228–1230.
56. Lieber CS, DeCarli LM. Recommended amounts of nutrients do not abate the toxic effects of an alcohol dose that sustains significant blood levels of ethanol. J Nutr 1989; 119:2038–2040.
57. Rao GA, Riley DE, Larkin EC. Dietary carbohydrate stimulates alcohol diet ingestion, promotes growth and prevents fatty liver in rats. Nutr Res 1987; 7:81–87.
58. Porta EA. Symposium on nutritional factors and oxidative stress in experimental alcoholic liver disease. J Nutr 1997; 127:893S–915S.
59. Lands WEM. Cellular signals in alcohol-induced liver injury: a review. Alcoholism Clin Exp Res 1995; 19:928–938.
60. Meagher EA, Lucey MR, FitzGerald GA. Oxidant injury in social drinking and alcoholic cirrhosis. Hepatology 1996; 24:444A.
61. Murray CJL, Lopez AD, eds. The Global Burden of Disease: A Comprehensive Assessment of Mortality and Disability from Diseases, Injuries, and Risk Factors in 1990 Projected to 2000. Cambridge: Harvard University Press, 1996.
62. Mennella JA, Gerrish CJ. Effects of exposure to alcohol in mother's milk on infant sleep. Pediatrics 1998; 101:E2.
63. Dawson DA. Correlates of past-year status among treated and untreated persons with former alcohol dependence: United States, 1992. Alcohol Clin Exp Res 1996; 20:771–779.
64. Project MATCH Research Group. Matching alcoholism treatments to client heterogeneity: Project MATCH three-year drinking outcomes. Alcohol Clin Exp Res 1998; 22:1300–1311.
65. Thakker KD. An overview of health risks and benefits of alcohol consumption. Alcoholism Clin Exp Res 1998; 22:285S–298S.
66. Lands WEM, Pawlosky RJ, Salem N. Alcoholism, antioxidant status, and essential fatty acids. In: Antioxidant Status, Diet, Nutrition and Health. Papas AM, ed. Boca Raton: CRC, 1998; 299–344.
67. Ringborg U. Alcohol and cancer risk. Alcoholism Clin Exp Res 1998; 22:323S–328S.
68. Thun MJ, Peto R, Lopez AD, Monaco JH, Henley SJ, Heath CW, Doll R. Alcohol consumption and mortality among middle-aged and elderly U.S. adults. N Engl J Med 1997; 337:1705–1714.
69. Gronbaeck M, Becker U, Johansen D, Tonnesen H, Jensen G, Sorensen TIA. Population based cohort study of the association between alcohol intake and cancer of the upper digestive tract. Br Med J 1998; 317:844–848.
70. Truelsen T, Gronbaeck M, Schnohr P, Boysen G. Intake of beer, wine, and spirits and risk of stroke. Stroke 1998; 29:2467–2472.
71. Rothman KJ. Research and prevention priorities for alcohol carcinogenesis. Environ Health Perspect 1995; 103(Suppl. 8):161–163.
72. Zumoff B. The critical role of alcohol consumption in determining the risk of breast cancer with postmenopausal estrogen administration. J Clin Endocrinol Metab 1997; 82:1656–1658.

73. Ginsburg ES, Gao X, Walsh BW, Gleason RE, Shea BF, Barbieri RL. The effects of ethanol on the clearance of estradiol in postmenopausal women. Fertil Steril 1995; 63:1227–1230.
74. Ginsburg ES, Mello NK, Mendelson JH, Barbieri RL, Teoh SK, Rothman M, Gao X, Sholar JW. Effects of alcohol ingestion on estrogens in postmenopausal women. JAMA 1996; 276:1747–1751.
75. Marmot MG, Elliott P, Shipley MJ, Dyer AR, Ueshima H, Beevers DG, et al. Alcohol and blood pressure: the INTERSALT study. Br Med J 1994; 308:1263–1267.
76. Rosenqvist M. Alcohol and cardiac arrhythmias. Alcoholism Clin Exp Res 1998; 22:318S–322S.
77. Camargo CA, Hennekens CH, Gaziano JM, Glynn RJ, Manson JE, Stampfer MJ. Prospective study of moderate alcohol consumption and mortality in US male physicians. Arch Int Med 1997; 157:79–85.
78. McElduff P, Dobson AJ. How much alcohol and how often? Population based case-control study of alcohol consumption and risk of a major coronary event. Br Med J 1997; 314:1159–1164.
79. Svarsudd K. Moderate alcohol consumption and cardiovascular disease: Is there evidence for a protective effect? Alcoholism Clin Exp Res 1998; 22:307S–314S.
80. Moore TJ. Prevention. In: Heart Failure: A Critical Inquiry into American Medicine and the Revolution in Heart Care. New York: Random House, 1989; 25–95.
81. Lands WEM. Lipid mediators in a paradigm shift: balance between omega-6 and omega-3. In: Egg Nutrition Conference Proceedings. Sim JS, ed. Wallingford, UK: CAB International, 1999; in press.
82. Balkau B, Eschwege F, Eschwege E. Ischemic heart disease and alcohol-related causes of death: a view of the French paradox. Ann Rev Epidemiol 1997; 7:490–497.
83. Pauly PJ. How did the effects of alcohol on reproduction become scientifically uninteresting? J Hist Biol 1996; 29:1–28.
84. Jones KL, Smith DW. Recognition of the fetal alcohol syndrome in early infancy. Lancet 1973; 2:999–1001.
85. Gordis E. Alcohol research and Social policy: an overview. Alcohol Health Res World 1996; 20:208–212.
86. Hilton ME. An overview of recent findings on alcoholic beverage warning labels. J Public Policy Marketing 1993; 12:1–9.
87. Toomey TL, Rosenfeld C, Wagenaar AC. The minimum legal drinking age: history, effectiveness, and ongoing debate. Alcohol Health Res World 1996; 20:213–218.
88. Allebeck P, Rydberg U. Risks and protective effects of alcohol on the individual. Alcoholism Clin Exp Res 1998; 22:269S.
89. Dufour MC. Risks and benefits of alcohol use over the life span. Alcohol Health Res World 1996; 20:145–151.
90. Taubes G. The (political) science of salt. Science 1998; 281:898–907.
91. McCarron DA. Diet and blood pressure: the paradigm shift. Science 1998; 281:933–934.
92. National Cholesterol Education Program. Report of the National Cholesterol Education Program Expert Panel on Detection, Evaluation, and Treatment of High Blood Cholesterol in Adults. Arch Int Med 1988; 148:36–69.
93. Consensus Development Panel. Lowering blood cholesterol to prevent heart disease. JAMA 1985; 253:2080–2086.
94. Ornish D, Scherwitz LW, Billings JH, Gould KL, Merritt TA, Sparler S, et al. JAMA Intensive Lifestyle Changes for Reversal of Coronary Heart Disease. JAMA 1998; 280:2001–2007.
95. Lands WEM, Culp BR, Hirai A, Gorman R. Relationship of thromboxane generation to the aggregation of platelets from humans: effects of eicosapentaenoic acid. Prostaglandins 1985; 30:819–825.
96. Ridker PM, Manson JE, Buring JE, Goldhaber SZ, Hennekens CH. The effect of chronic platelet inhibition with low-dose aspirin on atherosclerotic progression and acute thrombosis: clinical evidence from the Physicians' Health Study. Am Heart J 1991; 122:1588–1592.

22

Health Claims for Foods and Dietary Supplements in the United States and Japan

Annette Dickinson

1. INTRODUCTION

Although there is widespread scientific acceptance of the importance of diet in reducing the risk of chronic disease, there is continuing controversy about the extent to which statements about diet and health may appropriately be included in commercial product labeling and advertising. The United States and Japan have undertaken major initiatives in exploring mechanisms for harnessing the power of commercial product labeling to convey or reinforce government-sanctioned health messages about specific types of foods or food components. These two countries have developed very different approaches to the issue, illustrating the fact that there may be cultural and philosophical, as well as legal and scientific, considerations that affect public policy decisions about health claims for foods. A list of abbreviations used in this chapter appears in Table 1.

2. PUBLIC HEALTH RECOMMENDATIONS IN THE UNITED STATES

Scientific and public acceptance of the existence of a strong relationship between diet and health has been growing in the United States and worldwide. An early and influential compilation of data appeared in 1977, when the Senate Select Committee on Nutrition and Human Needs published its report, *Dietary Goals for the United States (1)*. The report included recommendations for dietary patterns that might decrease the risk of several killer diseases, such as cancer and heart disease (HD). Although there was opposition to the dietary goals from some quarters, the concept of public recommendations for dietary changes, leading to disease prevention, soon became firmly established.

Following publication of the Senate Select Committee report, Congress directed the Department of Health and Human Services and the U.S. Department of Agriculture to prepare a set of dietary guidelines for reducing the risk of chronic disease. The first edition of *Dietary Guidelines for Americans* appeared in 1980, and has been re-evaluated and republished, by Congressional directive, every 5 yr since that time *(2)*. The fifth edition was released in May 2000.

In 1979, the Surgeon General's Report on Health Promotion and Disease Prevention, *Healthy People*, set forth a broad agenda for preventive actions that could be taken to reduce health risks, including some general nutritional recommendations not dissimilar

From: *Primary and Secondary Preventive Nutrition*
Edited by: A. Bendich and R. J. Deckelbaum © Humana Press Inc., Totowa, NJ

Table 1
Abbreviations Used in This Chapter

Ca	Calcium
CDC	Centers for Disease Control and Prevention
CHD	Coronary heart disease
DSHEA	Dietary Supplement Health and Education Act (1994)
FAs	Fatty acids
FDA	Food and Drug Administration
FD&C Act	Food, Drug & Cosmetic Act
FDAMA	Food and Drug Administration Modernization Act (1997)
FOSHU	Food for Specified Health Uses (Japan)
FTC	Federal Trade Commission
GI	Gastrointestinal
HD	Heart disease
HT	Hypertension
Na	Sodium
NAS	National Academy of Sciences
NCI	National Cancer Institute
NLEA	Nutrition Labeling and Education Act (1990)
NRC	National Research Council
NTDs	Neural tube birth defects
OP	Osteoporosis
PHS	Public Health Service
RDA	Recommended Dietary Allowances
RDI	Reference Daily Intake
SG	Surgeon General

to those suggested by the Senate Select Committee *(3)*. This report ultimately led to the development of a series of wide-ranging U.S. action plans that call on federal, state, and local governments, and other organizations, to take cooperative action to measurably reduce recognized risk factors and increase health-promoting behaviors. Objectives were recently announced for the third decade of the program, *Healthy People 2010 (4)*.

In 1982, the National Research Council (NRC) published *Diet, Nutrition and Cancer*, outlining specific dietary recommendations for cancer reduction *(5)*. The report called for increased consumption of fruits and vegetables rich in antioxidant vitamins, cruciferous vegetables, and grains and other foods rich in fiber. It emphasized that these recommendations were aimed at increasing intakes of certain food groups or types of foods, not specific nutrients.

In 1988 and 1989, respectively, the Surgeon General's (SG's) report, *Nutrition and Health*, and the NRC's report, *Diet and Health*, again reviewed the data, and made broad recommendations regarding dietary habits that were likely to help reduce the risk of cancer, HD, hypertension (HT), diabetes, obesity, osteoporosis (OP), and other chronic diseases *(6,7)*.

In 1994, the Food and Nutrition Board of the National Academy of Sciences (NAS) began a new revision of the recommended dietary allowances for vitamins and minerals, for the first time using chronic disease prevention as one element of the underlying scientific basis for new recommendations *(8)*. That effort is ongoing, and has already resulted in three reports, one on calcium (Ca) and related nutrients; one on B-vitamins, including folic acid; and one on antioxidants. The first of these reports recommended substantial increases in intakes of Ca and vitamin D, in order to help reduce the risk of OP. The second approximately doubled the recommended dietary allowance (RDA) for folic acid, and further urged that women of childbearing age should get 0.4 mg (400 mcg) of synthetic folic acid, in addition to their usual dietary intake, in order to reduce the risk of having a baby with neural tube birth defects (NTDs). The third report on antioxidant nutrients was released in April 2000, raising recommendations for vitamins C and E only slightly and calling for more research on antioxidants and disease prevention.

Thus, public health policy regarding diet and health has been moving steadily forward in the United States, continuing to emphasize the potential for reducing the risk of chronic disease through dietary changes.

3. U.S. FOOD MARKETPLACE AND THE LAW

While the scientific community was in the process of uniting behind a set of common dietary recommendations, food marketing companies were constrained in their ability to make use of this information in labeling and advertising. As discussed below, disease-related statements in food labeling were officially viewed as inappropriate or illegal, and the food industry was accordingly restricted in promoting health benefits.

In 1984, the National Cancer Institute (NCI) was pursuing various educational programs to increase public awareness of dietary patterns that could reduce cancer risk. As part of this initiative, NCI entered into a joint national campaign with the Kellogg Company to promote diets high in fiber. Informational messages appeared prominently in the labeling of certain Kellogg high-fiber cereals. This government-sanctioned campaign marked the beginning of a change in U.S. policy that would eventually permit health claims on food labels. Before that policy developed, however, numerous marketers took up the theme of promoting high-fiber foods to reduce cancer risk, and such claims began to proliferate.

The U.S. Food, Drug and Cosmetic Act (FD&C Act) defines drugs in part as products "intended for use in the diagnosis, cure, mitigation, treatment, or prevention of disease in man or other animals." Under this law, claims relating to disease prevention were viewed historically as drug claims and were not permitted in food labeling. However, in 1984, faced with Kellogg cereals bearing NCI-supported claims about fiber and cancer, the Food and Drug Administration (FDA) entered into a public dialogue about the desirability of permitting health claims for foods, under certain conditions.

Several forces were at work during this period. The food industry was increasingly anxious to utilize the strong science base to promote foods with desirable characteristics. Consumer advocates were concerned that claims were getting out of control, and urged Congress to permit only those claims specifically authorized by FDA under strict guidelines. The Federal Trade Commission (FTC) released a 1989 report concluding that fiber claims in the marketplace had both increased consumer awareness of the relationship between fiber and cancer, and increased the number of high-fiber products available to the public *(9)*. Both of these outcomes were viewed as positive developments by the authors of the FTC report. The FDA was working its way toward guidelines or regulations on health claims, but some legal questions persisted about whether FDA had the authority to permit health claims for foods without a change in the statute.

In 1990, Congress passed the Nutrition Labeling and Education Act (NLEA), which gave FDA clear authority to permit health claims in food labeling, under certain conditions. NLEA also put mandatory nutrition labeling in place, and defined nutrient content claims, but neither of these aspects of NLEA are discussed here. A health claim is defined as a label statement characterizing the relationship of a nutrient or food component to a disease or health-related condition. Under the new law, foods with approved health claims are not considered drugs solely because their labeling contains a health claim, which by definition must mention a disease or health-related condition.

In order to approve an NLEA health claim, FDA must determine, "based on the totality of publicly available scientific evidence (including evidence from well-designed studies conducted in a manner which is consistent with generally recognized scientific procedures and principles), that there is significant scientific agreement, among experts qualified by scientific training and experience to evaluate such claims, that the claim is supported by such evidence." FDA must then issue a regulation describing the permitted claim, so that the claim accurately conveys the nutrient–disease relationship. NLEA specified that the claim should enable consumers "to comprehend the information provided in the claim and to understand the relative significance of such information in the context of a total daily diet."

NLEA provided FDA with a list of 10 health claims that the agency was required to evaluate initially, including four designated as claims for dietary supplements. The six core claims listed in NLEA related to fat and cancer, fat and HD, sodium (Na) and HT, fiber and cancer, fiber and HD, and Ca and OP. The four claims listed as dietary supplement claims were for antioxidant vitamins and cancer, folic acid and NTDs, omega-3 fatty acids (FAs) and HD, and zinc and immune function in the elderly.

4. U.S. HEALTH CLAIMS REGULATIONS

In January of 1993, FDA finalized regulations establishing general requirements for health claims (10). In order for a food to be eligible for a health claim, it must not contain disqualifying amounts of any risk nutrients, including total fat, saturated fat, cholesterol, or Na. Also, a serving of the food must naturally contain at least 10% of the recommended daily intake of vitamin A, vitamin C, iron, Ca, protein, or fiber. This provision, sometimes referred to as the "jelly bean rule," is intended to ensure that foods bearing health claims are products with some inherent nutritional value. If a health claim suggests that people should consume more of any substance (such as Ca or folic acid or fiber), FDA must make a determination that the substance is safe and lawful. Also, the substance must contribute taste, aroma, nutritive value, or a designated technical effect in foods, and must retain those qualities when consumed at levels high enough to justify the health claim. In the regulation authorizing a health claim, FDA provides model claims that may be used in product labeling. Marketers are not limited to the language of the model claim, but the language they use must convey certain information specified in the regulation.

In 1993, FDA issued separate regulations approving three health claims for foods low in certain components related to disease risk (11–13). These included claims for foods low in lipids, which may help reduce the risk of cancer; claims for foods low in saturated fat and cholesterol, which may help reduce the risk of coronary heart disease (CHD); and claims for foods low in Na, which may help reduce the risk of HT.

At the same time, FDA approved three health claims for foods which are naturally good sources of dietary fiber, soluble fiber, or two antioxidant vitamins (14–16). In all three cases, FDA argued that the available evidence indicated that diets high in these nutrients were protective against cancer and/or HD, but did not permit a determination that these nutrients were the cause of the protective effect. In other words, FDA concluded that fiber and antioxidant vitamins may be only markers for protective foods or disease-reducing food habits. Under these regulations, health claims about reducing cancer risk may be made for fruits, vegetables, and grains that are low in fat, and that are naturally good sources of dietary fiber, vitamin C, or vitamin A from β-carotene. Health claims may also be made about reducing the risk of CHD for fruits, vegetables, and grains that are low in fat, saturated fat, and cholesterol, and that contain at least 0.6 g soluble fiber/serving.

FDA declined to approve any health claims for specific fiber sources, in 1993, but the agency indicated that it would be willing to review health claim petitions based on sufficient evidence to show that specific fibers lower cholesterol. In 1997 and 1998, FDA approved petitions for health claims for oat fiber and psyllium fiber *(17,18)*. The oat claim is permitted for any foods (including dietary supplements) that contain a sufficient amount of oat bran, rolled oats, or whole oat flour to provide at least 0.75 g of β-glucan soluble fiber/serving. The psyllium claim is permitted for any foods (including dietary supplements) that contain at least 1.7 g psyllium fiber/serving. In 1999, FDA approved a health claim for soy protein, also on the grounds that it lowers cholesterol and therefore may reduce the risk of heart disease *(19)*. The claim is permitted for foods that are low in saturated fat and cholesterol and that contain at least 6.25 g per serving of soy protein.

In September 2000, the FDA approved a similar health claim for foods containing at least 0.65 g of plant sterol esters or at least 1.7 g of plant stanol esters *(20)*.

Also in 1993, FDA approved a Ca health claim, which may be used in the labeling of any food or dietary supplement that meets the general requirements for health claims, and contains at least 200 mg Ca/serving *(20a)*. The claim indicates that diets high in Ca may reduce the risk of OP.

In all of the 1993 regulations approving health claims, FDA relied heavily on the SG's *Nutrition and Health* report, the NRC's *Diet and Health* report, and the *Dietary Guidelines for Americans* as evidence of significant scientific agreement regarding specific diet and health relationships. Claims were disapproved for omega-3 FAs and HD, and for zinc and immune function in the elderly *(21,22)*.

In 1996, FDA approved a health claim petition for foods sweetened with sugar alcohols, relating to reduced risk of dental caries *(23)*. The rule permits the use of xylitol, sorbitol, mannitol, maltitol, isomalt, lactitol, hydrogenated starch hydrolysates, hydrogenated glucose syrups, or a combination of these. In 1997, erythritol was added to the list of sugar alcohols eligible for this health claim *(24)*.

The folic acid claim was the subject of particular controversy, and the delay caused by that controversy was eventually led to the development in 1997 of an alternative procedure for permitting health claims. In 1992, the U.S. Public Health Service (PHS) issued a recommendation urging women of childbearing age to obtain 0.4 mg folic acid daily, before conception and early in pregnancy, in order to reduce the risk of having a baby with a neural tube birth defect, such as spina bifida or anencephaly *(25)*. The development of this recommendation was led by scientists at the Centers for Disease Control and Prevention (CDC). Although the FDA, as part of the PHS, was a participating agency in making this recommendation, FDA declined in 1993 to authorize a health claim for folic acid *(26)*. The agency was considering requiring mandatory enrichment of grain products with folic acid and was concerned about potential safety issues if some individuals obtained additional folic acid from numerous resources, including foods and dietary supplements bearing health claims.

It was not until 1996 that FDA eventually approved a health claim for folic acid *(27)*. The agency indicated that the safety issues had been resolved, since an enrichment plan had been developed that would maintain total folic acid intake within safe ranges. The health claim is permitted in the labeling of any foods or supplements providing at least 10% of the reference daily intake (RDI) of folic acid. This relatively low level was selected as the basis for the claim in order to permit the claim to appear on the largest possible number of fruits and vegetables. Although this same low trigger level applies in defining the eligibility of a dietary supplement for this health claim, in fact, most dietary supplements containing folic acid provide the full RDI of 0.4 mg (400 mcg). The regulation also requires that dietary supplements bearing the folic acid health claim must meet disintegration and dissolution standards established by the U.S. Pharmacopeia, or must be shown to be bioavailable.

At the same time that the folic acid health claim was finalized, FDA also finalized a series of rules amending the Standards of Identity for enriched grain products that required mandatory addition of folic acid beginning in 1998 *(28)*. Products affected include enriched flour, corn meal, breads, rice, and pasta. The agency also amended the food additive rule on folic acid to define other permitted uses of folic acid in foods *(29)*. The rule permits breakfast cereals to contain up to 0.4 mg per serving of folic acid, and also permits addition of the vitamin to infant formula, medical foods, and foods for special dietary use; other addition of folic acid to foods is not allowed.

Table 2 is a summary list of the health claims currently approved by FDA.

5. FDAMA HEALTH CLAIMS

The FDA Modernization Act of 1997 (FDAMA) was a major legislative initiative with broad effects on the regulation of drugs and devices, and on FDA's approaches to priority-setting and stakeholder involvement in the decision-making process. Among its many provisions, FDAMA created an alternative route for permitting health claims for foods. The agency's delay in approving the folic acid health claim had been frequently and strongly criticized. It was argued that marketers should have been able to base a health claim on the 1992 PHS recommendation, even in the absence FDA approval of a formal health claim for folic acid. This argument found a sympathetic ear in Congress, and FDAMA contains a provision that permits manufacturers to make health claims based on authoritative statements by certain scientific bodies, including the National Institutes of Health, the CDC, and the NAS. Before making a health claim based on an authoritative statement by an appropriate scientific body, a company must notify FDA 120 d in advance. This provides an opportunity for FDA to evaluate the claim and, if it is found not to be valid, to deny it or require modifications to it.

In 1998, FDA denied an early petition for nine FDAMA health claims, mostly on the grounds that the statements cited were not "authoritative statements" of scientific bodies *(30)*. In 1999, FDA allowed the first FDAMA health claim to be utilized, which was a health claim submitted by General Mills, based on the NAS 1989 report, *Diet and Health*. The claim states that the consumption of whole grain foods is related to a reduced risk of HD and some cancers. Additional petitions for FDAMA health claims can be anticipated in the future.

6. COURT OF APPEALS DECISION

Some may be surprised to learn that government regulations (including FDA regulations) can raise constitutional issues, but in fact this can occur. The first amendment to

Table 2

NLEA Health Claims Approved by the U.S. Food and Drug Administration as of June 2000

Health claims for foods low in certain components
  Foods low in total fat and saturated fat: reduced cancer risk
  Foods low in saturated fat and cholesterol: reduced risk of CHD
  Foods low in Na: reduced risk of HT
Health claims for foods naturally containing certain components
  Foods that are good sources of fiber: reduced risk of cancer
  Foods that are good sources of soluble fiber: reduced risk of CHD
  Foods that are good sources of vitamin C or β-carotene: reduced risk of cancer
Health claims for specific food components, whether added or naturally occurring
  Foods high in Ca: reduced risk of osteoporosis
  Foods with folate or folic acid: reduced risk of having a baby with NTD
  Foods sweetened with sugar alcohols: reduced risk of dental caries
  Foods with whole oats or oat bran containing β-glucan: reduced risk of HD
  Foods with psyllium fiber: reduced risk of HD
  Food with soy protein: reduced risk of HD
  Food with sterol or stanol esters: reduced risk of HD

the U.S. Constitution guarantees freedom of speech, and the courts have held that this protection extends to commercial speech (such as labeling and advertising), as well as to individual speech. The government can prohibit false or misleading commercial speech, but is constrained in its ability to restrict speech that is truthful and not misleading. In the case of health claims, FDA does not permit claims unless they are supported by significant scientific agreement. Qualified health claims (health claims with disclaimers about the strength of the evidence) are not permitted, although they may truthfully state the degree of scientific support for the statement. Some have questioned whether this potential prohibition of truthful statements is legal under the first amendment.

Several parties brought suit against FDA for violating the first amendment in denying certain health claims. One case brought by a health-rights organization (National Council for Improved Health) and one case brought by an industry association (Nutritional Health Alliance) were found not to be eligible for substantive judicial review, since the appellants did not identify a particular proposed health claim that FDA had prevented them from making. A third case was brought by a coalition of petitioners including Durk Pearson and Sandy Shaw (authors who are also developers and marketers of some dietary supplement products), the American Preventive Medical Association (a health rights advocacy organization whose members are health care practitioners), and Citizens for a health rights advocacy organization whose members are consumers). In this case, known as Pearson vs. Shalala, a U.S. Court of Appeals ruled, in January 1999, that some aspects of FDA's current health claims approval process may violate the first amendment, as well as the Administrative Procedure Act (31). The court concluded that FDA must better define the term "significant scientific agreement," and must at least consider the appropriateness of permitting qualified health claims. For example, FDA rejected specific claims for antioxidants on the grounds that the evidence suggests a beneficial effect of certain types of foods, but the component responsible for the effect is not definitely known. The court suggested that, rather than ban the claim for antioxidant vitamins *per se*, FDA should consider adding a disclaimer such as: "The evidence is inconclusive because existing studies have been performed with foods containing antioxidant vitamins, and the effect on those foods on reducing the risk of cancer may result from other components in those foods."

In this ruling, the court relies on legal precedents that have been skeptical of regulations "that seek to keep people in the dark for what the government perceives to be their own good." The court suggested that more information, rather than less, may be the solution. At the same time, the court recognized that, when the evidence against a claim outweighs the evidence in its favor, FDA may well choose to ban it outright. That is, a disclaimer cannot salvage a claim that is basically misleading. Regulations denying substance-specific health claims for dietary fiber and cancer, antioxidant vitamins and cancer, and omega-3 FAs and CHD were remanded to FDA with instructions for reconsideration. Some aspects of the folic acid health claim must also be reconsidered. In December 1999 and January 2000, FDA announced its plan for implementing the court's decision, issued a guidance document better defining "significant scientific agreement," and re-opened the comment period on the four claims at issue *(32,33,34)*. Based on the comments submitted and the agency's own review of the scientific evidence, FDA will later determine whether a qualified claim can be permitted on any of the four topics under consideration. Whatever the outcome of FDA's further evaluation of these claims, the Pearson decision may have a substantial impact on the future regulation of health claims in the U.S.

7. CLAIMS FOR DIETARY SUPPLEMENTS IN THE UNITED STATES

Under NLEA, dietary supplements are eligible for health claims, and FDA has approved several claims that may be used in the labeling of dietary supplements, as well as foods containing certain nutrients or food components. Health claims potentially applicable to dietary supplements include those for Ca, folic acid, oat fiber, psyllium fiber and soyprotein. However, FDA's general requirements for health claims limit the types of substances that may be eligible for claims, in that the substances must have nutritive value. This requirement could potentially make some dietary supplement ingredients, such as St. John's Wort or echinacea, for example, ineligible for health claims.

The Dietary Supplement Health and Education Act of 1994 (DSHEA) defines dietary supplements and permits them to bear other types of claims, called "Statements of Nutritional Support" (DSHEA also has numerous other provisions that are not addressed here). Dietary supplements have always been considered as a subcategory of foods, and previously had been treated as foods for special dietary use, a category created in the 1938 FD&C Act.

DSHEA reaffirms that dietary supplements are foods, and provides a broad definition. A dietary supplement is defined as "a product (other than tobacco) intended to supplement the diet." Such products may contain vitamins, minerals, herbs or other botanicals, amino acids, or almost any other dietary substance that may be used to supplement the diet. Products may contain concentrates, metabolites, constituents, extracts, or any combination of the permitted types of ingredients. Dietary supplements may be in traditional dosage forms, such as tablets or capsules, or may be in the physical form of conventional foods, provided they are not "represented for use as a conventional food," and are not intended as the sole item of a meal or of the diet. There is considerable controversy regarding what types of label statements or vignettes can be considered to represent a product as a dietary supplement, compared to a conventional food.

Dietary supplement labeling is permitted under DSHEA to contain Statements of Nutritional Support. These statements may describe the role of a nutrient or dietary ingredient intended to affect the structure or function of the body, may characterize the documented mechanism for such an effect, may relate to general well-being, or may claim a benefit related to a classical nutrient deficiency disease (provided that the statement also discloses the prevalence of the deficiency in the United States). These statements may not claim to diagnose, mitigate, treat, cure, or prevent a specific disease or class of diseases.

In permitting statements describing the effect of a product on the structure and function of the body, DSHEA was building on the historical exemption of foods from one aspect of the drug definition. The relevant section of the drug definition in the FD&C Act states that drugs are "articles (other than food) intended to affect the structure or any function of the body of man or other animals." Thus, the 1938 law recognized that foods have effects on structure and function, and that such intended effects are not drug uses. However, in case law, FDA has argued that many statements about structure–function effects are implied disease claims.

DSHEA reaffirms the ability of dietary supplements and other foods to make structure–function statements. For clarity, a new sentence is added to the drug definition, specifically providing that a food, dietary ingredient, or dietary supplement, for which a truthful and not misleading Statement of Nutritional Support is made, is not a drug under the structure–function section of the drug definition, solely because of that statement. This sentence is parallel in structure and intent to the sentence added by NLEA in 1990, noting that a food for which an approved health claim is made is not a drug solely because of that claim.

DSHEA requires the manufacturer of any dietary supplement making a Statement of Nutritional Support to have substantiation that the statement is truthful, and not misleading. Also, the label should contain the following disclaimer, in order to avoid any implication that the statement is an FDA-authorized health claim or an FDA-approved drug claim: "This statement has not been evaluated by the Food and Drug Administration. This product is not intended to diagnose, treat, cure, or prevent any disease."

Marketers are required to notify FDA within 30 d, if they are making a Statement of Nutritional Support in labeling. According to a database compiled by AAC Consulting, FDA had received letters of notification from more than 400 companies regarding over 7000 Statements of Nutritional Support, as of April 2000 (35). The most commonly submitted statements relate to emotional or mental health, cholesterol or the heart, energy and strength, immune function, antioxidant effects, joints and bones, digestion or gastrointestinal (GI) function, weight loss, urinary function or prostate health, and women's health.

FDA does not evaluate or approve Statements of Nutritional Support, but it has responded to some letters of notification, indicating that the agency views the proposed statement as a disease claim or an unauthorized health claim. About 10% of the letters of notification have triggered FDA responses, called "courtesy letters" (to distinguish them from formal enforcement notices called "warning letters").

A few examples will serve to illustrate the current usage of Statements of Nutritional Support. In the area of immune function, Statements of Nutritional Support commonly appear on dietary supplements such as zinc or echinacea, indicating that the product supports a healthy immune system or enhances natural resistance. FDA has objected to any specific mention of diseases, such as colds, flu, sore throat, and bronchitis. Statements about supporting normal joint function or joint flexibility are commonly used for products, such as glucosamine and chondroitin sulfate, but FDA has objected to any specific reference to arthritis or rheumatism.

Statements of Nutritional Support may not be used in place of approved health claims. For example, statements relating to folic acid and NTD, or to Ca and OP, may only be made under the conditions described in the regulations approving these health claims, and must include the information specified in those regulations.

FDA's regulatory oversight of Statements of Nutritional Support has so far concentrated primarily on evaluating whether the statements legally qualify under DSHEA, and has not extended to probing the manufacturer's substantiation for the statements. Many Statements of Nutritional Support are clearly consistent with the recognized effects of certain nutrients or botanical ingredients, but there is substantial concern regarding the scientific basis of some label statements currently seen in the marketplace. Some groups have called for formal evaluation of the evidence supporting such statements. The Commission on Dietary Supplement Labels, in its 1997 report, emphasized the importance of ensuring that Statements of Nutritional Support are adequately substantiated, so that consumers are provided with scientifically valid information *(36)*. The Commission also suggested that summaries of the substantiation be made publicly available so that consumers and health professionals could better evaluate the claims being made.

Although it appears that Statements of Nutritional Support have to some extent accomplished the objective of better informing consumers about the uses of certain dietary supplements, there is concern regarding the blurring of traditional boundaries between permissible food claims and drug claims. In January 2000, FDA finalized regulations intended to better define the boundaries between permissible dietary supplement statements and impermissible disease claims *(37)*. The regulations permit statements about effects on the structure or function of the body, provided there is no implied disease claim. In the final rule, FDA provides numerous examples of permitted and prohibited claims, to illustrate the agency's view of what constitutes an implied disease claim. FDA's guidance for the most part is consistent with the agency's past comments as reflected in courtesy letters. Acceptable statements include claims relating to normal symptoms of the menstrual cycle or menopause (mild mood changes, cramps, hot flashes) and claims relating to mild memory problems or absentmindedness associated with aging. However, the agency finds that statements relating to benign prostatic hypertrophy would be considered disease claims, because the consequences are potentially more serious. Also, statements relating to lowering cholesterol or decreasing platelet aggregation would be considered to be implied claims about heart disease and thus not permitted. Statements about maintaining healthy function would generally be acceptable. One of the more surprising aspects of the final rule was FDA's determination that many approved claims for over-the-counter drug products are in fact statements about structure or function and not disease claims, and that such statements may be used for dietary supplements as well. These include statements about preventing nausea of motion sickness, relieving occasional sleeplessness, and soothing stress or nervous tension.

There is an inherent tension between providing consumers with meaningful information about the health benefits of foods and dietary supplements, and attempting to retain some legal or logical boundary to distinguish that information from the types of claims reserved for approved pharmaceutical products. With approved NLEA health claims specifically claiming to reduce the risk of serious chronic diseases, and with DSHEA Statements of Nutritional Support describing specific effects on the structure and function of the body, that tension is likely to continue into the foreseeable future. The food/drug distinction in the United States is no longer as sharp as it was even a decade ago, and it may become even more blurred as policymakers seek to provide consumers with more information, to enable them to more fully participate in efforts directed toward health promotion and disease prevention.

8. HEALTH CLAIMS IN JAPAN

In Japan, as in the United States, only pharmaceutical products traditionally could be formulated and labeled for health uses (38). As a scientific consensus began to emerge regarding the importance of food choices in modifying the risk of chronic disease, the concept of functional foods began to emerge. In 1984, 1988, and 1992, special study groups on functional foods were appointed by the Ministry of Education, Science, and Culture. Each group, consisting of top specialists in biochemistry, food chemistry, and agricultural chemistry, met for 2–3 yr, and produced recommendations relating to the functional effects of foods in the modulation of physiological systems. In 1988, the Ministry of Health and Welfare established an Office of Health Policy on Newly Developed Foods, which studied how best to systematize the regulation of functional foods.

In 1991, the Nutrition Improvement Law officially established a category of products known as Food for Specified Health Uses (FOSHU), which were eligible for health claims. FOSHUs are functional foods whose formulation and claims have been approved by the Minister of Health and Welfare, based on clinical evidence that the product promotes health. Such foods cannot bear statements relating to the prevention or treatment of disease, but may only bear claims regarding preserving or promoting health. Permitted claims included statements such as: "helps maintain a good gastrointestinal condition," "helpful for people concerned about high blood cholesterol level," and "suitable for people with mild hypertension." Statements such as these are considered to be sufficiently food-oriented to avoid conflict with the Pharmaceutical Affairs Law governing medicines in Japan.

FOSHUs that have been approved have included foods with functional ingredients, including oligosaccharides, lactobacillus, bifidobacteria, dietary fiber sources, peptides, sugar alcohols, and minerals. FOSHUs approved by the Ministry of Health and Welfare bear a graphic seal, and their labels must include information describing the functional effect, the amount to be used, and other directions for use. Contrary to health claims approval in the United States, the Japanese system does not confer FOSHU status generically for certain food ingredients or components. Rather, each individual product requires specific approval. In some instances, companies have even obtained separate approvals for different flavors of the same brand of the same product. Only conventional foods are eligible for designation as FOSHU. Products in the physical form of tablets or capsules are not eligible.

As of February 2000, there were over 170 FOSHU approved in Japan (39). Table 3 summarizes the approved products, categorized according to the functional component for which the claim is made. The claims listed in the table are simplified versions of the actual approved language. For example, the English translation of the full text of one approved claim for oligosaccharides is: "This product is suitable for those who are con-

Table 3
Foods for Specified Health Uses (FOSHU) Approved in Japan as of February 2000 *(39)*

No. products	Specified health use	Ingredients	Types of foods
124	Increase intestinal microflora, expecially bifidobacteria; provide fiber	Oligosaccharides, lactosucrose, lactobacillus, bifidobacterium, psyllium, indigestible dextrin polydextrose, guar gum, wheat bran	Yogurt, beverages, table sugar, candy, vinegar, cookies, cornflakes, cereals
23	For people concerned about cholesterol or triglycerides	Soy protein, psyllium, sodium alginate, chitosan, diacylglycerol, phytosterol, globin digest	Beverages, soy products, meat products, biscuits, cooking oils
10	To supplement intake of calcium or iron	Calcium citrate malate, casein phosphopeptide, heme iron	Soft drinks, tofu
9	For people with mild hypertension	Peptides, glycosides	Soft drinks, soup powder
5	Foods with low cariogenecity	Polyphenols, sugar alcohols	Candy, chocolate, chewing gum
3	For hyperglycemia	Indigestible dextrins	Beverages

cerned about their GI condition. It increases intestinal bifidobacteria and thus helps maintain a good intestinal environment."

There is a striking dissimilarity between the types of health claims approved in the United States and the types of conditions for which FOSHU are approved in Japan. In the United States, the majority of approved health claims relate to reducing the risk of cancer or HD. In Japan, the majority of FOSHU are approved for their effects on the GI tract, especially in affecting the nature of the microflora. In fact, many of the FOSHU statements are more comparable to DSHEA structure–function statements, than to NLEA health claims. In the United States, most foods for which health claims can be made are conventional foods that are major components of the diet (grains, fruits, vegetables), but some claims are permitted for fortified foods and dietary supplements. In Japan, many FOSHU claims are for specific food components delivered in the form of soft drinks or other beverages, but products in the form of tablets or capsules are not eligible. These differences reflect cultural and philosophical divergences in the two countries, more than legal differences, since the underlying food and drug laws are similar.

9. OUTLOOK FOR THE NEXT DECADE

After NLEA was passed in the United States, FDA initially approved a number of generic health claims, and is now moving in the direction of approving more substance-specific health claims, particularly involving fiber. Most of the approved health claims relate to reducing the risk of serious chronic diseases, such as cancer and HD. In 1997, FDAMA added an alternative method for allowing health claims, based on authoritative statements of certain scientific bodies. In January 1999, a Court of Appeals decision required FDA to better define "significant scientific agreement," and to reconsider whether some qualified health claims may be permitted under this standard. This evolution of events illustrates the pressure that is brought to bear on the system, once the basic legality of health claims for foods is accepted. Health claims will clearly continue to be part of the food marketing environment in the United States, and their scope is likely to expand.

DSHEA's provisions for Statements of Nutritional Support, for foods and dietary supplements, are in a sense a direct outgrowth of the overall policy to permit health claims in food and dietary supplement labeling. Statements of Nutritional Support could not have been created, except in the context of an existing policy permitting health claims. However, Statements of Nutritional Support are not subject to premarket evaluation by FDA or any other authoritative body, whereas health claims are. Health professionals and consumer advocacy groups are concerned about the soundness of some of the statements being used. There is a need for industry to be rigorous in adhering to the requirement for substantiation, and there is a need for FDA enforcement when statements are being made without adequate substantiation.

In considering the scientific evidence on diet and health, and in seeking ways to permit food manufacturers to convey meaningful information to consumers, Japan developed a regulatory system different from the one that evolved in the United States. It is product-specific, rather than generic, with separate approval being required for every product identified as a FOSHU. This system requires close communication and cooperation between manufacturers and local and national regulatory bodies, as is traditional in Japan. It may be said that these claims are essentially structure–function statements subject to a rigorous premarket clearance process.

Other countries will be watching the development of food claims policy in the United States and Japan, as they evaluate their own regulatory situation and the needs of their populations for health-related products and information. The European Union and Codex Alimentarius have so far not incorporated health claims or structure–function statements into their approaches to food labeling guidelines, but are beginning to discuss the possibility. Divergent national and international policies will inevitably have an impact on attempts to harmonize the global marketplace.

REFERENCES

1. Select Committee on Nutrition and Human Needs. Dietary Goals for the United States. Washington, DC: Government Printing Office, 1977.
2. Dietary Guidelines for Americans. Washington, DC: U.S. Department of Health, Education and Welfare and U.S. Department of Agriculture, 1980, 1985, 1990, 1995, and 2000.
3. U.S. Surgeon General. Healthy People: The Surgeon General's Report on Health Promotion and Disease Prevention. Washington, DC: U.S. Department of Health, Education and Welfare, 1979.

4. Office of Disease Prevention and Health Promotion. Healthy People 2010 (conference edition in two volumes). Washington, DC: U.S. Department of Health and Human Services, January 2000.

5. National Research Council. Diet, Nutrition, and Cancer. Washington, DC: National Academy Press, 1982.

6. U.S. Surgeon General. Report on Nutrition and Health. Washington, DC: U.S. Department of Health and Human Services, 1988.

7. National Research Council. Diet and Health: Implications for Reducing Chronic Disease Risk. Washington, DC: National Academy Press, 1989.

8. Food and Nutrition Board, Institute of Medicine. How Should the Recommended Dietary Allowances Be Revised? Washington, DC: National Academy Press, 1994.

9. Ippolito P, Mathios A. Health Claims in Advertising and Labeling: A Study of the Cereal Market. Washington, DC: Bureau of Economics, Federal Trade Commission, 1989.

10. Food and Drug Administration. Labeling: general requirements for health claims for food. Federal Register 1993; 58:2478–2536. (Codified in Section 101.14, Title 21, Code of Federal Regulations.)

11. Food and Drug Administration. Food labeling: health claims and label statements; dietary fat and cancer. Federal Register 1993; 58:2787–2819. (Codified in Section 101.73, Title 21, Code of Federal Regulations.)

12. Food and Drug Administration. Food labeling: health claims and label statements; dietary saturated fat and cholesterol and coronary heart disease. Federal Register 1993; 58:2739–2786. (Codified in Section 101.75, Title 21, Code of Federal Regulations.)

13. Food and Drug Administration. Food labeling: health claims and label statements; sodium and hypertension. Federal Register 1993; 58:2820–2849. (Codified in Section 101.74, Title 21, Code of Federal Regulations.)

14. Food and Drug Administration. Food labeling: health claims and label statements; dietary fiber and cancer. Federal Register 1993; 58:2537–2551. (Codified in Section 101.76, Title 21, Code of Federal Regulations.)

15. Food and Drug Administration. Food labeling: health claims and label statements; antioxidant vitamins and cancer. Federal Register 1993; 58:2622–2660. (Codified in Section 101.78, Title 21, Code of Federal Regulations.)

16. Food and Drug Administration. Food labeling: health claims and label statements; dietary fiber and cardiovascular disease. Federal Register 1993; 58:2552–2605. (Codified in Section 101.77, Title 21, Code of Federal Regulations.)

17. Food and Drug Administration. Food labeling: health claims; oats and coronary heart disease. Federal Register 1997; 62:3584–3601. (Codified in Section 101.81, Title 21, Code of Federal Regulations.)

18. Food and Drug Administration. Food labeling: health claims: soluble fiber from certain foods and coronary heart disease. Federal Register 1998; 63:8103–8121. (Codified in Section 101.81, Title 21, Code of Federal Regulations.)

19. Food and Drug Administration. Food labeling: health claims; soy protein and coronary heart disease. Federal Register 1999; 64:57699–57733. (Codified in Section 101.82, Title 21, Code of Federal Regulations.)

20. Food and Drug Administration. Food labeling: health claims; plant sterol/stanol esters and coronary heart diseases; interim final rule. Federal Register 2000; 65:54,685–54,739. (Codified in Section 101.83, Title 21, Code of Federal Regulations.)

20a. Food and Drug Administration. Food labeling: health claims; calcium and osteoporosis. Federal Register 1993; 58:2665–2681. (Codified in Section 101.72, Title 21, Code of Federal Regulations.)

21. Food and Drug Administration. Food labeling: health claims; omega-3 fatty acids and coronary heart disease. Federal Register 1993; 58:2682–2738. (Codified in Section 101.71, Title 21, Code of Federal Regulations.)

22. Food and Drug Administration. Food labeling: health claims; zinc and immune function in the elderly. Federal Register 1993; 58:2661–2664. (Codified in Section 101.71, Title 21, Code of Federal Regulations.)

23. Food and Drug Administration. Food labeling: health claims; sugar alcohols and dental caries. Federal Register 1996; 61:43,433–43,447. (Codified in Section 101.80, Title 21, Code of Federal Regulations.)

24. Food and Drug Administration. Food labeling: health claims; sugar alcohols and dental caries. Federal Register 1997; 62:63,653–63,655. (Codified in Section 101.80, Title 21, Code of Federal Regulations.)

25. Centers for Disease Control and Prevention. Recommendations for the use of folic acid to reduce the number of cases of spina bifida and other neural tube defects. MMWR 1992; 41(RR-14).

26. Food and Drug Administration. Food labeling: health claims and label statements; folic acid and neural tube defects. Federal Register 1993; 58:2606–2621.

27. Food and Drug Administration. Food labeling: health claims and label statements; folate and neural tube defects. Federal Register 1996; 61:8752–8781. (Codified in Section 101.79, Title 21, Code of Federal Regulations.)

28. Food and Drug Administration. Food standards: amendment of standards of identity for enriched grain products to require addition of folic acid. Federal Register 1996; 61:8781–8797. (Codified in Sections 136, 137, and 139 of Title 21, Code of Federal Regulations.)

29. Food and Drug Administration. Food additives permitted for direct addition to food for human consumption; folic acid (folacin). Federal Register 1996; 61:8797–8807. (Codified in Section 172.345, Title 21, Code of Federal Regulations.)

30. Food and Drug Administration. Food labeling: health claims; interim final rules. Federal Register 1998; 63:34,084–34,117.

31. U.S. Court of Appeals for the District of Columbia Circuit, No. 98-5043, Pearson et al. v. Shalala, decided January 15, 1999.

32. Food and Drug Administration. Food labeling: Health claims and label statements for dietary supplements; Strategy for implementation of Pearson court decision. Federal Register 1999; 64:67289–67291.

33. Food and Drug Administration. Guidance for industry: Significant scientific agreement in the review of health claims for conventional food and dietary supplements; availability. Federal Register 1999; 64:71794.

34. Food and Drug Administration. Food labeling: Health claims and label statements; Request for scientific data and information; reopening of comment period. Federal Register 2000; 65:4252–4253.

35. AAC Consulting Group. Dietary Supplement Notification List. Bethesda, Maryland, 1999.

36. Commission on Dietary Supplement Labels. Report of the Commission on Dietary Supplement Labels. Washington, DC: Superintendent of Documents, November 1997.

37. Food and Drug Administration. Regulations on statements made for dietary supplements concerning the effect of the product on the structure or function of the body; Final rule. Federal Register 2000; 65:999–1050.

38. Hosoya N. Health claims in Japan: foods for specified health uses and functional foods. Paper prepared for Codex Committee on Nutrition and Foods for Special Dietary Uses, Codex Alimentarius. Tokyo, Japan: Japan Health and Nutrition Food Association, September 1998.

39. Nakajima K. Japan health food and nutrition association. Functional claims for foods, presentation at symposium on marketing nutracenticals and functional foods in Asia. Singapore, January 2000.

23

Incorporating Preventive Nutrition into Medical School Curricula

Claudia S. Plaisted and Steven H. Zeisel

1. INTRODUCTION

Although the United States is thought to have one of the best health care (HC) systems in the world, in terms of both dollars and in human costs, it is overburdened with the expense of chronic diseases. In fact, for individuals over age 45 yr, chronic diseases supersede accidents as leading causes of death. As people age, the patterns of nutritional intake play a significant role in the onset and progression of these diseases: 5/10 leading causes of death have a strong relationship to poor diet *(1,2)*. The incidence of these diseases is highest among those who died after age 65 yr, but the comparative incidence of these diseases in those who died at relatively young ages, between 45 and 65 yr, is striking (Table 1). Surely, many of these deaths could have been prevented or delayed with adequate and timely nutrition intervention.

As the leaders of the HC team, physicians are uniquely positioned to emphasize to their patients the importance of nutrition in the prevention and management of chronic diseases. However, most physicians have little, if any, training in nutrition, and are ill-prepared to give specific advice on this topic to patients *(3,4)*. At some institutions, the medical school curriculum is changing (in an attempt to answer this public health crisis). In the future, more physicians need to be prepared to answer the challenge of preventing and managing chronic disease *(5)*. This chapter discusses the rationale behind, and methods for, incorporating preventive nutrition into medical school curricula.

2. CHRONIC DISEASE: A MAJOR PROBLEM FOR THE MODERN HC SYSTEM

Chronic disease is truly the scourge of the modern American HC system. Of deaths reported in 1993, a majority of individuals had a nutrition-related chronic condition (Table 2). About 90 million Americans suffer with a chronic disease *(7)*. Half of individuals in a mortality study had a heart attack or angina at the time of death *(2)*. Over 40% had hypertension. Cancer was present in about 33% of decedents. Although nonnutrition-related conditions appear on the list as well (Alzheimer's disease, asthma, arthritis, and so on), the top four on the list are diet-related, as are more than half of the total number of health conditions cited *(2)*.

Compounding the problem, the population subgroups with the highest incidence of chronic disease, particularly nutrition-related ones, have the poorest access to HC and the

From: *Primary and Secondary Preventive Nutrition*
Edited by: A. Bendich and R. J. Deckelbaum © Humana Press Inc., Totowa, NJ

Table 1
Deaths from Nutrition-Related Diseases in the United States

	Ages 45–65 yr		Ages 65 yr and over	
	No.	Rate/100,000	No.	Rate/100,000
Cancers	132,805	247.2	386,092	1140.2
Heart disease	102,510	190.8	612,886	1810
Cerebrovascular disease	15,526	28.9	140,938	416.2
Diabetes mellitus	12,678	23.6	46,194	136.4
Liver conditions	10,718	19.9	—	—

Adapted with permission from ref. 2.

Table 2
Number and Percent of Decedents Reported
to Have Had Selected Health Conditions
During Their Lifetime: United States, 1993

	No.	%
Hypertension	949,000	42.8
Heart attack	593,000	26.8
Angina pectoris	559,000	25.2
Stroke	444,000	20.0
Diabetes	411,000	18.6
Cancer	712,000	32.1
Cirrhosis of liver	86,000	3.9

Adapted with permission from ref. 6.

shortest life expectancy rates (8). In fact, although many Americans report their health as excellent or good (37 and 30%, respectively), these data do not represent minority or poor populations. Blacks were more likely to report poor health than whites, and those in the lowest income group were more than 7 times as likely to assess their health as poor than those with the highest income (9) (see Chapter 19).

In 1987, chronic diseases accounted for three-fourths of U.S. HC expenditures (7). The total estimated costs for chronic disease in 1990 were $659 billion ($425 billion in direct costs and $234 billion in indirect costs) (7). Obesity contributes significantly to many other chronic diseases, such as diabetes mellitus, heart disease, and certain cancers, and has been estimated to contribute $45.8 billion, or 6.8%, of preventable HC expenditures in 1990 (10).

Although much of the HC costs to the nation are put in terms of dollars, it is important to recognize the human costs of chronic disease as well, and to examine issues of quality of life. The February 1998 National Mortality Followback Survey report (1993 data) indicated that illness or injury kept 1/10 of decedents in bed for most of the last year of their lives (6). As the sum total of these costs is accounted for, the importance of disease prevention by improving nutrition becomes increasingly clear: The shortening of the length of functional limitations or illness at the end of the lifecycle is an added benefit (11).

3. THE ROLE OF PHYSICIANS IN PREVENTION

Americans look to their primary physicians as sources of reliable nutrition advice *(12)*. Although, in truth, the task of prevention needs to be shared across the spectrum of HC providers, the physician is likely to continue to be very influential in determining the priorities for HC delivery and research *(3,13)*. Limited physician awareness of nutrition has, in the past, resulted in iatrogenic malnutrition *(14)*. The number of physician visits in the United States is staggering. In 1995, Americans had an average of six physician contacts, including visits to the doctor's office, hospital, or phone contact, for a total of more than 1.5 billion physician contacts *(9)*. As the leaders of HC teams in the United States, physicians are uniquely positioned to convey the importance of prudent dietary choices to their patients, choices that can help the patients manage, or ultimately prevent, chronic diseases. In addition, dietary supplement sales amount to billions of dollars each year, and physicians are often expected to make recommendations to patients. Despite these roles, physicians historically have been poorly trained in nutrition. Of medical students graduating in 1990, almost two-thirds perceived that their nutrition training was inadequate *(13,15)*. This perception by medical students persists *(16)*. In 1991, the Association of American Medical Colleges reported that, of 128 U.S. medical schools, only 29 (23%) had a required nutrition course, and that was, on average, less than 6 h; 25% failed to offer nutrition education. Currently, there are calls for improved, systematic, scientifically strong, pervasive, and sustained efforts to create training programs that sufficiently prepare HC providers to take on the important task of prevention.

Most primary care physicians are providing inadequate preventive services, including nutrition screening, assessment, and counseling for cardiovascular disease risk reduction *(17–20)*. A number of factors hinder physicians from providing sound preventive nutrition care, including lack of nutrition training in medical school *(17,20,21)* and resulting lack of perceived self-efficacy concerning appropriate dietary interventions during medical practice *(22–24)*. Finally, skepticism abounds regarding the ability of patients to comply with dietary recommendations. At the authors' medical school at the University of North Carolina (UNC) at Chapel Hill, medical students were found to have a good understanding of the scientific basis of nutrition, but had many misconceptions as to practical information needed for dietary counseling *(21)*. The growing awareness of the need for inclusion of nutrition interventions as part of the prevention component of the physician's practice will only increase the need for a comprehensive core curriculum in nutrition for MSs, which includes information on nutrition and chronic disease.

4. WHAT DO MEDICAL STUDENTS NEED TO LEARN ABOUT NUTRITION?

Some practicing physicians currently undertake special residency programs or structured independent studies to learn nutrition. The majority of physicians currently practicing, however, teach themselves nutrition, or must learn about the advances and importance of preventive nutrition via reports in the scientific literature, or from continuing education seminars and conferences. It is difficult as a topic for credible preventive nutrition to compete with headlines touting the latest dramatic medical miracles or the whirlwind of activity around the changing HC system itself. Physicians, like any other individuals, are exposed not only to nutrition facts, but to a plethora of fraud and quackery, which often capitalizes on pseudobiochemical language to promote its legitimacy. Without adequate nutrition training, it can be difficult for any HC provider to discern fact from fiction when it comes to new alternative nutrition and botanical supplements or practices.

Physicians in training need to fully understand the biochemical basis explaining the relationship between nutrition and disease, and also how to communicate positive health messages to the patient. Further, since physician time is at a premium, physicians in training need to know how to effectively direct the patient to nutrition education services in both medical and community settings. Although it may be unreasonable to expect the physician to take on the role of the registered dietitian or health educator, physicians need to understand the importance of nutrition, emphasize it to patients, and facilitate patients getting the support and education they need.

Even if adequately trained in a well-understood area of nutrition, physicians are unlikely to succeed in practice unless readily usable nutrition intervention tools and office practice systems are in place that support a broader team and community approach to nutrition *(25–27)*. These tools and strategies must be taught to students when they are forming clinical habits, and they must be tailored to the knowledge, attitudes, and behaviors of patients, as well as to the practice environment and beliefs of the physician *(28–30)*.

5. THE CHANGING FACE OF MEDICAL EDUCATION

Parallel to the changes in the practice of medicine, there are changes in the approach to medical education (ME) in the United States. The federal government has considered plans for ensuring some training in nutrition and its relationship to human health for health professionals. Congress mandated that at least 50% of the physician pool be adequately trained in nutrition, in section 302, Public Law 1101-445/HR1608; The National Nutrition Monitoring And Related Research Act. The Dietary Supplements Health Education Act of 1994 and the Public Health Service's Year 2000 Objectives for the Nation also called for MS education in nutrition, but even following federal calls for action, physician education has changed little *(4,5)*. However, there are some encouraging signs. Data from surveys gathered by the authors' *Nutrition in Medicine* (NIM) team, at the UNC at Chapel Hill, indicate that, of responding medical schools (111 to date responding, of 119 surveyed), 62 plan to offer nutrition education using the NIM series of interactive computer-assisted educational software. Although the authors can provide approximations of the amount of nutrition education given to U.S. medical students, because of incomplete survey responses, the number of medical schools in the United States teaching nutrition to medical students cannot be absolutely quantified. Most schools offer more than 6 h of nutrition education to their medical students (Table 3). Methods for incorporating nutrition into the curriculum vary widely, as discussed later in this chapter. Although there has been some improvement during this decade, there is far more work to be done.

6. BARRIERS TO ADDING NUTRITION TO EXISTING CURRICULA

Although nutrition is an important topic of study, there is a valid argument that the existing medical curriculum is overburdened and struggling to fit within a 4-yr degree program. The high cost of ME impedes schools from lengthening training programs, despite the continually growing breadth and sophistication of material students must master. ME has traditionally been organized so that departments are assigned responsibility for design and implementation of specific components of the curriculum. Many

Table 3
Nutrition Education in U.S. Medical Schools:
Results NIM Annual Survey 1998–1999

	No. schools
Schools surveyed	119
Schools responding	111 (93.3% of schools surveyed)
Nutrition required[a]	53 (47.7%)
Nutrition optional[a]	9 (8%)
Hours of nutrition education	
0–5.9	12
6–15.9	23
15.9–29.9	18
≥30	12

Surveys mailed to all U.S. medical schools owning at least one copy of NIM modules in July 1998, and returned by July 13, 1999.

[a]Not all schools answered all questions on survey.

schools find the curriculum a hotly contested territory that contributes to the identities and funding allocations for these departments. Disciplines that are not well represented by the traditional departmental structure find it difficult to introduce or expand their time allocation in the curriculum. At most medical schools, nutrition is such an underrepresented discipline *(4)*.

A second significant barrier is that the primary role of nutrition in health is prevention. Traditionally, westernized medicine has focused on a systems approach, as opposed to a whole-person approach to health. Medical students have been taught to fix a health problem, rather than to prevent one. The scope of time for the practice of medicine lasted from minutes to hours, perhaps weeks to months in worst cases, but certainly not over a lifetime. To alter this scope from a crisis management mode to a public health approach requires a shift in the actual conceptual framework of medicine. Such large paradigm shifts often take time and are slow to progress.

A third barrier to the inclusion of nutrition in the core medical curriculum is a lack of qualified instructors. Because few physicians are adequately trained in nutrition themselves, there are not widely available individuals to share this expertise. The National Institutes of Health have begun modest efforts to redress this problem (a program to fund clinical nutrition specialists at 10 medical schools was begun in 1998). Larger universities can call upon academic departments of nutrition to fill this gap, where they are available, but that is not the situation at every school. Although, at some medical schools, the department of dietetics answers this educational need, these contributions often consist of isolated lectures.

Scientific discoveries have solidified a role for nutrition in medical practice. Medical students want more nutrition education, and have suggested core content *(16)*. The great increase in the health consumer's interest in nutrition and nutrition supplements has made it mandatory that physicians be able to give their patients sound nutrition advice. Changes in national priorities, including revision of the HC system so that it emphasizes prevention of diseases, are giving nutrition a more important role in medical schools. At the same time, medical schools are revising their curricula to reflect newer theories of education and a greatly expanded base of knowledge. A window in time is being entered when there is a special opportunity to introduce nutrition curricula within medical schools, innovative approaches can be identified that will grab the imagination of medical educators.

If nutrition is to be assigned a more prominent role in the national medical curriculum, models are needed that can be copied by other schools. The trend among medical schools is to increase curriculum content that focuses on problem-solving in a small group teaching setting (31), but at the same time, structured lecture time is being reduced. Increased allocation of the activities of medical students to primary care settings also presents problems and opportunities for teaching nutrition. Materials introduced must use innovative approaches that require a minimum of added contact hours (15). Proposed new curricula also need to present nutrition in a manner that expands academic influence beyond nutrition experts. Several such methods of instituting preventive nutrition education are available; all are in use at different schools. The rest of this chapter discusses various methods of education, their relative merits, and drawbacks.

7. NEW METHODS OF MEDICAL PREVENTIVE NUTRITION EDUCATION

7.1. Problem-Based Learning

In this method of instruction, students integrate textbook learning by application of information to practical cases to learn basic and clinical sciences. In this way, students synthesize knowledge, and focus on application of medical science as opposed to learning based on memorization. This has the benefit of providing a framework for the material as well as helping to humanize the facts of medicine. In part, problem-based learning (PBL) provides a role model for empowering the patient to investigate, learn more about their health, and make appropriate decisions, as the students themselves are empowered to do so in their own learning process. PBL is closer to real-life situations, because the material is case-based. It has been suggested that PBL also encourages self-directed, life-long learning (32), although disadvantages include higher costs for resources and staff time. PBL also focuses on health outcomes and evidence-based medicine as fundamental to appropriate HC.

PBL is fast becoming the primary mode of medical instruction in the United States and around the world (32,33). It is used in many medical schools, such as the UNC at Chapel Hill, Harvard, Emory, Duke University, Harvard, and Johns Hopkins.

7.2. Case-Based Learning

The University of Pennsylvania School of Medicine has pioneered an integrated, case-based curriculum, to implement a medical nutrition education program that can be used in lectures, small-group sessions, self-learning modules, and web-mounted format (34). In the first work of its kind, Morrison and Hark have compiled a series of patient cases as a way to stimulate student interest in nutrition. This case-based curriculum, which has been published as the textbook *Medical Nutrition and Disease (34)* is unique because it integrates nutritional concepts with clinical aspects of medicine, and it gives students the opportunity to learn about clinical medicine as early as their first semester of medical school.

Each chapter and case in *Medical Nutrition and Disease* was co-written by a multidisciplinary team of physicians and registered dietitians. The integrated, case-based approach offers a complete perspective on the medical and nutritional implications of various clinical scenarios, with emphasis on management of disease and prevention. Nutrition assessment and the life-cycle issues (pregnancy, pediatrics, geriatrics) are taught during year one. Teaching coincides with biochemistry and introduction to clinical medicine, in which history and physical exam skills are learned. Nutritional management of disease is integrated into the pathophysiology or systems courses during years one and two, and nutrition support is taught during the surgery clerkship. Nutrition during the life-cycle is covered during the pediatric, obstetrics, and family medicine clerkships.

The case studies create a role model that highlights the value of working within an interdisciplinary team of physicians, registered dietitians, and nurses. Further descriptions and examples of this program can be located at www.med.upenn.edu/nutrimed.

7.3. Self-Directed Study and Research/Residency Programs

Another possible method for nutrition education is independent study. Medical students (generally third or fourth year) can choose a research rotation that focuses on nutrition, or they can create an independent project to study their area of interest. In many university-based schools, medical students can earn a doctorate in a field such as nutrition, necessitating an extra 2 yr or more of medical school.

After graduation, there are limited opportunities in residency or fellowship programs to specialize in nutrition (through disciplines such as gastroenterology, endocrinology, or critical care medicine). According to a recent survey, twenty-two different nutrition fellowships are available currently in the United States. Responses to this survey, providing information about the primary teaching focus, number of positions, and eligibility requirements, as well as contact information, can be accessed on the American Society for Clinical Nutrition website at www.faseb.org/ascn/survey98.htm. Although some residency programs can provide excellent medical training, many are limited in scope; few traditional medical approaches teach the biochemical basis of nutrition and relate it to patient outcomes. Of notable exception are critical care fellowships, which feature training in nutrition support and total parenteral nutrition. Although nutritional biochemistry is fundamental to nutrition support programs, these fellowships still focus on disease crisis management, rather than prevention of that disease. However, many programs have opportunities for self-directed study and independent research, during which the physician can augment their education.

Regardless of the method of instruction in preventive nutrition, medical schools require the development of unique educational approaches that ultimately will have an impact on reducing chronic disease incidence, mortality, and morbidity. Schools require the development of educational techniques that quickly and effectively promote mastery of both nutritional biochemistry and the translation of this science into practical strategies for patient self-care. In order for it to be incorporated into the medical school curricula, this method must be cost-effective, and must be able to compete for the attention of students and instructors alike.

7.4. Computer-Assisted Instruction

To answer the demand for medical instruction that presents a reliable, consistent message and is flexible enough to be used in a variety of educational settings and formats, computer-assisted instruction (CAI) has been created. Lecture, problem-based learning, independent study, and specialized training programs can all benefit from computer technology.

7.4.1. Is Computer-Assisted Instruction Efficacious?

Computer-assisted diabetes education proved to be an efficient and effective method for teaching basic nutrition competencies to medical students *(35)*. The same was true for computer-assisted pediatric nutrition teaching *(36)*. In 1992, the American Cancer Society surveyed cancer education in U.S. medical schools, and called for high-quality, validated, computer-enhanced instruction as part of a national medical curriculum *(37)*. Computer programs have been successfully implemented for both undergraduate and graduate medical students *(38,39)* in pharmacology, pathology, anatomy, histology, and embryology, as well as for teaching medical procedures *(38–41)*. These programs use the computer to teach in a way that differs from normal lecture- or book-based curricula. One example, the patient simulation format, has been the most popular *(42–44)*. The National Board of Medical Examiners has developed a series of patient simulations that will be used on the National Board exams. Few programs in the field of nutrition currently combine the teaching of basic science and patient simulation, which is addressed later in this chapter.

Marion et al. *(45)* found that students using computer programs learned approximately as well as students experiencing traditional teaching, but the computer-taught groups spent less time learning the material. MacFayden *(39)* compared fourth-year students learning pharmacokinetics from a computer program or from lecture and reading. They found no difference in posttest scores. Overall time spent on the material was equivalent, but the computer group spent more time in initial learning, and less time studying for the test, than the other group. In contrast, Fincher et al. *(46)* found that students receiving computer instruction in electrocardiography had better posttest scores than those taught in seminars. The authors felt this was a clinically important difference. Another study *(43)* presented identical cases to students, either on computer or in a text. The computer group spent 43% less time to achieve the same level of mastery as the text group. A meta-analysis of 37 studies on the efficacy of CAI for health professionals *(47)* concluded that a majority of these studies favored CAI over conventional methods of instruction. For many reasons it is difficult to extrapolate from any of these studies the general efficacy of computer-enhanced instruction. The level of computer experience of subjects/students is variable, and has changed over time. Students entering medical school today have greater familiarity with microcomputers than did their colleagues of only a few years ago. The quality, sophistication, topic, and appropriateness of the teaching strategy chosen for the material are so different among software products that comparisons may not be valid. Most of the studies have tested programs on student volunteers. The resulting self-selected test population may not be representative for all medical students, and questions about appropriate control groups and other test design issues have not been sufficiently addressed.

Acceptance of CAI by students has generally been very good. In MacFayden's study *(39)*, the course received higher evaluations from students in the computer-based group than from those in the lecture-based group, and more students in the computer group rated the material's clinical relevance as good or better. The results of the study of Gjerde et al. *(48)* were not as favorable. Students rated CAI 3.56 on a 5-point scale, below self-directed study, laboratories, seminars, and slide-tapes. In an attempt to determine the reasons for students' opinions of computer programs, Xakellis et al. *(49)* asked second-year students to rate a group of software offerings. The students' perception of their learning was positively correlated with more student control over the program and higher level of feedback, and inversely correlated with frustration with the program–student interface.

In general, there are many advantages to CAI in medical schools. It grants the school or instructor great flexibility to use program modules in a variety of ways and to tailor the depth of the material to that school's or instructor's learning objectives for the students. Programs from different resources can be intermixed to create a customized learning experience. To ease the instructional burden, many CAI programs offer electronic exams (pre- and posttests, practice tests, final exams, electronic automated grading, web-based evaluation, and so on). CAI can allow the flexibility of distance education and individual instruction. Since CAI can capitalize on advanced computer graphics and programming, it can improve the learning experience itself. Enjoyable learning experiences can enhance retention. Programs can be designed to be interactive, self-paced, and to provide continuous user feedback. The primary disadvantages to CAI are the expense in creation of programs, the time required to create appropriate material and keep it updated, the cost of computer hardware at local schools, and the necessity for instructors to gain relative mastery over educating in the electronic age.

7.4.2. EXAMPLES OF CAI PROGRAMS

7.4.2.1. The NIM Series. One example of a successful CAI is the NIM series from the UNC at Chapel Hill, which was conceived, created, and edited in part by the authors of this chapter. The goal of the NIM series is to create an innovative, effective, flexible, and transportable nutrition curriculum. The NIM curriculum spans the preclinical and clinical training of physicians, incorporates the biochemical, clinical, and epidemiological elements of nutrition science, and includes preventive and therapeutic perspectives of nutrition. As the program modules are created, they are provided free of charge to all U.S. medical schools (for information, *see* the authors' website www.med.unc.edu/nutr). There are three topic series in the NIM programs (asterisked titles are released to medical schools as of this publication, the rest are in production for release in 2000–2002). Titles include: the Disease Series (*Nutritional Anemias*, Nutrition and Stress*, Nutrition and Cancer*, Diet, Obesity and Cardiovascular Disease**, and *Diabetes and Weight Management: Aberrations in Glucose Metabolism**); the Lifecycle Series (*Maternal and Infant Nutrition*, Nutrition and Growth**, and *Nutrition for the Second Half of Life*); and the Special Topics in Nutrition Series (*Nutrition Supplements and Fortified Foods*, and *Sports Nutrition*).

The authors' early studies on the teaching efficacy of the NIM series were promising, so we tested the <u>Nutrition and Cancer</u> program *(50)*. The entire UNC medical student class participated in the study during their first term in medical school. All students completed pretest questions, used the program during a 2-wk period, then completed posttest questions. A randomly drawn subset of these students (40 students recruited, of which 38 participated) completed retention test questions 3 months after completing the program. Pretest scores ($n = 163$) were 22% answers correct, posttest scores were 86% correct, and retention test scores remained high, at 61% correct ($n = 38$).

A survey conducted by the NIM team in the academic year 1998–1999 had a 93.3% response rate from schools surveyed (111/119 schools responding, as of July 1999). Of the schools responding, 55.9% ($n = 62$) implemented the NIM CAI programs, or reported concrete plans to implement them in the 1999–2000 academic year. Another 44.1% ($n = 49$) reported no concrete plans to implement the programs, or did not plan to

Table 4
Methods of Instruction: NIM Program Use in U.S. Medical Schools

How NIM CAI utilized	Total (% of schools using NIM)
Supplement course material	43 (74.1)
Entire course is devoted to NIM CAI	1 (1.7)
NIM CAI replace a course on that topic	2 (3.5)
NIM CAI replace lecture on topic	5 (8.6)
Other	7 (12.1)
Some schools use NIM CAI programs in multiple ways.	Used as interdisciplinary module (4 wk) Integrated into system-oriented, problem-based learning Available as independent study Provide nutrition component of course

($n = 58$, final survey data 1998–1999)
   Surveys mailed to all U.S. medical schools owning at least one copy of NIM modules in July, 1998, and returned by July, 1999. Schools were queried about medical school nutrition education and use of NIM or other nutrition education strategies.
   NIM CAI= Nutrition In Medicine computer-aided instruction.

implement them. Reasons for nonimplementation mostly resulted from curriculum time concerns, hardware concerns, or the fact that some schools had been unaware of the programs prior to the survey. Many of these schools agreed that they would like to consider using such CAI programs in the future.

In some cases, the fast turnover of teaching assignments in some medical schools created communication barriers, leaving new instructors unaware of teaching aids such as the NIM modules. Surveys indicate the schools who use CAI and the NIM program use them in a variety of ways, from a class supplement to a class replacement (Table 4). Survey results also suggest that schools using the NIM CAI programs teach more hours of nutrition education to their medical students than schools not implementing the programs (data not shown). Continuing surveys of the prevalence of nutrition education in medical schools will be conducted annually by the NIM project.

The National Cancer Institute (NCI) has been supporting innovative approaches through its R25 grant program. The NIM project was partially funded from this source. Other interesting NCI-funded efforts include those listed below. The curriculum for medical students developed at the University of California at Los Angeles School of Medicine created some novel written instructional materials. The multimedia program "Images of Cancer Prevention," developed at Eastern Carolina University, is for use with medical students and family medicine residents (51). As with many CAI programs, this one offers multiple levels of learning, as chosen by learner or instructor. Pre- and postuse performance evaluations in 155 students demonstrated its effectiveness in raising awareness of the nutrition–cancer link, in affecting the medical student's views on the role of the physician in nutrition counseling, and in increasing user confidence in this area. The team at Eastern Carolina University has also produced "Nutritional Management of Diabetes," a series of clinical cases available on CD-ROM (52). East Carolina University School of Medicine held a virtual seminar on nutrition education in medical schools in January 1999 which included a discussion of how to make room for nutrition in the curriculum, how to fund a nutrition education resource program, and what resources are available. Proceedings from this virtual seminar can be found at the website: www. PreventiveNutrition.com. The University of Nevada at Reno School of Medicine created a "Special Qualifications in Nutrition Program," which includes PBL components in all years of the medical curriculum. Finally, at the University of Alabama Birmingham, a training program was established that delivers courses, seminars, and research opportunities to medical and public health students. These institutions share the materials they developed with other medical schools.

8. CONCLUSIONS

The high cost of chronic disease coupled with the intimate relationship of those maladies to nutrition, make preventive nutrition necessary for incorporation into medical curricula. Because an overburdened educational system cannot continue to expand in scope without similarly expanding in educational strategies, alternative means of student education must be explored. CAI presents opportunities for efficient, cost-effective modes of teaching new information to students. With improvements in delivery of nutrition education to medical students, physician competency in nutrition knowledge can be enhanced, which ultimately can improve chronic disease prevention in the United States.

ACKNOWLEDGMENTS

This work was supported in part by grants from the National Institutes of Health (National Cancer Institute R25 5-53169, National Institute of Diabetes, Digestive Disease, and Kidney DK-56350 and Office of Dietary Supplements), U.S. Department of Agriculture (5-36322), American Institute for Cancer Research, Baxter Healthcare Corporation, Bristol-Myers Squibb, Clintec International, Dannon Institute, Kellogg, National Cattlemen's Beef Association, National Dairy Council, Nestle Clinical Nutrition, New York Community Trust, Quaker Oats Foundation, The University of North Carolina at Chapel Hill, and Wyeth-Ayerst Laboratories.

REFERENCES

1. McGinnis J, Foege W. Actual causes of death in the United States. JAMA 1993; 270:2207–2212.
2. Ventura S, Peters K, Martin J, Maurer J. Births and deaths: United States, 1996. Monthly Vital Statistics Report. Hyattsville, MD: National Center for Health Statistics, 1997:32–22.
3. Winick M. The nutritionally illiterate physician. J Nutr Ed 1988; 20:s12–s13.
4. Young EA. Nutrition education in US medical schools. Am J Clin Nutr 1997; 65:1558.
5. Havas S. The high cost of lost opportunities for prevention. JAMA 1997; 277:375–376.
6. National Center for Health Statistics. National Mortality Followback Survey—provisional data 1993. Centers for Disease Control and Prevention website, 1998.
7. Hoffman C, Rice D, Sung H-Y. Persons with chronic conditions: their prevalence and costs. JAMA 1997; 276:1473–1479.
8. Anderson R, Kochanek K, Murphy S. Advance report of final monthly statistics 1995. Monthly vital statistics report. Hyattsville, MD: National Center for Health Statistics, 1997; 45(Suppl. 2):19.
9. National Center for Health Statistics. Current Estimates from the National Health Interview Survey. Washington, DC: U.S. Public Health Service, 1995; 444.
10. Wolf A, Colditz G. Social and economic effects of body weight in the United States. Am J Clin Nutr 1996; 63:466S–469S.
11. Rogers A, Rogers R, Belanger A. Longer life but worse health? Measurement and dynamics. Gerontologist 1990; 30:640–649.
12. Hiddink G, Hautvast J, van Woerkum C, Fieren C, van't Hoff M. Consumer's expectations about nutrition guidance: the importance of primary care physicians. Am J Clin Nutr 1997; 65:1974S–1979S.

13. Feldman EB. Educating physicians in nutrition: a view of the past, the present, and the future. Am J Clin Nutr 1991; 54:618–622.
14. Roubenoff R, Roubenoff RA, Preto J, Balke CW. Malnutrition among hospitalized patients. A problem of physician awareness. Arch Intern Med 1987; 147:1462–1465.
15. Swanson AG. 1990 ASCN nutrition educator's symposium and information exchange. Am J Nutr Educ 1991; 53:587–588.
16. American Medical Student Association. Report of the American Medical Student Association's Nutrition Curriculum Project. Essentials of nutrition education in medical schools: a national consensus. Am J Clin Nutr 1997; 65:1559–1561.
17. Secker-Walker R, Morrow A, Kresnow M, Flynn B, Hochheiser L. Family physicians' attitudes about dietary advice. Fam Pract Res J 1991; 11:161–170.
18. Giles W, Anda R, Jones D, Serdula M, Merritt R, DeStefano F. Recent trends in the identification and treatment of high blood cholesterol by physicians. JAMA 1993; 269:1133–1138.
19. Glanz K, Tzirake C, Albright C, Fernandes J. Nutrition assessment and counseling practices. J Gen Inter Med 1995; 10:89–92.
20. Kushner R. Barriers to providing nutrition counseling by physicians: a survey of primary care practitioners. Prev Med 1995; 24:546–552.
21. Ammerman A, McGaghie W, Siscovick D, Maxwell K, Cogburn W, Simpson R. Medical students' knowledge, attitudes, and behavior about diet and heart disease. Am J Prev Med 1989; 5:271–278.
22. Mann K, Putnam R. Physicians' perceptions of their role in cardiovascular risk reduction. Prev Med 1989; 18:45–58.
23. Allen S, Harris I, Kofron P, Anderson DC, Bland CJ, Dennis T, Satran L, Miller WJ. A comparison of knowledge of medical students and practicing primary care physicians about cardiovascular risk assessment and intervention. Prev Med 1992; 21:436–448.
24. Bruer R, Schmidt R, Davis H. Commentary: nutrition counseling-should physicians guide their patients? Am J Prev Med 1994; 10:308–311.
25. Ockene J, Ockene I, Quirk M, Hebert JR, Saperia GM, Luippold RS, Merriam PA, Ellis S. Physician training for patient-centered nutrition counseling in a lipid intervention trial. Prev Med 1995; 24:563–570.
26. Helman A. Nutrition and general practice: an Australian perspective. Am J Clin Nutr 1997; 65:1939S–1942S.
27. Mant D. Effectiveness of dietary intervention in general practice. Am J Clin Nutr 1997; 65:933S–938S.
28. Ammerman A, DeVellis R, Carey T, Keyserling TC, Strugatz DS, Haines PS, Simpson RJ Jr, Siscovick DS. Physician-based diet counseling for cholesterol reduction: current practices, determinants, and strategies for improvement. Prev Med 1993; 22:96–109.
29. Baks J, Stafleu A, van Staveren W, van den Hoogen H, van Weel C. Long-term effect of nutritional counseling: a study in family medicine. Am J Clin Nutr 1997; 65:1946S–1950S.
30. Lazarus K. Nutrition practices of family physicians after education by a physician nutrition specialist. Am J Clin Nutr 1997; 65:2007S–2009S.
31. Bakemeier RF, Anderson JJB, Brooks CM, Cairoli VJ, Chamberlain RM, Gallagher RE, et al. Nutrition and cancer education objectives of the American Association for Cancer Education. J Cancer Ed 1989; 4:241–253.
32. Finucane P, Johnson S, Prideaux D. Problem-based learning: its rationale and efficacy. Med J Aust 1998; 168:445–448.
33. Devitt P, Palmer E. Computers in medical education 1: evaluation of a problem-oriented learning package. Aust NZ J Surg 1998; 68:284–287.
34. Morrison G, Hark L, eds. *Medical Nutrition and Disease*, 2nd ed. Malden, MA: Blackwell Science, 1999.
35. Engel SS, Crandall J, Basch CE, Zybert P, Wylie-Rosett J. Computer-assisted diabetes nutrition education increases knowledge and self-efficacy of medical students. Diabetes Educ 1997; 23:545–549.
36. Rodriguez MC, Larralde J, Martinez JA. Computer-assisted instruction in nutrition: a creative tool for medical education. Med Educ 1997; 31:229–331.
37. Gallagher RE, Bakemeier RF, Chamberlain RM, Kupchella CE, O'Donnell JF, Parker JA, Hill GJ, Brooks CM. Instructional methods and the use of teaching resources in cancer education curricula. J Cancer Ed 1992; 7:95–104.
38. Horn DL, Radhakrishnan J, Saini S, Pepper GM, Peterson SJ. Evaluation of a computer program for teaching laboratory diagnosis of acid-base disorders. Computers Biomed Res 1992; 25:562–568.

39. MacFayden JC, Brown JE, Schoenwald R, Feldman RD. The effectiveness of teaching clinical pharmacokinetics by computer. Clin Pharmacol Ther 1993; 53:617–621.

40. Merril JR, Notaroberto NF, Laby DM, Rabinowitz AM, Piemme TE. The ophthalmic retrobulbar injection simulator (ORIS): an application of virtual reality to medical education. Proc Ann Symp Comput Appl Med Care 1992; 702–706.

41. Trelstad RL, Raskova J. Teaching pathology without lectures through computer-based exercises, small-group discussions and reading. Proc Ann Symp Comput Appl Med Care 1992:781–782.

42. Harless WG, Duncan RC, Zier MA, Ayers WR, Berman JR, Pohl HS. A field test of the TIME patient simulation model. Acad Med 1990; 65:372–333.

43. Lyon HC Jr, Healy JC, Bell JR, O'Donnell JF, Shultz EK, Moore-West M, et al. PlanAlyzer, an interactive computer-assisted program to teach clinical problem solving in diagnosing anemia and coronary artery disease. Acad Med 1992; 67:821–827.

44. Perper EJ, Felciano R, Dev P. Real problems: a layered approach to constructing a patient simulation. Proc Ann Symp Comput Appl Med Care 1992:707–711.

45. Marion R, Niebuhr BR, Petrusa ER, Weinholtz D. Computer-based instruction in basic medical science education. J Med Educ 1982; 57:521–526.

46. Fincher R-ME, Abdulla A, Sridharan MR, Houghton JL, Henke JS. Computer-assisted learning compared with weekly seminars for teaching fundamental electrocardiography to junior medical students. South Med J 1988; 81:1291–1294.

47. Cohen PA, Dacanay LS. Computer-based instruction and health professions education. Eval Health Prof 1992; 15:259–281.

48. Gjerde CL, Xakellis GC, Shuldt SS. Medical student evaluation of self-selected learning modules. Fam Med 1993; 25:452–455.

49. Xakellis MD, Gjerde C. Evaluation by second-year medical students of their computer-aided instruction. Acad Med 1990; 65:23–26.

50. Kohlmeier M, Althouse L, Stritter F, Zeisel SH. Introducing cancer nutrition to medical students: instructional effectiveness of a computer-based curriculum. Am J Clin Nutr 2000; 71:873–877.

51. Kolasa K, Jobe A, Miller M. Images of Cancer Prevention, ver. 1.0. Eastern Carolina University: Interactive Design and Development, Blacksburg, VA 1997.

52. Kolasa K, Lasswell A, Lasswell W. Nutritional Management of Diabetes. ver. 1.0. Chapel Hill, NC: Health Sciences Consortium, 1997.

24

Preventive Nutrition
Throughout the Life Cycle
A Cost-Effective Approach to Improved Health

Adrianne Bendich and Richard J. Deckelbaum

1. INTRODUCTION

Nutrition can play a key and cost-effective role in decreasing risks of different chronic diseases. An increasing body of evidence suggests that there are far more commonalities relating to how nutrition reduces risk factors for varied chronic diseases than differences *(1)*. Different diets are not required to decrease risk of cancer, compared to cardiovascular disease (CVD). For example, as preventive nutrition strategies, increasing intake of fruits and vegetables has been linked to decreased prevalence of CVD, stroke, and also cancer *(2–11)*. Likewise, increased whole grain intake (compared to refined grains) has been associated with decreased prevalence of CVD, cancer, and also type II diabetes *(12–17)*.

Decreased fat intake, particularly saturated fat intake, is clearly linked to decreased serum cholesterol levels and decreased prevalence of CV complications, such as coronary artery disease *(18)*. Although recent studies place some doubt on the contribution of fat intake toward increasing risk of breast cancer, high levels of fat intake are still associated with the risk of some cancers, and perhaps type II diabetes *(1,19,20)*. Foods rich in other dietary components, including fiber, complex carbohydrates, and micronutrients, appear to decrease the risk of certain forms of cancer, as well as coronary heart disease and manifestations of diabetes *(12,13,21,22)*.

The major chronic diseases also share a number of common cellular and biochemical mechanisms in their pathogenesis *(1,23)*. For example, cell proliferation is common in both atherosclerosis and cancer, and is of importance to some of the complications associated with diabetes. Changes in signal transduction and gene expression relate to cancer, atherosclerosis, obesity, and diabetes. As well, DNA modifications likely contribute mechanistically to each of these disease classes. In examining the sets of nutrition recommendations aimed at reducing the risk of a number of chronic diseases, and developed by a number of different private and government organizations, the different recommendations show far more common themes and commonalities than differences. The recommendations of most nutrition and public health groups are very similar to the 1995 U.S. Dietary Guidelines of the U.S. Department of Health and Human Services and U.S. Department of Agriculture, which include the following recommendations (1995) *(17)*:

From: *Primary and Secondary Preventive Nutrition*
Edited by: A. Bendich and R. J. Deckelbaum © Humana Press Inc., Totowa, NJ

- Eat a variety of foods.
- Balance the food you eat with physical activity.
- Maintain or improve your weight.
- Choose a diet with plenty of grain products, vegetables, and fruits.
- Choose a diet low in fat, saturated fat, and cholesterol.
- Choose a diet moderate in sugars.
- Choose a diet moderate in salt and sodium.
- If you drink alcoholic beverages, do so in moderation.

1.1. Theory vs Reality

An important question is how to implement the current dietary recommendations for all population groups, regardless of their economic and educational status. Where will food fortification and micronutrient supplementation be of most benefit? The reality is that the majority of populations, both in the United States and elsewhere, do not follow dietary recommendations *(11,24–26)*. Given the available evidence that higher fruit and vegetable, as well as whole grain, intakes can have marked effects on reduction of chronic disease risk, it is likely that improved diets alone would be a major step forward in chronic disease risk reduction and economic cost. However, it is also clear that fortification and supplementation of certain nutrients has been associated with reduced risk of chronic diseases in populations that have not routinely consumed the highest intakes of recommended foods *(27–29)*. Thus, an inclusive approach of combining the best of many nutritional delivery systems, and including physical activity and smoking reduction, may provide a greater potential for cost-effective measures to reduce disease.

1.2. Objectives

The major objective of this chapter is to examine the wealth of data presented in the more than 50 chapters included in *Preventive Nutrition (23)* and this volume, *Primary and Secondary Preventive Nutrition*, as well as other relevant studies, and to look at the potential cost savings if these strategies were adopted. Highlighted are those nutritionally related interventions that can improve health, reduce disease risk, and save on health care costs. The goal, therefore, is to document the totality and consistency of the data, then attempt to quantify the savings that could be seen, once preventive nutrition strategies are put in place.

2. FROM CONCEPTION THROUGHOUT THE LIFE-SPAN

Each subheading includes data related to preventive nutrition interventions and/or epidemiological findings and then discusses the health economics potential. The discussion follows the life-span, and thus begins with the anticipation of conception and concludes with an examination of the diseases/conditions that most affect seniors. Emphases are placed on the role of nutrition in the prevention of birth defects and premature birth and the cost-effectiveness of nutritional interventions for osteoporosis (OP) prevention. The health economics information is based mostly on U.S. national databases on hospital costs. Globally, there will be many differences in the economic value of nutrition interventions, and these obviously also differ between countries at various stages of economic development and medical care availability.

2.1. Optimizing Pregnancy Outcomes

When *Preventive Nutrition* was published in 1997, the objectives of the researchers who wrote the chapters involved with optimizing pregnancy outcomes were to reduce the risk of birth defects *(30)* and premature birth *(31)*, so that infants' morbidity and mortality (M&M) would be decreased. Secondarily, there were also strategies that would reduce maternal M&M, and reduce the potential for paternal sperm DNA damage *(32)*, and, consequently, also improve neonatal health prospects. Now it appears that improvement in birth outcomes, especially decreasing prevalence of low birth weight (LBW), may also improve the health of newborns when they reach middle age and older *(33–36)*. Thus, the current economic predictions have not taken into account the potential reductions in health care costs that would be realized in the next half century or more. Nevertheless, the benefits of optimizing pregnancy outcomes to improve current neonatal and maternal health are more than sufficient to justify the nutritional interventions discussed below.

Birth defects are the leading cause of infant M&M in the United States. CV birth defects are the most common; neural tube birth defects (NTD) are the second leading defect. One important preventive nutrition finding of the twentieth century was that periconceptional use (use of the supplement prior to conception and during the first trimester) of a folic-acid-containing multivitamin/mineral supplement significantly reduced the occurrence of NTD. Another key finding was that supplementation with folic acid alone could more than halve the risk of having a second child affected by NTD.

In addition to showing that periconceptional use of multivitamins significantly reduced NTDs, Czeizel and Dudas *(37)* found that women who took the multivitamin containing 12 vitamins (including 800 µg folic acid, 4 µg vitamin B_{12}, 2.6 mg vitamin B_6, and 100 mg vitamin C and 15 IU vitamin E) had half the number of occurrences of CV birth defects as the women taking a matched placebo. In the UK's Medical Research Council (MRC) *(38)* trial for prevention of NTD recurrence, the multivitamin used contained only eight of the vitamins, and did not include vitamins E and B_{12}; it contained only 40 mg vitamin C and 1 mg vitamin B_6. Even though it contained 4 mg folic acid (5× the level in the Czeizel and Dudas trial), there was no decrease in CV birth defects in either the group taking folic acid alone or the group taking folic acid plus the multivitamins. CV birth defects were also not lowered in the group taking the multivitamins without folic acid, compared to the placebo group *(38)*.

The supplement used in the Czeizel and Dudas trial is more comparable to the typical one-a-day-type multivitamin/mineral supplement sold in the United States than the supplement used in the MRC trial. Thus, survey data from the United States suggest that lowered CV birth defect risk is associated with periconceptional use of multivitamin/mineral supplements that usually contain more of the vitamins and minerals found in the supplement that lowered CV birth defects.

Because CV birth defects are so prevalent, the total medical costs associated with this defect are high (about $50,000/patient; $3 billion/yr). Fortunately, the risk reduction associated with multivitamin use was high (about 50%) *(28,39)*, and thus the potential cost savings approached $1.5 billion/yr for hospitalization costs alone *(27)*. The cost savings are particularly great, because the balancing costs of the multivitamins are relatively low.

Unfortunately, there are few women (about 20%), even today, who take a multivitamin during the periconceptional period, before they have confirmed their pregnancy *(40)*. The cost savings would probably be much greater than $1.5 billion/yr because multivitamin use during the months before conception and throughout pregnancy has also been associated with significant reductions in the occurrence of NTD, renal birth defects, cleft lip and palate, and limb reduction birth defects *(41)*. Supplementation has also been associated with decreased risk of childhood brain tumors *(42)*.

Oakley *(43)* has suggested that the right advice to American women is to eat the best diets possible, and also take a multivitamin containing folic acid, to assure the birth-defect-preventive level of folic acid is consumed daily. This advice was given even after the U.S. Food and Drug Administration initiated its policy for fortification of enriched grain products and flour with folic acid. It appears that this level, which raises folic acid intakes, on the average, by 100 µg/d, may not be sufficient to prevent folic acid-responsive birth defects. Further verification of the need for intake of the 400 µg level of folic acid is seen in the recent study from China *(44)*. There was a fourfold reduction in NTD in the high-risk area and a 40% reduction in a lower-risk area, when women anticipating pregnancy took 400 µg supplemental folic acid during the periconceptional period.

2.2. LBW and Premature Birth Prevention

LBW and preterm delivery often occur simultaneously. Preterm delivery is defined as birth following less than 37 wk gestation; very preterm delivery is defined as less than 33 wk gestation. LBW is defined as less than 2500 g, and very LBW is less than 1500 g. Of all LBW infants born, 60–70% are also preterm. Preterm delivery associated with LBW is the second leading cause of infant hospitalization, and is also the second leading cause of infant mortality, following birth defects *(45)*. LBW is second only to CV birth defects in annual hospitalization costs, exceeding $2.5 billion/yr *(27)*. The vast majority of these costs are borne by public funds, and the affected mothers and children are often the least equipped to deal with this event. Preterm births are more prevalent in teens, those with less than a high school education, and those with the lowest incomes.

Scholl et al. *(46)* found, in a prospective, case–control study, that pregnant women in Camden, NJ, who took prenatal multivitamins during the first trimester, had a fourfold reduction in very preterm births and a twofold reduction in preterm births. Even if supplementation began in the second trimester, there was a significant twofold reduction in very preterm, as well as preterm, births. The risk of very low birth weight outcomes (which was highly correlated with preterm delivery) was dramatically reduced by 6–7-fold, when prenatal multivitamins were taken during the first two trimesters. LBW was also reduced significantly with supplementation. These results were found in women who were at high risk for preterm/LBW outcomes: They were poor, teens, and many had low weight gain during pregnancy. Prenatal supplements increased iron (Fe) and folate status significantly, but did not alter serum zinc (Zn) level. Previously, low Fe and/or folate status had been associated with increased risk of preterm and LBW *(31)*. Zn-containing multivitamins have also been shown to reduce preterm births in an intervention study *(47)*. Because there was such a dramatic reduction in preterm births in the women who took Zn- and (presumably) folic acid-containing prenatals, the cost savings were predicted to reach over $1.5 billion/yr *(27)*.

Recently, there have been links made between maternal diet during pregnancy, preterm birth, and CVD in offspring, 50 or more years after their birth *(33,34)*. It remains to be seen whether women who used supplements before and during pregnancy have children who, at middle age, have fewer chronic diseases, such as CVD. Thus, it appears certain that the cost savings associated with a program to provide folic-acid-containing multi-vitamins to all women of childbearing potential, before, as well as during, the entire pregnancy, would be far greater than that based on either CV birth defect or preterm birth reduction alone. Moreover, the reduction in pain and suffering for the newborn and parents is substantial.

2.3. Relevance of Data from Developed Countries to Developing Countries

In developing countries, premature births are a serious problem, and an additional problem is intrauterine growth retardation, which is often coincident with premature birth, but may also occur with term delivery. DeOnis et al. *(48)* reviewed the 12 nutrition-ally based interventions that have been examined for their potential to reduce the inci-dence of intrauterine growth retardation, and often preterm birth and LBW. Only one of the interventions, balanced protein/energy supplementation during pregnancy, signifi-cantly reduced the risk of LBW. The authors also suggest that many of the micronutrient supplementations that were reviewed are likely to prove beneficial, and larger cohorts are required to assure their efficacy. These micronutrients include vitamin D, folic acid, Zn, calcium (Ca), magnesium (Mg), and Fe. Ramakrishnan et al. *(49)* have also extensively reviewed both observational and intervention studies from developing and developed countries that examined the role of micronutrients in optimizing pregnancy outcomes. The authors remind us that, in developing countries, 1/5 infants are LBW (20%), com-pared to a rate of 6% in developed countries. Moreover, in developing countries, the majority of LBW infants are carried to term.

Thus, intrauterine growth retardation is a significant problem in developing countries, and impacts the potential physical and, probably, the mental growth of the child through-out their lifetime. Low maternal micronutrient intake of Zn, Ca, Mg, vitamin A, vitamin C and, possibly B-vitamins, copper, and selenium (Se) is associated with premature birth and LBW. Deficiency of iodine, folate, and/or Fe is also linked to adverse pregnancy outcomes.

Since the publication of the reviews cited above, two key papers have been published from large, well-controlled intervention studies in developing countries. West et al. *(50)* examined, in a placebo-controlled trial, the effects of weekly supplementation with either the recommended dietary allowance of preformed vitamin A or β-carotene, in over 20,000 pregnant women in Nepal. They found a significant, 40% reduction in maternal mortality. Women were provided the supplements before conception, and the relatively modest dose of vitamin A, in the form of β-carotene, appeared more effective than the preformed supplement of retinol. Low β-carotene status has been reported in cases of pre-eclampsia in women from developing countries, and, as discussed below, the antioxidant potential of β-carotene (compared to the much lower antioxidant potential of retinol) may have been involved in reducing maternal mortality in the study in Nepal.

The second critical study involved over 1000 HIV-infected pregnant women from Tanzania *(51)*. In this placebo-controlled trial, the pregnant women received placebo; β-carotene and preformed vitamin A; a multivitamin containing vitamins B_1, B_2, B_6, B_{12}, niacin, folic acid, and vitamins C and E; or the multivitamin plus β-carotene and retinol, from 12–27 wk gestation to birth. There was a 40% reduction in fetal death, 44% reduc-tion in LBW, 39% reduction in very preterm birth, and a 43% reduction in small-for-gestational-age outcomes in the groups supplemented with the multivitamin independent of the vitamin A. Additionally, mothers taking the multivitamin had significantly heavier babies than those not taking the multivitamin ($p = 0.01$). Even though the supplement did not contain Fe, the women in the multivitamin group had a significant increase in their hemoglobin levels, compared to those not taking the multivitamin. Because this study involved HIV[+] women, the investigators also measured the concentration of total T-cells (CD3), T-helper cells (CD4), and T-suppressor cells (CD8). HIV[+] pregnant women who took the multivitamin supplement had significant increases in total T-cells, which mostly resulted from increases in CD3 cells; CD8 cells also increased. Although vitamin A did not show an effect in this study, the HIV-infected women had low vitamin A status at the onset, and the level provided may not have been sufficient, and/or may have not been absorbed sufficiently to show an effect. It may also be that the vitamin A was administered too late in these pregnancies to see its effect. In the West et al. *(50)* study, vitamin A supplementation was started before conception. Vitamin A is critical for early embryonic growth. The critical finding in the Fawzi et al. *(51)* study was that a multivitamin supplement, containing modest doses of micronutrients, significantly improved birth outcomes at levels similar to that seen when poor non-HIV[+] women in the United States used multivitamins during their pregnancies *(46)*.

2.4. Reduction in Pre-Eclampsia and Other Adverse Effects of Pregnancy

Pre-eclampsia is defined as hypertension (HT) and proteinuria beginning during the second half of gestation. Approximately 5% of pregnant women develop this condition during pregnancy. Pre-eclampsia is the leading cause of maternal death, and accounts for more than 40% of premature births worldwide *(52–54)*. The costs associated with pre-eclampsia, therefore, would not only include 40% of the costs associated with the infant of a preterm delivery, but would also include the costs associated with maternal care.

Several mechanisms have been proposed for the initiation and progression of pre-eclampsia, including oxidative damage to the placenta and/or imbalance in blood pressure (BP) regulation. Because of the importance of micronutrients, such as vitamins C and E (and β-carotene, as mentioned above), as antioxidants and the association of low Ca status and high BP, these micronutrients have been studied in well-designed protocols, to determine their effects on pre-eclampsia.

Fourteen randomized clinical trials, which involved the use of Ca supplements during pregnancy, to determine effects on maternal BP and pre-eclampsia, were reviewed by Bucher et al. *(55)*. They concluded that Ca supplementation (usually 1500–2000 mg/d) led to a significant reduction in maternal systolic and diastolic BP, and 62% reduction in the risk of pre-eclampsia. The authors recommended that Ca supplementation be provided for all women at risk for pre-eclampsia. It should be noted that the populations included in this analysis had intakes of Ca of about 300–500 mg/d, well below recommended intake levels *(56,57)*.

Two important studies were published following that review. Levine et al. *(54)* randomized over 4500 pregnant women to either 2000 mg/d Ca or placebo, and found that there was no difference in the rate of pre-eclampsia between the groups (about 7%). It must be noted, however, that these women were not at increased risk for pre-eclampsia, and that they had dietary Ca intakes of over 1100 mg/d. In a recent re-evaluation of the data concerning Ca and risk of pre-eclampsia, DerSimonian and Levine *(53)* again found that Ca supplementation did not appear to further lower the risk of pre-eclampsia, but that, for high-risk pregnancies, Ca supplementation appeared to significantly lower the risk.

High-risk pregnancies include teens, women with pre-existing HT, and women carrying multiple fetuses.

One other study of interest has been published, which examined BP of the children of mothers who took Ca during pregnancy to prevent pre-eclampsia. Belizan et al. *(58)* showed that, at 7 yr of age, there was a significantly lower systolic BP in the group of children whose mothers had taken 2000 mg/d Ca during pregnancy. The greatest antihypertensive effect was seen in overweight children. As mentioned previously in Chapter 3, it is not possible to account for all of the savings that might accrue from Ca supplementation, if one limits the cost savings to those associated with pre-eclampsia alone. The greatest health care savings may not be seen until decades after the intervention.

As mentioned above, oxidative stress is another mechanism that has been examined in pre-eclampsia. Vitamin E is the major lipid-soluble antioxidant in serum, and vitamin C is the major water-soluble antioxidant in the blood. Wang et al. *(59)* found, and Jain and Wise *(60)* confirmed, that serum lipid peroxide levels were significantly higher and serum vitamin E levels were significantly lower in women with pre-eclampsia, compared to women with normal pregnancies.

Recently, Chappell et al. *(52)* enrolled 283 pregnant women at risk for pre-eclampsia in a placebo-controlled trial using daily supplements of vitamin C (1000 mg) and vitamin E (400 IU). There was a significant 61% reduction in risk of pre-eclampsia in the antioxidant-supplemented group. Those investigators hypothesized that antioxidants may stabilize the maternal endothelium and placenta, and thus reduce pre-eclampsia risk. They found that the plasma marker for endothelial activation, as well as the index for placental dysfunction, were significantly decreased in the supplemented group. The levels of the antioxidants used in the study were well above national recommended intake levels; therefore, the study also provides important data concerning the safety of high doses of antioxidants during pregnancy.

2.5. Adult Chronic Diseases

There is a critical convergence of the micronutrients discussed as preventive nutrition strategies related to pregnancy and those associated with reduction in risk of chronic diseases in adulthood. In fact, the origins of adult chronic disease may well be at conception, or very soon thereafter, so that the similarity in the list of essential nutrients may well be because these are required throughout the life-span. It is only now, when there is a critical mass of data, that one is able to see the connecting nutritional threads that run throughout life. Therefore, the authors now examine the parallel data from studies associating certain nutritional factors with reducing the risk of adult chronic diseases.

As detailed in Chapter 1, 5/10 leading causes of death in the United States are conditions that can be modified by diet. The major broad categories of nutrition-related chronic diseases include CVD, stroke, cancer, diabetes, and OP. Deterioration of visual and mental/neurological function could also be added to this list *(23)*. In trying to assign health-dollar costs to each of these individual categories, it is evident that these conditions overlap in terms of the cost of M&Ms. For example, a definable comorbidity of obesity is often type II diabetes, and the presence of insulin resistance or type II diabetes markedly increases risk for CVD *(61)*.

Nevertheless, in Preventive Nutrition, Blumberg reviewed costs that could be attributed to the different chronic diseases *(24)*. Examining the three leading causes of death, specifically, he estimated the annual economic costs of CVD, cancer, and stroke to be $138 billion, $104 billion, and $30 billion, respectively, a total exceeding $250 billion annually. Nutritional interventions that reasonably could delay the onset of CVD and stroke for 5 yr could result in annual health cost savings of $84 billion.

Bendich et al. *(23)* examined the cost savings that could be accrued if all U.S. adults daily took a supplement containing a minimum of 100 IU vitamin E. Based on intervention and epidemiological studies that found significant reductions in risk of heart attack in those who had used vitamin E *(4;* Chapter 7, this volume), it was predicted that universal intervention could lower annual hospital costs by over $5 billion, and lower overall costs associated with CVD complications by $20 billion (*see* Chapters 6 and 8).

In addition to antioxidants, such as vitamin E, there has also been a continued association of low B-vitamin status (especially folic acid and vitamins B_6 and B_{12}) with increased risk of CVD, stroke, and vascular dementia *(2,26,28,62,63)*. Multivitamin use has been associated with improved B-vitamin status and reduction in homocysteine levels, an important risk factor in CVD and related morbidities *(64)*. Although the cost-effectiveness of multivitamin supplementation has not been reported in the literature, this intervention could also prove to be a cost-saving health strategy.

Another major factor in increasing health care costs is the morbidity associated with obesity. In Chapter 11, this volume, Frier and Green suggest that the annual health care costs that can be attributed to obesity are over $99 billion in the United States. Again, the dissection of obesity costs from other factors that are associated with increased CVD and cancer remains to be determined. The association of obesity with hyperlipidemia, HT, and type II diabetes all contribute to increased risk for CVD and stroke *(61)*. Lack of physical activity is certainly another risk factor for both cancer and CVD *(65–67)*. Despite the difficulty in assigning exact dollar costs to each of these risk factors and diseases, it seems obvious that combining nutritional approaches with a healthy lifestyle can have a marked impact on reducing health care costs. Despite this, it has been estimated that, currently, only 0.25% of health care cost dollars go to prevention strategies that could be extremely cost-effective *(24)*.

Although it is difficult to determine the exact cost savings involved with a preventive nutrition strategy that could impact more than one disease condition, it is nevertheless worthwhile to examine the minimal health economic benefit of implementing such a strategy. The authors have chosen to examine in detail the data from well-controlled intervention studies that tested the hypothesis that nutritional intervention could reduce the risk of OP-related hip fracture, because there appears to be less overlap between OP and the other chronic degenerative diseases discussed. The authors are cognizant, however, that the intervention which was common among the studies reviewed (Ca) has been associated with reducing the risk of colon cancer *(68)*, and HT *(69)*, so that, even in this example, the economic benefits may well be underestimated.

2.6. Bone Health

More than six million U.S. adults have OP *(70)*, which is defined as having bones that are two standard deviations below the peak bone mineral density (BMD) seen in young adults *(71,72)*. OP is a known risk factor for hip fracture *(73)*. OP hip fractures pose enormous human and economic costs. The nearly 300,000 annual hip fractures in the United States have been estimated to cost the nation around $5.6 billion, based on hospital and other costs. Those with hip fractures experience increased risk of institutionalization and death *(74)*.

Supplemental Ca, with/without vitamin D, has been shown to reduce the risk of hip fractures *(75–77)*. These three placebo-controlled, double-blind studies have shown that Ca supplementation (with or without vitamin D) significantly reduced the risk of hip fracture in individuals over the age of 50 yr. Bendich et al. *(78)* conducted a meta-analysis from the risk reduction data presented in these three papers, and arrived at a Mantel-Haenzel combined relative risk estimate of 0.53 (95% CI, 0.31–0.90) for hip fractures. The pooled relative risk for all nonvertebral fractures, including hip, was 0.61 (CI, 0.46–0.80). Thus, in these three studies, there was a 47% reduction in the risk of hip fracture in those individuals who took supplemental Ca at levels that ranged from 500 to 1200 mg/d for up to 3.4 yr. At the same time, there was an additional benefit of a 39% reduction in all types of nonvertebral fractures.

Using the risk reductions seen in these studies, and U.S. national data on the hospital and certain other costs associated with hip fracture, the potential reduction in cost of care for hip fracture patients was calculated. Over 134,000 hip fractures and $2.6 billion could have been avoided, if all U.S. adults over 50 yr of age took 1200 mg supplemental Ca/d. Universal Ca supplementation was cost-effective for women over the age of 75 yr based on the need to take the supplemental Ca for 34 mo before the hip fracture reduction was seen. If, however, the assumption is made that the benefit would be seen after 12–14 mo of supplementation, as was seen in the Chapuy study *(75)*, then universal Ca supplementation becomes cost-effective for all U.S. men and women 65 yr and over.

The savings actually are greater, because the calculations did not include the cost savings associated with the reduction in the other classes of nonvertebral fractures. The costs associated with these events are not fully ascertainable, because many of those who break a wrist or other nonvertebral bone are often not hospitalized. Another key finding from this study was that Ca supplementation that commences in women over the age of 85 yr is very cost-effective, because the intervention data suggest that BMD can be lost less quickly, even at this age, if Ca supplementation is instituted.

Even though the cost analysis did not include vertebral fractures, it would appear that fractures of the spine would also be reduced in many older women who supplemented with 1200 mg/d Ca. Recker et al. *(79)*, in a placebo-controlled, double-blind study in women over 60 yr old, who consumed less than 1000 mg/d Ca, found that supplementation significantly reduced the risk of spine fractures, especially in women with a history of bone fractures.

The National Institutes of Health and the National Academy of Sciences recommend that postmenopausal women not taking estrogen replacement therapy (ERT), and those that are taking ERT should consume daily 1500 and 1200 mg/d, respectively, of elemental Ca *(56,57)*. The benefit of estrogen replacement and other antiresorptive therapies for OP prevention are predicated on the daily consumption of 1000 mg Ca *(80)* (*see* Chapter 18). However, data from a telephone survey of a representative sample of U.S. households revealed that the average daily intake of dietary Ca falls far short of the minimum recommended daily amount of 1000 mg. The telephone survey found that only half of the adults 60–94 yr of age drank one glass of milk, which provides 300 mg Ca, every day *(81)*. LeBoff et al. *(82)* measured the vitamin D and Ca status of postmenopausal women with hip fractures, and found that 50% had deficient vitamin D levels, and over 80% had low

Ca levels. Because vitamin D is required for Ca absorption, the authors suggest that the low Ca status was linked to the low vitamin D status. Thus, these data suggest that individuals at risk for hip and other fractures should increase their Ca as well as vitamin D intakes.

Cost-savings analyses are based on databases that capture the costs associated with certain events. Thus, when health economists are limited to hospitalization costs, it is not possible to determine the cost savings associated with reducing the occurrence of OP, because there are no hospital expenses associated with OP itself. It is well recognized that increasing bone mass during the years of bone growth and early adulthood is the best OP-preventive strategy. Yet, because there are so few hospitalizations of young people who fracture bones, universal Ca (and vitamin D) supplementation may not prove to be cost-effective. Recently, however, Singer et al. *(83)* documented the incidence of fractures in individuals 15–94 yr of age, in Edinburgh, Scotland. They reported that, between the ages of 15 and 49 yr, men had 2.9× the fractures as age-matched women; fractures of the wrist began to increase in women at 40 yr of age, before menopause, and that, over the age of 60 yr, women had 2.3× the risk of fractures as men. Although this study did not examine nutritional factors, other studies have linked increased risk of fractures in young adults with low intakes of Ca and other micronutrients and low sun exposure, as found in Scotland. It may be that the establishment of newer databases, that capture the total costs (loss of work, as well as medical costs) associated with fractures, will permit the evaluation of the cost-effectiveness of earlier nutritional interventions for improvement of bone health.

In addition to reducing the risk of OP, individuals over the age of 50 yr, who take Ca supplements at the level of about 1200 mg/d, may also be lowering their risk for colon cancer. Recently, the data from the Calcium Polyp Prevention Study, a double-blind, placebo-controlled study, were published *(68)*. The subjects had previously had one colon polyp removed prior to entering this study. Those that took 1200 mg Ca/d, for up to 4 yr, had significantly fewer recurrences of polyps than the placebo group. The mechanism of action of Ca in reducing the risk of colon cancer, by reducing the number of precancerous lesions, is thought to be via the reduction in bile acids that are considered carcinogenic (*see* Chapter 2).

One other potential benefit of Ca supplementation may be a reduction in BP in both men and women *(69)*. As described above, Ca supplementation lowered BP during pregnancy, and also reduced BP in male and female offspring of women who took Ca supplements during pregnancy *(55,58)*. Since high BP is a strong risk factor in stroke, and aggravates other CVDs, Ca supplementation may be very cost-effective in all of its biological functions.

In addition to Ca, antioxidant status has also been associated with hip fracture risk. Lifestyle factors, such as smoking, also increase the risk of hip fracture. Melhus et al. *(84)* found a threefold increased risk of hip fracture in women who were current smokers, and had the lowest intakes of either vitamin E or vitamin C, compared to nonsmoking women with the highest antioxidant intakes. If the smokers had the lowest intakes of both vitamins, the odds ratio increased to 4.9.

Smoking, independent of antioxidant status, has been shown to increase the risk of hip fracture, perhaps because of its association with decreased Ca absorption *(85)*. To complete the circle of life events, it is interesting to note that Jones et al. *(86)* found that maternal smoking during pregnancy resulted in their children having shorter stature that was linked to lower bone mass. It may well be that the children of smoking mothers are at greater risk for OP, because their bones did not accumulate the bone mass needed to prevent this disease in later life. Infant bone mass has been shown to be increased if mothers are supplemented with Ca during pregnancy. Koo et al. *(87)* showed that total bone mineral content was significantly greater in infants born to mothers supplemented with 2000 mg/d Ca during pregnancy, compared to women in the placebo group, who consumed less than 600 mg/d Ca.

3. KEY MICRONUTRIENTS FOR DISEASE PREVENTION

A number of vitamins and minerals have been consistently associated with preventing age-related chronic disease and, coincidentally, improving pregnancy outcomes. The list includes the antioxidant vitamins, C and E; the B-vitamins, folic acid, B_{12}, and B_6; and vitamin D; minerals associated with improved health outcomes for young and old include Ca, Mg, Fe, Zn, and Se. It should be noted that Fe, Zn, and Se are also required for the functioning of antioxidant enzymes. Copper and manganese also are required for some of the antioxidant enzymes, but, currently, there are less data available concerning the disease-preventing role of these specific minerals.

Most data associating micronutrients with disease prevention come from epidemiological studies. Findings suggest that individuals with the highest intakes of foods containing these micronutrients have the greatest reduced risk of disease. Some of the survey studies have included questions about dietary supplement use, and, in many cases, those with the highest intakes of the micronutrients from supplements also have lower risks of the major degenerative diseases. Those with the highest intakes of vitamins from naturally occurring sources, or from fortified foods, also have the highest total intakes, because they are often users of vitamin and/or mineral supplements.

For CVD prevention, there appears to be a link between antioxidant nutrients and the B-vitamins *(88)*. Although it is now well accepted that recommended intake levels, or higher, of folic acid, B_6, and B_{12} are required to lower homocysteine levels, new data suggest that high levels of vitamins E and C may also lower several of the CV risk factors associated with elevated homocysteine levels. Recent data also indicate that the antioxidant nutrients and the B-vitamins affect different aspects of the CV system, so that both classes of nutrients are needed for protection *(89)*. It appears that, in nature, evolution has required the human need for 13 essential vitamins and at least an equal number of minerals. It is only reasonable to find that these dietary components work best when all of their levels are optimized, and that not just a single "magic bullet" is at an optimal level.

4. CONCLUSIONS

Examples in this chapter provide ample evidence that there are important, simple, safe, and economically sound interventions that can be implemented to reduce disease risk throughout the life-span. Quoting from Blumberg's conclusion in his chapter *(24)* on "Public Health Implications of Preventive Nutrition," his counsel seems particularly appropriate at this time:

"Shifting the health care system from its current emphasis on treatment to prevention will take time. Even if such changes are implemented, more time will be required before its impact on chronic disease mortality will become apparent because of long latency periods, although a delay in the onset of clinical symptoms will be detected earlier.

The dividends of prevention in reducing the population illness burden and enhancing of the quality of life can be substantial. Efforts must be strengthened to encourage all segments of the population to adopt preventive nutrition strategies, not just those who are high risk. Food habits develop early in life, and this is a useful time to develop preventive nutrition behaviors, although an emphasis on older adults appears more critical at this juncture, since by 2004 the cost of health care for those over 65 is projected to constitute 50% of the total national health care bill. Together with an increase in physical activity and the cessation of tobacco use, dietary modification and improvements in nutritional status present us with the greatest potential for reducing the incidence of chronic disease, improving public health, and limiting the growth of health care expenditures."

REFERENCES

1. Deckelbaum RJ, Fisher EA, Winston M, Kumanyika S, Lauer RM, Pi-Sunyer FX, et al. Summary of a scientific conference on preventive nutrition: pediatrics to geriatrics. Circulation 1999; 100:450–456.
2. Beresford SAA, Boushey CJ. Homocysteine, folic acid, and cardiovascular disease risk. In: Preventive Nutrition: The Comprehensive Guide for Health Professionals. Bendich A, Deckelbaum RJ, eds. Totowa, NJ: Humana, 1997; 193–224.
3. Bostick RM. Diet and nutrition in the etiology and primary prevention of colon cancer. In: Preventive Nutrition: The Comprehensive Guide for Health Professionals. Bendich A, Deckelbaum RJ, eds. Totowa, NJ: Humana, 1997; 57–96.
4. Buring JE, Gaziano JM. Antioxidant vitamins and cardiovascular disease. In: Preventive Nutrition: The Comprehensive Guide for Health Professionals. Bendich A, Deckelbaum RJ, eds. Totowa, NJ: Humana, 1997; 171–180.
5. Comstock GW, Helzlsouer KJ. Preventive nutrition and lung cancer. In: Preventive Nutrition: The Comprehensive Guide for Health Professionals. Bendich A, Deckelbaum RJ, eds. Totowa, NJ: Humana, 1997; 109–134.
6. Fontham ETH. Prevention of upper gastrointestinal tract cancers. In: Preventive Nutrition: The Comprehensive Guide for Health Professionals. Bendich A, Deckelbaum RJ, eds. Totowa, NJ: Humana, 1997; 33–56.
7. Hertog MG, Bueno-de-Mesquita HB, Fehily AM, Sweetnam PM, Elwood PC, Kromhout D. Fruit and vegetable consumption and cancer mortality in the Caerphilly Study. Cancer Epidemiol Biomarkers Prev 1996; 5:673–677.
8. Howe GR. Nutrition and breast cancer. In: Preventive Nutrition: The Comprehensive Guide for Health Professionals. Bendich A, Deckelbaum RJ, eds. Totowa, NJ: Humana, 1997; 97–108.
9. Joshipura KJ, Asherio A, Manson JE, Stampfer MJ, Rimm EB, Speizer FE, et al. Fruit and vegetable intake in relation to risk of ischemic stroke. JAMA 1999; 282:1233–1239.
10. Kushi LH, Folsom AR, Prinaes RJ, Mink PJ, Ying W, Bostick RM. Dietary antioxidant vitamins and death from coronary heart disease in postmenopausal women. N Engl J Med 1996; 334:1156–1162.
11. Willett WC. Potential benefits of preventive nutrition strategies: lessons from the United States. In: Preventive Nutrition: The Comprehensive Guide for Health Professionals. Bendich A, Deckelbaum RJ, eds. Totowa, NJ: Humana, 1997; 423–440.
12. Jacobs DR, Meyer KA, Kushi LH, Folsom AR. Whole grain intake may reduce the risk of ischemic heart disease death in postmenopausal women: The Iowa women's Health Study. Am J Clin Nutr 1998; 68:248–257.
13. Jacobs DRR, Marquart L, Slavin J, Kushi LH. Whole grain intake and cancer: an expanded review and meta-analysis. Nutr Cancer 1998; 30:85–96.
14. Jarvi AE, Karlstrom BE, Granfeldt YE, Bjorck IM, Vessby BO, Asp NG. The influence of food structure on postprandial metabolism in patients with non-insulin-dependent diabetes mellitus. Am J Clin Nutr 1995; 61:837–842.
15. Lachance PA. Nutrient addition to foods: the public health impact in countries with rapidly westernizing diets. In: Preventive Nutrition: The Comprehensive Guide for Health Professionals. Bendich A, Deckelbaum RJ, eds. Totowa, NJ: Humana, 1997; 441–454.

16. Liu S, Stampfer MJ, Hu FB, Giovannucci E, Rimm E, Manson JE, Hennekens CH, Willett WC. Whole-grain consumption and risk of coronary heart disease: results from the Nurses' Health Study. Am J Clin Nutr 1999; 70:412–419.

17. U.S. Department of Health and Human Services and U.S. Department of Agriculture. Nutrition and Your Health: Dietary Guidelines for Americans, 4th ed. Washington, DC: US Government Printing Office, 1995; 402–519.

18. Holmes MD, Hunter DJ, Colditz GA, Stampfer MJ, Hankinson SE, Speizer FE, Rosner B, Willett WC. Association of dietary intake of fat and fatty acids with risk of breast cancer. JAMA 1999; 281:914–920.

19. Rozowski SJ, Moreno M. Effect of westernization of nutritional habits on obesity in Latin America. In: Preventive Nutrition: The Comprehensive Guide for Health Professionals. Bendich A, Deckelbaum RJ, eds. Totowa, NJ: Humana, 1997; 487–504.

20. Zhang S, Hunter DJ, Rosner BA, Colditz GA, Fuchs CS, Speizer FE, Willett WC. Dietary fat and protein in relation to risk of non-Hodgkin's lymphoma among women. J Natl Cancer Inst 1999; 91:1751–1758.

21. Calle EE, Thun MJ, Petrelli JM, Rodriguez C, Heath CW Jr. Body-mass index and mortality in a prospective cohort of U.S. adults. N Engl J Med 1999; 341:1097–1105.

22. Zhang S, Hunter DJ, Hankinson SE, Giovannucci EL, Rosner BA, Colditz GA, Speizer FE, Willett WC. A prospective study of folate intake and the risk of breast cancer. JAMA 1999; 281:1632–1637.

23. Bendich A, Deckelbaum RJ, eds. Preventive Nutrition: The Comprehensive Guide for Health Professionals. Totowa, NJ: Humana, 1997.

24. Blumberg J. Public health implications of preventive nutrition. In: Preventive Nutrition: The Comprehensive Guide for Health Professionals. Bendich A, Deckelbaum RJ, eds. Totowa, NJ: Humana, 1997; 1–17.

25. Krebs-Smith SM, Smicklas-Wright H, Guthrie HA, Krebs-Smith J. The effects of variety in food choices on dietary quality. J Am Diet Assoc 1987; 87:897–903.

26. Selhub J, Jacques PF, Rosenberg IH, Rogers G, Bowman BA, Gunter EW, Wright JD, Johnson CL. Serum total homocysteine concentrations in the third National Health and Nutrition Examination Survey (1991–1994): population reference ranges and contribution of vitamin status to high serum concentrations. Ann Intern Med 1999; 131:331–339.

27. Bendich A, Mallick R, Leader S. Potential health economic benefits of vitamin supplementation. West J Med 1997; 166:306–312.

28. Ross GW, Petrovitch H, White LR, Masaki KH, Li CY, Curb JD, et al. Characterization of risk factors for vascular dementia: the Honolulu-Asia Aging Study. Neurology 1999; 53:337–343.

29. Spencer AP, Carson DS, Crouch MA. Vitamin E and coronary artery disease. Arch Intern Med 1999; 159:1313–1320.

30. Czeizel AE. Folic acid-containing multivitamins and primary prevention of birth defects. In: Preventive Nutrition: The Comprehensive Guide for Health Professionals. Bendich A, Deckelbaum RJ, eds. Totowa, NJ: Humana, 1997; 351–371.

31. Scholl TO, Hediger ML. Maternal nutrition and preterm delivery. In: Preventive Nutrition: The Comprehensive Guide for Health Professionals. Bendich A, Deckelbaum RJ, eds. Totowa, NJ: Humana, 1997; 405–421.

32. Woodall AA, Ames BN. Nutritional prevention of DNA damage to sperm and consequent risk reduction in birth defects and cancer in offspring. In: Preventive Nutrition: The Comprehensive Guide for Health Professionals. Bendich A, Deckelbaum RJ, eds. Totowa, NJ: Humana, 1997; 373–385.

33. Barker DJ. Fetal origins of cardiovascular disease. Ann Med 1999; 1:3–6.

34. Klebanoff MA, Secher NJ, Mednick BR, Schulsinger C. Maternal size at birth and the development of hypertension during pregnancy: a test of the Barker hypothesis. Arch Intern Med 1999; 159:1607–1612.

35. Moore SE. Nutrition, immunity and the fetal and infant origins of disease hypothesis in developing countries. Proc Nutr Soc 1998; 57:241–247.

36. Yarbrough DE, Barrett-Connor E, Kritz-Silverstein D, Wingard DL. Birth weight, adult weight, and girth as predictors of the metabolic syndrome in postmenopausal women: The Rancho Bernardo study. Diabetes Care 1998; 21:1652–1658.

37. Czeizel AE, Dudas I. Prevention of the first occurrence of neural-tube defects by periconceptional vitamin supplementation. N Engl J Med 1992; 327:1832–1835.

38. MRC. Prevention of neural tube defects: results of the Medical Research Council Vitamin Study. MRC Vitamin Study Research Group. Lancet 1991; 338:13–17.

39. Botto LD, Khoury MJ, Mulinare J, Erickson JD. Periconceptional multivitamin use and the occurrence of conotruncal heart defects: results from a population-based, case-control study. Pediatrics 1996; 98:911–917.

40. MMWR. Use of folic acid-containing supplements among women of childbearing age: United States, 1997. MMWR 1998; 47:131–134.
41. Butterworth CE, Bendich A. Folic acid and the prevention of birth defects. Ann Rev Nutr 1996; 16:73–98.
42. Bunin GR, Cary JM. Diet and childhood cancer: preliminary evidence. In: Preventive Nutrition: The Comprehensive Guide for Health Professionals. Bendich A, Deckelbaum RJ, eds. Totowa, NJ: Humana, 1997; 17–32.
43. Oakley GP Jr. Eat right and take a vitamin. N Engl J Med 1998; 338:1060–1061.
44. Berry RJ, Li Z, Erickson JD, Li S, Moore CA, Wang H, et al. Prevention of neural-tube defects with folic acid in China. China-U.S. Collaborative Project for Neural Tube Defect Prevention. N Engl J Med 1999; 341:1485–1490.
45. MMWR. Preterm singleton births: United States, 1989–1996. MMWR 1999; 48:185–189.
46. Scholl TO, Hediger ML, Bendich A, Schall JI, Smith WK, Krueger PM. Use of multivitamin/mineral prenatal supplements: influence on the outcome of pregnancy. Am J Epidemiol 1997; 146:134–141.
47. Goldenberg RL, Tamura T, Neggers Y, Copper RL, Johnston KE, DuBard MB, Hauth JC. The effect of zinc supplementation on pregnancy outcome. JAMA 1995; 274:463–468.
48. deOnis M, Villar J, Gulmezoglu M. Nutritional interventions to prevent intrauterine growth retardation: evidence from randomized controlled trials. Eur J Clin Nutr 1998; 53:S83–93.
49. Ramakrishnan U, Manjrekar R, Rivera J, Gonzales-Cossio T, Martorell R. Micronutrients and pregnancy outcome: a review of the literature. Nutr Res 1999; 19:103–159.
50. West KP Jr, Katz J, Khatry SK, LeClerq SC, Pradhan EK, Shrestha SR, et al. Double blind, cluster randomised trial of low dose supplementation with vitamin A or beta carotene on mortality related to pregnancy in Nepal. The NNIPS-2 Study Group. Br Med J 1999; 318:570–575.
51. Fawzi WW, Masamanga GI, Speigelman D, Urassa EJ, McGrath N, Mwakagile D, et al. Randomised trial of effects of vitamin supplements on pregnancy outcomes and T cell counts in HIV-1 infected women in Tanzania. Lancet 1998; 351:1477–1482.
52. Chappell LC, Seed PT, Bailey AL, Kelly FJ, Lee R, Hunt BJ, et al. Effects of antioxidants on the occurrence of pre-eclampsia in women at increased risk: a randomized trial. Lancet 1999; 254:810–816.
53. DerSimonian R, Levine RL. Resolving discrepancies between a meta-analysis and a subsequent large controlled trial. JAMA 1999; 282:664–670.
54. Levine RJ, Hauth JC, Curet LB, Sibai BM, Catalano PM, Morris CD, et al. Trial of calcium to prevent preeclampsia. N Engl J Med 1997; 337:69–76.
55. Bucher HC, Guyatt GH, Cook RJ, Hatala R, Cook DJ, Lang JD, Hunt D. Effect of calcium supplementation on pregnancy-induced hypertension and preeclampsia: a meta-analysis of randomized controlled trials. JAMA 1996; 275:1113–1117.
56. Anonymous. Optimal calcium intake. NIH consensus development panel. JAMA 1994; 272:1942–1948.
57. Institute of Medicine Food and Nutrition Board. Dietary Reference Intakes for Calcium, Phosphorous, Magnesium, Vitamin D, and Fluoride. Washington, DC: National Academy Press, S-9, 1997.
58. Belizan JM, Villar J, Bergel E, del Pino A, DiFulvio S, Galliano SV, Kattan C. Long-term effect of calcium supplementation during pregnancy on the blood pressure of offspring: follow up of a randomised controlled trial. Br Med J 1997; 315:281–285.
59. Wang YP, Walsh SW, Guo JD, Zhang JY. Maternal levels of prostacyclin, thromboxane, vitamin E, and lipid peroxides throughout normal pregnancy. Am J Obstet Gynecol 1991; 165:1690–1694.
60. Jain SK, Wise R. Relationship between elevated lipid peroxides, vitamin E deficiency and hypertension in preeclampsia. Mol Cell Biochem 1995; 151:33–38.
61. Goldstein DJ. The management of eating disorders and obesity. Totowa, NJ: Humana, 1999.
62. Fassbender K, Mielke O, Bertsch T, Nafe B, Froschen S, Hennerici M. Homocysteine in cerebral macroangiography and microangiopathy. Lancet 1999; 353:1586–1587.
63. Ridker PM, Manson JE, Buring JE, Shih J, Matias M, Hennekens CH. Homocysteine and risk of cardiovascular disease among postmenopausal women. JAMA 1999; 281:1817–1821.
64. Jacques PF, Selhub J, Bostom AG, Wilson PW, Rosenberg IH. The effect of folic acid fortification on plasma folate and total homocysteine concentrations. N Engl J Med 1999; 340:1449–1454.
65. Blair SN, Brodney S. Effects of physical inactivity and obesity on morbidity and mortality: current evidence and research issues. Med Sci Sports Exerc 1999; 11(Suppl.):S646–662.
66. McTiernan A, Schwartz RS, Potter J, Bowen D. Exercise clinical trials in cancer prevention research: a call to action. Cancer Epidemiol Biomarkers Prev 1999; 8:201–207.

67. Pols MA, Peeters PH, Twisk JW, Kemper HC, Grobbee DE. Physical activity and cardiovascular disease risk profile in women. Am J Epidemiol 1997; 146:322–328.

68. Baron JA, Beach M, Mandel JS, van Stolk RU, Haile RW, Sandler RS, et al. Calcium supplements for the prevention of colorectal adenomas. Calcium Polyp Prevention Study Group. N Engl J Med 1999; 340:101–107.

69. McCarron DA, Reusser ME. Finding consensus in the dietary calcium-blood pressure debate. J Am Coll Nutr 1999; 18:398S–405S.

70. Looker AC, Orwoll ES, Johnston CC, Lindsay RL, Wahner HW, Dunn WL, et al. Prevalence of low femoral bone density in older U.S. adults from NHANES III. J Bone Miner Res 1997; 12:1761–1768.

71. Heaney RP. Osteoporosis: vitamins, minerals and other micronutrients. In: Preventive Nutrition: The Comprehensive Guide for Health Professionals. Bendich A, Deckelbaum RJ, eds. Totowa, NJ: Humana, 1997; 285–302.

72. Holick MF. Vitamin D. Totowa, NJ: Humana, 1999.

73. Marshall D, Johnell O, Wedel H. Meta-analysis of how well measures of bone mineral density predict occurrence of osteoporotic fractures. Br Med J 1996; 312:1254–1259.

74. Kleerekoper M, Avioli L. Evaluation and treatment of postmenopausal osteoporosis. In: Primer on the Metabolic Bone Diseases and Disorders of Mineral Metabolism. Favus M, ed. Philadelphia, PA: Lippincott-Raven, 1996; 264–271.

75. Chapuy M, Arlot M, Duboeuf F, Brun J, Crouzet B, Arnaud S, Delmas P, Meunier P. Vitamin D3 and calcium to prevent hip fractures in elderly women. N Engl J Med 1992; 327:1637–1642.

76. Dawson-Hughes B, Harris S, Krall E, Dallal G. Effect of calcium and vitamin D supplementation on bone density in men and women 65 years of age or older. N Engl J Med 1997; 337:670–676.

77. Reid I, Ames R, Evans M, Gamble G, Sharpe S. Long-term effects of calcium supplementation on bone loss and fractures in post-menopausal women: a randomized controlled trial. Am J Med 1995; 98:331–335.

78. Bendich A, Leader S, Muhuri P. Supplemental calcium for the prevention of hip fracture: potential health-economic benefits. Clin Ther 1999; 21:1058–1072.

79. Recker RR, Hinders S, Davies KM, Heaney RP, Stegman MR, Lappe JM, Kimmel DB. Correcting calcium nutritional deficiency prevents spine fractures in elderly women. J Bone Miner Res 1996; 11:1961–1966.

80. Nieves JW, Komar L, Cosman F, Lindsay R. Calcium potentiates the effect of estrogen and calcitonin on bone mass: review and analysis. Am J Clin Nutr 1998; 67:18–24.

81. Elbon S, Johnson M, Fischer J. Milk consumption in older Americans. Am J Pub Health 1998; 88: 1221–1224.

82. LeBoff MS, Kohlmeier L, Hurwitz S, Franklin J, Wright J, Glowacki J. Occult vitamin D deficiency in postmenopausal US women with acute hip fracture. JAMA 1999; 281:1505–1511.

83. Singer BR, McLauchlan GJ, Robinson CM, Christie J. Epidemiology of fractures in 15,000 adults: the influence of age and gender. J Bone Joint Surg Br 1998; 80:243–248.

84. Melhus H, Michaelsson K, Holmberg L, Wolk A, Ljunghall S. Smoking, antioxidant vitamins, and the risk of hip fracture. J Bone Miner Res 1999; 14:129–135.

85. Krall EA, Dawson-Hughes B. Smoking and bone loss among postmenopausal women. J Bone Miner Res 1991; 6:331–338.

86. Jones G, Riley M, Dwyer T. Maternal smoking during pregnancy, growth, and bone mass in prepubertal children. J Bone Miner Res 1999; 1:146–151.

87. Koo WWK, Walters JC, Esterlitz J, Levine RJ, Bush AJ, Sibai B. Maternal calcium supplementation and fetal bone mineralization. Obstet Gynecol 1999; 94:577–582.

88. Nappo F, De Rosa N, Marfella R, De Lucia D, Ingrosso D, Perna AF, Farzati B, Giugliano D. Impairment of endothelial functions by acute hyperhomocysteinemia and reversal by antioxidant vitamins. JAMA 1999; 281:2113–2118.

89. Woodside JV, Young IS, Yarnell JW, Roxborough HE, McMaster D, McCrum EE, Gey KF, Evans A. Antioxidants, but not B-group vitamins increase the resistance of low-density lipoprotein to oxidation: a randomized, factorial design, placebo-controlled trial. Atherosclerosis 1999; 144:419–427.

VII Nutrition-Related Resources

Books Related to Primary
and Secondary Preventive Nutrition

1. American Academy of Pediatrics Staff. 1998. Pediatric Nutrition Handbook, 4th edition. Elk Grove Village, IL: American Academy of Pediatrics.
2. Bendich, A.B., Deckelbaum, R.J. (eds.) 1997. Preventive Nutrition: The Comprehe sive Guide for Health Professionals. Totowa, NJ: Humana Press.
3. Berdanier, C.D. (ed.) 1996. Nutrients and Gene Expression: Clinical Aspects. Boca Raton, FL: CRC Press.
4. Berdanier, C.D. 1998. CRC Desk Reference for Nutrition. Boca Raton, FL: CRC Press.
5. Berdanier, C.D., Failla, M.L. 1998. Advanced Nutrition: Micronutrients. Boca Raton, FL: CRC Press.
6. Bray, G.A., Ryan, D.H. (eds.) 1999. Nutrition, Genetics, and Obesity, Pennington Center Nutrition Series Volume 9. Baton Rouge, LA: Louisiana State University Press.
7. Bogden, J.D. Klevay, L.M. 2000. Clinical Nutrition of the Essential Trace Elements and Minerals. Totowa, NJ: Humana Press.
8. Brody, T. 1998. Nutritional Biochemistry, 2nd edition. San Diego, CA: Academic Press.
9. Cadenas, E., Packer, L. (eds.) 1996. Handbook of Antioxidants. New York: Marcel Dekker.
10. Chernoff, R. 1999. Geriatric Nutrition: The Health Professional's Handbook, 2nd Edition. Gaithersburgh,MD: Aspen Publishers, Inc.
11. Cho, S.S., Prosky, L., Dreher, M. (eds.). 1999. Complex Carbohydrates in Foods. New York: Marcel Dekker, Inc.
12. Chow, C.K. (ed.) 1999. Fatty Acids in Foods and Their Health Implications, 2nd Edition. New York: Marcel Dekker, Inc.
13. Clifford, A.J., Muller, H-G. (eds.) 1998. Mathematical Modeling in Experimental Nutritional. New York: Plenum.
14. Combs, G.F. Jr. 1998. Vitamins: Fundamental Aspects in Nutrition and Health, 2nd edition. San Diego, CA: Academic Press.
15. Driskell, J. 1999. Sports Nutrition. Boca Raton, FL: CRC Press.
16. Eitenmiller, R.R., Landen, W.O., Jr. (eds.) 1999. Vitamin Analysis for the Health and Food Sciences. Boca Ranton, FL: CRC Press.
17. El-Khoury, A.E. (ed.) 1999. Methods for Investigation of Amino Acids and Protein Metabolism. Boca Raton, FL: CRC Press LLC.
18. Escott-Stump, S. 1998. Nutrition and Diagnosis-Related Care, 4th Edition. Hagerstown, MD: Lippincott Williams & Wilkins.

From: *Primary and Secondary Preventive Nutrition*
Edited by: A. Bendich and R. J. Deckelbaum © Humana Press Inc., Totowa, NJ

19. Garewal, H.S. (ed.) 1997. Antioxidants and Disease Prevention. Boca Raton, FL: CRC Press.

20. Gershwin, M., Keen, C.L., German, J.B. (eds.) 2000. Nutrition and Immunology: Principles and Practice. Totowa, NJ: Humana Press.

21. Gibson, G.R., Roberfroid, M.B. (eds.) 1999. Colonic Microbiota, Nutrition and Health. Boston, MA: Kluwer Academic.

22. Goldstein, D.J. (ed) 1999. The Management of Eating Disorders and Obesity. Totowa, NJ: Humana Press.

23. Heimburger, D.C., Weinsier, R.L. 1997. Handbook of Clinical Nutrition, 3rd Edition. St. Louis, MO: Mosby, Inc.

24. Hoffman-Goetz, L. (ed) 1996. Exercise and Immune Function. Boca Raton, FL: CRC Press.

25. Holick, M.F. (ed) 1999. Vitamin D: Physiology, Molecular Biology and Clinical Applications. Totowa, NJ: Humana Press.

26. Huang, Y., Sinclair, A. (eds.) 1998. Lipids in Infant Nutrition. Champaign, IL: AOCS Press.

27. Kessler, D.B., Dawson, P. (eds.) 1999. Failure to Thrive and Pediatric Undernutrition: A Transdisciplinary Approach. Baltimore, MD: Paul H. Brookes Publishing.

28. Kopple, J.D., Massry, S.G. (eds.) 1997. Nutritional Management of Renal Disease. Baltimore, MD: Williams & Wilkins.

29. Mann, J., Truswell, A.S., Truswell, S. (eds.) 1998. Essentials of Human Nutrition. New York: Oxford University Press.

30. McArdle, W.D., Katch, F.I., Katch, V.L. 1999. Sports and Exercise Nutrition. Philadelphia, PA: Williams & Wilkins.

31. McCormick, D.B. (ed). 1998. Annual Review of Nutrition. Palo Alto, CA: Annual Reviews Inc.

32. Miller, G.D., Jarvis, J.K., McBean, L.D. 1999. Handbook of Dairy Foods and Nutrition, 2nd Edition. Boca Raton, FL: CRC Press.

33. Miller, T.L., Gorbach, S.L. (eds.) 1999. Nutrition Aspects of HIV Infection. New York: Oxford University Press.

34. Morrison, G., Hark, L. 1999. Medical Nutrition and Disease, 2nd Edition. Malden, MA: Blackwell Science, Inc.

35. Nieman, D.C., Pedersen, B.K. (eds.) 2000. Nutrition and Exercise Immunology. Boca Raton, FL: CRC Press.

36. Oberleas, D., Harland, B.F., Bobilya, D.J. 1999. Minerals: Nutrition and Metabolism. New York: Vantage Press.

37. O'Dell, B.L., Sunde, R.A. 1997. Handbook of Nutritionally Essential Mineral Elements, Vol. 2. New York: Marcel Dekker Inc.

38. Papas, A. (ed). 1998. Antioxidant Status, Diet, Nutrition, and Health. Boca Raton, FL:CRC Press.

39. Peckenpaugh, N.J., Poleman, C.M. 1999. Nutrition Essentials and Diet Therapy, 8th Edition. Philadelphia, PA: WB Saunders Company.

40. Pence, B.C., Dunn, D.M. 1998. Nutrition and Women's Cancers. Boca Raton, FL: CRC Press.

41. Pennington, J.A.T., Bowes, A.D., Church, H. 1998. Bowes and Church's Food Values of Portions Commonly Used, 17th Edition. Philadelphia, PA: Lippincott.

42. Rugg-Gunn, A.J., Nunn, J.H. 1999. Nutrition, Diet, and Oral Health. Oxford[England]: Oxford University Press.

43. Sadler, M.J., Strain, J.J., Caballero, B. (eds.) 1998. Encyclopedia of Human Nutrition. San Diego, CA: Academic Press Inc.

44. Shils, M., Olson, J.A., Shike, M (eds.). 1998. Modern Nutrition in Health and Disease, 9th edition. Baltimore, MD: Williams & Wilkins.

45. Simopoulos. AP. 1997. Nutrition and Fitness. Basel, Switzerland: Karger, S., AG.

46. Simopoulos, A.P. (ed.) 1998. The Return of w3 Fatty Acids into the Food Supply. I. Land-Based Animal Food Products and Their Health Effects. Basel, Switzerland: Karger, S., AG.

47. Spallholz, J.E., Mallory Boylan, L., Driskell, J.A. 1999. Nutrition: Chemistry and Biology, 2nd Edition. Boca Raton, FL: CRC Press LLC.

48. Spiller, G.A. (ed.) 1996. Handbook of Lipids in Human Nutrition. Boca Raton, FL: CRC Press.

49. Stipanuk, M. (ed) 1999. Biochemical and Physiological Aspects of Human Nutrition. Philadelphia, PA: Saunders, W.B.

50. Taylor, A. (ed.) 1999. Nutritional and Environmental Influences on the Eye. Boca Raton, FL: CRC Press LLC.

51. Taylor, C.E. (ed) 1997. Nutritional Abnormalities in Infectious Diseases: Effects on Tuberculosis and AIDS. New York: Haworth Press.

52. Tarnopolsky M. (ed.) 1999. Gender Differences in Metabolism: Practical and Nutritional Implications. Boca Raton, FL: CRC Press.

53. Tsang, R.C., Nichols, B.L., Zlotkin, S.H., et al. (eds.) 1997. Nutrition During Infancy: Principles and Practice, 2nd Edition. Cincinnati, OH: Digital Educational Publishing.

54. Veith, W.J. (ed.) 1999. Diet and Health, 2nd Edition. Boca Raton, FL: CRC Press.

55. Wardley, B., Puntis, J.W.L., Taitz, L.S. 1997. Handbook of Child Nutrition, 2nd Edition. New York: Oxford University Press.

56. Watson, R.R. (ed.) 1997. Trace Elements in Laboratory Rodents. Boca Raton, FL: CRC Press.

57. Watson, R.R. (ed.) 1998. Nutrients and Foods in AIDS. Boca Raton, FL: CRC Press.

58. Watson, R.R., Mufti, S.I. (eds.) 1996. Nutrition and Cancer Prevention. Boca Raton, FL: CRC Press.

59. Willett, W. 1998. Nutritional Epidemiology, 2nd Edition. New York: Oxford University Press.

60. Wolinsky, I. (ed.) 1998. Nutrition in Exercise and Sport, 3rd Edition. Boca Raton, FL: CRC Press.

61. Wolinsky, I., Klimis-Tavantzis, D. (eds.) 1996. Nutritional Concerns of Women. Boca Raton, FL: CRC Press.

62. World Health Organization. 1996. WHO Publication: Trace Elements in Human Nutrition and Health. Albany, NY: WHO Publications Center USA.

63. Ziegler, E.E., Filer, L.J., Jr. (eds.). 1996. Present Knowledge in Nutrition. Washington, DC: ILSI Press.

Websites of Interest

http://www.ifst.org/
IFST (Institute of Food Science & Technology) is based in the UK, with members through-out the world, with the purpose of serving the public interest in the application of science and technology for food safety and nutrition as well as furthering the profession of food science and technology. Eligibility for membership can be found at the IFST home page, an index and a search engine are available.

http://www.nysaes.cornell.edu/cifs/start.html
The Cornell Institute of Food Science at Cornell University home page provides infor-mation on graduate and undergraduate courses as well as research and extension pro-grams. Links to related sites and newsgroups can be found.

http://www.blonz.com
Created by Ed Blonz, PhD, "The Blonz Guide" focuses on the fields of nutrition, foods, food science & health supplying links and search engines to find quality sources, news, publication and entertainment sites.

http://www.hnrc.tufts.edu/
The Jean Mayer United States Department of Agriculture (USDA) Human Nutrition Research Center on Aging (HNRC) at Tufts University. This research center is one of six mission-oriented centers aimed at studying the relationship between human nutrition and health, operated by Tufts University under the USDA. Research programs; seminar and conference information; publications; nutrition, aging, medical and science resources; and related links are available.

http://www.fao.org/
The Food and Agriculture Organization (FAO) is the largest autonomous agency within the United Nations, founded "with a mandate to raise levels of nutrition and standards of living, to improve agricultural productivity, and to better the condition of rural popula-tion," emphasizing sustainable agriculture and rural development.

http://www.eatright.org/
The American Dietetic Association is the largest group of food and nutrition profession-als in the US, members are primarily registered dietitians (RDs) and dietetic technicians, registered (DTRs). Programs and services include promoting nutrition information for the public; sponsoring national events, media and marketing programs, and publications (The American Dietetic Association); and lobbying for federal legislation. Also available

From: *Primary and Secondary Preventive Nutrition*
Edited by: A. Bendich and R. J. Deckelbaum © Humana Press Inc., Totowa, NJ

through the website are member services, nutrition resources, news, classifieds, and government affairs. Assistance in finding a dietitian, marketplace news, and links to related sites can also be found.

http://www.faseb.org/ain/hometest2.html
The American Society for Nutritional Sciences (ASNS) located in Bethesda, MD, is a research society facilitating, for example, animal and human nutrition studies, official publication (The Journal of Nutrition, available through nutrition.org), annual meetings, education and training opportunities, and professional networking. Categories for membership include the following: regular, associate, student, and emeritus.

http://www.faseb.org
The Federation of American Societies for Experimental Biology (FASEB) is a coalition of member societies with the purpose of enhancing the profession of biomedical and life scientists, emphasizing public policy issues. FASEB offers logistical and operational support as well as sponsoring scientific conferences and publications (The FASEB Journal).

http://www.ificinfo.health.org/
The International Food Information Council (IFIC) is a non-profit organization whose purpose is to provide access to health and nutrition resources, data, and information based on science to professionals, educators, journalists, government officials and others in order to facilitate the communication of health and nutrition information to consumers.

http://www.ifis.org/home.html
The International Food Information Service (IFIS) is a leading information, product and service provider for professionals in food science, food technology, and nutrition. IFIS publishing offers a wide range of scientific databases, including FSTA - Food Science and Technology Abstracts. IFIS GmbH offers research, educational training, and seminars.

http://www.ift.org/
The Institute of Food Technologists (IFT) is a membership organization advancing the science and technology of food through the sharing of information; publications include Food Technology and Journal of Food Science; events include the Annual Meeting and Food Expo. Members may choose to join a specialized division of expertise (there are 23 divisions); IFT student associations and committees are also available for membership.

http://www.veris-online.org/
The VERIS Research Information Service is a non-profit corporation, focusing on anti-oxidants, providing professionals with reliable sources on the role of nutrition in health. Data in VERIS publications, distributed without fee to those who qualify, is based on technical peer-reviewed journals. Quarterly written reports and newsletters, research summaries, annual abstract books, vitamin E fact book and educational programs are among the available VERIS publications and communications. Links to helpful web resources are also accessible.

http://www.osteo.org/

The National Institutes of Health Osteoporosis and Related Bone Diseases ~ National Resource Center (NIH ORBD-NRC) mission is to "provide patients, health professionals, and the public with an important link to resources and information on metabolic bone diseases, including osteoporosis, Paget's disease of the bone, osteogenesis imperfecta, and hyperparathyroidism. The Center is operated by the National Osteoporosis Foundation, in collaboration with The Paget Foundation and the Osteogenesis Imperfecta Foundation."

http://www.ag.uiuc.edu/~food-lab/nat/

The Nutrition Analysis Tool (NAT) is a free web based program designed to be used by anyone to analyze the nutrient content of food intake. Links to an "Energy Calculator" and "Soy Food Finder" are also available. NAT is funded by C-FAR at the University of Illinois.

http://www.calciuminfo.com

This is an online information source created, copyrighted, and maintained by SmithKline Beecham Consumer Healthcare Research and Development. The nutritional and physiological role of calcium is presented in formats designed for healthcare professionals, consumers, and kids. References and related links, educational games for kids, calcium tutorials, and a calcium calculator are easily accessible.

http://vm.cfsan.fda.gov/

The Center for Food Safety and Applied Nutrition (CFSAN) is one of five product-oriented centers implementing the FDA's mission to regulate domestic and imported food as well as cosmetics. An overview of CFSAN activities can be found along with useful sources for researching various topics such as food biotechnology and seafood safety. Special interest areas, for example, advice for consumers, women's health, and links to other agencies are also available.

http://www.bcm.tmc.edu/cnrc/

The Children's Nutrition Research Center (CNRC) at Baylor College of Medicine is one of six USDA/ARS human nutrition research centers in the nation, assisting healthcare professionals and policy advisors to make appropriate dietary recommendations. CNRC focuses on the nutrition needs of children, from conception through adolescence, and of pregnant and nursing women. Consumer news, seminars, events, and media information are some of the sections available from this home page.

http://www.dsqi.org/

The Dietary Supplement Quality Initiative (DSQI) is designed to educate consumers on the health benefits, safety, standards and regulations, and labeling of dietary supplements. Industry news, interviews, editorials, and DSQI resources and services provide useful tools for consumers, practitioners, producers and distributors.

http://www-sci.lib.uci.edu/~martindale/Nutrition.html
Martindale's Health Science Guide-2000, "The Virtual Nutrition Center", provides a large volume of information. The Nutrition Overview lists resources such as travel warnings and immunization, on-line nutrition calculators, nutrition journals, literature and patent searches, conferences, and dictionaries. Nutrition Interactive allows access to databases, courses and tutorials. All sections are accessed through a single site, use caution when printing!

http://www.usda.gov
The United States Department of Agriculture (USDA) provides a broad scope of service to the nation's farmers and ranchers. In addition, the USDA ensures open markets for agricultural products, food safety, environmental protection, conservation of forests and rural land, and the research of human nutrition. Affiliated agencies, services and programs are accessible through this website.

http://www.nalusda.gov/
The National Agriculture Library (NAL), a primary resource for agriculture information, is one of four national libraries in the US and a component of the Agriculture Research Service of the US Department of Agriculture. Access to NAL's institutions and resources are available through this site.

http://www.fns.usda.gov/fns/
The Food and Nutrition Service (FNS) administers the US Department of Agriculture's (USDA) 15 food assistance programs for children and needy families with the mission to reduce hunger and food insecurity. Details of nutrition assistance programs and related links can be found.

http://www.agnic.org/
The Agriculture Network Information Center (AgNIC), established through the alliance of the National Agriculture Library (NAL) and other organizations, provides public access to agriculture-related resources.

http://www.who.int/nut/welcome.htm
The World Health Organization (WHO) has regarded nutrition to be of fundamental importance for overall health and sustainable development. The Global priority of nutritional issues, activities, mandates, resources, and research are presented in detail.

Nutritional Science Journals
Brown CM. Where to find nutritional science journals on the World Wide Web. J Nutr 1997;127:1527–32

http://annurev.org/series/nutrition/nutrition.htm
Annual Review of Nutrition

http://www.faseb.org/ajcn
American Journal of Clinical Nutrition

http://www.erlbaum.com/1065.htm
Nutrition and Cancer

http://www.faseb.org/asns/journal/journal/html
The Journal of Nutrition

http://www.crcpress.com/jour/catalog/foods.htm
Critical Reviews in Food Science and Nutrition

http://www.cup.org/Journals.JNLSCAT/pns/pns.html
Proceedings of the Nutritional Society

http://www.stockton-press.co.uk/ijo/index.html
International Journal of Obesity

http://www.wiley.com/Home.html
International Journal of Eating Disorders

http://www.cup.org/Journals/JNLSCAT/nut/nut.html
The British Journal of Nutrition

http://www.ilsi.org/dnutrition.html
Nutrition Reviews

http://www.peakcom.com/clinnutr.org/jabs.html
Journal of Parenteral and Enteral Nutrition

http://www.hbuk.co.uk/ap/journals/ap.htm
Appetite

http://www.stockton-press.co.uk/ejcn/index.html
European Journal of Clinical Nutrition

http://www.lrpub.com/journals/j1013.htm
Journal of Pediatric Gastroenterology and Nutrition

http://www.eatright.org/journaltoc.html
Journal of the American Dietetic Association

http://www.elsevier.nl:80/inca/publications/store/5/2/5/0/1/3/
Journal of Nutritional Biochemistry

http://www.karger.com/journals/anm/anm jh.htm
Annals of Nutrition and Metabolism

http://www.hscsyr.edu/ñutrition/
Nutrition: The International Journal of Applied and Basic Nutritional Sciences

http://www.elsevier.nl/inca/publications/store/5/2/5/4/8/3/
Nutrition Research

http://www.mcb.co.uk/liblink/nfs/jourhome/htm
Nutrition and Food Science

http://www.tandf.co.uk/journals/carfax/09637486.html
International Journal of Food Sciences and Nutrition

http://167.208.232.26/catalog/wbs-prod.pl?1051-2276
Journal of Renal Nutrition

http://www.ajnd.org/au/index.html
Australian Journal of Nutrition and Dietetics

INDEX